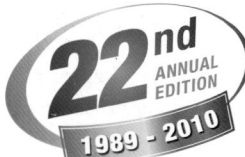

Contents

Alcoholic Drinks (w. Alcohol Counts)	25
Baking Ingredients	32
Bars (Breakfast, Granola, Nutrition)	33
Beverages: Cocoa, Hot Chocolate	37
Coffee & Coffee Drinks	37
Fruit & Vegetable Juices	40
Milk (Plain, Flavored, Mixes)	46
Non-Dairy (Soy, Rice/Cereal/Nut)	48
Protein, Energy, Diet Shakes	50
Soda/Soft Drinks	52
Tea & Iced Tea Drinks	55
Bread & Bread Products, Bagels	56
Breakfast Cereals (Hot & Cold)	59
Cakes, Donuts, Muffins, Pastries	65
Candy, Chocolate, Gum	70
Cheese & Cheese Products	78
Chicken ~ *See Poultry*	
Condiments, Salsa, Pickles	82
Cookies, Crackers	83
Crispbreads, Matzo	90
Cream & Creamers	91
Desserts (Puddings, Gelatin Desserts)	92
Eggs, Egg Substitutes, Egg Dishes	93
Fats, Butter, Spreads, Oils, Mayonnaise	95
Fish, Shellfish	97
Flour, Grains	100
Fruit (Fresh/Packaged/Dried/Snacks)	101
Ice Cream & Frozen Yogurt/Novelties	105
Meals, Entrees, Sides: Cans/Packaged	113
Frozen	119
Meats: Beef, Lamb, Pork, Game	125
Sausages/Franks/Hot Dogs	129
Lunch/Deli Meats & Sausages	130
Milk ~ *See Beverages*	
Nuts, Seeds, Peanut Butter	133
Pancakes & Waffles	134
Pasta & Noodles, Macaroni	135
Pies (Fruit), Pie/Pastry Crusts	136
Pizza: Ready-To-Eat	137
Frozen	138
Poultry (Chicken, Turkey, Duck, Goose)	140
Recipe Dishes (CalorieKing.com)	142
Rice & Rice Dishes	143
Salads	144
Salad Dressings	145
Sauces & Gravy	148
Snacks (Popcorn, Chips, Pretzels)	152
Soups	156
Soy Products, Tofu	162
Spices, Herbs, Seasonings	163
Supplements: Food/Vitamins/Cough	163
Sugar, Sweeteners, Honey, Jam	164
Syrups, Dessert Toppings	164
Vegetables (Fresh, Frozen, Canned)	165
Yogurt, Yogurt Drinks	169

Eating Out:

Cafeteria, Sandwiches	172
Fair/Carnival/Stadium Foods	173
Restaurant & International Foods	175

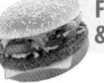

Fast-Food Chains & Restaurants	182-270
A-Z Food Index	294-302

EXTRA DIET GUIDES & COUNTERS

Diabetes Guide	16-20
Alcohol Guide	25
Caffeine Guide & Counter	39
Fats & Cholesterol Guide	271-275
Fiber Guide & Counter	276-281
Protein & Iron Guides & Counter	282-287
Salt & High Blood Pressure with Sodium Counter	288-293
Weight Control Guide	2-14

Weight Control Tips

✅ Eat Sensibly

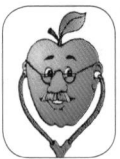

- Avoid fad diets. Eat 3 sensible meals daily with adequate fruit and vegetables.
- Limit portion size. Limit fats and high-fat foods, sugar, soda and alcohol. *(Sample Meal Plan ~ Page 11)*

✅ Exercise Daily

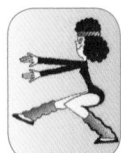

- Get active and exercise every day!
- Include muscle-strengthening exercises. You'll lose more fat and keep it off. You'll also feel and look better, and you can eat a little more! *(Exercise Guide ~ Page 12)*

✅ Reshape Eating Behaviors

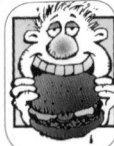

- Be aware of eating habits and behaviors that lead to overeating.
- Also focus on social and emotional situations that lead you to snack compulsively. *(Extra Notes ~ Page 14)*

✅ Keep a Food & Exercise Journal

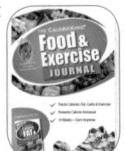

- A journal helps you see exactly what you eat and drink, and how much you exercise. *(Extra Notes ~ Page 15)*
- An excellent motivator and proven weight loss aid. Keeps you honest!

✅ Arrange Moral Support

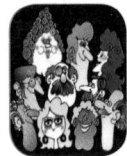

Gain the support of family and friends. Get extra professional help if required, from your doctor, dietitian, psychologist, exercise trainer, or diet club. Beware of family saboteurs who discourage you from adopting a healthier lifestyle!

DOCTOR CHECK-UP

Ask your doctor to check your blood pressure, blood sugar and blood cholesterol levels.

HEALTHY WEIGHTS
~ MEN & WOMEN ~
(Over 18 Years)

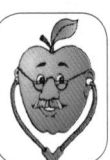

Based on weights with least risk of disease or death from heart disease, diabetes, stroke and cancer.

Based on Body Mass Index of 20-25

BMI calculated as: $\dfrac{\text{Weight (kg)}}{\text{Height (m)}^2}$

Height (No Shoes) Ft Ins		Healthy Weight Range (Pounds)
4'7"	~	86-108
4'8"	~	88-110
4'9"	~	92-114
4'10"	~	97-121
4'11"	~	99-123
5'0"	~	101-127
5'1"	~	105-132
5'2"	~	110-136
5'3"	~	112-140
5'4"	~	114-145
5'5"	~	119-149
5'6"	~	123-156
5'7"	~	127-158
5'8"	~	129-162
5'9"	~	134-167
5'10"	~	138-173
5'11"	~	143-178
6'0"	~	145-182
6'1"	~	149-187
6'2"	~	156-193
6'3"	~	158-198
6'4"	~	162-202
6'5"	~	170-211
6'6"	~	172-215
6'7"	~	175-220

Body Fat Distribution & Health

Moderate amounts of body fat do not compromise health. However, excess fat above the hips carries a far greater health risk than fat on or below the hips - better to be a 'pear-shape' than an 'apple-shape'.

Abdominal obesity greatly increases the risk of developing diabetes, heart disease, high blood fats, hypertension, stroke, sleep apnea, arthritis and some cancers. So-called **'cellulite'** carries no extra health risk.

Waist Circumference directly reflects the increased health risk of abdominal obesity. Waist size associated with a high health risk:
Men ~ Over 40 inches **Women** ~ Over 35 inches

Body Mass Index (BMI)

BMI is a general (but not specific) indicator of body fatness. Although BMI alone is not diagnostic, the higher the BMI, the greater the health risk of developing diabetes, high blood pressure and heart disease. BMI does not apply to heavily muscled persons. BMI is used in a different way for children.

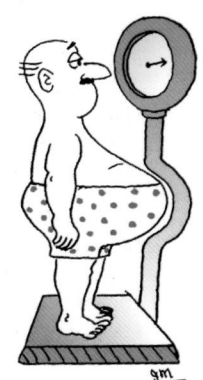

Abdominal obesity greatly increases the risk of ill-health and earlier death.

Check Your BMI: Find your height (no shoes) - look across the row to the weight nearest your own. Then track down to BMI.

Ht	WEIGHT (LBS) ~ ADULTS													
5'1"	100	106	111	116	122	127	132	137	143	148	153	158	185	211
5'2"	104	109	115	120	126	131	136	142	147	153	158	164	191	218
5'3"	107	113	118	124	130	135	141	146	152	158	163	169	197	225
5'4"	110	116	122	128	134	140	145	151	157	163	169	174	204	232
5'5"	114	120	126	132	138	144	150	156	162	168	174	180	210	240
5'6"	118	124	130	136	142	148	155	161	167	173	179	186	216	247
5'7"	121	127	134	140	146	153	159	166	172	178	185	191	223	255
5'8"	125	131	138	144	151	158	164	171	177	184	190	197	230	262
5'9"	128	135	142	149	155	162	169	176	182	189	196	206	236	270
5'10"	132	139	146	153	160	167	174	181	188	195	202	207	243	278
5'11"	136	143	150	157	165	172	179	186	193	200	208	215	250	286
6'0"	140	147	154	162	169	177	184	191	199	206	213	221	258	294
6'1"	144	151	159	166	174	182	189	197	204	212	219	227	265	302
6'2"	148	155	163	171	179	186	194	202	210	218	225	233	272	311
6'3"	152	160	168	176	184	192	200	208	216	224	232	240	279	319
6'4"	156	164	172	180	189	197	205	213	221	230	238	246	287	328
BMI	19	20	21	22	23	24	25	26	27	28	29	30	35	40

BMI Classification:

BMI Below 19
Underweight

BMI 19-24.9
Healthy Weight
(Low Health Risk)

BMI 25-29.9
Overweight
(Moderate Health Risk)

BMI 30-40
Obese (High Health Risk)

BMI Over 40
Morbid Obesity
(Very High Risk)

Interactive BMI Calculator
www.calorieking.com

Calories & Weight Loss

Calories in Food

Calories in food are derived from protein, fat and carbohydrate. Alcohol also provides calories. Vitamins, minerals and water provide no calories.

Calorie Values Per Gram

Fat/Oil	~ 9 Calories
Carbohydrate	~ 4 Calories
Protein	~ 4 Calories
Alcohol	~ 7 Calories

Note that fats have over double the calories of protein and carbohydrate. The higher the fat content of food, the higher the calories.

Sample Calculation

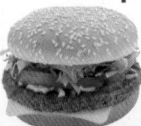

QUARTER POUNDER® WITH CHEESE has 510 calories derived from:

26g Fat (x 9 cals/gram)	=	234
40g Carbohyd.(x 4 cals/gram)	=	160
29g Protein (x 4 cals/gram)	=	116
Total Calories	=	510

Calorie Levels for Weight Loss

Start with a calorie-controlled diet that allows a moderate weight loss of ½ - 1 pound per week. Weight loss is usually much greater in the first few weeks due to extra fluid losses.

Note: It is better to increase exercise rather than lessen food calories too drastically.

Suggested Calories for Weight Loss

Women:	Non-active 1000 - 1200
Active	1200 - 1500
Men:	Non-active 1200 - 1500
Active	1500 - 1800
Teenagers:	1200 - 1800

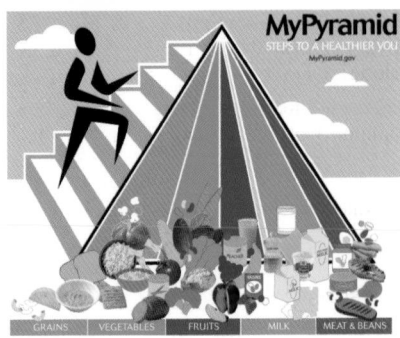

MyPyramid
STEPS TO A HEALTHIER YOU
MyPyramid.gov

GRAINS   VEGETABLES   FRUITS   MILK   MEAT & BEANS

The MyPyramid symbol **represents the recommended proportion of foods from each food group and focuses on the importance of making smart food choices in every food group, every day. Daily physical activity is also important.** *(More info: www.MyPyramid.gov)*

Examples of Single Serving Sizes

Grains (Eat 6 servings per day):
- 1 slice whole-grain bread (1 oz)
- ½ bun, small bagel or English muffin
- 4 small crackers or 1 tortilla
- 1 oz ready-to-eat whole-grain cereal
- ½ cup cooked cereal, rice or pasta

Vegetable (Eat 3-5 servings per day):
- 1 cup raw leafy vegetables
- 1½ cups raw chopped vegetables
- ½ cup cooked vegetables
- ½ - ¾ cup vegetable juice

Fruits (Eat 3-5 servings per day):
- 1 medium apple, orange, banana
- ½ cup canned fruit (in own juice)
- ¼ cup dried fruit
- ¾ cup fruit juice (unsweetened)
- ¼ medium avocado

Milk (2-3 servings per day):
- 1 cup (8 fl.oz) milk/soy (enriched)/yogurt
- 1½ oz cheese or ½ cup cottage cheese

Meat & Beans (Eat 2-3 servings per day):
- 2-3 oz (cooked) lean meat/poultry/fish
- 2 eggs **or** 7 oz tofu **or** ¼ cup nuts
- 1 cup (cooked) dried beans **or** chickpeas
- 4 Tbsp peanut butter **or** ½ cup nuts/seeds

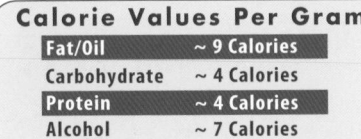

Portion Size Counts!

Food portion size is critical to controlling calorie intake for weight control.

Super-sized food servings have become more common when eating out and in the home. This can mean a day's worth of calories being consumed in one meal; or a snack being equivalent to a full meal.

It is easy to underestimate portion size of foods and drinks, and unwittingly consume excess calories – even if the fat content is low or even zero!

To more accurately estimate portion size of different foods, weigh and measure your food with food scales, measuring spoons and cups. Better control of calories will result.

For a visual idea of portion sizes, visit www.CalorieKing.com. See examples (fries and cola) on this page.

Allow for Extra Calories in Packaged Food

The actual weight of packaged foods is usually 5-10% more than the label net weight (the minimum legal weight) - and in some cases up to 50% more. However, manufacturers calculate the calories based on the net weight. For actual calories, weigh the product and calculate the extra calories.

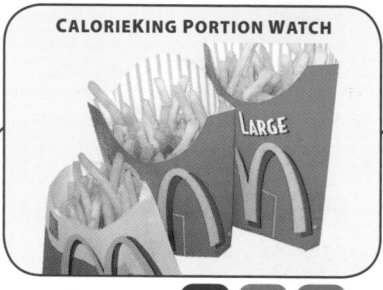

Basic 'Tools of the Trade'

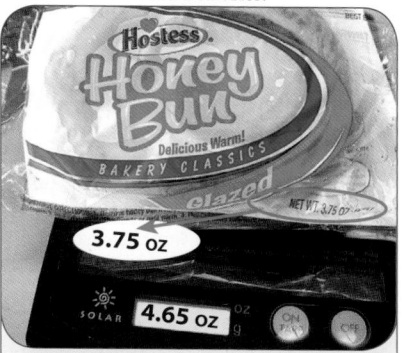

Actual weight of this bun is 24% more than the stated net weight.

CALORIEKING PORTION WATCH

Fries	Cal	Fat	Carb
Small	250	13	30
Medium	380	20	47
Large	570	30	70

CALORIEKING PORTION WATCH

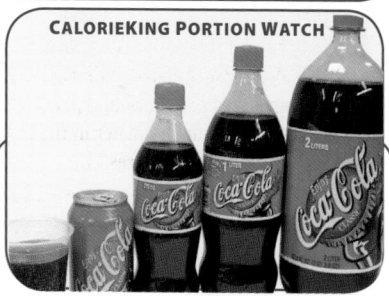

Cola	Cal	Fat	Carb
8 fl.oz Cup	100	0	25
12 fl.oz Can	150	0	37
20 fl.oz Bottle	250	0	63
1 Liter Bottle	400	0	100
2 Liter Bottle	800	0	200

Recommended Fat Intake

Americans consume too much fat with many getting over 40% of total daily calories from fat – either as fat or oil, or as fat in foods and drinks. A range of 20-30% is healthier.

Fat Intake - Healthy Ranges		
Children	~	30-60g
Teenagers (Active)	~	40-80g
Women	~	30-60g
Men: Active	~	40-80g
Heavy Activity/Athlete	~	80-120g

MAXIMUM DESIRABLE FAT INTAKE (Daily)

Calories	Fat	% Fat Cals
1200 cals	30g fat	23%
1500 cals	40g fat	24%
1800 cals	50g fat	25%
2000 cals	60g fat	27%
2200 cals	70g fat	28%
2500 cals	80g fat	29%
3000 cals	100g fat	30%
4000 cals	135g fat	30%

Percentage Fat Calories Formula:
$$\frac{\text{Grams of Fat Per Serving} \times (900)}{\text{Total Calories Per Serving}}$$

Fat Percent Content

(Grams of fat per 100 grams of food)

Don't be fooled by promotion of foods claiming to have a low percentage of fat. It's serving size and total grams of fat that count.

Examples: Whole Milk with 3.5% fat sounds low (3.5g fat/100ml) but an 8 fl.oz cup contains 8g fat; and 2 cups contain 16g fat.

Ice cream with 10% fat seems high, yet a regular scoop (3 fl.oz) has only 5g fat.

(Low-fat ice cream has less than 2g fat/serving.)

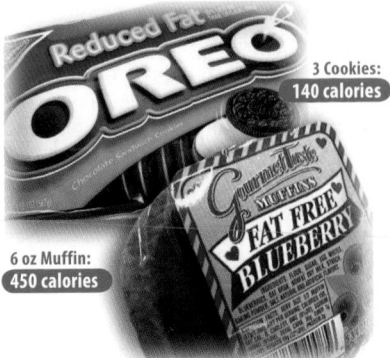

3 Cookies: 140 calories

6 oz Muffin: 450 calories

Reduced fat & fat-free foods are not necessarily low calorie. Portion size is still important.

It is a mistake to think that eating low-fat or fat-free foods allows you to eat double the quantity. You can end up with even more calories than eating smaller amounts of regular fat products.

Also fat-free but high in calories are soda drinks, fruit juices, beer, alcoholic spirits, sugar and candy. Bread, rice and pasta also have negligible fat.

Total Calories Count!

Ultimately, it is food portion size and total calories that count whether from fat, carbohydrate or protein. Remember, cows get fat on grass!

FOOD LABEL MEANINGS

FDA Nutrition Claim Definitions
(All are on a Per Serving Basis)

Low Calorie: 40 Calories or less

Light or Lite: One third fewer calories or, 50% or less fat than regular product

Fat-Free: Less than half a gram of fat

Low-Fat: 3 grams or less of fat

Reduced Fat: 25% less fat than regular product

Fewer or Less Calories: At least 25% fewer calories than regular product

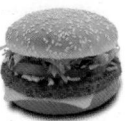

Meats, Poultry, Fish

- Choose **lean cuts** of meat with little marbling. **Trim all visible fat** from meat and remove the skin from poultry. Removal of fat after cooking, is okay (to prevent dryness). Choose 'extra lean' ground beef.
- **Avoid high-fat meat products** such as salami, bacon, sausage and franks.
- **Broil or bake. Avoid frying in oil.** Allow casseroles to cool and skim off surface fat.
- **Avoid fried fish**, frozen fish in batter and canned fish in oil.

Fats & Oils

- **Use minimal amounts** of all types of fat and oil. All are high in calories.
- **Choose** 'light' and 'reduced fat' spreads but still use sparingly.
- Use minimal amounts of oil when stir-frying. Use no-stick sprays like Pam.

Salad Dressings & Sauces

- **Avoid regular mayonnaise and oil dressings.** Choose 'light', 'reduced fat' or 'fat-free' brands.
- **Choose** low-fat or fat-free sauces (mainly tomato-based). Avoid 'pesto', 'alfredo', 'cheese' and 'creamy' sauces.

Milk, Cheese

- **Choose** low-fat or nonfat milks and yogurts. **Avoid** full-cream milk, cream, Half & Half.
- **Cheese:** Choose fat-free, and low-fat cheese. Part-skim ricotta is still high in fat. Low-fat cottage cheese is a good choice. Cheese substitutes can still be high in fat.

Snacks, Cookies, Candy

- **Avoid** high-fat snacks such as potato chips, corn/tortilla chips, cheese puffs, buttered popcorn, chocolate and carob bars.

Desserts/Sweets

- **Avoid high-fat desserts**, such as cake, pie, pastries, cheesecake, full-fat puddings.
- **Choose** fresh fruits, fresh fruit salad, canned fruit in water pack, low-fat ice cream. Use low-fat yogurt in place of cream.

Fast-Foods & Take-Out

Check the Fast-Foods Section of this book for actual fat and calorie counts.

- **Avoid deep-fried chicken,** french fries, and onion rings.
- **Pizzas:** Avoid sausage/pepperoni. Choose vegetarian topping and modest quantity of cheese. Eat a moderate serving. Eat extra salad and fresh fruit.
- **Hamburgers:** Choose medium size, lower fat burgers. Avoid bacon. Have a side salad (with fat-free dressing).
- **Delis:** Choose sandwiches/bread rolls, pitas with low-fat fillings and plain salad. Limit meat/cheese to small portions.
- **Coffees:** Avoid large sizes of latte and frappuccino. Request nonfat milk and no whipped cream. Avoid cookies and pastries.

Extra Information: www.CalorieKing.com

FRYING ADDS FAT!

The greater the surface area of potato exposed to fat or oil, the higher the fat content and calories.

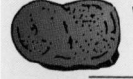

Whole Potato (3 oz)
0g Fat, 65 Cals

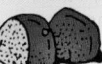

Roast Potato (3 oz)
5g Fat, 155 Cals

Fries (Large cut, 3 oz)
12g Fat, 220 Cals

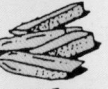

Fries (Small, 3 oz)
15g Fat, 265 Cals

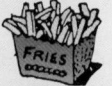

Potato Chips (3 oz)
30g Fat, 450 Cals

Carbohydrates ~ Friend or Foe?

Naturally-Friendly Carbs

- **Carbohydrate foods in their more natural forms** (not overly processed) are essential to good health. They are the main source of fuel for the body, and also provide important vitamins, minerals, antioxidants and fiber – all of which help protect against heart disease, diabetes, hypertension, constipation-related ailments and many other diseases.

- Carbohydrates even help the body produce serotonin, the 'feel good' brain chemical that helps control appetite and overeating. Too little serotonin can lead to mood swings and depression.

Carbohydrates are found in different forms in food as:

- Sugars in fruit, sugar cane, milk
- Starches in whole grains, legumes, nuts, seeds and vegetables
- Dietary fiber (See Fiber Guide ~ Page 276)
  Glycemic Index & Diabetes ~ Page 20

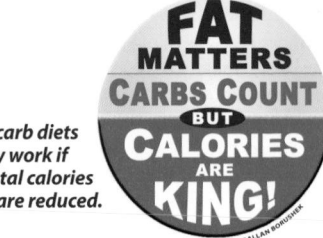

Low-carb diets only work if total calories are reduced.

FAT MATTERS
CARBS COUNT
BUT
CALORIES ARE KING!

RECOMMENDED CARBOHYDRATE INTAKE

Calories (Daily)	Carbohydrate (Grams)	Percent Carbohydrate Calories
1200 cals	120g	40%
1500 cals	170g	45%
1800 cals	210g	47%
2000 cals	250g	50%
2500 cals	345g	55%
3000 cals	450g	60%

How Much Do We Need?

- As shown in the chart, well-balanced diets above 2000 calories contain 50-60% of total calories from carbohydrates.

- At lower calorie levels used for weight control (1200-1500 calories), carbohydrates account for as little as 40% of total calories. This is because protein calories have nutritional priority.

- Carbohydrates & Diabetes ~ *See Page 20*

Low-Carbohydrate Diets

- Popular low-carbohydrate diets are extreme in their recommendations to initially cut carb intake to as little as 20 grams per day – the amount in 1 thick slice of bread, or 1 medium apple, or 1 small potato.

  This greatly increases the risk of nutritional deficiencies and compromises health, particularly if fat intake is excessive through fatty meats, high-fat dairy products, and fried foods.

- While overweight Americans do need to reduce carbohydrate intake, it should be done **sensibly as part of reducing portion size and total calories.**

- Simply eating 'low-carb' food products without regard to portion size, calories or fats, will do little to promote weight loss or good health.

- **Low-carb diets (and indeed any diet) only work if total calories are reduced.**

- Refined sugars should be one of the first targets in moderating carb intake.
  Extra Info ~ www.CalorieKing.com

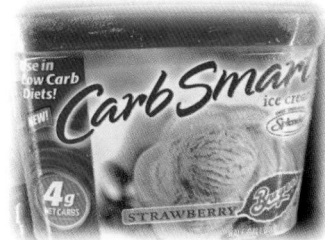

Lower carbohydrate products may still be high in calories and fat.

- Many overweight, inactive people consume over 500 calories of refined sugars per day, either self -added or as part of food products. This is equivalent to over 30 level teaspoons – a significant amount in weight control terms. Halving this amount would be reasonable and worthwhile.

  Note: Naturally occurring sugars in fruits, vegetables and milk are fine when consumed in normal recommended amounts. These foods are also rich in other nutrients.

  Refined sugar is referred to as having 'empty calories' because it supplies calories but negligible nutrients and no fiber.

- **Most sugar in our diet is 'hidden'** in processed foods such as soft drinks, fruit drinks, candy, cookies, cake, jam, sauces, ice cream, desserts, canned foods, and breakfast cereals.

  Certainly enjoy moderate quantities of these foods, but for serious weight control, look for 'low calorie', 'diet' or 'sugar-free'.

  However, be careful not to substitute sugar-rich foods with high-fat foods which might boost calories even more!

- Be aware that sugar comes in different forms such as sucrose, glucose, fructose, malt, high-fructose corn syrup, molasses, honey and maple syrup. Check the label.

- **Sugar alcohols such as sorbitol,** mannitol and maltitol are carb-based and have ½ - ¾ the calories of regular sugar. While not counted as sugar on food labels, they do add to the carb count. Excess amounts can cause bloating, gas and diarrhea.

- **Sugar-free sweeteners** such as *Equal, DiabetiSweet, NutraSweet, Splenda, Sweet'n Low* and *Stevia* make it easy to reduce sugar in drinks and recipes. Use only in moderation. **Note:** Most recipes can be adapted to contain less sugar with little effect on taste or quality.

Extra Info ~ www.CalorieKing.com

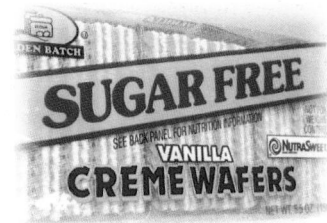

Sugar-free snacks and foods may be higher in fat and calories than the regular product.

Example ~ Creme Wafers (3):
Regular ~ 115 cals, 6g fat
Sugar-Free ~ 160 cals, 10g fat

SUGAR CONTENT OF SOME COMMON FOODS

	Teaspoons of Sugar
Coca Cola or *Pepsi*, 12 fl.oz	10
20 fl.oz size	17
Iced Tea, sweetened, 12 fl.oz	8
Chocolate Milk, 12 fl.oz	6
Honey Smacks Cereal, 1 oz	4
Popcorn, caramel, 1 cup	3.5
Chocolate Bar, 1.5 oz	6
M&M's 1.7 oz pkg	7
Muffin, large, 4 oz	6
Choc Chip Cookie, 1 oz	2
Donut, iced	6
Apple Pie, 1 piece	7
Jell-O, ½ cup	4.5
Jam, 1 Tbsp, 20g	2.5
Syrup, maple, 1 Tbsp	3

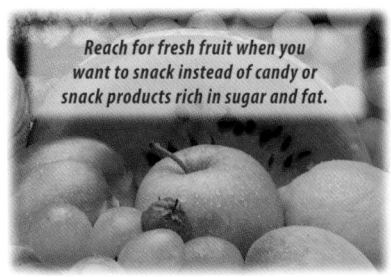

Reach for fresh fruit when you want to snack instead of candy or snack products rich in sugar and fat.

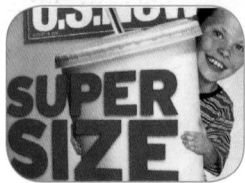

The XL Generation

Some 15% of American kids and adolescents are overweight; and childhood obesity has doubled over the last 20 years. Diabetes, high blood pressure and high cholesterol are major problem areas for overweight children and adolescents, as are depression, low self-esteem, sleep apnea and bone joint problems.

To address this problem, cooperation is required between kids, parents, schools and government. Weight control is a family and community affair.

Five Simple Tips To Get Started:

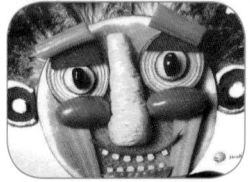

❶ Watch Soda Intake

Limit soda and sugary drinks to one serving on the weekends. Soda should not be an everyday beverage – water should be. When at restaurants or using a soda fountain, choose small servings with ice or choose diet soda instead. Schools should provide water and restrict access to soda as should parents when eating out or in the home!

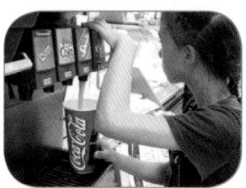

❷ Cut back on Fast-Foods and Eating Out

Many more calories are consumed when you eat out. Healthy meals prepared at home are best for the whole family.

❸ Say "No" to Super-Sizing

When meals are upsized, loads more calories are consumed. Choose sensible portion sizes when eating out and at home. Use smaller plates and choose smaller packages.

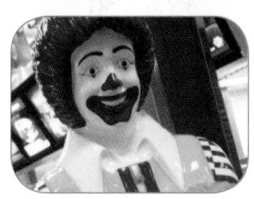

❹ Limit Between-Meal Snacking

Watch out for high-fat and high-calorie snacks – they can have more calories than a meal! Keep your eye on portion sizes and limit salty snack foods and candy to parties and special occasions. Choose fresh fruit, vegetables, nuts and low-fat milk instead.

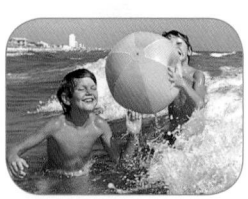

❺ Get Moving ~ Watch Less TV

Kids need at least 60 minutes of physical activity every day. It's critical for their fitness, and greatly lessens the risk of obesity.

Encourage kids to be active out of school hours. Wearing a pedometer can be highly motivational for kids to move more – as can playing dance video games such as *Dance Dance Revolution*. *Wii Fit (Nintendo)* is also useful as a fitness motivator.

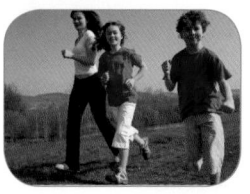

Limit TV and non-active computer games to just one hour per day. Also limit the accompanying snacks! Include exercise in family activities.

Extra information and tips ~ www.CalorieKing.com

Sample Meal Plan - 1400 Calories

**For Healthy, Overweight Persons ~ Not for Persons With Any Medical Condition
~ Please Check With Your Doctor & Dietitian ~**

Breakfast (approx. 300 cal)

	1 Small Fruit or ½ oz Dried Fruit
Plus	Cereal: 1½ oz Dry (high fiber)
	or 1 cup cooked Oatmeal
Plus	½ oz Almonds/Seeds
Plus	Milk (from daily allowance) or Yogurt (low-fat)

Daily Milk Allowance (approx.160 calories)
2 cups Non-Fat Milk or 1½ cups Low-fat (1%) Milk
or equivalent Soy Drink, Yogurt, Cheese, Tofu

Fat Allowance (140 calories; 15g Fat)
4 tsp Fat or 6-8 tsp Diet Margarine or 3 tsp Oil
or 1½ Tbsp Mayonnaise or ½ medium Avocado
or 1½ Tbsp Peanut Butter or 30g Nuts/Seeds

Breakfast ~ Choice 2

	1 Small Fruit
Plus	2 Eggs (no added fat)
	or 2 oz Cheese (low-fat)
	or 4 oz Cottage Cheese (low-fat)
	or 2 oz Lean/Canadian Bacon
Plus	1 Tomato
Plus	1 Slice Whole-Grain Toast

Lunch (approx. 440 calories)

	2 slices Whole-Grain Bread (2 oz)
	or 4 Crispbreads/Crackers or 6" Pita
Plus	2 oz lean Meat, Chicken or Turkey
	or 3½oz Tuna (in water) or 2½ oz Salmon
	or 1 oz Cheese or ½ cup (4 oz) Cottage Cheese
	or ½ cup (4 oz) Ricotta Cheese (low-fat)
	or ½ cup (4 oz) Fruit Yogurt (low-fat)
	or ½ cup (4 oz) Bean Salad
Plus	Large Salad (Oil-free dressing)
Plus	1 small Fruit or ½ oz Dried Fruit

Dinner (approx. 360 calories)

	Soup (fat-free)
Plus	3 oz lean Meat (cooked weight)
	or 4 oz Chicken Breast (no skin)
	or 3 oz Chicken Thigh/Leg (no skin)
	or 5 oz Fish (grilled, no fat)
	or ¾ cup (6 oz) Beans (Soy, Kidney, Pinto etc)/Lentils
	or Low-fat Entree (e.g. Lean Cuisine)
Plus	1 small Potato or ½ cup Rice/Pasta/Sweet Corn
	or 1 slice Whole-Grain Bread
Plus	2-3 servings Vegetables/Salad
Plus	1 small Fruit + Diet Gelatin Dessert

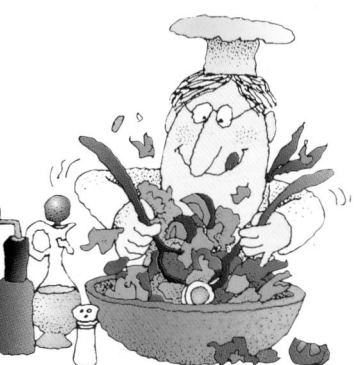

Between Meals
Water, Coffee, Tea, Diet drinks,
Fruit from main meals; Raw vegetable pieces, Milk from Daily Allowance

Exercise & Weight Control

- Persons who exercise regularly lose more weight and keep it off longer than non-exercisers.

- Exercise also improves general health and well-being. Mood, confidence and self-esteem are enhanced by a sense of control and accomplishment.

- **Exercise increases the metabolic rate** of the body even for hours after exercise - a good way to 'wake up' a sluggish metabolism and burn extra fat. Exercise compensates for any decrease in metabolic rate with increasing age and also in some heavy smokers who stop smoking.

- **Strength training** further builds muscle and aids body reshaping. You can also eat a little more food! Note: Each extra pound of muscle burns an extra 50 calories daily ~ even while you sleep! Weight from exercised muscles is okay. It is surplus fat (particularly abdominal fat) that is potentially harmful to health.

- **Avoid injury** by beginning with walking, low impact aerobics, or weight-supported exercise (e.g. swimming, cycling). Avoid competitive sports.

- **How Much?** Start with 10 - 20 minutes/day and progress to 30 - 60 minutes/day.
  Also walk up stairs instead of using elevators. Take a brisk walk at lunch. Use an exercise bike, treadmill or stair machine while watching TV. Walk the dog.

- **How Often?** While aerobic fitness requires only 3 - 4 sessions weekly, **weight control is a daily event which requires daily exercise.**

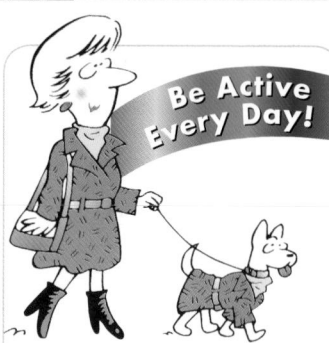

Be Active Every Day!

Brisk walking each day is a safe and effective way to keep trim and fit. Try it – you'll like it!
Strength-training with light weights helps to retain or rebuild muscle tissue. It enhances weight control.

FATNESS VS FITNESS

An overweight but fit person can be healthier than a thin, unfit person.

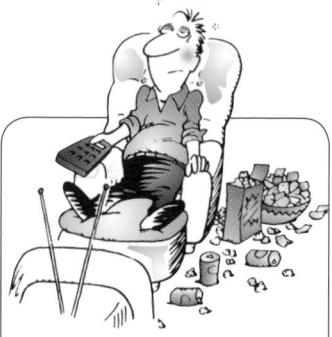

TV CAN BE FATTENING!

- Many adults and children spend over 20 hours per week watching TV or at the computer (playing games or 'surfing') – at the same time as eating high-calorie snacks and drinks.

- Are you a TV couch potato or computer addict? Limit your TV and computer hours and plan healthy physical activities.

- At home, limit kids to just one hour daily for TV and computers. Kids need at least 60 minutes of physical activity every day.

Too little exercise and too much food are the main contributors to middle-age spread.

Daily exercise and sensible eating can minimize middle-age spread. Include some strength-training to retain or build muscle.

Calories Used in Exercise

LIGHT	MODERATE	HEAVY
130 lbs ~ 3 Cals/Min	130 lbs ~ 5 Cals/Min	130 lbs ~ 8 Cals/Min
170 lbs ~ 4 Cals/Min	170 lbs ~ 6 Cals/Min	220 lbs ~ 12 Cals/Min
220 lbs ~ 5 Cals/Min	220 lbs ~ 7 Cals/Min	170 lbs ~ 10 Cals/Min

LIGHT	MODERATE	HEAVY
Walking, slow	Walking, brisk	Walking (power), Jogging
Cycling, light	Cycling, moderate	Cycling (vigorous), Spinning
Frisbee playing	Swimming, crawl	Swimming, strenuous
Gardening, light	Weight-training, light	Weight-training, heavy
Golf, social	Tennis, moderate	Wrestling/Judo, advanced
Tennis, doubles	Racquetball, beginners	Racquetball, advanced
Housework, cleaning	Aerobics, light	Tae Bo, Kick Boxing
Calisthenics, light	Football, touch	Football, training
Bowling	Basketball, Baseball	Basketball (Pro)
Ping-pong, social	Walking Downstairs	Climbing Stairs
Ice Skating, light	Snow Skiing (downhill)	Skipping Rope
Aquarobics, light	Shovelling snow	Skiing (cross country)
Skate Boarding	Dancing (ballroom)	Aquarobics, advanced
Line/Square Dancing	Rowing, moderate	Dancing (strenuous), Zumba
Tai Chi, Yoga	Volleyball, competitive	Rowing, vigorous
Volleyball		Martial Arts

Note: Only those sports or activities that are sustained over a period of time (e.g running) qualify for heavy exercise. Stop-start sports such as tennis are considered 'moderate'.

Interactive Calculations ~ www.CalorieKing.com/tools

WALKING PROGRAM

USE DISTANCE, STEPS OR TIME

Weeks	Distance	Steps Pedometer	Time
1-2	1 mile	2000	20 mins
3-5	1.5 miles	3000	18 mins
6-8	2 miles	3500	35 mins
9-10	2.5 miles	4500	45 mins
11+	3.5 miles	6000	60 mins

10,000 STEPS PER DAY

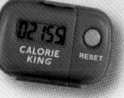

A pedometer can motivate you to be more active. It clips to your belt or waist band and registers each step.

Aim for 8,000 - 10,000 steps per day, instead of an average of only 3,000 - 4,000 steps.

For Extra Information:
www.CalorieKing.com

Reshaping Eating Behaviors

- Eating is a behavior that is largely controlled by people with whom we live or socialize, places in which we carry out our lives, and our emotions. Become aware of those situations that commonly lead to extra food being eaten.

- We may also be unaware of 'bad' eating habits that can lead to excess calorie intake; e.g. eating quickly, large mouthfuls, eating when tense or bored, finishing a large serving of food when not hungry.

Tips to help uncover and correct those 'bad' eating habits:

- **Don't eat while engaged in other activities;** for example, watching TV, reading. Eat only at the table, not at the fridge or while standing.

- **Don't eat quickly.** Chewing slowly allows time to register a feeling of fullness. Don't use fingers, only utensils. Cut food into smaller pieces. Don't load your fork until the previous mouthful is finished.

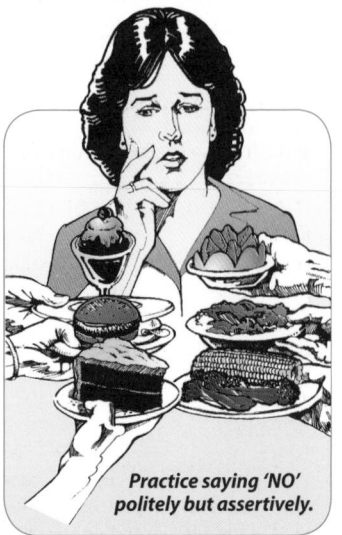

Practice saying 'NO' politely but assertively.

- **Don't purchase problem high calorie foods.** Shop from a set list to prevent impulse buying. Avoid shopping with children.

- **Buy snack foods** in the smallest package. The larger the serving size or package, the more you are likely to eat or drink.

- **Plan meals in advance. Stick to a set menu.**

- **Plan a strategy to avoid uncontrolled eating** and drinking at social events, or when your emotions urge you to binge.

  Rehearse repeatedly in your mind exactly what you will do in such situations. Remind yourself several times each day that you are in charge of your actions and that you can be strong-willed. Seek counseling or coaching on various strategies.

- **Promise yourself** that when you feel the urge to snack, you will engage in some activity that will distract you away from food (e.g. go for a walk, brush your teeth, phone a friend.)

  If you eat out of boredom, find some new hobby or interest that gets you out of the house. Even enroll in an adult education class.

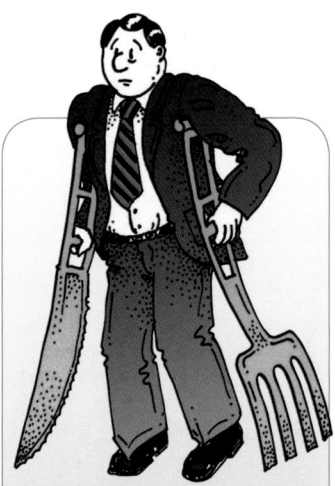

Do you use food as an emotional crutch? If so, professional counseling may be helpful.

The food journal is the most powerful proven aid for dieters. Persons who keep a food and exercise journal not only lose more weight, they also keep it off. Here are some of the reasons:

- **Recording your eating and exercise habits** jolts you into realizing just what you do eat and drink each day; and also whether you exercise sufficiently.

- **Helps you identify problem foods** and drinks with excessive calories and fat.

- **Helps identify moods**, situations and events that lead to excessive eating of unwanted calories. You can then plan to overcome or avoid them.

- **Prevents 'calorie amnesia'**, the forgetfulness that leads to rebound weight gain after successful weight loss. Recording puts you back on the right track.

- **Helps you develop greater self-discipline.** You will think twice about overindulging if you have to record it - especially if someone checks your journal regularly. It certainly keeps you honest!

- **Motivates you** to carefully plan your meals and to exercise each day.

- **Serves as a check system** for your doctor, dietitian or counselor to assess your progress and make recommendations.

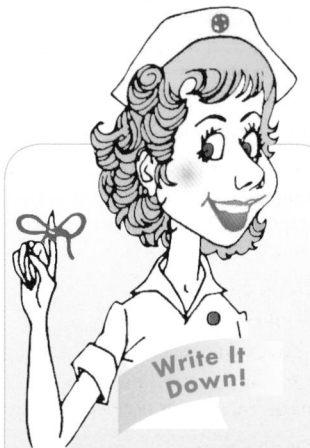

Write It Down!

"Keeping a journal gives me feedback on exactly what I eat and drink each day.

It helps prevent 'calorie amnesia' and reminds me to exercise each day.

It's a 'must' for successful weight control!"

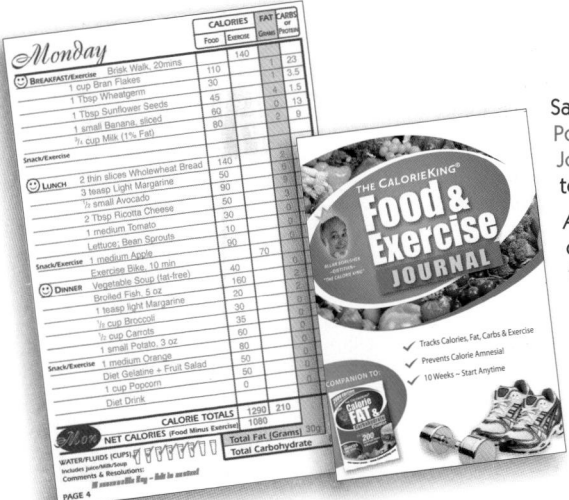

Sample Page from The Pocket Food & Exercise Journal, a 10-week journal to record food and exercise.

At day's end, exercise calories are deducted from food calories.

Includes Weekly Summary Page & Progress Checklist.

EXTRA DETAILS

~ SEE PAGE 302

What is Diabetes?

Diabetes is a disorder whereby the body cannot use carbohydrates (sugar and starches) properly.

- **After digestion**, sugar and starches are changed into **glucose** – the simplest form of sugar vital for body energy and growth.
- **Insulin** is the hormone which acts like a key that opens the door to body cells and allows glucose to enter.
- **Without enough insulin**, glucose builds up in the blood and passes into the urine. High blood glucose levels lead to frequent urination, extreme thirst, and tiredness.
- **Untreated diabetes increases the risk of damage to nerves and blood vessels.** This, in turn, increases the risk of heart disease, stroke, blindness, kidney damage, foot ulcers and gangrene (with amputation), impotence and other complications.

≈ **Body Cell**

Glucose

Insulin Key

Insulin acts like a key. It opens the door to body cells and allows glucose to enter.

People with type 1 diabetes and some with type 2 have too few or no keys and require insulin injections.

Others (primarily type 2) make enough insulin but the body doesn't use it as well as it should – particularly if obese and inactive.

SYMPTOMS OF DIABETES

- Frequent urination
- Extreme thirst
- Unusual hunger
- Rapid weight loss
- Extreme fatigue
- Blurred vision
- Skin infections that are slow to heal
- Tingling/numbness in feet

Note: Diabetes can be present even with no symptoms.

DON'T IGNORE DIABETES
IT'S A SERIOUS DISEASE!

TYPE 2 DIABETES

- Occurs in 90% of diabetes cases
- Occurs mainly in adults - particularly in overweight and inactive persons
- Insulin is produced but body cells resist its action and glucose cannot enter cells
- Usually treated with meal planning and physical activity. Sometimes requires medication (pills or insulin)

TYPE 1 DIABETES

- Occurs in 10% of diabetes cases
- Usually in children and young adults
- Pancreas produces little or no insulin. Daily insulin injections (or use of an insulin pump) are necessary, as well as: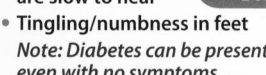
  - Matching pre-meal insulin to the amount of carbohydrate eaten
  - Weight control and regular physical activity

GESTATIONAL DIABETES

- Occurs in some women during pregnancy
- Usually disappears after the baby's birth
- Women who have had gestational diabetes still have a high risk of developing type 2 diabetes within 5 to 10 years
- Requires weight control, a healthy lifestyle and regular medical checks

Are You At Risk for Diabetes?

Pre-Diabetes ~ An Early Warning!

Pre-diabetes means that your blood glucose levels are higher than normal, but not high enough to be called diabetes.

If you have pre-diabetes, you have a higher risk for getting diabetes later on.

The good news is that you can start taking steps to prevent diabetes by making healthy lifestyle changes – such as losing weight if overweight, and being more physically active.

WHAT'S YOUR RISK?

Find out if you're at risk for diabetes by answering the following questions:

☐ I have been told I have pre-diabetes

☐ I have a family history of diabetes

☐ I am African American, Latino American, Asian American, Native American or a Pacific Islander

☐ I have had gestational diabetes (diabetes during pregnancy)

☐ I am over age 45

☐ I am overweight

☐ I get little or no physical activity

☐ My waist is larger than: 35 inches (for a woman) or 40 inches (for a man)

☐ My blood pressure is higher than 130 over 85

☐ My HDL (good cholesterol) is too low

☐ My triglycerides (blood fats) are too high

✔ **CHECK YOUR RESULT**

- **If you've put a check mark in two or more of the boxes, you may be more likely to develop type 2 diabetes.**
- **Talk with your healthcare provider to see if you should have a blood test for diabetes.**

BLOOD GLUCOSE CLASSIFICATION OF DIABETES	
Normal:	**Below 100 mg/dl***
Pre-Diabetes:	100-125 mg/dl*
Diabetes:	**Over 125 mg/dl***

(*Fasting Blood Glucose)

KNOW YOUR BGL
(Blood Glucose Level)
Everyone over the age of 45 should have a blood glucose test every three years

Importance of Weight Control

- **Type 2 diabetes** is more common in people who are overweight.
- **Being overweight** means that your insulin doesn't work as well to control blood glucose levels.
- **Losing just 10 to 20 pounds** can help you better manage your diabetes and lower your risk for heart disease.
- **Keys to weight control include:**
  - Following a healthy eating plan
  - Controlling food portions
  - Being physically active most days of the week
  - Keeping food records
  - Setting realistic goals
- **Work with a registered dietitian** who can help you reach a weight that's good for you.

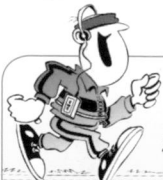

KEEP MOVING!
Every day, do at least 30 minutes of moderate intensity exercise.
(even in 5-minute sets)

It's the key to improving insulin action. Add muscle strength training 3-4 times a week to double the benefits.

Managing Diabetes

Don't battle diabetes alone. Establish a partnership with your doctor, dietitian, certified diabetes educator, and pharmacist.

Extra Support: • *Joslin Diabetes Center*
  • *American Diabetes Association*
  • *American Association of Diabetes Educators*
  • *Juvenile Diabetes Research Foundation*
  • *National Diabetes Education Program*

Hints to keep blood glucose within safe limits:

• **Control your food intake.** Know what and when you will eat. Seek referral to a dietitian for expert advice.

• **Exercise regularly.** It assists weight control and can improve sensitivity of body cells to insulin. Plan physical activity into your daily routine.

• **Monitor your blood glucose** at home and work with a blood glucose meter. It will help you become familiar with your blood glucose patterns, and the effects of food, activity and medication.

• **Take insulin or oral medication as prescribed.** If on insulin, know what action to take if hypoglycemia (low blood glucose) occurs. Also educate your family and friends.
More Info: www.joslin.org

Be Heart Smart ~ Know Your ABC's

If you have diabetes, you are at a higher risk for heart attack and stroke than someone without diabetes. But you can fight back!

Be smart about your heart!
Take control of the ABC's of diabetes and live a long and healthy life. Talk to your healthcare provider about your ABC targets.

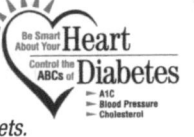

National Diabetes Education Program

Ⓐ is for A1C
The A1C (A-one-C) test – short for hemoglobin A1C – measures your average blood glucose (sugar) over the last 3 months.
Suggested target: below 7%

Ⓑ is for Blood Pressure
High blood pressure makes your heart work too hard. **Suggested target: below 130/80**

Ⓒ is for Cholesterol
Bad cholesterol, or LDL, can build up and clog your arteries. **Suggested target: below 100**

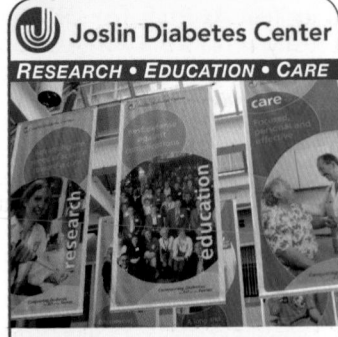

Joslin Diabetes Center
RESEARCH • EDUCATION • CARE

Joslin Diabetes Center, an affiliate of Harvard Medical School, is the world's largest diabetes research center, diabetes clinic and provider of diabetes education.

MORE INFORMATION
www.joslin.org or call 800-344-4501

Blood glucose meters and insulin pumps can greatly improve control of diabetes

BLOOD GLUCOSE METERS (EXAMPLES)

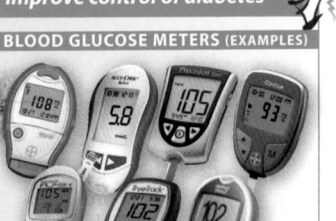

INSULIN PUMPS (EXAMPLES)

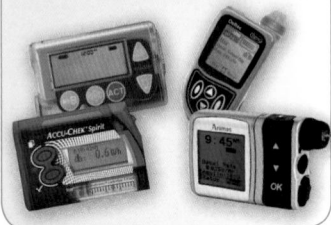

Guidelines for choosing a healthy diet apply equally to people with or without diabetes. Eating a wide variety of foods that are mainly low in fat, low in refined sugars, and high in fiber, is recommended.

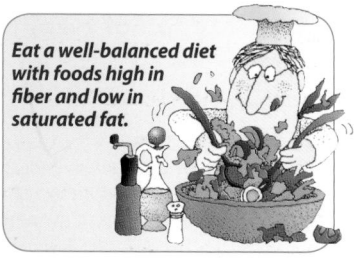

Eat a well-balanced diet with foods high in fiber and low in saturated fat.

However, actual food quantities, as well as when you eat, will also influence control of blood glucose. Your dietitian will individualize a meal plan to suit your food preferences, lifestyle and medical status. Here are a few tips:

- **Maintain a healthy weight.** If overweight, even a modest weight loss plus daily physical activity can help manage blood glucose in type 2 diabetes.

- **Don't skip meals.** If you take insulin or an oral hypoglycemic agent, regular meals are important.

- **If on insulin,** eat meals at the same time each day. Eat a similar amount of food at each meal. Eating about the same amount of carbohydrate over the day will make best use of insulin and prevent wide variations in blood glucose levels.

- Know how much carbohydrate you should eat at your meals and snacks each day.

- **Choose whole-grain breads, cereals and pasta.** Eat fresh fruits, vegetables and legumes. These foods contain more fiber and slow the release of glucose into your blood after a meal.

- **Limit foods high in saturated fat, trans fat and cholesterol.** Enjoy fish, soy foods, and other foods rich in omega-3 fats. *(Extra Notes: Page 271)*

- **Limit sugars and foods high in added sugar** particularly if overweight. Small amounts of sugar as part of a meal may occasionally be okay. Check with your dietitian. *(Extra Notes: Page 9)*

- **Read the Nutrition Facts label** on foods. Check the serving size, total fat and total carbohydrate.

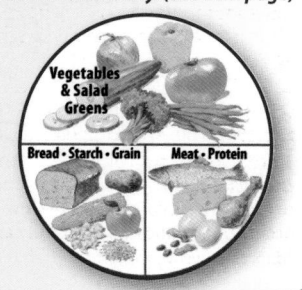

The Plate Method is an easy way to eat healthfully. (See next page)

Vegetables & Salad Greens

Bread · Starch · Grain

Meat · Protein

ALCOHOL TIPS

- **If you drink alcohol, have only moderate amounts:**
  Men ~ 1-2 drinks/day
  Women ~ 1 drink/day
  For some people, safe drinking will mean no alcoholic drinks at all.
  (Also see Alcohol Guide ~ Page 25)

- **Drink along with your food** – especially if you use insulin or diabetes pills.

- **Do not omit any carb food** in exchange for an alcoholic drink. However, non-alcoholic beers (12 fl oz) count as one carb exchange.

- **Alcohol increases the risk of hypoglycemia** (low blood sugar) and drug interactions if you take insulin and certain types of diabetes pills.

- **Check with your doctor and dietitian.**
  Extra Info: www.joslin.org

The Plate Method — An Easy Way to Eat Healthfully

The plate method is a helpful tool to guide your food choices until you see a dietitian for your own meal plan.

For a healthy meal:

- **Fill half of your plate** with non-starchy vegetables (broccoli, green beans, carrots).
- **Fill a quarter of your plate** with carbohydrate (whole-grain bread, pasta, potato, brown rice).
- **Fill the other quarter of your plate** with 3-4 ounces of lean meat, poultry, or fish.
- **Use 1-2 teaspoons of tub margarine** or a heart-healthy vegetable oil.
- **Add** a small piece of fruit or 8 ounces of skim/low-fat milk or yogurt.

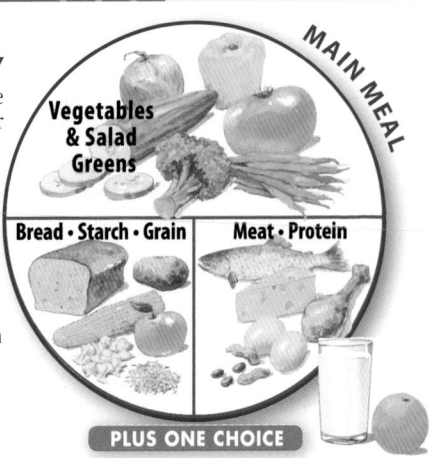

MAIN MEAL

Vegetables & Salad Greens

Bread · Starch · Grain   Meat · Protein

PLUS ONE CHOICE

Milk, Fruit, Dessert or other Carb Food

How Much Carbohydrate Should You Eat?

A dietitian can best determine how much carbohydrate you need at each of your meals, based on your lifestyle, food preferences, and overall diabetes control.

Until you see a dietitian, aim to keep the amount of carbohydrate you eat the same at each of your meals.

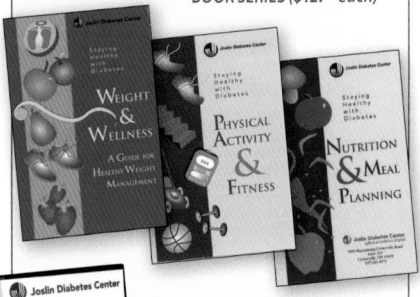
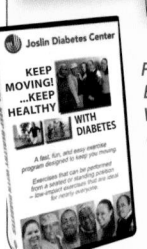
CARB CHOICES MEAL PLAN
One Carb Choice = 15 Grams of Carb

The amount in: 1 slice Bread **or** ¾ cup Cereal (unsweetened) **or** 1 small Potato **or** 1 small Fruit

 Breakfast
- Eat 2-3 carb choices (30-45 grams)
- Include a low-fat protein source such as egg whites or skim milk.

Lunch and Dinner
- Eat 3-4 carb choices (45-60 grams carb)
- Include fruit and non-starchy vegetables. Choose small portions of low-fat protein foods.

Snacks: If needed, eat 1-2 carb choices (15-30 grams carb).

Carb Type Affects Blood Glucose

The various forms of carbohydrate affect blood glucose levels in different ways. It is difficult to predict the effect of particular foods, sugars, or meals, simply by their carbohydrate content.

Thus the same amount of carbohydrate from different foods may affect blood sugar levels very differently. Many factors affect the rate of digestion and absorption – particularly the type of sugar, starch, and fiber; the degree of processing and cooking (which increases digestion rate); and the amount of protein and fat (which slow stomach emptying and digestion).

Glycemic Index (GI)

The GI is a method of ranking carbohydrate foods on a scale (0-100) according to how they affect blood glucose levels. (See next column). The higher the GI value, the greater the food's ability to rapidly raise blood glucose levels, and the more insulin needed by the body (not desirable).

Eating low-GI foods may lead to better control of blood glucose and insulin levels (which in turn lowers the risk of damage to blood vessels and nerves). The slower digestion of low-GI foods may also help to delay hunger pangs and benefit weight control.

Note: Choosing low-GI foods is not a license to eat unlimited amounts. Calorie restriction and portion control for weight control is of prime importance.

- GI is not meant to be used by itself without regard to portion size, and other dietary recommendations for healthy eating. Foods are not good or bad on the basis of their GI.

- While GI may be a helpful tool for some people with diabetes, what is most important is to control the total amount of carbohydrate that you eat.

Extra Info: *www.joslin.org*
www.glycemicindex.com

LOWER-GLYCEMIC FOODS

Slower-Acting Carbohydrates
These foods are more slowly digested and absorbed. They help maintain more even blood glucose levels, as long as excessive amounts are not eaten. Use these foods regularly but still limit portion size for weight control.
Examples:
- Dried beans, peas, lentils
- Nuts and seeds
- Whole-grain breads
- Bran cereals, oats
- Sweet corn, barley, buckwheat
- Whole-grain pasta, basmati rice
- Fresh fruit: apples, avocados, bananas (firm), cherries, grapefruit, grapes, olives, oranges, peaches, pears, plums. Fresh juices.
- Vegetables: broccoli, yam, sweet potatoes, salad greens
- Milk, yogurt, soy drinks
- Dark chocolate
- Sugar alcohols (sorbitol, maltitol)

HIGHER-GLYCEMIC FOODS

Quicker-Acting Carbohydrates
These foods more rapidly raise blood glucose levels. Eat only in moderation.

- White bread, rice cakes, bagels, croissants, doughnuts
- Low-fiber cereals: Cornflakes, *Rice Krispies, Froot Loops*
- White potatoes, white rice
- Watermelon, ripe bananas, cantaloupe, pineapple
- Soda, sugar-sweetened sports and energy drinks
- Sugar, candy, popcorn (plain)
- Ice cream (low-fat), frozen yogurt

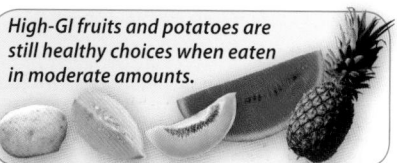

High-GI fruits and potatoes are still healthy choices when eaten in moderate amounts.

Calcium's Role in the Body

Calcium plays a vital role in nerve and muscle function, clotting of blood, enzyme regulation, insulin secretion and overall bone strength. Bones and teeth store 99% of the body's calcium.

The calcium level in blood is kept at a steady level by the continual exchange of calcium between blood and bone. When insufficient calcium is obtained from food the body draws calcium out of the bones.

This bone loss over a period of years may lead to **osteoporosis** – thinning of the bones (porous bones).

The bones become weak, brittle and easy to fracture, particularly the bones of the wrist, hips and spine. Loss of height and curvature of the spine may also result, as may periodontal disease - the deterioration of the jaw bones that support the teeth.

Common in Women & Men

While osteoporosis also occurs in men, women are particularly vulnerable (1 in 4 by age 60). They have about 30% less bone than men, and a greater bone loss at menopause when oestrogen levels drop. Slender framed women are at greater risk. (A woman in her eighties can have lost up to two thirds of her skeleton.)

Insufficient dietary calcium during pregnancy and breastfeeding will see bone reserves drawn upon, increasing the risk of osteoporosis in later years.

Hip fractures account for 300,000 hospitalizations each year. One in 5 older Americans with hip fracture die within a year – and 1 in 5 end up in a nursing home.

Causes of Osteoporosis

The major factors associated with the bone loss of osteoporosis appear to be:

- hormone changes of menopause
- inadequate dietary intake of calcium and other bone nutrients such as magnesium, vitamin D, zinc and protein
- insufficient exercise (weight bearing - such as walking, cycling ~ 30-60 minutes daily)
- family history of osteoporosis

Other contributing factors may include:

- excessive cola (regular or diet) and alcohol intake
- cigarette smoking
- some drug medications (e.g. steroids, thyroid)

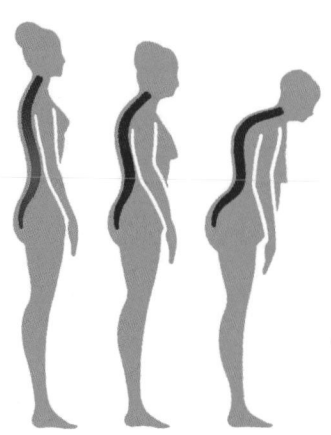

As osteoporosis progresses after menopause, vertebrae may collapse causing the spine to curve and shoulders to hunch.

RECOMMENDED DAILY INTAKE OF CALCIUM

Children:	1-3 yrs	~	500mg
	4-8 yrs	~	800mg
	9-12 yrs	~	1300mg

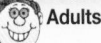

Teenagers:			
	13-18 yrs	~	1300mg

Adults:	19-50 yrs	~	1000mg
	51+ yrs	~	1200mg

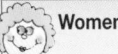

Women:		
Pre-menopausal	~	1000mg
Menopausal (beginning)	~	1200mg
Post-menopausal	~	1500mg
Pregnant & Breast-feeding		
14-18 yrs	~	1300mg
19+ yrs	~	1000mg

Early Prevention Important

Gradual loss of bone begins in the thirties after maximum bone mass is reached. The stronger the bones at that time, the less trouble is likely to occur later. The earlier that prevention or treatment begins the greater the benefit. **The key to prevention is to build strong, dense bones early in life. By age 16, some 80% of peak bone mass is already reached.**

Young women may lessen the risk by:

* eating high-calcium foods as well as adequate fruits, vegetables, whole grains and nuts
* drinking less soda, and more milk
* not engaging in extreme dieting that results in menstrual period cessation (via less estrogen)
* taking regular exercise and not smoking

Good Dietary Sources of Calcium
(Eat 3-4 servings a day of calcium-rich foods)

* Milk, Yogurt, Cheese
* Flavored Milk Drinks & Fruit Smoothies
* Ice Cream (low-fat), Frozen Yogurt (low-fat)
* Soy Drinks (calcium-enriched)
* Orange Juice (calcium-fortified)
* Tofu (with calcium coagulant), Miso, Tempeh
* Canned Salmon or Sardines (with edible bones)
* Breakfast Cereals (calcium-enriched): *Total, Wheaties*
* Broccoli, Dried Beans, Baked Beans
* Almonds, Brazil nuts, Hazelnuts, Seeds

Calculating Calcium From Food Labels

The calcium content of packaged foods and drinks is shown in the Nutrition Facts label as a percentage of the DRI (dietary reference intake) of 1000 mg calcium.

To convert this percentage into milligrams of calcium, simply multiply the percent figure by 10 (or add a zero). Examples: 5% = 50 mg calcium; 35% = 350 mg calcium.

Food Calcium Counter ~ www.CalorieKing.com

Calcium Supplements

Because absorption of dietary calcium decreases with age, prescribed high doses of calcium (1500-2000mg/day) may benefit persons with osteoporosis - as well as vitamin D (preferably in D3 form, not D2), vitamin K, magnesium and zinc. Check with your doctor.

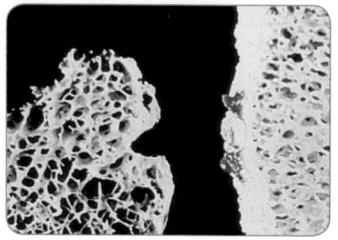

▲ Osteoporotic Fragile Bone   ▲ Healthy Dense Bone

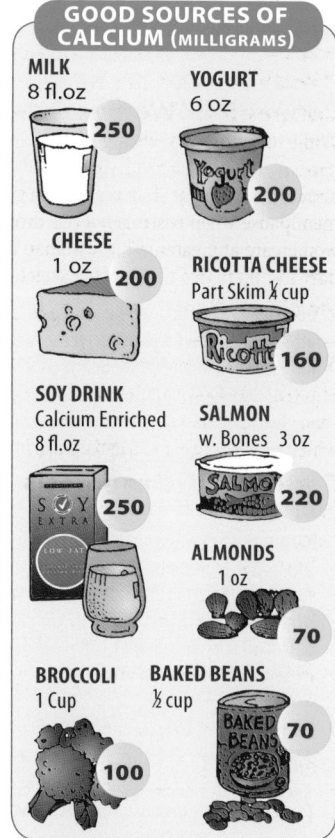

GOOD SOURCES OF CALCIUM (MILLIGRAMS)

MILK 8 fl.oz — 250

YOGURT 6 oz — 200

CHEESE 1 oz — 200

RICOTTA CHEESE Part Skim ¼ cup — 160

SOY DRINK Calcium Enriched 8 fl.oz — 250

SALMON w. Bones 3 oz — 220

ALMONDS 1 oz — 70

BROCCOLI 1 Cup — 100

BAKED BEANS ½ cup — 70

» Calorie and fat values have been rounded off.
Calories ~ to the nearest 5 or 10 calories.
Fat ~ to nearest half gram. **Note:** Trace amounts of fat (less than 0.3 grams) have been treated as zero.

» **Carbohydrate figures** in this book are for total carbohydrate, and not **Net Carbs** (which deducts fiber, polydextrose and sugar alcohols from total carbs).

» Because manufacturers' figures on labels are rounded off, figures in this book may differ slightly from the label. Serving sizes may also vary.

IMPORTANT DISCLAIMER

* The authors and publishers of this book are not physicians and are not licensed to give medical advice. This book is not a substitute for professional advice. Users should consult their medical professional before making any health, medical or other decisions based on the material contained herein.

* This book is a compilation of original material from other sources intended for educational purposes only. Because food manufacturers constantly change their products, only they are the authoritative source for food's most current nutritional information.

* Persons using the information herein for any medical purposes, such as matching insulin dosage to carbohydrate intake, should not rely solely on the accuracy of figures herein and should independently check food labels or contact the food manufacturer for the latest data.

* Because nutrition data for food products is subject to change, users should consult the most recent edition of this book, and the author's website www.calorieking.com for the most up-to-date information.

* **WARRANTY DISCLAIMER:**
THE AUTHOR AND PUBLISHER DISCLAIM ANY LIABILITY ARISING DIRECTLY OR INDIRECTLY FROM THE USE OF THIS BOOK. THE INFORMATION HEREIN IS PROVIDED "AS IS" AND WITHOUT ANY WARRANTY EXPRESSED OR IMPLIED. ALL DIRECT, INDIRECT, SPECIAL, INCIDENTAL, CONSEQUENTIAL OR PUNITIVE DAMAGES ARISING FROM ANY USE OF THIS INFORMATION IS DISCLAIMED AND EXCLUDED.

This information is also provided subject to Family Health Publications' Terms and Conditions found at the website, www.calorieking.com/terms and incorporated herein.

C ~ Calories
F ~ Fat (grams)
Cb ~ Carbohydrate (grams)

Abbreviations

tsp	= teaspoon
Tbsp or T	= Tablespoon
oz	= ounce(s)
c	= cup
fl.oz	= fluid ounce(s)
g	= gram(s)
avg	= average
pkg	= package

Volume Measures

(All measures are level)

3 tsp	= 1 Tbsp
2 Tbsp	= 1 fl.oz
½ cup	= 4 fl.oz
1 cup	= 8 fl.oz
2 cups	= 1 Pint
2 Pints	= 1 Quart

Note: 8 oz weight is not the same as 8 fl oz volume (space occupied). Dense foods weigh more per set volume. Examples:
1 cup popcorn weighs ½ oz
1 cup milk weighs 8½ oz
1 cup pudding weighs 10 oz

Metric Conversion

½ oz	= 14 grams
1 oz	= 28.4 grams
2 oz	= 57 grams
3½ oz	= 100 grams
1 fl.oz	= 30 mls
1 cup (8 fl.oz)	= 240 mls
33 fl.oz	= 1 liter (volume)

INFORMATION SOURCES
• U.S. Dept. of Agriculture
• Food Manufacturers
• Food Industry Boards & Councils
• Author extrapolations

FEEDBACK WELCOME!
Please contact the author with your queries and suggestions.
feedback@calorieking.com

● **Health Hazards: Excessive alcohol intake** contributes to obesity, high blood pressure, stroke, heart and liver disease, some cancers, and even impotence. **Concentration and short-term memory** are reduced as well as athletic performance.

Other alcohol hazards include fetal alcohol syndrome, stomach upsets, menstrual problems, depression, snoring, sleep problems, work absenteeism, impaired judgement, and social/family problems.

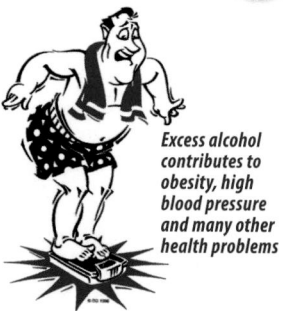

Excess alcohol contributes to obesity, high blood pressure and many other health problems

● **Alcohol contributes to obesity** through its high calories and by lessening the body's ability to burn fat. Fat storage is promoted, particularly in the belly - a health danger zone. Alcohol can also stimulate the appetite.

● **Alcohol is potentially more harmful while dieting.** Blood sugar levels may drop with resultant fatigue and further impairment of concentration, reflexes and driving skills - and maybe even the dieter's resolve!

HOW TO CALCULATE ALCOHOL CONTENT

Percent alcohol on label refers to alcohol volume (ml alcohol/100ml).
Note: 100ml = 3½ fl.oz

To convert to grams (weight) of alcohol, multiply the percent volume by 0.8 – since 1 ml of alcohol weighs only 0.8 grams.

EXAMPLE:
12 fl.oz Can Beer (5% alcohol)
5% alc. volume
= 5% of 12 fl.oz = 0.6 fl.oz
= 18ml alcohol (Note: 1 fl.oz = 30ml)
Weight (18ml x 0.8) = 14.4g alcohol

LOWER RISK ALCOHOL LIMITS

 WOMEN:
No more than
1 drink per day

 MEN:
No more than
2 drinks per day
(Over 65 ~ 1 drink)

(At least 2 days a week should be alcohol-free)

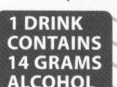
1 DRINK CONTAINS 14 GRAMS ALCOHOL
➤ 12 fl.oz Regular Beer (5% Alc.)
➤ OR 14 fl.oz Light Beer (4.2% Alc.)
➤ OR 5 fl.oz Wine (12% Alc.)
➤ OR 1½ fl.oz Spirits (80 Proof)

Note: You cannot save daily drinks for one occasion.
Binge drinking is particularly harmful ~ 4 drinks
for males or 3 drinks for females (within 2 hours).

For some people, **safe drinking** means no alcohol at all. Even one drink may impair driving skills, particularly if tired. For women who drink frequently, breast cancer risk is increased by 9% for each drink after the first drink.

GOVERNMENT WARNINGS!

(1) According to the Surgeon General, women should not drink alcoholic beverages during pregnancy because of the risk of birth defects.

(2) Consumption of alcoholic beverages impairs your ability to drive a car or operate machinery, and may cause health problems.

● **It is advisable not to drink at all if you are:**
* pregnant, trying to conceive or breastfeeding
* taking medication or have liver or heart disease (unless approved by your doctor or pharmacist)
* planning to drive, use machinery or play sports
* studying or needing to concentrate
* a child or adolescent

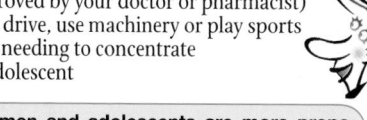
Women and adolescents are more prone to alcohol's ill-effects due to their lower body weight, smaller livers and lesser capacity to metabolize alcohol. As we age, our ability to handle alcohol decreases.

EXTRA INFORMATION
Alcohol & Diabetes ~ See Page 19
Alcohol & The Heart ~ See Page 274
Tips to Avoid Harmful Drinking ~ p. 31

Quick Guide

Alc ~ Alcohol (Grams)
Cb ~ Carbohydrate

Beer

Beer Contains Zero Fat	C	Alc	Cb
Regular Beer (5% Alc. Vol.)			
7 fl.oz Glass	80	8.5	4
12 fl.oz Bottle/Can/Glass	140	14	10
16 fl.oz Bottle/Can	185	19	13
22 fl.oz Bottle	260	25	18
24 fl.oz Can	280	28	20
32 fl.oz Bottle	370	35	28
40 fl.oz Bottle	470	46	35
50 fl.oz Football	590	57	50
Light Beer (4.2% Alc. Vol.)			
7 fl.oz Glass	65	7	4
12 fl.oz Bottle/Can/Glass	110	12	7
16 fl.oz Bottle/Can	145	16	9
22 fl.oz Bottle	200	22	13
24 fl.oz Can	220	24	14
Non-Alcoholic Brews			
(Less than 0.5% alcohol by volume)			
Average All Brands, 12 fl.oz	70	1	14

Beer Brands

Per 12 fl.oz Serving — **Alc** ~ Alcohol (Grams)
Percentage alcohol listed is by volume - not by weight.

	C	Alc	Cb
Aguila (3.9%)	125	11	11
Amber Ice (5.3% alcohol)	130	15	6
Amstel Light (3.5%)	100	10	5
Anheuser World Select (5%)	165	15	15
Anchor Steam (4.6%)	155	13	16
Artic Ice (5.3%)	150	15	8
Artic Ice Light (3.9%)	100	11	6
Asahi Super Dry (5.2%)	150	15	11
Aspen Edge Low Carb (4.1%)	95	12	3
Augsburger Bock (4.9%)	170	14	17
Bass (5.51%)	140	16	13
Beck's (5%)	145	14	12
Beck's Premier Light (2.3%)	65	6.5	4
Big Sky (4.8%)	150	14	12
Big Sky Light (4.5%)	105	13	5
Black Label (5.6%)	155	15	11
Blackhook Porter (4.9%)	160	14	14
Blatz (4.6%)	145	13	13
Blatz LA (2.3%)	75	7	6
Blatz Light (3.9%)	110	11	8
Blonde (4.3%)	140	12	10
Blue Moon, Belgian (5.4%)	170	15	14
Bud Dry (5%)	130	14	8

Brands (Cont)

Per 12 fl.oz Serving — **Alc** ~ Alcohol (Grams)

	C	Alc	Cb
Bud Light (4.2%)	110	12	7
Bud Ice (5.5%)	125	15	4
Bud Ice Light (4.2%)	110	12	7
Bud Light Lime (4.2%)	115	12	8
Budweiser (5%)	145	14	11
Budweiser Select (4.3%)	100	12	3
Busch (4.6%)	135	13	10
Busch Ice (5.9%)	170	16	13
Busch Light (4.1%)	95	12	4
Carling (4.4%)	140	13	10
Carlsberg (5%)	135	13	10
Castlemaine XXXX (4.7%)	140	13	9
Cerveza Aquila (3.9%)	125	11	11
Chelada Budweiser (5%)	370	28	40
Chelada Bud Light (4.2%)	300	24	31
Colt 45 Malt (5.6%)	160	15	11
Coors (4.9%)	150	14	12
Coors Extra Gold (5%)	155	14	13
Coors Light (4.2%)	105	12	5
Corona Light (4.1%)	105	12	5
Dos Equis Lager (5%)	130	14	9
Fosters Lager (5%)	145	14	11
Genesse: Regular (4.5%)	150	12	14
Genny Light (3.6%)	95	10	6
George Killian's Irish Red (5%)	160	14	15
Goebel (4.1%)	130	11	12
Goebel Light (3.9%)	110	11	8
Grolsch: Blonde (2.8%)	120	8	16
Light (3.6%)	95	11	6
Premium (5%)	145	14	10
Guinness Draught (4.2%)	125	12	10
Guinness Extra Stout (5.8%)	175	17	14
Hamm's: (4.7%)	145	13	12
Special Light (3.9%)	110	12	8
Harp (4.5%)	150	12	13
Heineken: (5%)	150	14	12
Special Dark (5.2%)	175	15	16
Premium Light (3.5%)	100	10	7
Icehouse (5.0%)	135	14	9
Icehouse Light (5%)	125	14	7
Jacob Best Ice (5.8%)	160	16	11
Keystone: Ice (5.9%)	145	16	6
Light (5%)	105	12	6
Premium (4.4%)	110	12	6
Killarney's Red Larger (5%)	200	14	23
Killian's Irish Red (4.9%)	165	14	14
King Cobra (5.6%)	135	16	5
Kirin Ichiban (5%)	150	14	12
Kirin Light (3.2%)	95	9	8

Brands (Cont)

Beer Contains Zero Fat

Per 12 fl.oz Serving

Alc ~ Alcohol (Grams)
Cb ~ Carbohydrate

	C	Alc	Cb		C	Alc	Cb
Labatt: Blue (5%)	155	14	10	Olympia Gold Light (2.2 %)	70	6	6
Blue Light (4%)	110	11	8	Pabst (4.3%)	145	13	12
Lech (4.9%)	145	14	11	Pabst Blue Ribbon (4.7%)	145	14	12
Leinenkugel's: Original (4.7%)	150	13	14	Pabst Light (3.9%)	110	11	8
Light (4.2%)	110	11	6	Pabst Extra Light (2.2%)	70	6	6
Lone Star: Regular (4.7%)	135	14	12	Pearl Light (2.2%)	70	6	6
Light (3.9%)	110	11	9	Pete's Wicked Ale (5.3%)	175	15	17
Lowenbrau Dark/Special (4.9%)	160	14	15	Piels (4.3%)	125	12	9
Magic Hat #9 (4.6% alc)	155	13	14	Pilsner (5% alc)	140	14	9
Magnum Malt Liquor (5.6%)	160	16	11	Red Dog (5%)	150	14	14
Meister Brau (4.5%)	130	13	12	Red Hook ESB (5.7%)	180	17	16
Memphis Brown (4.6%)	120	13	6	Red Hook India Pale Ale (4.7%)	180	13	19
Michelob: Larger (5%)	165	14	15	Red Stripe Jamaican Ale (5.0%)	155	14	14
Light (4.3%)	125	12	9	Rolling Rock (4.5%)	130	13	10
Ultra (4.2%)	85	12	2.5	Samuel Adams: Lager (4.9%)	180	13	19
Amber (5%)	115	14	3.5	Summer Ale (5.3%)	160	15	14
AmberBock (5.2%)	155	15	12	Sam Adams Light (4.6%)	120	11	10
Honey Lager (4.9%)	180	14	19	Sapporo Draft (3.9%)	135	11	14
Porter (5.9%)	195	16	18	Schaefer (4.6%)	145	13	12
Mickey's Malt Liquor (5.6%)	160	16	11	Schaefer Light (3.9%)	110	11	8
Miller Chill, 100 Cal, (4.2%)	100	13	4	Schlitz (4.6%)	145	13	12
Miller Genuine Draft: (4.7%)	145	14	13	Schlitz Light (3.9%)	110	11	8
Light 64 (2.8%)	65	8	2.5	Schmidt's (4.6%)	145	13	13
Miller High Life (4.7%)	145	14	13	Schmidt's Light (3.9%)	110	11	8
Miller High Life Light (4.2%)	110	13	7	Sheaf Stout, 5.8%	190	16	19
Miller Lite (4.2%)	95	13	3	Sierra Nevada: Pale Ale (5.6%)	175	16	14
Milwaukee's Best: (4.3%)	130	13	12	Bigfoot (9.6%)	295	28	25
Ice (5.9%)	145	16	7	Porter (5.6%)	195	16	19
Light (4.2%)	100	13	4	Silver Thunder (5.9%)	165	17	11
Minnesota's Best (4.9%)	140	14	10	Skyy Sport (5%)	160	14	15
Molson: Canadian (5%)	135	14	11	Sol Cerveza Especial (4%)	125	11	11
Ice (5.6%)	160	16	11	Southpaw Light (5%)	125		7
Light (4%)	120	11	9	St Pauli Girl (4.9%)	135	14	9
Molsons XXX (7.3%)	210	21	15	Stella Artois (5.2%)	155	15	14
Moosehead (5%)	125	14	14	Stroh's (4.6%)	145	13	12
Natural Ice (5.9%)	160	17	9	Stroh's Light (3.9%)	115	11	7
Natural Light (4.2%)	95	12	3	Tecate (4.7%)	155	13	16
Negra Modela (5%)	155	14	14	Tequiza (4.5%)	130	13	9
Newcastle Brown Ale (4.5%)	140	12	13	Tsingtao (4.7%)	155	13	16
Northstone Amber Ale (4.9%)	150	14	8	Warsteiner Verum/Dunkel (5%)	155	13	13
Olde English "800" (5.9%)	160	16	11	Weinhard's: Pale Ale (4/6%)	150	13	13
Old Milwaukee (4.6%)	145	13	13	Hefeweízen (4.9%)	155	14	12
Light (3.9%)	110	11	8	Wheat Hook (4.8%)	150	14	12
Ice (5.9%)	180	16	15	Widmer: Hefeweizen (4.9%)	155	13	16
Old Style (4.7%)	145	14	12	Zeigenbock Amber (4.4%)	145	12	13
Old Style Light (4.2%)	115	12	7				
Old Style LA (2.2%)	70	6	6				

Home-Brewed Beer: Similar to regular beers, according to alcohol content.

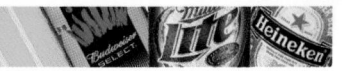

Alc ~ Alcohol (Grams) **Cb** ~ Carbohydrate

Non-Alcoholic Brews

Less Than 0.5% Alcohol
Average All Brands
(Busch NA, Coors NA, Haake Beck,
Kaliber, Kingsbury, O'Douls,
Old Milwaukee NA, Pabst NA,
Stroh's NA, Texas Select)

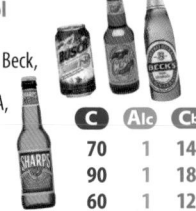

	C	Alc	Cb
12 fl.oz Can/Bottle	70	1	14
O'Doul's Amber, 12 fl.oz	90	1	18
Sharp's 12 fl.oz	60	1	12

Cider (Alcoholic)

	C	Alc	Cb
Hardcore Crisp Hard Cider (6%)	190	17	19
Hornsby's: Draft Cider (6%)	170	17	16
Hard Apple Cider (5.5%)	200	16	27
Woodchuck (5%) Amber, 12 fl.oz	200	15	21
Dark & Dry, 12 fl.oz	180	15	17
Granny Smith, 12 fl.oz	165	15	11
Wyder's: *Per 11.5 oz Bottle*			
Apple (4%)	155	11	12
Peach (5%)	175	12	16
Pear (5%)	130	12	15
Raspberry (4%)	140	11	16

Quick Guide

Table Wines
Average All Varieties (11.5% Alc.)
(Wine Contains Zero Fat)

	C	Alc	Cb
4 fl.oz 1 small wine glass OR ½ large wine glass	90	11	3
6 fl.oz (¾ large wine glass)	135	16	4
8 fl.oz (1 large wine glass)	180	22	6
½ Carafe/Bottle, 375ml	290	34	10
1 Bottle, 750ml	580	68	20

Table Wines

	C	Alc	Cb
Red: Claret/Burgundy/Chianti, 4 fl.oz	80	11	2
Sparkling Reds, 4 fl.oz	90	11	3
Rose: Medium, 4 fl.oz	80	11	2
White: *Per 4 fl.oz*			
Dry (Chablis/Hock/Riesling)	75	11	1
Zinfandel Sweet (Moselle/Sauterne), 4 fl.oz	85	11	2
Sparkling, 4 fl.oz	95	11	4

Table Wines (Cont)

	C	Alc	Cb
Champagne: *Per 4 fl.oz Serving*			
Average 1 glass, 4 fl.oz	85	11	2
w. Orange Jce (3:1 orange)	75	8	4
w. Orange Jce (1:1 orange)	65	5	7
Cold Duck 4 fl oz	108	11	8
Mulled Wine *(Gluhwein),* 4 fl.oz	180	14	20
Non-Alcoholic Wine, avg., 4 fl.oz	50	0	12
Reduced Alcohol Wine (6%):			
Average all types, 4 fl.oz	50	0	12
Sake: Rice Wine (16% alc.), 4 oz	125	15	5

Flavored Wines

Average All Brands (6% alcohol)
(Examples: Arbor Mist, Wild Vines, Boones)

	C	Alc	Cb
1 small wine glass, 4 oz	80	6	10
1 large wine glass, 8 oz	160	11	20
1 bottle, 750 ml (25.4 fl.oz)	510	36	64

Dessert Wines

	C	Alc	Cb
Madeira (18% alc), 2 oz	85	9	5
Marsala (18%), 2 oz	110	9	11
Port, Muscatel (18%), 2 oz	85	9	5
Sherry (18%), 2 oz			
Dry, 1 Sherry glass	65	9	0.5
Sweet/Cream, average	85	9	5
Vermouth: Dry (18%), 2 oz	65	9	0.5
Sweet (15%), 2 oz	85	7	8

Cooking Wines

	C	Alc	Cb
Average All Brands			
Red/White: 2 Tbsp, 1 oz	20	3	1
1 cup, 8 oz	160	22	12
Marsala, 2 Tbsp, 1 oz	35	4	2
Sherry, 2 Tbsp, 1 oz	40	4	2

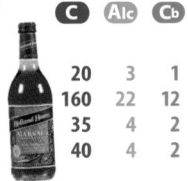

COOKING WITH WINE
For alcohol to evaporate, sufficient heat and cooking
time (at least 30 minutes) is required.
Red and white table wines would
then contain negligible residual calories.
Sweetened wines (marsala/sherry)
would contain 10 calories per 1 fl.oz.
Flambé Desserts: Only surface alcohol is burned
off, so negligible reduction in alcohol or calories.

Quick Guide · Alc ~ Alcohol (Grams)

Spirits/Liquors

Includes Bourbon, Brandy, Gin, Rum, Scotch, Tequila, Vodka, Whiskey.
Note: All spirits with same alcohol proof have similar calories and zero fat.

Average All Brands	C	Alc	Cb
80 Proof (40% Alcohol by Volume):			
1 fl.oz	65	9.5	0
1½ fl.oz (1 shot)	100	14	0
3 fl.oz (Double shot)	200	29	0
½ Bottle, 350 ml	810	120	0
1 Bottle, 700 ml (24 fl.oz)	1620	240	0
86 Proof (43% Alc): 1 fl.oz	70	10	0
1½ fl.oz (1 shot)	105	15	0
1 Bottle, 700 ml (24 fl.oz)	1750	250	0
100 Proof (50% Alc): 1½ fl.oz	120	18	0

Flavored Spirits ~ Average All Brands			
Includes Malibu Rum; Captain Morgan (Original)			
70 Proof (35% Alc): 1½ fl.oz	105	13	1
3 fl.oz (Double shot)	210	26	3
Parrot Bay (21%), avg., 1½ fl.oz	100	8	12
Southern Comfort (35%), 1½ fl.oz	100	13	3

Shochu (Soju) ~ Izakaya Lounges			
Average all types (20% alc), 2 fl.oz	65	9	0

Hard Lemonade & Sodas

	C	Alc	Cb
Henry's Hard L'ade (5%), 12 fl.oz	285	14	46
Mike's Hard Lemonade (5.2%):			
11.2 fl.oz bottle	240	13	38
16 fl.oz bottle	345	19	54
Light (4%), 11.2 fl.oz	100	10	6
Mike's Hard Iced Tea (5%), 11.2 fl.oz	195	13	27
Rick's Spiked (5.2%), 12 fl.oz	250	14	39
Twisted Tea: Half & Half (5%) 12 fl.oz	250	14	37
Hard Iced (5%): All flavors	220	14	30
Light (4%), 12 fl.oz	115	11	9
Original (5%):, 12 fl.oz bottle	220	14	30
24 fl.oz can	440	28	60
Zima (4.9%), avg. all flav., 12 fl.oz	185	14	22

Alcoholic Energy Drinks (with Caffeine)

	C	Alc	Cb
Sparks: *Per 16 fl.oz Can*			
Sparks (6%)	340	23	47
Sparks Light (6%)	180	23	5
Sparks Plus (7%)	385	26	49
Tilt Green (8%), 16 fl.oz	460	30	64
Tilt Orange (6.6%), 16 fl.oz	410	25	46

Coolers & Premix Cocktails

Ready-To-Drink
Zero Fat Unless Indicated

	C	Alc	Cb
Arbor Mist: Blenders,			
all flavors (12.5%), 4 fl.oz	100	11	14
Bacardi Silver: *Per 12 fl.oz*			
Fruit Flavors (5%)	240	14	36
Silver O³/Raz (5%)	240	14	36
Silver Mojito (5%)	230	14	33
Ready to Pour, (1.75 liter bottle)			
Bahama Mama (10%), 4 fl.oz	130	13	16
Hurricane (12.5%), 4 fl.oz	144	12	16
Rum Island Ice Tea (12.5%), 4 fl.oz	150	12	16
Bartles & Jaymes			
Malt Based Coolers (3.9% alc.): *Per 12 fl.oz*			
Classic Original; Blue Hawaiian	190	11	29
Black Cherry; Berry; Peach	220	11	33
Raspb./Strawb. Daquiri	215	11	36
Margarita/Pina Colada	260	11	47
Other flavors, avg.	230	11	39
Wine Cooler (5% alc.): *12 fl.oz*			
Classic Original	200	14	29
Blue Hawaiian; Exotic Berry, avg.	230	14	33
Other flavors, average	240	14	38
Captain Morgan Parrot Bay (5% Alc),			
Average all flavors, 12 fl.oz	250	14	37
Daily's *(Ready-To-Drink):*			
Bag-In-Box Cocktails (6.9%),			
Bloody Mary, ½ cup, 4 fl.oz	70	6	6
Other flavors, 4 fl.oz	110	6	15
Frozen Pouches (5%), 10 fl.oz	280	11	44
Jack Daniels Country Cocktails:			
Average all flavors, 6.8 fl.oz	170	10	25
Jack Daniels Hard Cola (5%) 12 oz	234	14	34
Jose Cuervo Margaritas (5.9% alc)			
Premix (9.95%), Strawb./Lime, 1½ oz	50	3.5	7
Minis (5.9%), 200ml bottle	180	10	27
Sauza Diablo (5%), 12 fl.oz	260	14	40
Seagram's Coolers (5%)			
Average all flavors	240	14	35
Skyy Blue (5%), 12 fl.oz	280	14	45
Stolichnaya Citr. (5%), 12 fl.oz	240	14	36
Smirnoff Ice (5%), 330ml	220	13	33
Black Ice (5.5%), 12 fl.oz	240	19	36
TGI Friday's: *Per 3 fl.oz*			
On The Rocks: Margarita (7.5%)	90	6	14
Long Island Ice Tea (15%)	130	11	14
Mudslide (10%)	200	8	18
Blenders (12.5% alc): *Per 3 fl.oz*			
Mudslide (12.5%)	120	8.5	15
Orange Dream (12.5%)	120	8.5	15
Strawberry Shortcake (12.5%)	115	8.5	12

29

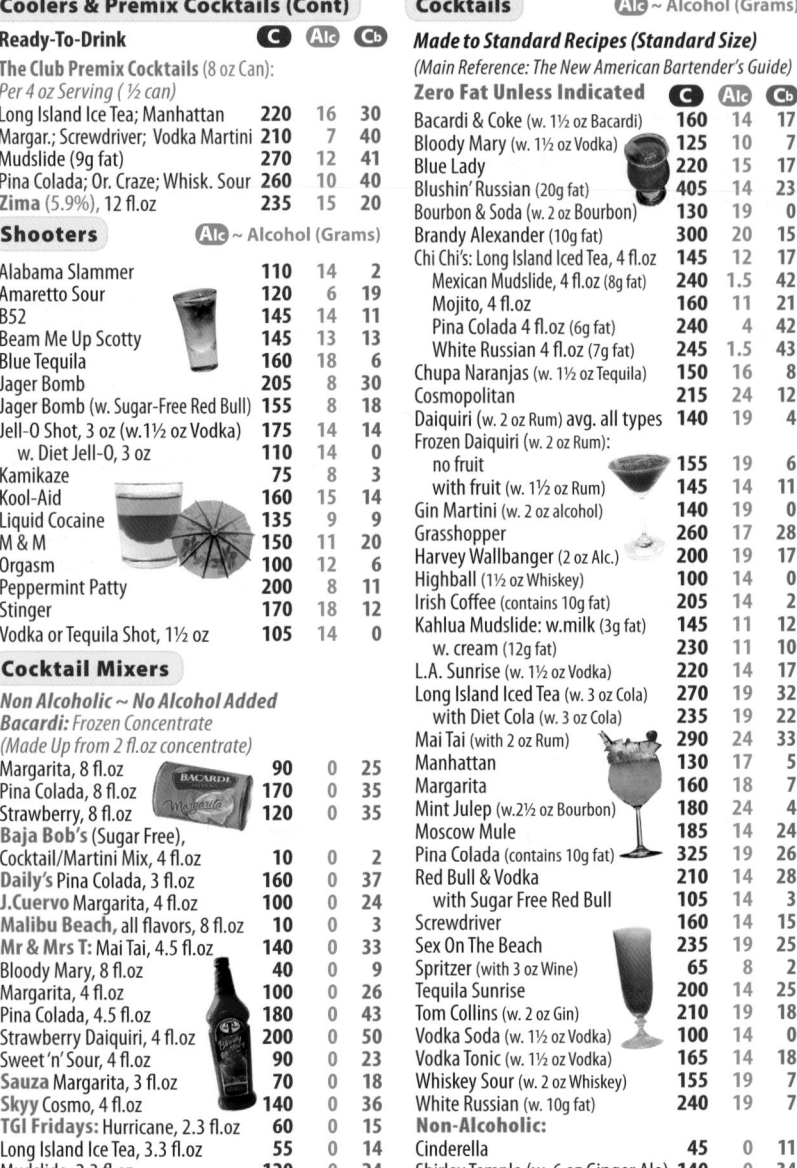

Coolers & Premix Cocktails (Cont)

Ready-To-Drink | **C** | **Alc** | **Cb**

The Club Premix Cocktails (8 oz Can):
Per 4 oz Serving (½ can)

	C	Alc	Cb
Long Island Ice Tea; Manhattan	220	16	30
Margar.; Screwdriver; Vodka Martini	210	7	40
Mudslide (9g fat)	270	12	41
Pina Colada; Or. Craze; Whisk. Sour	260	10	40
Zima (5.9%), 12 fl.oz	235	15	20

Shooters — Alc ~ Alcohol (Grams)

	C	Alc	Cb
Alabama Slammer	110	14	2
Amaretto Sour	120	6	19
B52	145	14	11
Beam Me Up Scotty	145	13	13
Blue Tequila	160	18	6
Jager Bomb	205	8	30
Jager Bomb (w. Sugar-Free Red Bull)	155	8	18
Jell-O Shot, 3 oz (w.1½ oz Vodka)	175	14	14
w. Diet Jell-O, 3 oz	110	14	0
Kamikaze	75	8	3
Kool-Aid	160	15	14
Liquid Cocaine	135	9	9
M & M	150	11	20
Orgasm	100	12	6
Peppermint Patty	200	8	11
Stinger	170	18	12
Vodka or Tequila Shot, 1½ oz	105	14	0

Cocktail Mixers

Non Alcoholic ~ No Alcohol Added
Bacardi: *Frozen Concentrate*
(Made Up from 2 fl.oz concentrate)

	C	Alc	Cb
Margarita, 8 fl.oz	90	0	25
Pina Colada, 8 fl.oz	170	0	35
Strawberry, 8 fl.oz	120	0	35
Baja Bob's (Sugar Free),			
Cocktail/Martini Mix, 4 fl.oz	10	0	2
Daily's Pina Colada, 3 fl.oz	160	0	37
J.Cuervo Margarita, 4 fl.oz	100	0	24
Malibu Beach, all flavors, 8 fl.oz	10	0	3
Mr & Mrs T: Mai Tai, 4.5 fl.oz	140	0	33
Bloody Mary, 8 fl.oz	40	0	9
Margarita, 4 fl.oz	100	0	26
Pina Colada, 4.5 fl.oz	180	0	43
Strawberry Daiquiri, 4 fl.oz	200	0	50
Sweet 'n' Sour, 4 fl.oz	90	0	23
Sauza Margarita, 3 fl.oz	70	0	18
Skyy Cosmo, 4 fl.oz	140	0	36
TGI Fridays: Hurricane, 2.3 fl.oz	60	0	15
Long Island Ice Tea, 3.3 fl.oz	55	0	14
Mudslide, 2.3 fl.oz	120	0	24

Cocktails — Alc ~ Alcohol (Grams)

Made to Standard Recipes (Standard Size)
(Main Reference: The New American Bartender's Guide)

Zero Fat Unless Indicated | **C** | **Alc** | **Cb**

	C	Alc	Cb
Bacardi & Coke (w. 1½ oz Bacardi)	160	14	17
Bloody Mary (w. 1½ oz Vodka)	125	10	7
Blue Lady	220	15	17
Blushin' Russian (20g fat)	405	14	23
Bourbon & Soda (w. 2 oz Bourbon)	130	19	0
Brandy Alexander (10g fat)	300	20	15
Chi Chi's: Long Island Iced Tea, 4 fl.oz	145	12	17
Mexican Mudslide, 4 fl.oz (8g fat)	240	1.5	42
Mojito, 4 fl.oz	160	11	21
Pina Colada 4 fl.oz (6g fat)	240	4	42
White Russian 4 fl.oz (7g fat)	245	1.5	43
Chupa Naranjas (w. 1½ oz Tequila)	150	16	8
Cosmopolitan	215	24	12
Daiquiri (w. 2 oz Rum) avg. all types	140	19	4
Frozen Daiquiri (w. 2 oz Rum):			
no fruit	155	19	6
with fruit (w. 1½ oz Rum)	145	14	11
Gin Martini (w. 2 oz alcohol)	140	19	0
Grasshopper	260	17	28
Harvey Wallbanger (2 oz Alc.)	200	19	17
Highball (1½ oz Whiskey)	100	14	0
Irish Coffee (contains 10g fat)	205	14	2
Kahlua Mudslide: w.milk (3g fat)	145	11	12
w. cream (12g fat)	230	11	10
L.A. Sunrise (w. 1½ oz Vodka)	220	14	17
Long Island Iced Tea (w. 3 oz Cola)	270	19	32
with Diet Cola (w. 3 oz Cola)	235	19	22
Mai Tai (with 2 oz Rum)	290	24	33
Manhattan	130	17	5
Margarita	160	18	7
Mint Julep (w.2½ oz Bourbon)	180	24	4
Moscow Mule	185	14	24
Pina Colada (contains 10g fat)	325	19	26
Red Bull & Vodka	210	14	28
with Sugar Free Red Bull	105	14	3
Screwdriver	160	14	15
Sex On The Beach	235	19	25
Spritzer (with 3 oz Wine)	65	8	2
Tequila Sunrise	200	14	25
Tom Collins (w. 2 oz Gin)	210	19	18
Vodka Soda (w. 1½ oz Vodka)	100	14	0
Vodka Tonic (w. 1½ oz Vodka)	165	14	18
Whiskey Sour (w. 2 oz Whiskey)	155	19	7
White Russian (w. 10g fat)	240	19	7
Non-Alcoholic:			
Cinderella	45	0	11
Shirley Temple (w. 6 oz Ginger Ale)	140	0	34

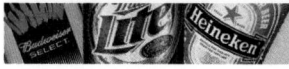

Liqueurs/Cordials · **C** **Alc** **Cb**

Per 1 fl.oz

	C	Alc	Cb
Advocaat (36 Proof; 2g fat)	85	4	9
Alizé: Cognac	70	11	2
Gold/Red Passion	105	4.5	11
Amaretto (56 Proof)	110	6	17
Baileys Irish Cream (34 Proof; 5g fat)	95	4	5
Lite (30 Proof; 2g fat)	75	4	7
Benedictine (80 Proof)	90	10	5
Chambord (33 Proof)	105	5	11
Chartreuse (80 Proof)	100	10	7
Cherry Brandy (48 Proof)	80	6	9
Coffee Liqueur (53 Proof)	90	6	11
Cointreau (80 Proof)	100	10	7
Creme de Cacao (54 Proof)	100	6	15
Creme de Menthe (60 Proof)	120	7	14
Curacao (70 Proof)	95	8	6
Drambuie (80 Proof)	105	10	9
Frangelico (48 Proof)	80	6	9
Galliano (80 Proof)	100	10	8
Grand Marnier (80 Proof)	100	10	7
Kahlua (53 Proof)	90	6	11
Kirsch (68 Proof)	80	8	6
Midori (42 Proof)	80	5	11
Ouzo (80 Proof)	105	11	11
Pernod (80 Proof)	75	10	2
Sambuca (84 Proof)	100	10	7
Schnapps (80 Proof)	100	10	7
Southern Comfort (70 Proof)	80	10	3
Starbucks Coffee Liqueur (40 Proof)	80	4	13
Tia Maria (64 Proof)	90	8	9
Triple Sec (60 Proof)	80	7	4

Liqueur Coffee & Hot Drinks

Per Standard Drink

	C	Alc	Cb
Liqueur Coffee, avg. all types	200	10	10
Egg Nog	270	10	25
Hot Toddy, w. 2 oz liquor	200	19	17
Irish Coffee, w. 2 Tbsp whip. crm	80	7	4
Mulled Wine (Glühwein), 5 oz	175	14	6

Flavorings/Syrups

	C	Alc	Cb
Angostura Bitters, ¼ tsp	3	0	0
Ginger Ale, 8 fl.oz	80	0	22
Grenadine/Cassis, 2 Tbsp, 1 oz	70	0	17
Lime/Lemon Juice, 2 Tbsp, 1 oz	10	0	2
Maraschino Cherry, 1 small	8	0	2
Pure Lemon Extract (70%) avg., 1 oz	145	20	0
Sugar Syrup, 2 Tbsp, 1 oz	70	0	17
Sour Mix, 2 Tbsp, 1 oz	10	0	2
Tonic Water, 8 fl.oz	90	0	22
Vanilla Extract, (35%), avg., 1 oz	80	10	3.5

TEN HINTS TO AVOID HARMFUL DRINKING

1. **Add up the alcohol** you typically drink each day and on social occasions. How does this compare with 'low risk' amounts?

2. **Compare the alcohol content** of different drinks and select the lowest. Request half ounces of alcohol in cocktails and mixed drinks. Dilute them and keep topping off with non-alcoholic drinks.

3. **Go easy on 'Light' beers.** At 4% alcohol, on average, they are still high in alcohol compared to regular beer (5% alcohol).

4. **Try low alcohol or non-alcohol** alternatives such as fruit juices and mineral water. Take your own to parties.

5. **Before drinking alcohol,** quench your thirst with water and non-alcoholic drinks – particularly after vigorous exercise or sports.

6. **Slow the rate of drinking.** Chugging or drinking fast is the major cause of illness and death from alcohol poisoning.

7. **Avoid drinking in 'rounds'.**

8. **Have a non-alcoholic 'spacer'** between drinks (e.g. mineral water, orange juice).

9. **Don't drink on an empty stomach.** Food slows the rate of alcohol absorption.

10. **Keep track of the number of drinks** and know when to stop. Stick to a set limit.

Note: • Alcohol can be very dangerous when taken with prescription or street drugs or when you are very tired.

Extra Info: www.CalorieKing.com

"The doctor told him to cut down to just one glass a day."

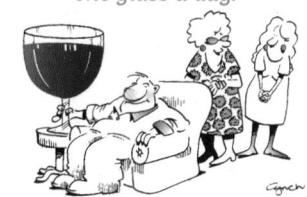

Baking Ingredients

	C	F	Cb
Almond Paste:			
(Marzipan), 2 Tbsp 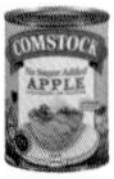	170	7	24
Apple Pie Filling,			
Sweetened, 9.4 oz	240	0	60
Also See Page 136			
Baking Powder: Regular, 1 tsp	5	0	2
Cream of Tartar, 1 tsp 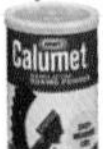	10	0	2
Baking Mix *(Bisquick)* :			
Original, ⅓ cup, 1½ oz	160	5	26
Heart Smart, ⅓ cup, 1½ oz	140	2.5	27
Batter Mix *(Golden Dipt)*, ¼ c. mix	100	0	23
Blueberries, 1 cup, 5 oz	85	0.5	21
Butter/Margarine, ½ c., 4 oz	815	92	1
Stick, *Land O' Lakes*, ½ oz 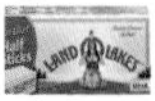	100	11	0
Carob Flour, ½ cup	115	0.5	46
Chocolate Baking Bars: *Average all Brands*			
Sweet *(Baker's)*: 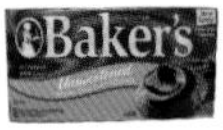			
1 oz portion	120	7	16
4 oz bar	470	28	64
Semi-sweet, 1 oz	140	9	16
Bittersweet, 1 oz	140	12	14
White Baking 1 oz	160	9	16
Unsweetened, 1 oz	140	14	8
Grated, 1 cup, 4½ oz	660	69	39
Chocolate Baking Chips: *Average all Brands*			
Milk Choc./Semi Sweet 1 oz	140	8	18
½ cup, 3 oz 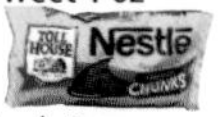	420	24	54
1 cup, 6 oz	840	48	108
Mini Kisses *(Hershey)*, 1 pce	5	0.5	1
Cocoa Powder, Baking: *Nestle*, 1 T.	15	1	3
⅓ cup, 1 oz 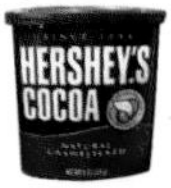	85	5	17
Hershey's, 1 Tbsp	20	0.5	3
⅓ cup, 1 oz	115	3	17
Coconut, dried:			
Unsweet., 1 oz	190	18	7
Sweetened/flaked, 1 oz 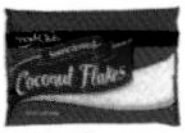	130	8	15
½ cup, 1.3 oz	195	12	22
Toasted *(Baker's)*, 1 oz	170	13	13
Coconut Cream/Milk: *See Page 91*			
Cornstarch, 1 Tbsp	30	0	7
Eggs: Large (1)	75	5	0
Jumbo (1)	90	6	0.5
Egg White: 1 Egg White	15	0	0
½ cup (4 egg whites), 4 oz	60	0	1
Flour, white: 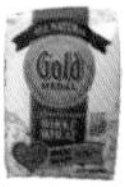			
1 Tbsp, 0.3 oz	25	0	5.5
1 cup, 4.2 oz	400	1	88
Whole Wheat, 1 cup, 4.2 oz	400	2	84

	C	F	Cb
Flavor Extracts: *Average all Brands*			
Imitation, 1 tsp 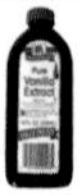	10	0	2
Pure Extract, 1 tsp	10	0	0.5
Almond, Vanilla, 1 tsp	10	0	0.5
Fruit Pectin: Swtnd, ¼ tsp	5	0	1
Unsweetened, ¼ tsp	0	0	0
Gelatin, dry, ¼ oz pkg	20	0	0
Golden Dipt, Batter Mix 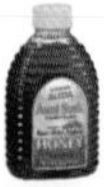			
¼ cup mix, 1 oz	100	0	23
Honey, ½ cup, 6 oz	515	0	140
Lemon/Orange Peel, ¼ cup	25	0	6
Lighter Bake *(Sunsweet)* 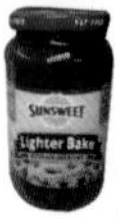			
(Butter & Oil replacement)			
1 Tbsp, ½ oz	35	0	9
¼ Cup, 2.7 oz	140	0	36
Milk: Whole, 1 cup, 8 fl.oz 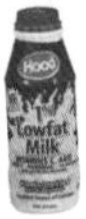	150	8	12
2%, 1 cup, 8 fl.oz	120	5	12
1%, 1 cup, 8 fl.oz	100	2.5	12
Fat-Free, 1 1 cup, 8 fl.oz	90	0.5	13
Pastry ~ *See Page 136*			
Pie Crusts ~ *See Page 136*			
Pie Fillings: 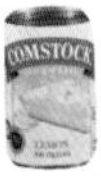			
Fruits ~ *See page 136*			
Lemon Creme, ⅓ cup	130	1.5	28
Mincemeat, 3½ oz	190	5	45
Pumpkin, 1 cup, 9.3 oz 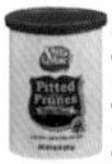	270	1.5	60
Prune Puree, ¼ cup, 3 oz	220	0	55
Raisins, ½ cup, 2.8 oz	240	0.5	63
Rennin, 1 pkg (11g)	10	0	2
Soy Milk ~ *See Pages 48-49* 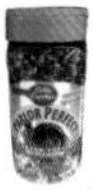			
Sprinkles, all types, 1 tsp	20	1	3
Sugar: 1 Tbsp, ½ oz 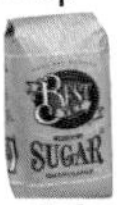	55	0	14
1 oz	110	0	28
1 cup, 7 oz	775	0	195
1 lb, 16 oz	1760	0	454
Sweeteners & Sugar Substitutes ~ *See Page 164*			
Vinegar, avg. all types, 1 oz	5	0	1
Whey, sweet, dry, 1 oz	100	0.5	21
Yeast: Active, dry, ¼ oz pkg	21	0	3
Bakers, compressed, 1 oz 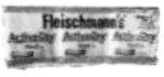	30	0.5	5
Fleischmann's, 0.6 oz pkg	0	0	0

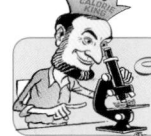

For Full Nutritional Data & Product Updates
~ See Author's Website
www.CalorieKing.com

Note: Actual weight of bars is usually 5-10% more than label Net Wt. Weigh bar and allow extra calories.

Breakfast Bars

	C	F	Cb
Atkins, Day Break:			
Apple Crisp; Fruit Crumble, avg	130	5	17
Choc. Chip; Cranberry, avg	140	5	16
Cinnamon Bun	160	8	18
Peanut Butter Fudge	150	7	14
Barbara's Bakery: Nature's Choice	140	2	28
Fruit & Yogurt, 1.1 oz	150	3	28
dotBAR: *Per 2 oz Bar*			
Iced Oatmeal Blueberry	220	5	29
Iced Oatmeal Strawberry	220	5	29
Note: Carb figures include 11 grams of sorbitol and maltitol sweeteners			
General Mills: Milk 'n Cereal Bars,			
Cinnamon Toast Crunch, 1.6 oz	180	4	32
Honey Nut Cheerios, 1.6 oz	160	4	28
Health Valley: Bar, avg., 1.3 oz	130	2.5	26
Cereal Tarts, all flav. 1 bar, 1.4oz	150	3	29
Kellogg's: All-Bran Bar, 1.2 oz	130	2.5	30
Crunch Cereal Bar, avg., 1 oz	110	2	22
Smart Start Bars, 1.4 oz	150	2.5	30
Fiber Plus, Chewy Bars	130	5	25
Pop Tarts: French Toast (1)	220	8	35
Fruit/Frosted, avg., 1.8 oz	200	5	37
Low-Fat, all flavors, 1.8 oz	190	3	39
Go Tarts, avg., 1.2 oz	140	4.5	24
Splitz, average all flavors, 1.7 oz	200	6	35
Market Pantry *(Target),* Bar, 1.4 oz	140	3	26
Nature's Path: Crispy Rice, avg.	110	3	20
Toaster Pastries, 1.8 oz	210	5	37
Nutri-Grain Bars			
Cereal Bars, avg., 1.3 oz	140	3	26
Fruit & Nut Bar, 1.1 oz	120	3.5	22
Yogurt Bars, avg., 1.3 oz	140	3	26
Post, Honey Bunches of Oats Bar	140	4	24
Quaker: Breakfast Cookies (1), 1.7 oz	170	4.5	33
Fruit Flavor Crisp Bar, 1.3 oz	130	2.5	26
Muffin Bars, 1.3 oz	130	3.5	26
Granola Bars: *See Page 36*			
Slim-Fast: Fruit Crisp, 1.3 oz	180	4.5	29
Muffin Bar, 1.2 oz	140	5	20
South Beach Living *(Kraft)*			
High Protein Cereal Bars, avg., 1.23 oz	140	5	15
Special K Cereal Bars, avg., 0.8 oz	90	1.5	18
Bliss Bar, Mocha	90	2	17
Toaster Strudel:			
Fruit flavors, avg.	190	9	26
Boston Cream Pie	210	9	29
Cream Cheese	200	11	23
Trader Joe's: Fig, 1.3 oz	120	2	24
Apple, Blueb./Strawb., avg.	140	2.5	28

Sports & Diet Bars

	C	F	Cb
ABB, Steel Bar, 2.3 oz	260	4	36
AdvantEdge *(EAS)*			
Carb Control:			
Crisp Bar, 2.1 oz	240	8	27
Nutrition Bar, avg., 2.1 oz	230	8	27
All-Bran Fiber Bars, avg., 1.4 oz	130	2.5	30
Apex:			
Fix Crisp Bar: Chocolate, 1.4 oz	150	3.5	23
Oatmeal Raisin, 1.03 oz	150	3	23
Peanut Butter, 1.4 oz	160	4	21
Fit Fruit Fuel Bars: Apple Pie, 1.3 oz	200	2	37
Blueberry Cobbler	210	3.5	36
Strawberry Struedel	200	2	36
Atkins:			
Advantage: Caramel flavors, avg.	170	10	21
Choc. Fudge Brownie	170	9	19
Choc. Peanut Butter	240	12	22
Granola flavors, avg.	200	8	18
Marshmallow Mudslide	210	10	19
S/Mores	220	9	27
Endulge: Caramel Nut Chew	130	8	17
Choc. P'nut Butter Cups (2)	160	13	18
P'nut Caramel Cluster	140	9	12
Attune Bars:			
Chocolate Probiotic Wellness Bars: *Per 0.7 oz Bar*			
Blueberry Vanilla	100	7	9
Chocolate Crisp	90	6	12
Dark Chocolate	80	6	11
Mint Chocolate	100	7	12
Granola Probiotic, avg, 1.4 oz	170	7	23
Balance: Balance Bars, 1.76 oz	200	7	23
Balance Bar Bare:			
Sweet & Salty, avg.	210	9	23
Trail Mix, avg., 1.8 oz	210	7	23
Carb Well: Caramel 'n Choc., 1.7 oz	190	7	23
Chocolate Fudge, 1.7 oz	190	6	23
Chocolate Peanut Butter, 1.7 oz	200	8	22
100 Calorie Bar, avg.	100	4	14
Balance Gold, avg.	210	6	23
Barbara's Bakery:			
Crunchy Granola, 1.5 oz	190	8	27
Fruit & Yogurt Bar, 1.1 oz	150	3	28
Bariatrix Proti-Bar: (15g Protein)			
Caramel Nut, 1.42 oz	150	5	15
Biochem: Greens & Whey Bar, 2.1 oz	280	12	26
Raw Foods & Whey Bar, 2.1 oz	200	4	37
Bumble Bar: Original/w. Nuts 1.6 oz	230	15	20
Awsome Apricot, 1.4 oz	180	11	18
Lushus Lemon, 1.6 oz	210	15	21
Tasty Tropical, 1.58 oz	190	12	17
CarbRite Diet *(Doctor's),* avg., 2 oz	190	3.5	23

Note: Actual weight of bars is usually 5-10% more than label Net Wt. Weigh bar and allow extra calories.

Bars (Cont)

	C	F	Cb
Cascadian Farms *(General Mills)*			
Chewy Granola Bar, avg., 1.23 oz	140	4	25
Harvest Berry, 1.3 oz	130	2	26
Multi Grain, 1.3 oz	130	2	27
Clif Bars: Regular, avg., 2.4 oz	230	3	45
Clif Kid, 1.26 oz	130	3.5	23
Builder's, avg., 2.39 oz	270	8	30
Luna Bar, average, 1.69 oz	180	4	27
Mojo Bar: Avg., 1.58 oz	200	10	30
Dipped, avg., 1.6 oz	210	10	22
Nectar Bar, average, 1.58 oz	150	5	29
Z Bar, P'nut Butter, 1.27 oz	130	3.5	23
Curves: Apple Streusel	100	1.5	19
Chocolate Peanut, 25g	100	3.5	18
Detour *(Next Proteins):* 2.8 oz bar	320	9	32
Biker Bars, average, 1.76 oz	210	7	25
Core Strength, average, 1.76 oz	200	7	20
Lean Muscle, 3.17 oz	370	12	33
Lower Sugar, 3 oz	340	9	34
Oatmeal Whole Grain, 4.28 oz	460	12	58
Original, 1.5 oz	180	6	16
Runner Bars, 1.76 oz	200	3.5	29
Yoga, 1.6 oz	190	3.5	28
dotSTICK: *Breakfast Bars ~ Page 33*			
Protein Stick (12g Protein):			
Iced Peanut Butter Delight	190	6	26
Iced Lemon Vanilla Cream	190	6	26
Dr Soy: Chocolate/Peanut, 1.76 oz	190	5	25
Healthy Snacker, avg., 1.7 oz bar	180	6	27
Dr Weil, Fruit & Nut:			
Banana Manna, 1.6 oz	180	6	29
Choc Walnut, 1.6 oz	190	10	24
Goji Moji, 1.6 oz	170	4.5	29
Pistachio, 1.6 oz	190	7	27
EAS Advantage Edge			
Carb Control, average, 2.12 oz	230	8	27
EAS: Champions Energy Bar	160	4.5	26
EAS Myoplex			
Deluxe Bar, avg., 3.17 oz	340	9	35
Lite , P'nut Caramel, 1.9 oz	190	6	25
AdvantEdge *(Carb Control),* 2.11 oz	240	8	27
(Carbs include 17g sugar alcohol)			
Elevate Me!, avg. all flav.,3 oz	230	4	33
Extend Bar, 1.4 oz	150	3	21
Fi-Bar Nectar Granola Bars, 1 oz	120	2	26
Chewy & Nutty Bar, 1.2 oz	140	4	23
First Endurance, EFS Bar, 2.32 oz	250	6	40
General Mills, Fiber One Granola, avg.	150	4.5	28

Per Bar	C	F	Cb
GeniSoy: Genisoy Bars, 2.2 oz	240	5.5	35
Natural Choice, 1.6 oz	160	3	25
Protein Crunch	150	5	18
Ultra Bar, 1.6 oz	160	2	27
Glenny's: Light 'n Crispy, ½ oz	65	2.5	9
Slim Carb: Double Fudge, 1.3 oz	100	3	20
Slim 1, 1.06 oz	100	3	20
Glucerna: Meal Replacement, 2 oz	220	7	34
Snack Bar, 1.3 oz	150	4	25
Mini Snack Bar (1)	80	2.5	12
GNC ProCrunch:			
Choc Crisp	260	7	35
Cookies n' Cream	250	4.5	36
Peanut Butter Crunch, 2.3 oz	260	7	34
Pro Crunch Lite, 1.2 oz	140	1.5	4
Gnu Foods:			
Banana Walnut	140	4	30
Cinn. Raisin; Orange Cranberry	130	3	32
Choc. Brownie; P'nut Butter, avg.	140	4.5	30
Health Valley Fruit/Granola, avg.	110	1.5	22
Herbalife: Protein Deluxe!, 1.23 oz	140	4	15
Shapeworks Protein Bar, 1.41 oz	150	7	15
Hershey's Smart Zone, avg, 50g	205	7	22
HMR Benefit Bar	160	4	25
Jenny Craig: Oat & Honey,1.78 oz	170	4.5	32
Choc Chip Snack Bar, 1.21 oz	140	3	23
Peanut Butter, 1 oz	150	5	19
Joy Ride Bars, avg., 2.8 oz	340	12	27
Kashi, GoLean Chewy, avg, 2.75 oz	290	6	48
GoLean Crunchy!:			
Chocolate Almond	170	5	27
Chocolate Peanut	180	5	30
Other Flavors, avg.	160	3	28
GoLean Roll!, avg., 1.94oz	190	5	28
TLC: Crunchy Granola Bar, 1.42 oz	180	6	26
Chewy Granola Bar, avg., 1.3 oz	140	5	19
Cereal Bars, all varieties, 2 oz	110	3	21
Fruit & Grain Bars, avg.	120	3	22
Keribar, Apple P'nut Butter, 1.4 oz	160	6	21
Kind Fruit & Nut Bars			
Almond & Apricot	170	11	16
In Yogurt	210	13	19
Almond & Coconut	190	14	14
Banana & Oatbran	160	7	23
Fruit & Nut in Yogurt	210	13	20
Macadamia & Apricot	190	14	15
Sesame & Peanuts in Choc.	230	15	19
Walnut & Date	150	7	22
Kind Plus:			
Antioxid./B-Complex/Calcium, avg.	190	13	20
Omega-3: Almond & Cashew	150	9	18
Protein: Almond, Waln./Macad.	210	15	11

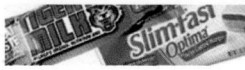

Bars (Cont)	C	F	Cb
Per Bar			
Kudos: Chocolate Chip, 1 oz	120	3.5	20
Peanut Butter, 1 oz	130	6	18
M&M's; Snickers, average, 0.84 oz	100	3	17
Larabar:			
Apple Pie	180	10	23
Banana Bread	220	11	28
Cherry Pie	190	8	28
P'nut Butter Cookies	210	13	23
Lean Body: Cookie Bar, 3.25 oz	360	13	30
Gold, 3 oz	330	7	36
Hi Pro Granola Bar, 2.85 oz	330	16	26
Rockin' Roll, 2.5 oz	290	16	25
Lindora: Mocha Nut/Cinn. Crisp	160	4.5	15
Other varieties, average	150	5	19
Live Active *(Kraft),* Granola Bars			
Avg. all flavors, 1¼ oz	140	4	26
Live Bright *(Kellogg's),* avg., 1.23 oz	150	5	20
Luna: Bars, avg., 1.69 oz	180	4.5	27
Sport, Moons Chews, avg., 1.1 oz	100	0	24
Sunrise, avg., 1.69 oz	180	4.5	27
Tea Cakes, avg., 1.4 oz	140	2	28
Marathon *(Snickers):* Energy, 2 oz	210	6	29
Low Carb, average, 1.7 oz	170	7	19
Protein, average, 2.8 oz	290	9	37
Market Pantry *(Target)*			
Chewy Granola, 1 oz, average	100	3	17
Sweet & Salty Bar, 1.3 oz, avg.	155	6.5	22
Medifast: Maintenance Bar, 1.5 oz	160	5	20
Crunch, 1.13 oz	110	3	12
Met-Rx: Big 100, avg., 3.5 oz	370	5	52
Big 100 Colossal:			
Crispy Apple Pie	400	10	47
P'nut & Butter: Caramel Crunch	400	12	44
Pretzel	420	12	48
Super Cookie Crunch	410	14	43
Big 100 Brownies, avg.	400	13	41
MLO Bio Protein: 2.85 oz	315	6.5	43
Xtreme, 3.2 oz	370	8	43
Mojo Bars: *See Clif*			
Muscle Milk, 2.57 oz	300	11	28
Muscle Tech:			
Nitro-Tech: Choc. Caramel Nut	310	12	25
Smores; Peanut Butter	270	6	42
Strawberry Cheesecake	290	7	32
Nabisco: HoneyMaid Bars, 1.32 oz	150	6	24
100 Calorie Granola Bars:			
Chips Ahoy, 1 bar	100	1.5	22
Nutter Butter, 1 bar	100	1.5	22
Oreo, 1 bar	100	2	21
Nature Valley Granola Bars			
Chewy w. Yogurt coating, 1.4 oz	140	3.5	26
Crunchy, average, 1.5 oz	180	6	29
Heart Healthy: Honey Nut, 1.4 oz	160	4	28
Oatmeal Raisin, 1.4 oz	150	2	30
Trail Mix, average, 1.3 oz	140	4	25

Per Bar	C	F	Cb
Nature's Path			
Granola Bars, average, 1.2 oz	160	5	26
Optimum Energy, avg., 1.98 oz	220	6	36
Weil: Banana Manna, 1.6 oz	180	6	29
Goji Moji, 1.6 oz	170	4.5	29
NiteBite (Time-release Glucose Bar)			
Choc. Fudge; P'nut Butter, 0.9 oz	100	3.5	15
Nutiva: Hempseed, 1.4 oz	210	14	11
Flax Chocolate, 1.4 oz	200	12	19
NutriSystem:			
Dessert Bars: Blueberry Lemon	160	5	26
Chocolate Raspberry	200	7	25
Granola Bars: Cranberry	150	2	27
Apple: Choc. Chip Cranberry	140	3	25
Nutrilite *(Quixtar):*			
Fruiji Bar, 1.4 oz	130	0	30
Meal Bars: Blueb. Crunch, 1.8 oz	200	7	26
Cherry Almond, 1.8 oz	200	6	26
Chocolate Crisp, 1.8 oz	190	6	26
Lemon Twist, 1.8 oz	200	7	27
Snack Bar: Caramel Creme, 0.9 oz	100	2.5	16
Cranberry Crunch, 0.9 oz	100	3	15
Fudge Brownie, 0.9 oz	100	3.5	9
Odwalla Energy Bars			
Choc. Chip Peanut/Crunch, avg.	240	7	37
Strawberry Pomegranate	220	4	44
Super Food, 2.2 oz	230	4.5	43
Other varieties, average, 2.2 oz	240	6	41
Oh Yeah! *(ISS),* 3 oz	380	19	31
One Way, avg, 3 oz	340	12	29
Optifast: P'nut Butter,			
45g (1.59 oz) bar	160	4	23
Performance, 65g	230	2.5	43
PowerBar: Energize, avg.	210	3.5	42
Harvest: WholeGrain	250	5	42
Dip'd, avg., 2.3 oz	250	5	42
Nut Naturals, 1.6 oz	210	10	28
ProteinPlus, 2.75 oz	300	6	39
Recovery	260	10	30
Pria Bars: 110 Plus, avg., 1.7 oz	110	3	16
Protein Plus: Choc. Brownie	360	11	33
Cookies n Cream	300	6	38
Reduced Sugar, Choc. P'Nut	270	9	30
Triple Threat, avg., 2 oz	230	8	30

Bars (Cont)

	C	F	Cb
Power Crunch, average, 1.3 oz	220	12	10
PR Bar average, 1.78 oz	200	6	22
Premier: Premier Protein, 2.5 oz	290	9	23
Odyssey Bar, avg., 2.8 oz	330	10	30
Twisted Bar, avg., 1.6 oz	190	6	21
Promax: Cookies 'N Cream, 2.64 oz	270	4.5	38
Choc Peanut Crunch, 2.64 oz	280	7	37
Double Fudge, 2.64 oz	270	7	37
70 Calorie Bars, 0.66 oz	70	2	10
Proti 15, Choc P'nut, 1.48 oz	160	5	16
Pure Protein:			
1.76 oz Bars, avg.	200	5	18
2.75 oz Bars, avg.	300	8	30
Pure Fit, average, 2 oz bar	230	6	26
Quaker Chewy Granola Bars			
Chewy (Regular): Avg. 0.86 oz	100	3	18
Peanut Butter/Chocolate	100	3	18
Chewy Dipps:			
Choc Chip	140	5	22
Peanut Butter	150	7	19
Snack Bars:			
Chewy Granola 25% Less Sugar	100	3.5	17
Chewy 90 Cal Granola, 0.86 oz	90	1.5	19
Mini Delights: Peanut Butter (1), 0.7 oz	90	4	13
White Choc. Drizzle (1), 0.7 oz	90	3.5	15
True Delights, average all flavors	140	4.5	24
Rebar: Original, 1.75 oz	160	0	38
Energy: Seeds n' Greens, 1.75 oz	180	8	29
Supplement, Caramel Flav., 1.75 oz	200	8	21
Revival Soy Bars (Direct):			
Chocolate Temptation	270	7	32
Apple Cinnamon; Marshm. Krunch	225	3	30
Peanut Pal	240	6	28
Low Carb, average all flavors	235	8	31
Slim-Fast Bars:			
Original Breakfast & Lunch Bars:			
Dutch Chocolate, 1.2 oz	140	5	20
Peanut Butter, 1.2 oz	150	6	19
Meal Bar, Choc. Cookie Dough, 2 oz	220	5	36
High Protein:			
Meal Bar, avg., 1.7 oz	195	7	20
Snack Bar, average, 1 oz	105	3.5	15
Lower Carb, Snack Bars, avg., 1 oz	120	4.5	18
Optima: Meal Bars, avg., 2 oz	220	5	35
Snack Bar, avg., 1 oz	120	4	20

Per Bar	C	F	Cb
Snickers Marathon	220	7	29
South Beach Living			
Fiber Fit Granola Bars, avg., 1.23 oz	120	4	25
High Protein Cereal Bars, avg., 1.23 oz	140	5	15
Snack Bars, avg., 1 oz	100	4	14
SoyJoy Bars, avg., 1.07 oz	140	6	16
Solo GI, average, 1.78 oz	200	7	26
South Beach Diet			
Meal Replacement,			
avg. all flav., 2.11oz	220	7	26
Special K			
Protein Meal, avg., 1.59 oz	180	5	25
Protein Snack Bars, avg., 1 oz	110	3	16
Spiru-tein (Nature's Plus), 1.4 oz	150	1.5	19
Supreme, 1.8 oz	170	4.5	21
Steel Bar (ABB), avg., 2.47 oz	270	5	35
Supreme Protein: Per 1.8 oz			
Caramel Nut Choc	200	8	17
Peanut Butter Crunch	200	9	13
Think: ThinkFruit,			
P'nut Goji, 1.76 oz	210	11	26
Other flavors, avg., 1.76 oz	190	8	29
ThinkGreen: Blueberry Noni, 1.76 oz	180	5	29
P'nut Butter Choc., 1.76 oz	200	8	28
ThinkThin: Avg., all flavors, 2.1 oz	240	8	27
Bites, avg., 2 pces, 1.37 oz	150	5	18
Tiger's Milk:			
Protein Rich, 1.25 oz	140	5	18
Peanut Butter, 1.25 oz	150	6	18
King Size, avg., 1.94 oz	225	9	28
Trader Joe's:			
Chewy Granola Bars, 6-Packs:			
Chocolate Chip, 1.23 oz	140	4	24
Vanilla Almond, 1.23 oz	130	4	21
Fruit & Nut Bars:			
Choc. Chip, 1.6 oz	170	4.5	31
Trail Mix, 1.6 oz	200	6	37
Tri-O-Plex: avg., 4.2 oz	430	16	45
Duo: Bursting Peanut Butter, 3.5 oz	300	10	36
Caramel Peanut Butter, 3.5 oz	340	8	45
U-Turn Protein, 2.8 oz	300	8	26
Usana:			
Nutrition Bar: Oatmeal Raisin, 1.96 oz	190	3	22
Peanut Butter Crunch, 1.45 oz	160	4.5	20
Vyo-Pro (AST) Choc. Brownie, 2.2 oz	220	7	27
Zoe's, Omega-3's, Choc.Delight	190	7	27
Zone Perfect			
Classic, avg., 1.76 oz	210	7	24
Dark Chocolate, avg., 1.58 oz	190	6	22
Fruitified: Apple Cinn., 1.76 oz	180	2	2
Banana Nut, 1.8 oz	200	6	24
Blueberry, 1.8 oz	190	4	25
Snack Size, avg., all varieties, 0.7 oz	80	2.5	9

Cocoa & Hot Chocolate

	C	F	Cb
Cocoa (8 fl.oz cup):			
w. Whole Milk	205	8.5	22
w. Nonfat Milk	145	1	23
Tall (12 fl.oz): w. Whole Milk	280	12	26
w. Nonfat Milk	185	1	28
Hot Chocolate:			
8 fl.oz cup: w. Whole Milk	180	7	26
w. Nonfat Milk	140	2	17
Tall (12 fl.oz): w. Whole Milk	260	10	36
w. Nonfat Milk	190	2	37
Cinnabon, Mochalatta Chill, 16 oz	450	18	66
Swiss Miss Mixes, avg., 1 packet	120	2.5	22

Cocoa - Chocolate Mixes

Add extra cals/fat/carbohydrate for milk

	C	F	Cb
Carnation Breakfast Drinks: *See Page 50*			
Ghirardelli			
Choc Mocha, 4 Tbsp, 1.4 oz	130	1.5	33
Double Chocolate, 4 Tbsp, 1.4 oz	140	0.5	35
White Mocha, 2 T., 0.8 oz	100	0	24
Hershey's			
Cocoa, unsweetened, 1 T, 5g	10	0.5	3
Horlicks, Malt Extract, 1 oz	90	1	18
Land O' Lakes: *Per 1¼ oz Pkg*			
Choc.Mint/Raspb./Supreme	140	3.5	26
Nestle: *Per Single Serve Pkg*			
French Vanilla, 1 envelope	120	3	22
Milk Chocolate, 2 Tbsp	80	2.5	15
Carb Select: Fat-Free Hot Cocoa	25	0	5
w. Marshmallows	35	0	8
Rich Chocolate	80	3	15
No Sugar Added	50	0	10
Dble Choc Meltdown	140	3.5	28
Nesquik Powder (Nestle): *Per 2 Tbsp*			
Choc.; Strawberry, 25% less sugar	60	0	15
Chocolate, No Added Sugar	35	1	7
Ovaltine Cocoa Mixes, avg., 4 Tbsp	80	0	20
Swiss Miss: *Per Single Serve Pkg*			
Milk Chocolate: Made with water	120	2.5	23
Made with milk	210	6	31
w. Marshmallows, made w. water	120	2	23
Made with milk	210	6	33
Choc. Sensation	150	3.5	28
Mocha Cappuccino	120	2	24
Sensible Sweets	25	0	4
Pick Me Up, 1 oz	110	2	23
Fat-Free	50	0	10
Marshmallow Lovers	70	0	13

Instant Coffee

	C	F	Cb
Powder/Granules: Regular or Decaffeinated			
1 level tsp	2	0	0.5
1 rounded tsp	4	0	1
Ground, 3 tsp	7	0	1
Brewed/Percolated, 1 cup, 8 fl.oz	4	0	1
Coffee With Milk/Cream/Creamers:			
Per Cup Coffee (8 fl.oz):			
Black	4	0	1
w. Whole Milk: Dash, 1 T.	15	0.5	2
2 Tbsp, 1 fl.oz	25	1	2
w. 2% Milk, 2 Tbsp	20	0.5	2
w. 1% Milk, 2 Tbsp	20	0.5	3.5
w. Fat Free Milk, 2 Tbsp	15	0	3
w. Half & Half, 2 Tbsp	50	3	2
w. ¼ cup, 2 fl.oz	90	6	3
w. Cream (light coffee), 2 Tbsp	65	6	2
w. *Coffee Mate:* Liquid, reg., 1T.	20	1	2
Liquid Fat Free, 1 Tbsp	25	0	5
Powder, 1 heaping tsp	15	1	2
Sugar ~ Add Extra: 1 heaping tsp	25	0	6
Single portion, 1 package	25	0	6
Sweeteners: *Equal/Splenda/Sweet N Low*			
Powder, pkg	0	0	0

Flavored Coffee Mixes

	C	F	Cb
Chicory: Instant Coffee, 1 tsp	5	0	1
Coffee Essence, 1 tsp	15	0	4
Caffé D'Vita: Mixes, 3 tsp	60	1.5	11
Sugar Free Mixes, 2 tsp	35	2	3
General Foods Int'l:			
Average, ½ oz	60	3	10
Sugar-free, avg, 1 tsp	30	2.5	3
Cappuccino Coolers, ½ oz	60	0	15
Hills Bros:			
Cappuccino, Fr. Vanilla			
3 Tbsp, 1 oz	120	4.5	19
Jakada (Folgers):			
Cappuccino, 3 tsp	80	2	16
Mocha Latte, 3 Tbsp	90	2.5	15
Nescafé: Average all flavors	75	2.5	10

Coffee Shops/Restaurants

Per 8 fl.oz Cup (Unless Indicated)

	C	F	Cb
Coffee (Regular/Percolated/Filtered)	5	0	0
Americano Drip Coffee, 1 cup	7.5	0	1
Cafe Au Lait: 1 cup, 8 fl.oz	60	3.5	5
Nonfat Milk, 1 cup, 8 fl.oz	35	0	5
Caffe Latté:			
8 fl.oz cup: w. Whole Milk	110	6	9
w. 2% Milk	100	3.5	9
w. Nonfat Milk	70	0	10
12 fl.oz: w. Whole Milk	180	9	14
w. Nonfat Milk	100	0	15
16 fl.oz: w. Whole Milk	220	11	18
w. Nonfat Milk	130	0	19
Cafe Mocha (Mochaccino): 1 cup	150	6	20
12 fl.oz	230	9	31
16 fl.oz	290	12	41
Cappuccino:			
8 fl.oz cup: w. Whole Milk	90	3.5	7
w. 2% Milk	80	3	8
w. Nonfat Milk	50	0	8
12 fl.oz: w. Whole Milk	110	6	9
w. 2% Milk	90	3.5	9
w. Nonfat Milk	60	0	9
16 fl.oz: w. Whole Milk	140	7	11
w. 2% Milk	120	3.5	11
w. Nonfat Milk	80	0	12
Mocha (with cream):			
8 fl.oz: w. Whole Milk	200	11	22
w. Nonfat Milk	160	6	22
12 fl.oz: Whole Milk	290	15	33
w. Non-fat Milk	230	8	34
Iced Mocha (no cream):			
12 fl.oz: w. Whole Milk	170	6	26
w. Nonfat Milk	130	2	27
Espresso: Single (Solo)	5	0	1
Doppio (Double)	10	0	2
Espresso con Panna,			
(w. dollop whipped cream), solo	30	2.5	2
Espresso Macchiato, solo	10	0	1
Frappuccino: Tall, 12 fl.oz	180	2.5	37
Grande, 16 fl.oz	240	3	48
Frappuccino Mocha			
(w. Cream): Tall, 12 fl.oz	280	11	43
Grande, 16 fl.oz	380	15	57
Iced Latte: *Similar to Caffe Latte*			
Starbucks: *See Fast-Foods Section*			

Coffee Substitute Mixes

	C	F	Cb
Roasted Cereal Beverages: (No Caffeine)			
Cafix Instant Beverage, 1 tsp	5	0	1
Kaffree Roma *(Morningstar Farms),*			
1 tsp	10	0	2
Postum, Instant Hot Beverage, 1 tsp	10	0	3
Revival Soy "Coffee", 1 Tbsp	0	0	0
Teeccino Caffe, 1 tsp	10	0	2

Irish & Liqueur Coffees

Irish Coffee (no sugar)	175	10	0
Liqueur Coffee, average 1 fl.oz	100	5	7

Coffee Extras

Chocolate (Cocoa) Topping, ½ tsp	5	0	1
Flavored Syrups: Regular, 2 Tbsp	80	0	20
Sugar-free, 2 Tbsp	0	0	0
Half & Half Cream, 2 Tbsp	40	3.5	1
Single Serve Cup, ⅜ fl.oz T.	15	1.5	0.5
Light Whipped Cream, 2 T.	15	1.5	1
Marshmallows, miniature (2)	5	0	1
Sugar: 1 pkg, 5 g	20	0	5
1 level tsp, 4g	15	0	4
1 heaping tsp, 6g	25	0	6
Equal/Splenda/Sweet 'N Low, pkt	0	0	0

Coffee Shop ~ Cakes, Cookies

	C	F	Cb
Cookies:			
Biscotti, 1 oz	140	6.5	18
Chocolate Chip, 3 oz	350	15	54
Oatmeal Raisin, 3 oz	350	12	56
Peanut Butter, 3 oz	410	25	39
White Choc. Macadamia, 3⅓ oz	420	20	55
Cakes/Pastries:			
Almond Croissant, 5 oz	620	35	67
Apple Danish, 5 oz	450	18	67
Banana Walnut, 4½ oz	410	17	60
Brownie, 3 oz	390	24	42
Bundt, Chocolate, 4 o	440	21	61
Carrot Cake, 4 oz	400	22	45
Chocolate Cake, 5 oz	530	28	65
Crumble Coffee Cake, 4½ oz	500	25	65
Cupcake, 3 oz	330	16	43
Pound Cake, 3 oz	330	17	40
Cinnamon Roll, 6 oz	500	15	83
Doughnuts: Sugared, 1¾ oz	220	11	27
Glazed, 2 oz	250	12	34
Pretzel, large, 4 oz	290	5	52

Bottled Coffee (Chilled)

Ready-To-Drink: Per Bottle

Caribou: Espresso, 12 fl.oz	100	0.5	22
Regular; Vanilla, 12 fl.oz	120	1.5	23
Deerfield Farms: Per 11 oz Bottle			
Chai Latte, Reg./Vanilla, average	220	6	37
Full Throttle Coffee & Energy ~ *See Page 50*			
Java Monster Energy ~ *See Page 51*			
Kahlúa Cappuccino Shake 10.5 fl.oz	130	2	24
Main St Cafe			
French Vanilla Ice Latte, 12 fl.oz	190	1.5	34
Shock Coffee: Triple Latte, 15 fl.oz	150	3.5	27
Triple Mocha, 15 fl.oz can	150	3.5	28
Starbucks: *Per Bottle*			
Frappuccino: Caramel, 9.5 fl.oz	200	3	37
Coffee: 9.5 fl.oz	200	3	37
13.7 fl.oz bottle	290	4.5	53
Mocha: Regular, 13.7 fl.oz	260	4.5	47
Dark Choc.: 13.7 fl.oz	280	4.5	51
13.7 fl.oz bottle	265	5	51
Light: 9.5 fl.oz	100	3	12
Vanilla: 9.5 fl.oz	200	3	37
13.7 fl.oz bottle	295	4.5	55
DoubleShot: Espresso & Crm, 6.5 fl.oz	140	6	18
Light Espresso & Cream, 6.5 fl.oz	70	4	6
Energy + Coffee, all flavors, 15 fl.oz	210	2.5	18
Iced Coffee, 11 fl.oz can	100	1	23
Tully's: *Per 12 fl.oz*			
Caramel	620	15	118
Creme	390	14	63
Espresso	380	14	60
Mocha	460	14	78

CALORIE KING TIP!

Reduce the Calories in Your Coffee:

- Request non-fat milk in place of whole or 2% milk
- Downsize to 8 fl.oz or 12 fl.oz
- Avoid cream on frappuccinos
- Replace sugar with *Equal, Splenda Stevia* or *Sweet 'N Low*
- Avoid syrup add-ons

CAFFEINE COUNTER

Moderate caffeine intake is not harmful to healthy adults. However, frequent large amounts (over 350mg/day) may cause dependency ('caffeinism') and adversely affect health. To be safe, limit caffeine to 200mg/day. Avoid if pregnant; breast feeding; a child under 8; have sleep problems or heart arrhythmia.

Caffeine (mg)	
Coffee: Instant, Weak, 1 level teaspoon	30
Medium, 1 rounded teaspoon	60
Strong, 1 heaping teaspoon	100
Decaffeinated, 1 round teaspoon	2
Bags (*Folgers*), 1 bag (6-8 fl.oz)	115
Ground, 1 Tbsp, 6g	60
Bottled (Ready-To-Drink), 9.5 fl.oz	70
Coffee Shop: Brewed, 8 fl.oz	110-150
Cappuccino: 1 cup, 8 fl.oz	75
Tall, 12 fl.oz	110
Large, 16 fl.oz	150
Decappuccino (decaffeinated)	5
Espresso: Regular/Solo	75
Double (Doppio) Espresso	150
Iced Coffee, 12 fl.oz	140
Latte, 1 cup, 8 fl.oz	75
Mocha, 1 cup, 8 fl.oz	90
Hot Chocolate, 8 fl.oz	15
Tea (Black/Green): Weak, 1 cup	20
Medium Strength, 1 cup	40
Strong, 1 cup	70
Decaffeinated Tea	0-5
Herbal Tea	0
Iced Tea, Tall Glass/Can, 12 fl.oz	25-30
Soft Drinks: *Per 12 fl.oz Can*	
Coca-Cola, Pepsi (Reg./Diet)	35
Diet Coke; TAB; RC Cola (Regular)	45
Dr. Pepper (Reg./Diet) *Sunkist* Orange	40
Pepsi One; Mtn Dew; Mellow Yellow; Surge	55
Pepsi Max (Reg./Diet) *Sun Drop* (Reg./Diet)	70
7-Up, Fanta, Sprite, Fresca, Diet Rite Cola	0
Energy Drinks (with added caffeine):	
(AMP, Adrenaline Rush, Full Throttle Monster, No Fear, Red Bull, Rockstar)	
Average all brands: 8 fl.oz	80
16 fl.oz	160
Chocolate Bars: Milk Chocolate, 2 oz	20
Dark Chocolate, 2 oz	30
Cocoa/Hot Choc. Mix, 1 oz pkt	5
Chocolate Milk, 1 cup, 8 fl.oz	2
Choc Chip Cookies, 2 medium, 2 oz	6
Chocolate Syrup, 2 Tbsp, 1.4 oz	5
Medicinals: *Excedrin,* Extra Strength (2)	130
NoDoz Maximum, 1 tablet	200

Extensive Caffeine Counter ~ www.CalorieKing.com

Quick Guide

	C	F	Cb
Orange Juice			
Average ~ Fresh or Sweetened:			
½ Cup, 4 fl.oz	55	0	13
Small Glass, 6 fl.oz	85	0	19
Regular Glass, 8 fl.oz	110	0.5	26
8¾ fl.oz Box	120	0.5	28
10 fl.oz Bottle	140	0.5	32
11½ fl.oz Can	160	0.5	37
16 fl.oz Bottle	225	1	52
20 fl.oz Bottle	280	1	64
64 fl.oz/½ Gallon	895	4	206

Juices ~ Generic

Average All Brands: Per 8 fl.oz Unless Indicated

	C	F	Cb
Aloe Vera Juice, unsweet., 2 oz	10	0	0
Apple Juice: 8 fl.oz	120	0	29
10 fl.oz Bottle	145	0.5	36
16 fl.oz	235	0.5	58
Carrot Juice: Fresh, 6 fl.oz	35	0	8
Sweetened, 6 fl.oz	75	0	17
Cranberry Juice, Cocktail/Blend	140	0	34
Fruit Blends, average, 8 fl.oz	110	0	27
Fruit Nectars, average, 8 fl.oz	140	0	36
Grape Juice, 8 fl.oz	155	0	38
Grapefruit Juice, 8 fl.oz	95	0	22
Lemon/Lime Juice: 1 Tbsp	3	0	1
1 cup, 8 fl.oz	50	0.5	16
Concentrate, 1 tsp	0	0	0
Noni Juice: *Tahitian*, 2 Tbsp, 1 fl.oz	5	0	1
Tahiti Traders, 1 fl.oz	20	0	5
Passion Fruit Juice (Fresh):			
Purple, 1 cup, 8 fl.oz	125	0	34
Yellow, 1 cup, 8 fl.oz	80	1.5	14
Papaya/Peach Nectar, avg., 8 fl.oz	140	0	36
Pear Nectar, 8 fl.oz	150	0	40
Pineapple Juice, 8 fl.oz	130	0	32
Pomegranate Juice, 8 fl.oz	160	0	40
Prune Juice, 8 fl.oz	180	0	45
Strawb./Raspberry Juice, 8 fl.oz	100	0	23
Tangerine Juice, 8 fl.oz	105	0.5	25
Tomato Juice, 8 fl.oz	40	0	10
Vegetable Juice, 8 fl.oz	45	0	11
Wheat Grass Juice: 1 fl.oz 'Shot'	5	0	1
2 fl.oz 'Shot'	15	0	2

Quick Guide

	C	F	Cb
Fruit Smoothies (Jamba Juice; Smoothie King)			
Average All Brands			
Fruit Only: 8 fl.oz	115	0.5	29
12 fl.oz	175	1	43
16 fl.oz	230	1	58
24 fl.oz	350	1	78
Fruit + Non-Fat Milk/Soy:			
12 fl.oz	135	0	29
16 fl.oz	155	0	37
24 fl.oz	265	1	59
Fruit + Non-Fat Frozen Yogurt/Sherbet:			
12 fl.oz	200	0	47
16 fl.oz	265	0	63
24 fl.oz	395	0	95

Juice Brands

Per 8 fl.oz Unless Indicated

	C	F	Cb
Apple & Eve			
Naturally Cranberry	130	0	32
Cranberry Grape	140	0	34
Cranberry/Raspberry	120	0	30
Fruitables, avg all flavors, 6.75 fl.oz	70	0	16
Bolthouse			
100% Juices: Carrot, 8 fl.oz	70	0	14
Clementine	110	0	29
Vedge	60	0	12
Lemonade, Prickly Pear	140	0	34
Fruit Smoothies:			
Berry Boost	110	0	30
Blue Goodness	170	0	41
C-Boost	150	0	36
Green Goodness	140	0	33
Strawberry Banana	120	0	29
Bossa Nova: *Per 10 fl.oz Bottle*			
Acai Juice: Original	115	0	28
w/ Blueb./ Mango/Raspb./P'Fruit	110	0	27
Other Juices,			
Acerola/Goji/Mangostein, average	105	0	26
Bright & Early (Minute Maid)			
Orange Juice (Chilled/Frozen)	110	0	29
Campbell's			
Tomato Juice: 5.5 fl.oz can	30	0	7
8 fl.oz	50	0	10
Capri Sun			
Juice Drink, 25% Less Sugar: *Per 6.75 fl.oz Pouch*			
Coastal Cooler; Mountain Cooler	70	0	19
100% Juice, avg., 6.75 fl.oz	100	0	24

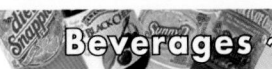

Beverages ~ Fruit & Vegetable Juices

Juice Brands (Cont)

	C	F	Cb
Chiquita Smoothies:			
Average all flavors,			
4 oz concentrate (8 oz reconst'd)	120	0	28
12 oz Can (concentrate)	360	0	84
Clamato			
Tomato Cocktails, average, 8 fl.oz	50	0	11
Crystal Geyser			
Juice Squeeze: Per Bottle (12 fl.oz)			
Blackberry Pomegranate	170	0	43
Ruby Grapefruit	150	0	36
Average other flavors	140	0	32
Dannon			
Frusion Smoothie, avg., 7 fl.oz	180	2.5	35
Light & Fit, 7 fl.oz bottle	70	0	14
Dole			
100% Fruit Juice Blends: *Per 6 fl.oz Can*			
Pineapple	110	0	26
Pineapple Orange/Banana	100	0	25
Chilled, 100%: *Per 8 fl.oz*			
Orange Peach Mango	120	0	29
Pina Colada	120	0	29
Pineapple Juice	130	0	30
Pineapple Orange Banana	120	0	30
Average other flavors	120	0	29
Frozen Concentrates 100%:			
Average all flavors, ¼ cup	125	0	31
Single Serve, 100%: *Per 15.2 fl.oz Bottle*			
100% Apple, no sugar added	210	0	51
100% Blends:			
Grape, no sugar added	300	0	74
Orange, no sugar added	210	0	51
Pineapple Peach Mango	240	0	58
Strawberry Kiwi	230	0	58
Five Alive *(Minute Maid):*			
Frozen Concentrate, prep'd, 8 fl.oz	110	0	29
Florida's Natural			
Orange	110	0	27
Ruby Red Grapefruit	90	0	22
Frützzo: *Per 12 fl.oz Bottle*			
(No Added Sugar)			
Pomegranate 100%	210	0	52
With Acai/Cherry	210	0	51
Blueberry/Raspberry	195	0	48
Yumberry 100%			
Natural	150	0	33
Organic	120	0	25
with Other Juices, avg.	165	0	39

	C	F	Cb
Fuze: *Per 16 fl.oz*			
Refresh, avg. all flavors	180	0	48
Slenderize, avg.	15	0	3
Vitalize, all flavors	200	0	50
Vitamin Tea	120	0	30
Goya Nectar			
Apricot/Pear Nectar, 12 fl.oz	220	0	56
5% Juice: Guanabana, 12 fl.oz	230	0	57
Passion & Pineapple, 12 fl.oz	220	0	55
Hansen's			
Juice Slam: *Per 6.75 fl.oz Box*			
Awesome Apple	90	0	23
Other flavors	120	0	29
Organic, 1 Pouch	100	0	24
Junior Juice, 4.23 oz box	60	0	15
Natural (64 fl.oz Bottles): *Per 8 fl.oz*			
Apple, Strawberry	120	0	28
Black Grape, Pomegranate Cocktail	160	0	39
White Grape	140	0	36
Organic Blends, avg.	110	0	27
Fruit Smoothies, avg., 12 fl.oz	175	0	44
Low-Carb, avg., 12 fl.oz	40	0	9
Light Juice Cocktails, avg., 8 fl.oz	40	0	9
Hawaii's Own			
Frozen Concentrate: *Per 8 fl.oz, Prepared*			
100% Juice, average all varieties	100	0	28
Hi-C Juice Drinks: Average, 8 fl.oz	120	0	32
6.75 fl.oz box, average	100	0	27
Blast, 6 fl.oz pouch	100	0	26
Hood: Apple, 8 fl.oz	120	0	31
Fruit Punch; Orange	120	0	30
Jamba Juice: *See Fast-Foods Section*			
Juicy Juice (Nestle): *Per .75 fl.oz Box*			
Grape	100	0	25
Average other flavors	100	0	24
4.23 fl.oz box, average	70	0	15
Kerns All Nectars			
Canned Juice: *Per 11.5 fl.oz Can*			
Pear	220	0	54
Pineapple Coconut	280	8	53
Other flavors, average	210	0	52
Kool Aid			
Jammers	90	0	24
Jammers 10	10	0	2
Kroger Smoothies, avg., 10 fl.oz	280	3.5	53
L & A: All Cherry, 8 fl.oz	180	0	45
Grape Juice Plus	160	0	40
Mixed Berry	120	0	30
Prune Juice	180	0	41
Average other varieties	140	0	32

Juice Brands (Cont) | C | F | Cb |

Lakewood Organic: *Per 8 fl.oz*	C	F	Cb
Acai Amazon Berry	125	0	28
Banana Strawberry	115	0	28
Blueberry Blend	120	0	30
Cranberry Lemonade	80	0	20
Fruit Garden: Summer/Green, avg.	100	0	20
Blue/Purple/Red Pomegr., avg.	110	0	24
Goji	90	0	20
Lemonade	85	0	21
Pomegranate Blends, avg.	125	0	32
Pure: Apple	105	0	26
Blueberry	125	0	31
Carrot	90	0	20
Pink Grapefruit	90	0	22
Prune	220	0	55
Super Veggie	55	0	12
Light: Lemonade	40	0	15
Other flavors, avg.	60	0	21

(Note: Carbs include Erythritol natural sweetener)

Langers: *Per 8 fl.oz*			
100% Juice (No Sugar Added):			
All Pomegranate	140	0	34
Apple Cider	120	0	28
Apple Juice	120	0	28
Mixed Berry	120	0	30
Pineapple Coconut	140	3	28
Red Grape Juice	160	0	40
White Grape Juice	160	0	40
Diet Low-Carb (25-50% Juice):			
Diet Apple Juice Cocktail	60	0	14
Diet Cranberry	30	0	8
Diet Pomegranate	40	0	9
Juice Cocktails (27% Juice)			
Blueberry Cranberry	135	0	34
Cranberry Berry	135	0	34
Cranberry Grape	165	0	41
Cranberry Raspberry	150	0	36
Pomegranate	140	0	34
Pomegranate Blueb./Cranb.	140	0	34
Strawberry Peach (20% Juice)	120	0	30
White Cranberry	120	0	28
White Cran-Raspberry	120	0	28

Minute Maid	C	F	Cb
Orange Juice: 100%, 8 fl.oz	110	0	27
15.2 fl.oz bottle	210	0	51
Light, 42%, 8 fl.oz	50	0	13
Heart Wise; Kids Plus	110	0	27
Pineapple, Orange, Apple, 8 fl.oz	120	0	29
Enhanced: *Per 8 fl.oz*			
Pomegranate Blueberry	120	0.5	31
Pomegranate Lemonade	110	0	28
Tropical Punch	100	0	28
Juices to Go, average, 11.5 fl.oz	155	0	45
Boxed Juices, average, 6.75 fl.oz	90	0	22
Frozen Concentrates, *8 fl.oz Prepared*			
Average all varieties	120	0	29
MonaVie Acai Blends			
Original/Active, 4 fl.oz	120	2	20
Mott's			
100% Apple Juice: *Per 8 fl.oz*			
Original	120	0	29
Natural	110	0	27
100% Juice Singles: *Per 14 fl.oz*			
Apple	200	0	48
Fruit/Grape Medley	230	0	54
Sunkist Orange Sensation	210	0	50
Veggie Blend	90	1	15
100% Juice Boxes: Avg. all flavors			
6.75 fl.oz box	100	0	24
4.23 fl.oz box	60	0	15
Mott's Plus Light,			
All flav., 8 fl.oz	130	0	15
Mott's Plus for Kids, 8 fl.oz	130	0	31
Mott's For Tots (47-54% Juice),			
All flavors, 6.75 fl.oz box	50	0	13
Naked Juice: *Per 8 fl.oz Unless Indicated*			
Just Juice (100%): O-J	110	0	27
Tangerine Scream	110	0	25
Protein Zone: Banana Choc.	240	1.5	39
P'apple, Coconut & Banana	220	2	34
Antioxidants:			
Cherry Pomegranate Power	140	0	34
Pomegranate Blends, avg.	160	2	35
Bare Breeze, avg. all flavors	130	0	31
Probiotics, avg., 10 fl.oz	180	0	43
Well Being: Berry Blast	130	0	29
Black & Blueberry	130	0	31
Mighty Mango	150	0	36
Strawberry Banana	120	0	29
Tropical	130	0	31

Juice Brands (Cont)   C   F   Cb

Naked Juice (Cont)
Superfood Smoothies:

	C	F	Cb
Acai Machine	160	3	31
Blue Machine	170	0	40
Gold/Green Machine, avg.	140	0	32
Power C	120	0	29
Red Machine	170	4.5	31

Nantucket Nectars
Juice Cocktails: *Per 17.5 fl.oz Bottle*

	C	F	Cb
Big Cranberry	285	0	70
Carrot Orange Mango	260	0	60
Grapeade	305	0	72
Other varieties, avg.	260	0	65

100% Juice: *Per 17.5 fl.oz Bottle*

	C	F	Cb
Apple	260	0	65
Peach Orange	285	0	70
Pineapple Orange Banana	305	0	74
Pomegranate Cherry	265	0	63
Premium Orange Juice	240	0	57
Nectar Lemonade, 17.5 fl.oz	240	0	61

Newman's Own

	C	F	Cb
Lemonade (Reg./Pink), 8 fl.oz	110	0	27
Fruit Juice Cocktail: Gorilla Grape	140	0	34
Orange Mango Tango	150	0	37
Razzma Tazz Raspberry	120	0	28

Northland
100% Juice: *Per 8 fl.oz*

	C	F	Cb
Cranberry/Blackberry; Raspb.	140	0	34
Cranberry Grape	140	0	36

Ocean Spray: *Per 8 fl.oz*
Juice Cocktails:

	C	F	Cb
Cranberry Juice Cocktail	120	0	30
with Calcium	130	0	31
Grapefruit Tangerine	110	0	28
Ruby Red Grapefruit	110	0	28

100% Juice Blends:

	C	F	Cb
Cranberry & Concord Grape	150	0	37
Cranberry Blueberry	140	0	36
Cranberry Blends	140	0	35

Juice Drinks:

	C	F	Cb
CranApple	130	0	32
CranGrape	120	0	31
CranRaspberry/Strawberry	110	0	27
Light Juice Drinks, all flavors	40	0	10

Diet Juice Drinks:

	C	F	Cb
Cranberry Spray	5	0	2
Cranberry Grape Spray	5	0	2

Odwalla *Per 16 fl.oz Bottle*

	C	F	Cb
B Berrier; Quencher	260	0	60
Carrot Juice	140	0	30
Mo'Beta	300	0	74
Mojito Mambo	100	0	28
Poma Grand Pomegranate	320	0	80
Pomegranate Strawberry	100	0	28
Strawberry Lemonade	220	0	56
Super Protein, average	350	8	48

Smoothies:

	C	F	Cb
Blueberry B Monster	280	0	68
C Monster	300	0	72
Mango Tango	300	2	68
Strawberry Banana	260	0	62
Strawberry C Monster	320	0	76

Orange Julius
Originals, Orange:

	C	F	Cb
Small, 16 fl.oz	130	0.5	33
Medium, 20 fl.oz	160	0.5	41
Large, 32 fl.oz	260	1	65

Smoothies: *See Fast-Foods Section*

Pom Wonderful
100% Juice: *Per 8 fl.oz*

	C	F	Cb
Blueberry; Pomegranate	160	0	40
Cherry	150	0	38
Mango; Tangerine	140	0	35

R.W. Knudsen: *Per 8 fl.oz*

	C	F	Cb
Natural Juices: 100% Apple	120	0	30
Cranberry Raspberry	130	0	32
Grape	150	0	37
Guava Strawberry	120	0	28
Hibiscus Cooler	100	0	25
Kiwi Strawberry	120	0	29
Razzleberry	120	0	30
Rio Red Grapefruit	140	0	35
Other varieties, average	120	0	30
Sparkling Juice, avg., 8 fl.oz	120	0	30
Nectars: Coconut	140	5	27
Papaya; Peach	130	0	31
Boysenberry, average	130	0	31
Very Veggie, Orig., 8 fl.oz	50	0	11
Simply Nutritious: Mega C	140	0	34
Average other varieties	125	0	30

Spritzers, 100% Juice: *Per 12 fl.oz Bottles*

	C	F	Cb
Black Cherry	180	0	46
Mango Fandango	170	0	42
Red Raspberry; Tangerine	200	0	47

Juice Brands (Cont) C F Cb

	C	F	Cb
Ralphs			
Lemonade (Premium Juice), 8 fl.oz	110	0	29
Orange Juice, 8 fl.oz	120	0	30
Pineapple Juice, 8 fl.oz	130	0	33
ReaLemon - ReaLime (Borden)			
Lemon/Lime Juice (from concentrate)			
1 teaspoon	0	0	0
2 Tbsp, 1 fl.oz	8	0	2.5
Santa Cruz (Organic)			
Apple Juice;	120	0	30
Concord Grape; White Grape	160	0	40
Orange Mango	130	0	32
Strawberry Kiwi	120	0	30
Tropical Blend	140	0	33
Average other varieties	100	0	24
Nectars: Cranberry	110	0	27
Passionfruit	130	0	40
Average other varieties	120	0	30
Sodas: *Per 12 fl.oz*			
Cherry	140	0	34
Concord Grape	150	0	36
Lemonade, Champagne Style	100	0	26
Raspberry/Strawberry Lemonade	100	0	24
Juice Boxes: *Per 8 fl.oz*			
Lemon	120	0	29
Orange; Grape, average	100	0	24
Tropical Punch	110	0	27
Seismic Super Juices *(Quixtar): Per 12 fl.oz Bottle*			
Citrus/Berry	200	0	49
Low Sugar Cherry	60	0	15
Simply Orange			
Lemonade; Limeade	120	0	31
Orange Juice, all varieties	110	0	26
Snap·E· Tom			
Tomato & Chili Cocktail, 6 fl.oz	40	0	7
Snapple			
Fruit Drink Blends, 8 fl.oz	120	0	29
Grapeade; Orangeade, 8 fl.oz	120	0	29
Lemonade, all types, 8 fl.oz	110	0	28
Diet: Cranberry Raspberry	10	0	2
100% Juiced,			
(added vitamins), 11.5 fl.oz	160	0	40
Ssips			
Juice Drinks, avg., 6.75 fl.oz box	105	0	26
Stonyfield Farm: *Per Bottle (10 fl.oz)*			
Peach Smoothie	230	3	41
Wildberry; Strawberry Smoothie	230	3	39
SunnyD			
Baja Juice: *Per 12 fl.oz Bottle*			
Orange	190	0	46
Orange Berry	190	0	46
Orange Pineapple	190	0	46
Red Punch	170	0	43

	C	F	Cb
SunnyD (Cont)			
SunnyD Blends: *Per 8 fl.oz*			
Fruit Punch	120	0	29
Mango; Smooth Style	130	0	32
Tangy Original Style	120	0	29
Reduced Sugar (35% less)	60	0	15
With Calcium	140	0	35
Orange Fused Drinks, (5% Juice):			
Mango; Peach	80	0	20
Pineapple; Strawberry	80	0	20
Sunsweet			
Prune Juice/w. Pulp, 8 fl.oz	180	0	43
Tampico: Citrus Punch, 1 c.	110	0	25
Mango/Trop. Frt. Punch, 1 cup	110	0	28
Tang			
Pouches, avg. all flavors (1)	90	0	24
Mix: *Prepared as Directed*			
Regular (2 T. dry), 6 fl.oz	110	0	27
Sugar Free, 8 fl.oz	5	0	0
Trader Joe's			
Refrigerated: *Small 16fl.oz Bottle:*			
Carrot Juice	160	2	33
Mango Smoothie	150	0	30
Protein w. Pzazz	440	4	68
Strawberry Smoothie	240	0	58
Watermelon Juice	160	0	54
Organic, *32/64.oz Bottle: Per 8 fl.oz*			
100% Pomegranate	140	0	35
Apple Juice	120	0	30
Concord Grape Juice	160	0	39
Cranberry	70	0	18
Grapefruit Sunset; Lemonade	120	0	30
Mango Nectar	130	0	32
Pink Lemonade	130	0	32
Strawberry Lemonade	120	0	29
White Grape Juice	160	0	40
All Natural Pasteurized, *32/64 fl.oz Bottle: Per 8 fl.oz*			
100% Cranberry	70	0	18
Just Blueberry	130	0	24
Just Pomegranate	160	0	40
Mango PassionFruit	130	0	32
Omega Orange Carrot	110	0	26
Pomegranate Blueberry	140	0	34
Joe's Kids: *Per 6.75 oz Box*			
100% Juice: Apple	90	0	23
Apple Grape	100	0	24
White Apple	120	0	30
10% Juice, Lemonade	90	0	22
Sparkling Juices, *750ml/25.4 fl.oz Bottle: Per 8 fl.oz*			
Blueberry	120	0	30
Cranberry	140	0	35
Pomegranate	130	0	31

Juice Brands (Cont)   C   F   Cb

Per 8 fl.oz Unless Indicated

Tree Top

	C	F	Cb
Apple Reserve/Fruit Punch	120	0	30
Apple Berry/Grape	120	0	30
Apple/Spiced Cider	120	0	29
Fiber Rich: Apple	140	0	35
Apple Apricot/Orange Banana	160	0	37
Grapefruit	130	0	30
Orange	120	0	28
Orchard Blends	130	0	31
Boxes: Average, 6.8 fl.oz	100	0	26
Chilled Juices: Grape	155	0	38
Cranberry; Cranberry Cocktail	140	0	34
Orchard Berry/Apple, avg.	115	0	29
Essentials: Fiber, 8 fl.oz	120	0	29
Healthy Heart	120	0	26
Healthy Kids	110	0	26
Immunity Defense; Low Acid	110	0	26
Light 'n Healthy varieties	50	0	13
Non-Refrigerated Juice Drinks:			
100% Fruit Punch	135	0	32
100% Grape	150	0	38
100% Orange; Apple; Ruby Red	110	0	27
100% Pineapple Orange	130	0	32
Light 'n Healthy, average	50	0	14
Refrigerated Juice Drinks:			
Average all flavors, 8 fl.oz	130	0	32
Light varieties, avg., 8 fl.oz	10	0	2
Twisters: Average, 8 fl.oz	120	0	29
20 fl.oz bottle	300	0	74
Fruit Smoothies, avg., 11 fl.oz	220	0	54

Tropicana

	C	F	Cb
Pure Premium Orange Juice, 8 fl.oz	110	0	26
Trop50 Orange, 42% Juice, 50% Less Sugar			
All varieties, 8 fl.oz	50	0	13

V8® Juices & Drinks

	C	F	Cb
V8 100% Vegetable Juice:			
5.5 fl.oz can	30	0	7
8 fl.oz cup	50	0	10
11.5 fl.oz can	70	0	14
12 fl.oz bottle	75	0	15
V-8 Splash, average, 8 fl.oz	70	0	19
V-8 Splash Smoothies: Strawb. 8 fl.oz	90	0	20
Tropical Colada, 8 fl.oz	100	0	21
Diet V-8 Splash, all flavors, 8 fl.oz	10	0	3
Fusion, all flavors, 8 fl.oz	120	0	28
12 fl.oz bottle	180	0	42

Per 8 fl.oz Unless Indicated   C   F   Cb

Veryfine

	C	F	Cb
Apple Juice (100%)	110	0	27
Orange Juice (100%)	120	0	28

Walnut Acres: *Per 8 fl.oz*

	C	F	Cb
Organic: Apple	110	0	29
Apricot; Raspberry	130	0	32
Cherry	140	0	34
Cranberry	110	0	26
Incredible Vegetable	50	0	12
Mango Nectar	120	0	29

Welch's: *Per 8 fl.oz*

	C	F	Cb
100% Grape/Red Grape	170	0	42
100% White Grape/Peach			
8 fl.oz	160	0	39
14 fl.oz bottle	280	0	68
100% Orange Juice	120	0	30
Cocktails (Refrig'd/64 fl.oz Ctn):			
Healthy Tropical w. Calcium, 8 fl.oz	110	0	27
Strawberry Breeze, 8 fl.oz	130	0	33
Other flavors, avg., 8 fl.oz	145	0	36
Light Juices (52 fl.oz Bottle),			
All flavors, 8 fl.oz	50	0	13
Naturals: All flavors,			
10oz bottle	100	0	26
11.5 fl.oz can	120	0	30
Sparkling Juice Cocktail, 8 fl.oz	160	0	40
Concentrates (100% Juice),			
All flavors, ¼ cup, 2 fl.oz	160	0	41

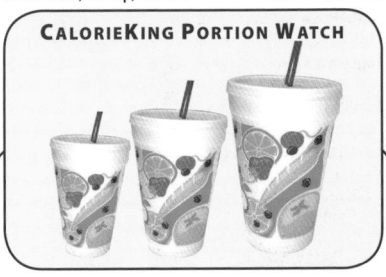

CALORIEKING PORTION WATCH

ORANGE JUICE	C	Cb
8 fl.oz	110	26
16 fl.oz	220	52
24 fl.oz	330	78
32 fl.oz	440	104

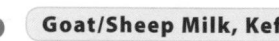

Quick Guide **C** **F** **Cb**

Cow's Milk ~ *Average All Brands*
Whole (3.25% fat):

	C	F	Cb
2 Tbsp, 1 fl.oz	20	1	1.5
1 Cup, 8 fl.oz	150	8	12
1 Large Glass, 12 fl.oz	220	12	17
1 Pint, 16 fl.oz	295	16	22
1 Quart, 946 ml	590	32	44

Reduced-Fat (2% fat):

	C	F	Cb
2 Tbsp, 1 fl.oz	15	0.5	1.5
1 Cup, 8 fl.oz	120	5	12
1 Large Glass, 12 fl.oz	180	7.5	18
1 Pint, 16 fl.oz	245	10	23
1 Quart, 946 ml	490	20	46

Light/Low-Fat (1% fat):

	C	F	Cb
2 Tbsp, 1 fl.oz	13	0.3	1.5
1 Cup, 8 fl.oz	100	2.5	12
1 Large Glass, 12 fl.oz	150	4	18
1 Pint, 16 fl.oz	205	5	25
1 Quart, 946 ml	410	10	49

Fat Free/Skim:

	C	F	Cb
2 Tbsp, 1 fl.oz	10	0	1.5
1 Cup, 8 fl.oz	90	0.5	13
1 Pint, 16 fl.oz	180	1	26
w. Oatrim Fiber (for replacement), 1 cup	85	0	12

Buttermilk: *Average All Brands*

	C	F	Cb
Reduced-Fat (2%), 1 cup	120	5	10
Low-Fat (1%): 1 cup	100	2.5	12

Lactose-Free: Per 8 fl.oz
Lactaid 100:

	C	F	Cb
Whole	150	8	12
2% Reduced-Fat	130	5	12
1% Low-Fat	110	2.5	13
Fat-Free	80	0	13
Calcium-Fortified	80	0	13

Dairy Ease:

	C	F	Cb
Whole	160	9	11
2% Reduced-Fat	130	5	12
Fat-Free	90	0	12

Lower Carb Dairy Drinks: Per 8 fl.oz
Carb Countdown (Hood):

	C	F	Cb
Whole	130	8	3
2% Reduced-Fat, 1 cup	90	5	3
Fat-Free, 1 cup	45	0	3

Goat/Sheep Milk, Kefir **C** **F** **Cb**

Goat's Milk (Meyenberg):

	C	F	Cb
Whole, 1 cup, 8 fl.oz	140	7	11
Light/Low-Fat (1%), 8 fl.oz	100	2.5	11
Evaporated, reconst., 8 fl.oz	150	8	11

Kefir (Cultured Milk):

	C	F	Cb
Nancy's: Plain, 8 fl.oz	110	3	14
Fruit flavors, avg, 8 fl.oz	180	2.5	34
Trader Joe's: Plain, 8 fl.oz	110	2.5	8
Strawberry, 8 fl.oz	160	2	21
Sheep's Milk: Whole, 1 cup	265	17	13

Canned & Dried Milk

Condensed:

	C	F	Cb
Reg. 2 Tbsp, 1 fl.oz	130	3	23
Low-Fat (*Eagle*), 2 Tbsp	120	1.5	23
Fat-Free (*Eagle*), 2 Tbsp	110	0	24

Evaporated:

	C	F	Cb
Whole, 2 Tbsp	40	3	3
Whole, ½ cup	170	10	13
Low-Fat (*Carnation*), 2 Tbsp, 1 oz	25	0.5	3
½ cup, 4 fl.oz	115	2.5	14
Fat-Free, 2 Tbsp, 1 oz	25	0	4

Dried:

	C	F	Cb
Whole, ¼ cup, 1 oz	160	9	12
Skim/Non-Fat, ⅓ cup	80	0	12
Made-up, 1 cup, 8 fl.oz	80	0	12
Buttermilk (sweet cream), 1 oz	110	2	14
Non-Fat, 1 Tbsp	25	0	3
Malted (*Carnation*), dry, 1 Tbsp	30	0.5	6

Soy/Non-Dairy Drinks ~ *See Page 48*

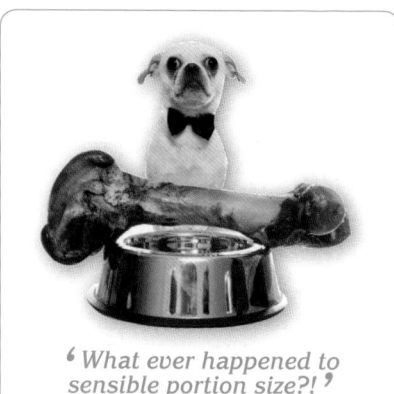

' What ever happened to sensible portion size?! '

Quick Guide

Chocolate Milk **C** **F** **Cb**
Average All Brands: Per Cup (8 fl.oz)

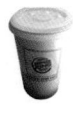

	C	F	Cb
Whole Milk (3.3%): 1 cup	210	8	26
1 Pint	415	17	52
Reduced-Fat (2%), 1 cup	190	5	30
Low-Fat (1%), 1 cup	160	2.5	26

Brands ~ Flavored Milk

Ready-To-Drink: Per 8 fl.oz Cup Unless Indicated

	C	F	Cb
Albertson's, Choc Milk, low-fat	200	2.5	34
Alta Dena: Chocolate	260	9	37
Low-Fat Chocolate	200	3	32
Cool Moos: Chocolate, 8 fl.oz	180	2.5	32
Strawberry, 8 fl.oz	160	2.5	27
Dean's Milk Chug: *Per 12 fl.oz Bottle*			
Chocolate; Cookies & Cream	420	12	68
Vanilla	440	11	68
Hood: Chocolate	230	9	31
Low-Fat (1%), Chocolate	170	3	28
Horizon Organic: Choc., Low-Fat	170	3	27
Reduced-Fat Vanilla, avg., 1 cup	190	4.5	30
Kroger			
Choc Milk, Low-Fat, 1%, 8 fl.oz	180	2.5	33
Muscle Milk (*Cytosport*) (Hi Prot.):			
Chocolate, 17 fl.oz	330	16	13
Avg. other flavors, 17 fl.oz	310	12	16
Nesquik: Choc.,16 fl.oz	400	10	64
Banana, 16 fl.oz	400	10	60
Choc. Fat Free, 16 fl.oz	320	0	64
Reduced Fat:			
Double Choc., 16 fl.oz	400	10	60
Very Vanilla, 16 fl.oz	400	10	60
Prairie Farms, Choc., 16 fl.oz bottle	220	8	29
Quaker Milk Chillers, 14 fl.oz bottle	245	9	32
Ralphs, Chocolate, Low-Fat, 8 fl.oz	210	2.5	36
Skinny Cow, Fat-Free Chocolate, 1 c.	150	0	26
Starbucks, Strawb. & Creme, 9.5 fl.oz	230	6	38
Yoo-Hoo:			
Choc Drink, 6½ fl.oz box	105	1	29
Choc., 16 fl.oz pkg	260	2	56
Lite Choc., 9 fl.oz bottle	70	1	15

Shakes **C** **F** **Cb**

Burger King:	C	F	Cb
Chocolate:			
Value, 12 fl.oz	310	7	52
Small, 16 fl.oz	445	15	78
Medium, 22 fl.oz	660	20	118
Large, 32 fl.oz	975	31	175

Other flavors ~ *See Page 193*

McDonalds:	C	F	Cb
Average all flavors:			
12 fl.oz cup	430	10	75
16 fl.oz cup	570	13	101
21 fl.oz cup	760	18	132
32 fl.oz cup	1140	26	200

Nutrition/Meal Shakes ~ *See Page 50*

Smoothies

Smoothies **C** **F** **Cb**
Made Up Ready-To-Drink
(8 fl. oz Milk/Soy + Fruit): *Per 12 fl.oz*
Average all types:

	C	F	Cb
w. Whole Milk	300	8	50
+ Ice Cream, 1 scoop	400	13	62
with Non-Fat Milk	240	0	50

Fruit Smoothies ~ *See Page 40*
Freshens; Jamba Juice; TCBY: See Fast-Foods

Bottle Coffee Drinks ~ *See Page 39*

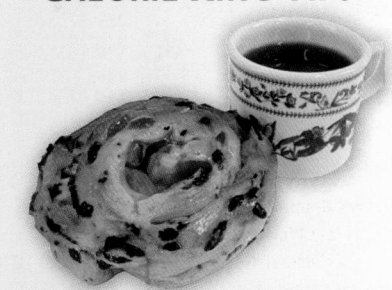

CALORIE KING TIP!

'Low-Fat' does not mean 'Low-Calorie'.
This low-fat Apricot Sticky Bun
has only 2g fat but has
over 400 calories!

Rice & Cereal Drinks

Per 8 fl.oz Cup	C	F	Cb
Almond Breeze (Blue Diamond)			
Original	60	2.5	8
Chocolate	120	3	22
Vanilla	90	2.5	16
Almond Dream			
Original Enriched	50	2.5	6
Unsweetened	30	2.5	1
Amazake, Original	150	0	34
Better Than Milk			
Rice Vegan Mix:			
Orig., 2 Tbsp powder, 19g	100	2.5	16
Van., 2 Tbsp powder, 19g	75	2	15
Cacique:			
Horchata Rice Drink	160	3.5	31
Don Jose:			
Horchata Rice Drink	140	4	25
Cereal Match	100	3	17
Eden Blend, Rice & Soy	120	3	18
Kern's Horchata, 8 fl.oz	140	3	26
Pacific			
Rice Drinks: Multigrain	160	2	30
Low-Fat Plain/Vanilla	130	2	27
Organic Oat: Original	130	2.5	24
Vanilla	130	2.5	25
Nut Drinks: Hazelnut Original	110	3.5	18
Almond: Original Low-Fat	60	3	9
Vanilla Low-Fat	90	2.5	16
Organic: Original	60	2.5	8
Choc., Single Serve	100	3	19
Vanilla, Single Serve	70	2.5	11
Unsweetened: Original	35	2.5	2
Vanilla	40	2.5	3
Rice Dream			
Organic: Carob	150	2.5	30
Heartwise: Original	130	2	27
Vanilla	140	2	30
Horchata	160	2.5	32
Vanilla/Vanilla Enriched	130	2.5	27
Original/Original Enriched	120	2.5	23
Supreme: Chocolate Chai	160	3	35
Vanilla Hazelnut	140	2.5	29
Trader Joe's:			
Rice Drinks:			
Original, Organic	120	2.5	23
Vanilla	130	2.5	26
Organic Almond, Vanilla	70	2.5	11
WestSoy: Plain Rice	110	2.5	20
Vanilla Rice	110	2.5	20

Note: Rice/Oat/Nut drinks are very low in protein. Unless enriched with protein (and calcium), they are not suitable for infants as a substitute for milk or calcium-enriched soy drinks.

Soy Milk ~ Ready-To-Drink

Per 8 fl.oz Cup	C	F	Cb
365 Organic (Whole Foods):			
Original	90	3.5	10
Plain, unsweetened	70	3.5	5
Chocolate	150	3.5	24
Vanilla	100	3.5	11
Edenblend, Organic	140	3.5	19
Edensoy: Original	140	5	14
Carob; Chocolate, average	175	4	28
Vanilla	160	3	25
Light: Original	100	2	15
Vanilla	110	1	22
Extra Original	140	4	14
Extra Vanilla	150	3	23
8th Continent:			
Soymilk: Original	80	3	7
Chocolate	140	3	22
Vanilla	100	3	11
Light, Original	50	2	2
Fat-Free: Original	60	0	8
Vanilla	70	0	11
Kidz Dream Smoothie			
Berry Blast	100	2	17
Orange Cream	120	2	21
Lifeway			
SoyTreat, Peach/Strawberry	160	4	23
Naturally Preferred (Ralph's/Kroger)			
Regular, Plain	90	3.5	10
Low-Fat: Plain; Vanilla	100	2.5	11
O Organics (Safeway):			
Plain	90	3.5	10
Chocolate	150	4	23
Vanilla Soy	100	3.5	11
Odwalla:			
Super Protein: Original	190	1	35
Vanilla Al'Mondo	190	6	25
Protein Monster, Vanilla	200	3.5	24
Pacific: Select Plain, Low-Fat	70	2.5	9
Select Vanilla, Low-Fat	80	2.5	11
Organic, Original Unsweetened	90	4.5	4
Ultra (Extra Protein/Calcium): Plain	120	4	11

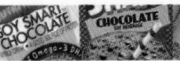

Soy Milk ~ Ready-To-Drink

Per 8 fl.oz Cup

	C	F	Cb
Silk			
Plain, 11 fl.oz	140	6	12
Chocolate	200	5	32
Light: Chocolate	120	1.5	22
Plain	70	2	8
Vanilla	80	2	10
Plus DHA Omega-3	110	5	8
Plus for Bone Health	100	3.5	11
Unsweetened	80	4	4
Vanilla, 11 fl.oz	140	5	16
Vanilla Plus Fiber	100	3.5	14
Very Vanilla	130	4	19
Slim-Fast (Soy-Based) ~ *See Page 52*			
Soy Dream			
Original; Enriched	100	4	8
Vanilla	120	4	14
Classic: Original	130	4	16
Vanilla	140	4	18
Chocolate Enriched	150	4	21
Vanilla Enriched	120	4	14
So Nice:			
Natural	70	4	3
Original	80	3	7
Chocolate	150	3	24
Strawberry	110	3	15
Omega Plus: Original	110	4	10
Vanilla	130	4	15
Trader Joe's:			
Soy Milk: Original	90	2	13
Vanilla	100	2	16
Extra Organic: Original	120	3	17
Chocolate	120	3	17
Vanilla	130	3	19
Organic Unsweetened	90	4.5	4
Soy Essential	90	4	6
Chocolate Soy Milk, 8 fl.oz box	130	2.5	23
Vitasoy			
Chocolate Banana	130	4	21
Peppermint Chocolate	140	4	24
Plain	110	4	11
Chocolate	160	4	24
Strawberry Banana	140	4	19
Vanilla	120	4	13

Soy Milk ~ Ready-To-Drink (Cont)

Per 8 fl.oz Cup

	C	F	Cb
Vitasoy (Cont):			
Light: Chocolate	100	2	17
Original	60	2	5
Vanilla	70	2	8
Unsweetened: Original	80	4	5
Single Serve Bottle:			
Plain, 11.5 fl. oz	140	6	12
Chocolate, 11.5 fl. oz	230	6	33
Vanilla, 11.5 fl. oz	160	5	18
WestSoy			
Lite: Plain	70	2	10
Vanilla	90	2	14
Low-Fat: Plain	110	2.5	20
Vanilla	120	1.5	21
Non-Fat: Plain	70	0	10
Vanilla	80	0	12
Longevity, Plain	90	3.5	10
WestSoy Plus:			
(25% Less Sugar):			
Plain	90	3.5	7
Vanilla	100	3.5	10
Soy Shakes, Chocolate/Vanilla, avg.	170	3.5	29
Soy Slender: Plain	60	3	3
Other flavors, average	70	3	4
Unsweetened:			
Organic/Almond	90	4.5	5
Vanilla/Chocolate	100	4.5	6

Soy Powder Mix

1 oz (¼ cup) mix makes 8 fl.oz Cup

	C	F	Cb
Soy Protein Isolate, 1 oz dry	95	1	0
Better Than Milk:			
Original, 2 Tbsp	100	2.5	16
Vanilla, 2¾ Tbsp	80	2	8
Light, 2 Tbsp	75	2.5	7
Genisoy (Powder Shakes):			
Per 3 Rounded Tbsp			
Plain; Natural: 1 oz	110	1.5	0
Ultra-XT, 1.3 oz	130	1.5	5
Chocolate: 1.2 oz	130	0.5	16
Ultra-XT, 1.4 oz	150	1	20
Vanilla: 1.2 oz	130	1	17
Ultra-XT, 1.4 ox	150	1	20
Now, Soy, ¼ cup, 22g	90	4	5
Revival Soy Shakes: *Per Packet*			
Plain; Unsweetened	100	1.5	2
Vanilla Pleasure	220	2	31
Flavors, average	230	2	33
Whole Foods			
Choc.w. Spirulina, 1 oz	110	0	11
Vanilla w. Spirulina, 1 oz	110	0	11

Energy/Protein Drinks

	C	F	Cb
180 Energy/180 Blue, 8.2 fl.oz	120	0	33
Blue Low-Calorie, 8.2 fl.oz	15	0	4
24-7 Energy, 16 fl.oz can	260	0	60
5-hour Energy, 2 fl.oz	4	0	1
ABB Energy: Turbo Tea, 18 fl.oz	150	0	38
Adrenalyn Stack, 18 fl.oz	25	0	6
Ripped Force, 18 fl.oz	90	0	23
Hi-Pro: Extreme Body, 15 fl.oz	250	2	9
Pure Pro, 22 fl.oz	150	0.5	2
Pure Pro Shake, 11 fl.oz	160	0.5	5
Power: Blue Thunder, 22 fl.oz	290	0.5	40
Extreme XXL, 22 fl.oz	980	1	197
Accelerade, all flav., 20 fl.oz	200	0	38
Acai, A/oxid. Smoothie, 11 oz	180	5	34
AdvantEdge (EAS):			
Carb Control, 11 fl.oz	110	3	4
AllSport, all flav., 20 fl.oz	150	0	40
AMP Energy Drink, 16 fl.oz	220	0	58
Overdrive, 16 fl.oz	220	0	58
Relaunch/Elevate, 16 fl.oz	220	0	58
Arizona: All City, 16 fl.oz	200	0	56
Caution Energy, 8.3 fl.oz	120	0	30
Green Tea Energy, 16 fl.oz	200	0	32
Atkins: Advantage Shake, 11 oz can	160	9	3
Bally Total Fitness, Whey Pro, 1 scoop	100	1.5	2
Blast, 8.3 oz	120	0	29
Bariatrix Shakes, 1 serving	100	2	6
Proti 15 Drinks, avg., 1 pkg	75	1	4
Read-To-Serve, 1 box	120	4	4
Bawls Guarana, 10 fl.oz	120	0	32
Blue Sky:			
Blue Energy, 8.3 fl.oz	120	0	30
Blue Sport, 16 fl.oz	90	0	24
Body Fuel (w. NutraSweet), 1 scoop	80	0	20
Bolthouse: Per 15.2 fl.oz			
Perfectly Protein:			
Mocha Cappuccino	340	5	55
Vanilla Chai Tea	305	6	48
Boost: High Protein, 8 fl.oz	240	6	33
Nutritional Energy, 8 fl.oz	240	4	41
Boost Plus, 8 fl.oz	360	14	45
Boost Smoothie, 8.25 fl.oz	240	3	44
Glucose Control, 8 fl.oz	190	7	16
Kid Essentials, 8.25 fl.oz	245	9.5	33
Carnation Instant Breakfast			
Powder: 1 envelope, 1.3 oz	130	1	27
Carb Conscious, 1 envelope, 21g	150	1	24
Ready-To-Drink, avg., 11 fl.oz	260	5	41
Celebrity Juice Diet, 4 fl.oz	60	0	14
CeraSport: Liquid, 11 fl.oz	70	0	17
Champion Lyte, Sports Drink	0	0	0

	C	F	Cb
Champion Nutrition			
Heavywt Gainer 900, 4 sc., 5.4 oz	630	10	101
Ultramet: Original, 1 pkt, 2.7 oz	280	2	24
Ultramet Lite, 1 pkt, 2 oz	190	1	17
Ultramet Low Carb, 1 pkt, 2 oz	230	6.5	6
Clif Shot Energy Gel, 1.1 oz pkt	100	0	24
Cocaine Energy, 8.4 fl.oz can	70	0	18
Curves Protein Drink:			
Chocolate; Vanilla, 2 scoops	100	1.5	8
made with skim milk, 8 fl.oz	190	2	23
CytoSport Muscle Milk, 2 scoops	300	12	16
Designer Whey Protein, Van. Praline., 1 s.	100	2	3
dotFIT: Pre & Post Workout,			
Creamy Choc., 2 scoops, 2¼ oz	240	3	35
Creamy Vanilla, 2 scoops, 2¼ oz	240	2.5	35
FirstString: Choc., 4 scoops, 5.2 oz	570	6	89
Vanilla Blast, 4 scoops, 5.2 oz	570	7	86
WheySmooth: Choc., 2 scps, 2¼ oz	240	4.5	12
Vanilla Creme, 2 scoops, 2¼ oz	240	4.5	11
Drank, Anti Energy, 8 fl.oz serve	110	0	27
EAS ~ See AdvantEdge/Myoplex			
Endura (Unipro), 2 scoops, 1.3 oz	120	0	30
Ensure: High Protein, 8 oz bottle	230	6	31
Ensure Fiber/Regular, 8 fl.oz can	250	6	42
Ensure Plus, 8 fl.oz bottle	350	11	50
High Calcium, 8 fl.oz	220	6	31
Enterex Glucose Control, 8 fl.oz	235	9	27
FRS Energy, Orange, 11.5 fl.oz	140	0	35
Fruit₂0 (Veryfine)	0	0	0
Full Throttle			
Energy: Original, 16 fl.oz	220	0	57
Blue Demon/Fury, 16 fl.oz	220	0	57
Coffee & Energy:			
Caramel/Vanilla, 15 fl.oz	260	0	45
Mocha, 15 fl.oz	280	0	50
Hydration + Energy, 16 fl.oz	140	0	35
Fuze: Slenderize, 8 fl.oz	10	0	2
Refresh, 8 fl.oz	90	0	25
Vitalize, 8 fl.oz	100	0	25
Gatorade			
Thirst Quencher:			
(Lemon/Lime, AM, Fierce, Rain)			
1 Cup, 8 fl.oz	50	0	14
12 fl.oz Bottle	75	0	20
20 fl.oz Bottle	125	0	32
32 fl.oz Bottle	200	0	52
Carbohydrate Energy, 12 fl.oz bottle	320	0	79
Endurance (Powder), made up, 8 fl.oz	50	0	14
G2 (Low Calorie), 1 cup, 8 fl.oz	25	0	7
20 fl.oz bottle	70	0	17
Nutrition Shake, all flavors, 11 oz	360	8	54
Protein Recovery Shake, 11 oz	270	1.5	45
Genisoy: Ultra XT, 3 Tbsp	150	1	20
Protein Powder, 3 Tbsp	130	1.5	17

	C	F	Cb
Glaceau: Smartwater	0	0	0
Vitaminenergy, 16 oz can	100	0	26
Vitaminwater, 20 fl.oz	125	0	31
Glucerna Shakes: 8 fl.oz	200	7	27
Snack Shakes, 8 fl.oz	140	5	19
GNC Lean Shake, 2 scoops	180	2	30
GNC Pro Performance:			
24 Hour Pro Complex,1.4 oz	150	5	7
100% Whey Protein, 1 oz	120	1.5	5
50 Gram Slam, Van., 15 fl.oz	240	1	8
Mass XXX, Strawb., 7 oz	750	5	126
Weight Gainer 2200 Gold, Choc., 17 oz	1840	30	402
Wheybolic Extreme 60, Van., 2.9 oz	270	1	6
GU Energy Gel, avg., 1 packet	100	0	25
Guru Energy: Regular, 8.3 oz can	100	0	25
Lite, 8.3 oz can	10	0	2
Hammer Gel, avg. all flav., 2 T., 1¼ oz	90	0	23
Hansen's: Energy Pro	120	0	32
Rumba, 8 fl.oz	120	0	28
Herbalife: Shapeworks Mix, 2 sc, 25g	90	1	13
with 8 fl.oz non-fat milk	180	1	26
HMR, 70 Plus, 1 package	110	0.5	13
Hollywood Celebrity Diet, ½ cup	100	0	25
Jarrow: Whey Protein, 1 scoop	100	1	5
Berry High, 1 scoop, 6g	20	0	5
Muscle Optimeal, 2 scoops	180	2	18
Java Monster Energy: *Per 15 fl.oz Can*			
Lo-Ball/Mean Bean	95	3	10
Loca Moca	190	0	48
Orig./Irish/Nut-Up/Russian	190	3	32
Jolt: Cola, 16 fl.oz can	200	0	52
Blue Raspberry, 16 fl.oz	240	0	60
Jones, Energy,16 fl.oz	260	0	64
Kashi GoLEAN Shakes, 2 scoops	220	1	32
Knudsen: ReCharge, 8 fl.oz	70	0	18
Simply Nutritious, 8 fl.oz	130	0	30
Kombucha, Wonder Drink, 8.5 fl.oz	60	0	16
La Brada			
Drink: Lean Body, RTD, 17 fl.oz	260	9	9
Powders: Lean Body, 79g	330	8	24
Lean Body Mass 60, 6 oz	610	7	76
Breakfast, 92g	360	7	35
Carb Watchers, 65g	250	4.5	12
Lipovitan B3, 8.6 fl.oz	130	0	30
Liquid Ice, 8.3 fl.oz	130	0	32
Liquid Lightening, Reg., 8.4 fl.oz	95	0	23
Max Velocity:			
Reg., 8.45 fl.oz can	120	0	30
16 fl.oz can	240	0	60
Sugar Free: 8.45 fl.oz can	10	0	0
Met-Rx:			
Colossal RTD 15Z, 15 fl.oz can	380	14	28
Meal Replacement, 1 pkt, avg	250	2	21
Protein Plus, Choc., 2 scoops	220	1.5	7
Metabolol: Endurance, 2 scp, 52g	200	5	24
GlyProXTS, 1 scoop, 6g	20	0	4
Met, 2 scoops, 66g	260	3	40
Met Max, mix, 2 scoops, 62g	230	2.5	11
MLO Mus-L Blast, Choc., 4 scoops	570	3.5	112
Monster Energy: 16 fl.oz can	200	0	54
Lo-Carb, 16 fl.oz can,	20	0	5
M-80, 8 fl.oz can	90	0	23
Mixxd (with Juice), 16 fl.oz	220	0	54
MRM: Low Carb Protein, 1 sc. 30g	120	2.5	2
Iso-bolic, 1 scoop, 1 oz	115	1.5	2
Metabolic Whey, 1 scoop, 30g	115	2	2
Muscle Milk (Hi Protein):			
Chocolate: 17 fl.oz	350	17	17
14 fl.oz bottle	230	9	12
Other flavors, avg., 14 fl.oz	220	9	11
Lite, Chocolate, 14 fl.oz bottle	160	4.5	10
Muscle Tech: Meso-Tech Comp. 1 pkt	280	3	32
Mass Tech Weight Gain, 5 scoops	870	4	168
Nitro Tech Hard Core, RTD, 15 fl.oz	195	1	6
Myoplex: Original Shake, 17 fl.oz	300	7	20
Carb Control, 11 fl.oz	150	3.5	5
Deluxe Powder, 1 pkt, 3.4 oz	330	3	29
Lite (Ready to Drink), 11 fl.oz pkg	170	2	20
Lite Powder, 1 pkt, 2 oz	180	2	24
Naturade: Power Shake, 1 scoop	100	1	10
Protein Veg Booster, avg., ⅓ c. dry	100	1.5	1
Total Soy, Orig., 2 scoops, 1.3 oz	150	1	21
Nature's Best: Isopure, 20 fl.oz	260	0	25
Isopure Endurance, 3 scoops	320	0	60
Carbo Power, 16 fl.oz	400	0	100
Zero Carb, 2 scoops, 2.1 oz	220	1	3
Pro Smoothie, 15 oz	240	1.5	7
No Fear: 16 fl.oz	260	0	68
Sugar Free, 16 fl.oz	20	0	2
Noni: Tahitian/Pacific, 2 Tbsp	10	0	3
Noni Juice, 1 Tbsp	10	0	3
Liquid Hawaiian/Tahiti, 1 Tbsp	30	0	8
Nutrament (Nestle), 12 fl.oz	360	10	52
Nutri•15•Fast, 8 fl.oz pkg	160	3	19
Nutrilite			
Protein Shakes, 11.5 fl.oz	170	6	6
Sports Drinks, Regular, 16 fl.oz	120	0	28
Whey Protein: Choc., 1.27 oz pkg	130	2	5
Odwalla Serious Energy, 15.2 fl.oz	305	0	74
Optifast 800:			
Ready To Drink Shakes, 8 oz	160	3	20
Powder 800 Formula, 1 pkg	160	3	20
High Protein Powder, 1 pkg	200	6	10

Energy/Protein Drinks (Cont)

	C	F	Cb
Optimum Nutr.: 100% Whey, 1.1 oz	120	1	3
100% Oats & Whey, 1 scoop, 1.85 oz	200	1.5	22
100% Soy Protein, 1.1 oz Scoop	120	1.5	1
Piranha Energy (EAS), 8.4 oz	140	0	35
PowerAde			
Regular: 12 fl.oz bottle	85	0	23
20 fl.oz bottle	160	0	30
PowerAde Zero	0	0	0
PowerBar			
Endurance, 1 scoop, 0.7 oz	70	0	17
Power Gel, avg., 1.5 oz pkg	115	0	27
Pro-Cal 100 (R-Kane), 1 pkt	100	1.5	7
Propel Fitness Water,			
all flavors, 23.7 oz bottle	30	0	6
Red Bull Energy, 8.3 fl.oz	110	0	27
12 fl.oz can	160	0	40
Sugar-Free, 8.3 fl.oz	10	0	3
Red Devil Energy Drink, 16 fl.oz	230	0	58
Redline Energy	0	0	0
Resource (Nestle): Breeze, 8 fl.oz	250	0	54
Benefiber Juice, 4 oz	70	0	18
Diabetishield, 8 fl.oz	150	0	30
Health Shake: 4 fl.oz	200	4	35
No Added Sugar, 4 oz	200	9	22
Shake Plus, 8 fl.oz	480	16	69
Shake, Thickened, 6 fl.oz	270	6	45
Revenge Pro (Champ. Nutr.), 1 oz	100	0.5	20
Pro-Score 100, 2 scoops	160	2	3
Revival Soy Mix: Plain Soy, 1 pkg	100	1.5	2
Chocolate Day Dream, 1 pkg	240	2.5	36
Other varieties, avg., 1 pkg	225	2	33
Rhino's Energy Drink, 100ml	50	0	11
Rip It Energy Fuel, Citrus X, 16 fl.oz	260	0	66
Rite Aid: Nutritional, 8 fl.oz	250	6	40
Plus, 8 fl.oz	350	11	50
Rockstar:			
Energy Drink, 16 fl.oz	280	0	62
Punched, 16 fl.oz	260	0	64
Sugar Free, 16 fl.oz	20	0	0
Rush Energy Lite: 8 fl.oz	0	0	0
Regular, 8 fl.oz	120	0	30
Sav-on Nut'l: Plus, 8 oz	350	11	50
Equaline Advance, 8 oz	250	6	40
High Protein, 8 oz	230	6	31
Slim-Fast Shake (Ready To Drink):			
Original, 11 fl.oz	220	3	40
High Protein, 11 fl.oz	190	5	24
Easy To Digest, 11 oz	180	5	26
Optima Shake, 11 fl.oz can	185	6	24
Low Carb Diet, avg., 11 oz	185	9	6
Powder Shake Mix: 1 scoop, 26g	110	3	18
w. 8 fl.oz fat-free milk	200	5	30

	C	F	Cb
Snapple: Antioxidant Water			
Average all flavors, 20 fl.oz bottle	125	0	31
SoBe: *Per Can/Bottle*			
Adrenaline Rush, 16 fl.oz	260	0	62
Courage, 20 fl.oz	280	0	70
Elixir 3C: *Per 20 fl.oz*			
Cranberry Grapefruit	260	0	65
Orange-Carrot	230	0	58
Pomegranate-Cranberry	250	0	63
White Concord Grape	300	0	75
Energy: 20 fl.oz	270	0	67
Lean, all flavors, 20 fl.oz	25	0	2
Life Water: All flav., 20 fl.oz	100	0	42
O-Cal, all flavours	0	0	6
Lizzard Fuel, 20 fl.oz	300	1	73
Tsunami, 20 fl.oz	250	0	61
Power, 20 fl.oz	260	0	67
Synergy, all flavors, 11.5 fl.oz can	120	0	30
Sparks (Alcoholic) ~ *Page 29*			
Spiru-Tein: Powder, 1 scp, 34g	100	0	10
Steaz Energy, 12 fl.oz	130	0	34
Diet Berry Energy, 12 fl.oz	60	0	14
The Sports Club/LA, PTS Protein Powder,			
Choc/Mocha/Van., 2 sc., 1.4 oz	130	4	7
Trader Joe's: Energy, 8 fl.oz can	130	0	33
Enhanced Water, 20 fl.oz	120	0	30
Twin Lab: Ultra Fuel, 16 fl.oz	400	0	100
Energy Fuel, 250ml can	0	0	0
Vault: Citrus/Red, 20 fl.oz	290	0	78
Vault Zero, 8 fl.oz	0	0	0
Venom Energy: 16 fl.oz	240	0	58
Low Carb, 16 fl.oz	50	0	8
Verve Energy, 8.3 fl.oz can	70	0	18
Sugar Free	5	0	1
Vitamin Water ~ *See Glaceau*			
Weider (Powders)			
Creatine ATP, ½ cup, 1.7 oz	210	0	37
Mega Mass 4000, 1½ cups	570	3.5	105
Muscle Builder, 1½ oz	170	1	21
Pure Pro Shake: Chocolate, 11.5 fl.oz	170	0.5	7
Vanilla, 11.5 fl.oz	160	0	6
Ultra Whey Pro, ⅓ cup, 1 oz	110	1.5	6
Weight Gainer, 4 scps, 3.4 oz	380	2	67
Worldwide: Carbo Rush, 20 fl.oz	285	0	60
Size Up, 22 fl.oz	1000	0	190
Supercharged Tea, 20 fl.oz	15	0	4
Pure Protein Shakes:			
21g Protein, 11 fl.oz	110	1	5
35g Protein, 11 fl.oz	170	1	3
XS (Quixtar), Energy Drink, 8.4 oz	10	0	1
Zola Acai, 12 fl.oz pkg	190	2.5	44
Energy Smoothie, 12 fl.oz	190	1.5	42

Quick Guide

Cola Drinks
Average All Brands
Includes *Coca-Cola* and *Pepsi*

	C	F	Cb
8 fl.oz Cup/Can	100	0	26
12 fl.oz Can	150	0	39
16 fl.oz Bottle	200	0	52
20 fl.oz Bottle	250	0	65
24 fl.oz (Pepsi)	300	0	84
1-Liter Bottle (34 fl.oz)	400	0	100
2-Liter Bottle (68 fl.oz)	800	0	200

Other Soda Drinks (Average All Brands)

	C	F	Cb
Club Soda, 12 fl.oz	0	0	0
Cream Soda, 12 fl.oz	190	0	48
Diet/Low Cal Drinks, 12 fl.oz	5	0	1
Ginger Ale, 12 fl.oz	125	0	31
Lemon Lime, 12 fl.oz	150	0	37
Orange, 12 fl.oz	180	0	45
Pink Lemonade, 12 fl.oz	180	0	45
Root Beer, 12 fl.oz	150	0	39
Tonic Water, 12 fl.oz	125	0	2
Mineral Water: Plain, 12 fl.oz	0	0	0
Sweetened/flavored, 12 fl.oz	150	0	37
w. Fruit Juice, 12 fl.oz	120	0	30
Soda Water/Seltzer: Plain/Diet	0	0	0
Sweetened/flavored, 12 fl.oz	155	0	39
w. Fruit Juice, 12 fl.oz	160	0	40
Soft Frozen Lemonade, 12 fl.oz	300	0	75

Fountain, Movie Theater & Take-Out

Average All Flavors

	C	F	Cb
Small Cup, 12 fl.oz: No Ice	160	0	40
With ⅓ Ice	120	0	30
Regular, 16 fl.oz: No Ice	215	0	53
With ⅓ Ice	160	0	40
Medium, 22 fl.oz: No Ice	295	0	73
With ⅓ Ice	220	0	55
Large, 32 fl.oz: No Ice	430	0	105
With ⅓ Ice	320	0	80

(Note: ⅓ Cup of Ice = ¼ Cup Liquid)

Soft Drinks Brands

Per 12 fl.oz Unless Indicated

	C	F	Cb
A&W:			
Float, 11.5 fl.oz bottle	260	1.5	64
Root Beer	180	0	46
Diet Cream Soda/Root Beer	0	0	0
Albertson's: Max Cola	165	0	44
Lemon Lime	150	0	41
Other flavors, average	180	0	48

Soft Drink Brands (Cont)

Per 12 fl.oz Unless Indicated

	C	F	Cb
Barq's: Root Beer	165	0	45
Floatz, 12 fl.oz	190	0	51
Big Red, 12 fl.oz	150	0	38
Blue Sky: Cola; Orange Cream	160	0	43
Black Cherry	140	0	37
Grape; Lemon Lime	130	0	36
Raspberry; Root Beer, avg.	165	0	44
Bubble Up, 12 fl.oz	160	0	42
Cactus Cooler, 12 fl.oz	150	0	40
Canada Dry: Club Soda	0	0	0
Ginger Ale, all flavors	135	0	38
Tonic Water	135	0	36
Capri Sun:			
Roaring Waters, 6.75 fl.oz	35	0	9
Sport, all flavors, 6.75 fl.oz	60	0	16
Coca-Cola: *Per 12 fl.oz*			
Classic/Caffeine Free	145	0	41
Diet Coke, all flavors	0	0	0
Cherry Coke/Vanilla Coke	155	0	42
Coca-Cola Zero	0	0	0
Country Time, Lemonade, 12 fl.oz	135	0	36
Crush:			
Orange/Grape: 12 fl.oz	190	0	47
20 fl.oz bottle	320	0	80
Strawberry, 20 fl.oz	290	0	72
Diet Orange, 20 fl.oz	35	0	9
Dad's: Orange Cream Soda, 12 fl.oz	180	0	46
Root Beer, 12 fl.oz	165	0	41
Diet Rite, Pure Zero	0	0	0
Dr Pepper: Regular	150	0	40
Cherry Vanilla	150	0	39
Diet, all flavors	0	0	0
Fanta, all flavors	175	0	48
Fresca: Orig. Citrus	0	0	0
Blackcherry Citrus	0	0	0
Peach Citrus	0	0	0
GuS, average all flavors	95	0	23
Hansen's: Diet Soda	0	0	0
Natural Cane Sugar:			
Creamy Root Beer	160	0	40
Pomegranate	130	0	32
Hawaiian Punch, Fruit Juicy Red	180	0	45
Henry Weinhard's: Root Beer	170	0	43
Cream flavor, average	175	0	42
Hires, Root Beer	170	0	45
IBC: Root Beer	160	0	43
Cherry Limeade	170	0	44
Cream Soda; Black Cherry	180	0	48
Icee: Coca-Cola; Barq's	100	0	27
Minute Maid: Fruit Punch	175	0	45
Lemonade	100	0	25

B Beverages ~ Soft Drinks ◊ Soda

Per 12 fl.oz Unless Indicated	C	F	Cb
Jolt Cola, 16 fl.oz	200	0	52
Cherry Cola, 16 fl.oz	180	0	46
Grape, Orange, 16 fl.oz	210	0	52
Ultra Citrus, 16 fl.oz	10	0	0
Jones Soda: Cola, 16 fl.oz	260	0	64
Whoopass, 16 fl.oz	200	0	52
Other flavors, average	185	0	46
Mello Yello, Regular	175	0	48
Minute Maid: Fruit Punch	160	0	44
Lemonade Reg./Pink			
12 fl.oz can/bottle	150	0	42
20 fl.oz Bottle	275	0	70
Orangeade	160	0	43
Mountain Dew:			
Live Wire; Code Red	180	0	47
Diet flavors	0	0	0
Mug Root Beer	150	0	39
Natural Brew: Vanilla, Cream	170	0	42
Ginseng Cola; Ginger Ale	170	0	42
Root Beer	180	0	44
Nehi, Royal Crown Peach	190	0	51
Orangina: 10 fl.oz bottle	120	0	32
Pepsi: Regular/Blue/Caffeine Free	150	0	42
Diet Pepsi; Jazz	0	0	0
One, 12 fl.oz	2	0	0
Wild Cherry; Vanilla	150	0	42
Perrier, Carbonated Water	0	0	0
Pibb Xtra	145	0	39
RC Cola, Regular	165	0	45
Reed's, Ginger Brew,			
avg. all varieties	145	0	38
7•UP: Regular	150	0	39
Cherry, Gold	150	0	39
Diet varieties, 12 fl.oz	0	0	0
7•UP Plus, 12 fl.oz	15	0	3
Safeway/Vons: Go 2 Cola	160	0	44
Cherry Cola	160	0	43
Ditto Lemon Lime	160	0	40
Parker's Cream Soda	170	0	42
Parker's Root Beer	170	0	47
Santa Cruz, Sparkling, average	135	0	32
Schweppes: Seltzer	0	0	0
Tonic Water; Ginger Ale, average	130	0	35
Shasta: Cream Soda	190	0	47
Cherry Cola; Doc Shasta	160	0	39
Club Soda; Diet, all flav.	0	0	0
Fr. Punch, Pineapple; Or.	200	0	50
Ginger Ale	130	0	32
Other flavors, average	175	0	45

Per 12 fl.oz Unless Indicated	C	F	Cb
Sierra Mist, Lemon Lime	150	0	39
Sprite: Regular	145	0	40
Zero	5	0	0
Squirt, Citrus Burst	150	0	40
Stewarts: Root Beer	160	0	41
Grape; Orange 'n Cream	190	0	48
Sun Drop: Regular, 20 fl.oz bottle	325	0	81
Cherry Lemon, 20 fl.oz bottle	300	0	78
Sunkist: Orange	190	0	52
Diet Sunkist	0	0	0
Sunkist Float, 11.5 fl.oz	230	1.5	55
TAB, 12 fl.oz	0	0	0
Thomas Kemper: Root Beer	160	0	41
Other flavors, average	160	0	40
Trader Joe's:			
Sparkling:			
French Berry Lemonade,			
1 cup, 8 fl.oz	130	0	31
1 Bottle, 33.8 fl.oz	520	0	124
Lime Ade, 1 cup, 8 fl.oz	110	0	27
1 Bottle, 33.8 fl.oz	440	0	108
Pink Lemonade, 8 fl.oz	130	0	31
1 Bottle, 33.8 fl.oz	520	0	124
Mojito: 8 fl.oz	110	0	26
25.4 fl.oz bottle	340	10	80
Refreshers Blueberry, 12 fl.oz	150	0	37
Vernor's, Ginger Ale	150	0	39
Virgil's Root Beer	160	0	40
Walgreens: Grape Soda, 20 fl.oz	300	0	84
Cola; Lemon Lime, 20 fl.oz	225	0	65
Root Beer, 20 fl.oz	225	0	65
Welch's: Soda, 12 fl.oz	190	0	51
Sparkling Juice (Cocktail)	320	0	80
365 Organic (Whole Foods):			
Spritzers, all flavors	110	0	27

Powdered Soft Drink Mix

Per 8 fl.oz Prepared, Unless Otherwise Stated	C	F	Cb
All-Bran Fiber Drink Mix, 17 fl.oz Prepared			
Pink Lemonade, 1 pkt	20	0	12
(Note: Carbs include Polydextrose)			
Capri Sun, Sport ½ pk	25	0	6
Cool Splashers, 8 fl.oz	60	0	16
Country Time: Lemonade	60	0	16
Other flavors, average	80	0	19
Lite	35	0	9
Crystal Light, 8 fl.oz	5	0	0
Flavoraid, ⅛ pkg	0	0	0
Kool-Aid: All flavors	60	0	16
Unsweetened, 6 fl.oz	0	0	0
Propel, ½ pkg	10	0	3
Tang: Regular, 2 Tbsp. 0.9oz	100	0	24
Sugar Free	0	0	0

Quick Guide

Teas	C	F	Cb
Regular: Bag, Loose or Instant			
Brewed, 1 cup, 8 fl.oz	2	0	0.5
(Add extra for sugar/milk)			
Herbal: Average all varieties, 1 cup	2	0	0
Bigelow, *all flavors*	0	0	0
Celestial Seasonings:			
All flavors	0	0	0
Bubble Tea, average, 12 fl.oz	175	0	41
Chai Tea: *Cafe D' Vita,* 2 Tbsp	120	3.5	21
Starbucks: *See Fast-Foods Section*			

Iced Tea	C	F	Cb
Average All Brands			
Sweetened: 8 fl.oz	100	0	25
12 fl.oz	150	0	38
16 fl.oz	200	0	50
Unsweetened: 8 fl.oz	2	0	0

Iced Tea Mixes

Per 1 Cup Made-Up

4C Iced Teas:			
Sweetened, avg. all flavors	70	0	18
Totally Light, all flavors	0	0	0
All-Bran Fiber Drink Mix, 1 pkt	20	0	12
(Note: Carbs include Polydextrose)			
Crystal Light Sugar Free	5	0	0
Lipton: Instant, unsweetened	0	0	0
Instant Raspberry	80	0	19
Lemon	70	0	18
Peach/Raspb, Sugar Free	5	0	1
Iced Tea To Go	0	0	0
Nestea			
Lemonade Tea, 1⅓ Tbsp	60	0	15
Lemon flavored Iced Tea, 1⅓ Tbsp	60	0	15
Sugar Free Lemon Iced Tea, 2 tsp	5	0	2
Unsweetened Tea, 2 tsp	0	0	0

Bottled & Canned Teas

Arizona: *Per 8 fl.oz Cup*	C	F	Cb
Black with Ginseng	60	0	15
Green Tea(s)/Asian Plum	70	0	18
Diet Green Tea (w. Sorbitol)	5	0	2
Extra Sweet Tea	90	0	23
Peach/Raspberry	70	0	18
24 fl.oz Cans: Avg all flavors	270	0	68
Fuze, all flavors, 16 fl.oz	120	0	30
Gold Peak, Lem. ,16.9 fl.oz bottle	170	0	46
Hansen's: Green Tea, 16 fl.oz	120	0	30
Peach/Pomegr. Green, 16 fl.oz	180	0	44

Bottled & Canned Teas (Cont)

Honest Tea: *Per 16.9 fl.oz*			
Black Forest Berry/Peach/Lori's Lemon	65	0	17
Lipton Brisk			
Avg. all flavors, 12 fl.oz can	130	0	33
20 fl.oz bottle	215	0	55
Lipton Iced Tea			
Lem./White w. Raspb., 16.9 fl.oz	120	0	32
Grean Tea w. Citrus:			
16.9 fl.oz bottle	160	0	42
20 fl.oz bottle	200	0	53
Diet, all flavors	0	0	0
Nantucket, Lemon Tea 17.5 fl.oz	175	0	48
Nestea Iced Tea			
Lemon Sweetened: 12 oz can	125	0	31
16.9 oz Bottle	180	0	45
20 oz Bottle	210	0	52
Diet Green/Lemon	0	0	0
Minute Maid,			
Pomegranate Tea, 8 fl.oz	110	0	28
Pom Pomegranate:			
Pomegranate Tea, 16 fl.oz	140	0	34
Lychee Green, 16 fl.oz	140	0	36
Light flavors, 16 fl.oz	70	0	34

Note: Carbs figure for Light flavors includes Erythritol natural sweetener which has negligible calories.

Sbarro, Lemon, 16 fl.oz Bottle	180	0	48
Shasta, Lemon, 16 fl.oz	140	0	35
Snapple: Iced Tea Blends, all flav., 16 fl.oz	200	0	50
Black Teas, avg., 17.5 fl.oz	75	0	19
Diet/Unsweetened Teas	0	0	0
Green/White, 17.5 fl.oz	130	0	32
Red Tea, 17.5 fl.oz	80	0	14
SoBe: Green, 20 fl.oz	250	0	63
Dragon; Zen Tea, 20 fl.oz	270	0	70
Special K20 Protein Water			
Iced Tea, 16 fl.oz	50	0	12
Ssips, Lemon Iced, 6¾ fl.oz	80	0	21
Steaz: Peach/Mint. 16 fl.oz	80	0	20
Sparkling Organic Green, 16 fl.oz	135	0	35
TeaZazz: Original, 20 fl.oz	50	0	12
Green Tea Lemon, 20 fl.oz	60	0	15
Peach Tea, 20 fl.oz	50	0	12
Trader Joe's: *Per 8 fl.oz*			
Organic Tea & Lemonade	100	0	25
Pomegranate Green Tea	60	0	15
Unsweetened *(Kettle/Green)*	0	0	0
Turkey Hill: Iced Tea, 16 fl.oz	180	0	44
Fruit flavors, avg., 16 fl.oz	220	0	55
365 Organic *(Whole Foods):*			
Berry Black Tea, 16 fl.oz	60	0	14
Lemon Green Tea, 16 fl.oz	40	0	10
White Jasmine Tea, 16 fl.oz	30	0	8

Note: Most breads have similar calories on a weight basis. However, volume may vary.

For example, 1 oz of bread may equal 1 slice regular bread or 2 slices of a lighter bread.

It is best to weigh bread used and calculate using: 1 oz bread = 70 calories, 14g carb.

Quick Guide

Bread	C	F	Cb
White or Wheat ~ Average Per Slice			
Thin or Light, ¾ oz	50	0.5	10
Sandwich slice, 1 oz	70	1	14
Thick or Large slice, 1½ oz	105	1.5	21
Thick/Home-made, 2 oz	140	2	28
Extra Thick/Home-made, 3 oz	210	3	42
Whole Loaf, 16 oz	1120	16	224
Whole Loaf, 24 oz	1680	24	336
With Seeds or Nuts:			
Sandwich slice, 1½ oz	130	5	18
Thick slice/Home-made, 2½ oz	215	8	30
Toast ~ Has same calories as bread used			
1 Slice (1 oz fresh)			
w. 2 tsp regular spread	140	9	12
w. 2 tsp "light" spread	105	5	12
w. 1 Tbsp regular spread	170	12	12
w. 1 Tbsp "light" spread	120	7	12

Breads

	C	F	Cb
12-Grain, 1½ oz slice	110	1.5	22
Batard (8 oz), thick slice, 2 oz	150	0.5	28
Bran style/Dark, 1 oz slice	70	1	14
Bread w. Soy Isoflavones, 1.2 oz	80	2.5	13
Buttermilk, average, 1½ oz slice	110	1	22
Caraway Rye, 2 oz slice	150	2	28
Challah, ¾ oz slice	85	1.5	17
Chapati, 1 oz	110	3	18
Ciabatta, 1 slice, 2 oz	130	1	26
Cornbread, average, 1 pce, 3 oz	220	6	37
Cracked Wheat Sourdough, 1½ oz	130	0.5	27
Croissants: *See Page 113, 173*			
Crustless Bread, regular slice ¾ oz	40	0.5	8.5
Crusts Only, regular slice, ¼ oz	30	0	7
English Toasting, slice, 2 oz	140	1.5	27
'Enriched' Breads, average, 1 oz sl.	60	1	12
Flax & Sunflower Round, 1.2 oz	90	2	18

Breads (Cont)

	C	F	Cb
Foccacia: Plain, 2 oz portion	150	2.5	28
Cheese & Garlic; Pesto, 2 oz	160	6	21
Tomato & Olive, 2 oz	150	5	21
French Stick/Baguette, 1 oz slice	70	1	15
French Toast, 1 slice, 1.6 oz	140	2	26
Sticks *(Aunt Jemima)*, 1 pce, 1 oz	90	2	17
Garlic Bread/Toast:			
Small slice + 1 tsp spread, ¾ oz	80	5	7
Med. slice + 2 tsp spread, 1½ oz	160	10	14
Thick slice + 3 tsp spread, 1.8 oz	220	14	20
Pepperidge Farm, 1 slice, 1.4 oz	160	10	15
Hemp Bread, 1.2 oz	95	2	12
Italian Bread, 2 oz slice	140	1	28
Light Bread, avg., 0.8 oz slice	40	0.5	8
Lower Carb (higher Protein/fiber),			
average all brands, 1 oz	60	1.5	9
MultiGrain, 1 slice, 1.3 oz	60	1.5	17
Nut/Health Nut, 1.35 oz slice	90	1.5	18
Oatmeal/Oatbran Bread, 1½ oz	90	0.5	19
Pita: Average all types,			
Small (4" diam) 1.1 oz	90	0	18
Large (6½" diam) 2 oz	140	1.5	27
Extra Large (9" diam) 4 oz	300	1.5	60
Popovers (1), no butter	130	2	18
Poppyseed (Vienna), 0.8 oz sl.	55	1	10
Pumpernickel: Large slice, 1.35 oz	80	0	15
Cocktail/Party size	30	0.5	6
Raisin Bread, 1 oz slice	80	1.5	14
Raisin Walnut, 1 oz slice	70	0.5	15
Roman Meal, 1.1 oz slice	80	1	15
Rye: Average, 1 thin slice, 1 oz	80	1	14
1 thick slice, 2 oz	150	2	25
Cocktail size, 0.4 oz	25	0.5	4
Sandwich Bread, 1 oz slice	70	1	12
Sandwich Pockets, 2 oz	140	1.5	27
Sourdough, 1½ oz slice	120	1	25
Sourdough French, 1 oz	75	0	14
Spelt, 1.6 oz	130	1	26
Sprouted 7-Grain, 1.5 oz slice	110	0.5	18
Squaw, 1.1 oz slice	85	0.5	13
Sweet Hawaiian Bread, 1.3 oz	110	2	19
Tacos/Tortillas: *See Page 179*			
Turkish/Middle Eastern, 1 oz sl.	80	1.5	16
Wheat-Free Breads: Spelt, 1.6 oz	130	1	26
Brown Rice w/ Fruit Juice, 1.5 oz	110	2	21
Healthseed Rye, 1.6 oz	90	1	20
Kamut, 1.2 oz	80	2	16
Millet, 1.5 oz	100	1	20

Bread Brands

	C	F	Cb
Ener-G: Gluten-Free Breads			
Brown Rice Bread, 1 slice, 1.3 oz	130	6	18
Light Brown Rice, 1 slice, ¾ oz	50	2	7
Corn Loaf, 1 slice, ¾ oz	40	1.5	8
Light Tapioca, 1 slice, ¾ oz	45	1.5	7
Ezekiel: Low Sodium (1), 1.2oz	30	0.5	15
Sesame (1), 1.2 oz	80	0.5	14
Francisco International			
French (1), 1.6 oz	120	1	23
Sourdough,1 sl., 1¾ oz	110	0	22
Nature's Path: *Per 2 oz Slice*			
Manna: Carrot Raisin; Millet Rice	130	0	27
Cinnamon Date	150	0	29
Fruit & Nut	140	1	27
Sun Seed	160	2	29
Whole Rye	150	0	32
Oroweat: *Per Slice*			
100% Whole Wheat, 1.3 oz	90	1	18
Sandwich Thins, 1 roll	100	1	20
9 Grain DHA, 1.3 oz	110	1.5	19
Health Nut, 1.3 oz	100	2	18
Pepperidge Farm: *Per Slice*			
100% Whole Wheat, Very Thin	110	2	20
15 Grain, Small Slice	80	1.5	13
Farmhouse Soft Hearty White	120	1.5	22
Light Style, average	45	0	9
Raisin/Cinnamon Swirl	80	1.5	15
Frozen Breads, Garlic Bread:			
Crusty Slice, 2.5"	170	7	24
Prem. Roasted, 1 sl.	150	7	18
Texas Toast, avg., 1 sl.	150	7	18
Sara Lee: *Per Slice*			
Delightful Wheat, 0.8 oz	45	0.5	9
Honey Wheat, 1 oz	80	1	14
Hearty & Delicious:			
100% Multigrain (1), 1.5 oz	120	1.5	21
100% Whole Wheat & Hon., 1.5 oz	120	1.5	21
Sunflower Seed (1), 1.5 oz	130	2	23
Soft & Smooth, 100% Wh. Wheat, 1 oz	70	1	12
45 Calories, 1 slice	45	0	9
Schwan's, Frozen: *Per Serving*			
Chse Stuffed Breadsticks w. Sce, 2 oz	160	7	18
Five Chse Garlic French Bread (1), 3.3 oz	330	20	26
Fr. Baguette Bread, ¼ loaf, 1.7 oz	130	0	25
Southern Style Biscuits (1), 2.2 oz	190	9	23
Trader Joe's: *Per Slice*			
Fat-Free Multi-Grain, 1.1 oz	70	0	15
Gourmet White, 1.5	120	3.5	19
Seeded Harvest, 1 oz	65	1	12
Sprouted Rye, 1.2 oz	90	1	15
Wonder: Classic White S'wich, 1 slice, 1 oz	60	0.5	13
Light Wheat, 1 slice, ¾ oz	40	0.5	9

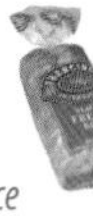

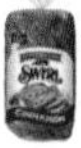

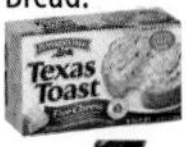

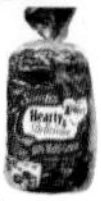

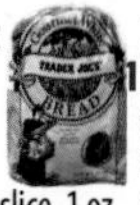

Bread Rolls & Buns

	C	F	Cb
6" Roll, Plain, average 2½ oz	200	1	38
Brown 'n Serve, average, 1 oz	70	1	13
Ciabatta Roll, 3½ oz	230	4	41
Dinner Rolls:			
1 small, 1 oz	90	1.5	17
1 medium (3" diam),1½ oz	110	1	23
Frankfurter/Hot Dog: 1¼ oz	110	1.5	21
1½ oz size	130	2	25
French: 1 med, 1.3 oz	110	1.5	22
1 large, 3 oz	230	2.5	42
Hamburger: Regular, 1½ oz	110	1.5	22
Large, 3 oz	210	3	40
Hoagie/Submarine, Plain, 2⅓ oz	200	1	38
Kaiser Roll:			
Small, 2 oz	200	2.5	35
Large, 3½ oz	350	4	61
Onion Roll, 2.4 oz size	180	2.5	34
Party Roll, 0.6 oz	45	0.5	9
Sandwich Roll:			
Small, 2½ oz	190	1.5	37
6" size, 4 oz	300	2.5	57
Sourdough Roll, 1¼ oz	110	1	21
Wheat Roll:			
Small, 1.2 oz	100	1	17
Medium, 1¾ oz	130	1.5	23
Large, 3½ oz	260	3	46

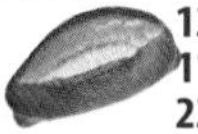

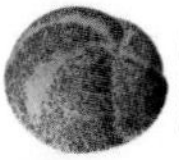

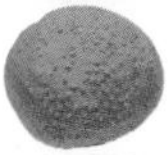

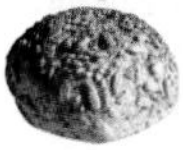

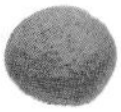

Breadsticks, Croutons

	C	F	Cb
Breadsticks: Salt Sticks, plain, 1 oz	110	1	20
Fresh baked (1), 2 oz	180	2.5	34
Stella D'oro: Sesame (1)	50	2	7
Original, 1 piece	45	1	7
Croutons: Seasoned, 2 Tbsp, ¼ oz	35	1.5	4
9 small or 6 large, ¼ oz	35	1.5	4
Zesty Italian (Pepp. Farm), 6 croutons	30	1	5
Fat-Free *(Pepp. Farm),* 2 Tbsp	30	0	5

Bread Products

	C	F	Cb
Bread Crumbs, dry:			
Plain or seasoned, 1 oz	110	1.5	20
1 cup, 3½ oz	385	5	70
Corn Flake Crumbs, 1.1 oz	120	0	29
Graham Cracker Crumbs, 1 oz	110	2.5	20
Keebler, 3 Tbsp, ½ oz	70	1.5	13
Bread Dough: Frozen, 1 slice, 2 oz	140	2	26
Refrigerated, French, 1" slice	60	1	13
Wheat/White, 1" slice	80	2	14
Coating Mixes: Avg., 2 Tbsp., 1 oz	100	0.5	20
Stuffing: Average, dry mix, 1 oz	110	1	10
Prepared, ½ cup, 4 oz	180	9	11

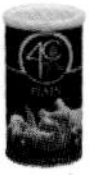

Quick Guide

Bagels
Average All Brands

	C	F	Cb
Plain/Onion:			
1 mini/bagelette, 1 oz	75	0.5	15
1 small bagel, 2 oz	145	1	29
1 medium bagel, 3 oz	230	1.5	45
1 large bagel, 4 oz	285	2	56
Bagel Chips *(New York Style)*,			
4 slices, ¾ oz	100	4.5	12
Pizza Bagel Bites, 4 pces, 3.1 oz	200	6	29
Bagel Bites *(Ore-Ida)*, 4 pces	200	6	29
Bagel Crisps *(New York Style)*, 7 pces	140	6	17

Bagel Brands

	C	F	Cb
Controlled Carb Gourmet			
High Fiber Bagel (1), 2 oz	160	5	22
Individual Wrapped (1), 2 oz	80	6	18
Zero Net Carbs (1), 2 oz	120	2	14
Costco Bakery: Plain, 4 oz	300	1	61
Everything, 4 oz	330	3.5	62
Enjoy Life, all types, 3.2 oz	275	6	50
Lenders: Original, plain, frozen, 2 oz	140	0.5	29
New York, plain, frozen, 3.3 oz	230	1	47
Premium, plain, refrigerated, 2.9 oz	210	1.5	42
Sara Lee: Mini, average, 1.3 oz	100	0.5	19
Plain	270	1.5	57
Blueberry, 3.7 oz	290	1.5	61
Cinnamon Raisin, 3.7 oz	280	1.5	60
Everything, 3.7 oz	300	4	55
Onion, 3 oz	230	1.5	50
Western: All flavors, avg., 2 oz	110	0	25

Fast-Food Stores: *See Page 182*

Bagel Spreads

	C	F	Cb
Cream Cheese:			
Plain: 2 Tbsp, 1 oz	80	8	2
2 oz mini-tub	160	16	4
Reduced Fat: 2 Tbsp, 1 oz	60	5	2
2 oz mini-tub	120	10	4
Flavors: Lox, 1 oz	75	6	1
Raisin Walnut, 1 oz	90	6	8
Strawberry, 1 oz	60	3	7
Sundried Tomato, 1 oz	80	7	2
Vegetable, 1 oz	60	6	1

English Muffins

Average All Brands

	C	F	Cb
Plain/Whole Wheat:			
Regular, 2 oz	133	1.5	26
Heavier, 2.5 oz	155	2	31
Super Size, 3.2 oz	190	2	38
Raisin-Cinnamon, 2.2 oz	140	1	29

Note: Actual weight of packaged muffins can be 10-15% heavier than stated net weight.

Rice Cakes

	C	F	Cb
Reg. size, avg.1 cake, 9g	35	0	7.5
Hain, Mini, plain, 10 pieces	70	2	12
Lundberg, all types, 18.5g each	70	0.5	14
Quaker, Apple Cinnamon, 13g each	50	0	11

Taco Shells & Tortillas

	C	F	Cb
Tacos: Mini Size (1)	25	1.5	2
Regular size, all types (1)	50	2	7
Large (1)	90	4	13
Salad Shell, flour *(Del Oro)*, 1.4 oz	230	17	10
Tortilla (Soft Taco), each	85	2	15
Corn Tortilla: 6", 1 oz each	55	0.5	11
Flour Tortilla: 8", 1.75 oz	145	3	26
Low-Fat	110	1.5	22
Burritos, 1 tortilla, 2.3 oz	190	5	32
Low-Fat	110	1.5	22
Tostada Bowl (Rio Rancho), 6" 1.25 oz	180	9	22
Tostada Shells, each	55	3	6
La Tortilla Factory			
Fat Free Flour Tortillas:			
Burrito size, 2.5 oz	120	0.5	34
Soft Taco, 1.8 oz	90	0	24
Low Carb Tortillas:			
Large, 1.26 oz	80	3	18
Original; Flavors, 1.26 oz	50	2	11
Mission Foods			
Tortillas: *Per 6" Tortilla*			
Carb Balance (1), 1.5 oz	110	2.5	18
Flour, 1.73 oz	150	3.5	25
Multi-Grain, 1.7 oz	140	4	23
White Corn, 1.15 oz	70	1	14
96% Fat-Free Burrito, 1.7 oz	130	2	25

Crispbreads & Matzos ~ Page 90

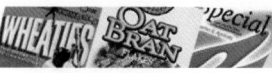

Quick Guide

Cooked Cereals

	C	F	Cb
Buckwheat Groats, roasted:			
Dry, ½ cup, 3 oz	285	2	61
Cooked, 1 cup, 6 oz	155	1	34
Bulgur: Dry, ½ cup, 2½ oz	240	1	53
Cooked, 1 cup, 6½ oz	150	0.5	34
Corn/Hominy Grits:			
Dry: ¼ cup, 1.4 oz	145	0.5	31
3 Tbsp, 1 oz	110	0.5	23
Cooked, ¾ cup, 6½ oz	110	0.5	23
Instant, 1 pkt, dry, 0.8 oz	75	0	18
w. Imitation Bacon Bits, 1 oz	100	0.5	22
Cream of Rice, ckd, ¾ cup, 6½ oz	95	0	21
Cream of Wheat:			
Regular, ckd, ¾ cup, 6½ oz	100	0.5	21
Quick, ckd, ¾ cup, 6½ oz	95	0.5	20
Instant, ckd, ¾ cup, 6½ oz	110	0.5	24
Farina: Cooked, ¾ cup, 6 oz	85	0	18
Millet, dry, ¼ cup, 1¾ oz	190	2	36
Oat Bran: Raw, ⅓ cup, 1 oz	70	2	19
Cooked, ½ cup, 3¾ oz	45	1	13
Oatmeal: Dry, ⅓ cup, 1 oz	105	1.5	18
Regular, ckd, ¾ cup, 6 oz	110	2	19
1 cup, 8 oz	145	2.5	25
Instant: Regular, dry, avg., 1 oz	105	1.5	18
Flavored, dry, average, 1½ oz	150	2	32
Wheat Hearts, 1 oz dry, ¾ c. ckd	110	0.5	24

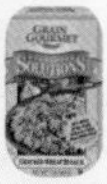

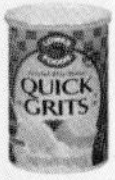

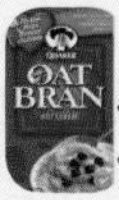

Brans, Wheat Germ, Add-Ons

	C	F	Cb
Bran: Wheat, unprocessed,			
1 Tbsp, 3g	5	0	2
Rice Bran: Raw, 1 Tbsp, 5g	15	1	2.5
¼ cup, 1 oz	95	6	15
Oat Bran: Raw, 1 Tbsp, 5g	10	0.5	4
⅓ cup, 1 oz	70	2	19
Wheat Germ: Raw, 1 Tbsp, ¼ oz	25	0.5	4
¼ cup, 1 oz	105	3	15
Fruit: Dried, average, 1 oz	70	0	18
Banana, ½ medium	55	0	14
Prunes in Syrup (5), 3 oz	90	0	23
Honey, 1 Tbsp, ¾ oz	65	0	17
Lecithin Granules, 1 Tbsp, 10g	55	4	0.5
Nuts, Almonds (6), ¼ oz	40	4	1.5
Bee Pollen Granules, 1 T., 8g	25	1	2
Psyllium Husks, 1 Tbsp, 5g	15	0	4

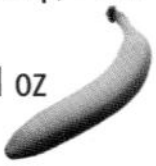

Hot/Cooked Cereals ~ Brands

Per Serving

	C	F	Cb
Albers Grits, ¼ cup, 1.4 oz	140	0.5	31
Bobs Red Mill-10 Grain, ¼ c., 40g	140	1	28
Country Choice Oats, 1 pouch, avg.	110	2	19
Dr McDougall's			
Oatmeal: *Per Package*			
& Barley, Peach Raspb., 3 oz	300	4	62
& Wheat, Apple Cinn., 2.32 oz	250	3	50
Organic, Maple 4 Grain, 2.57 oz	260	3	52
Organic Instant Oatmeal: *Per Packet*			
Original, 1 oz	120	2	21
Light Apple Cinnamon, 1.95 oz	120	1.5	24
Light Maple Brown Sugar, 1.34 oz	150	2	28
4 Grains w. Maple Sugar, 2.2 oz	220	2	44
Erewhon: Barley Plus, ¼ c., 1.7 oz	170	1	37
Brown Rice Crm, ¼ cup, 1.6 oz	170	1	36
Instant Oatmeal, 1.2 oz pkg, avg.	130	2.5	25
McCann's Instant Irish Oatmeal			
Apple & Cinnamon, 1.23 oz	130	1.5	27
Maple & Brown Sugar, 1.5 oz	160	2	32
Original, 1 oz pkg	100	1.5	18
Steel Cut Oats, ¼ cup, 1.4 oz	150	2.5	27
Nabisco: Cream of Wheat, Farina, 1 oz	120	0	23
Malt-O-Meal: Orig., 3 T., 1.2 oz	130	0.5	27
Maple Brown Sugar, ¼ cup	170	0	37
Natures Path: Apple Cinn.1.7 oz	210	2.5	40
HempPlus, 1 pkt, 40g	160	4	40
Average other varieties	200	4	40
Quaker: Oatbran, 1¼ cup, 2 oz	210	3	43
Instant Oatmeal: *Per Package*			
Regular, 1 oz	100	2	19
Bakery Favorites, avg., 1½ oz	160	2	33
Cinnamon Pecan, 1 pkt, 40g	180	4	33
Fruit and Cream, avg. all flavors	130	2.5	26
Honey Nut, 1 cup, 1.5 oz	170	3.5	31
Maple Brown Sugar, 1.9 oz ctn	160	2	33
Take Heart, avg., 1 pkt, 1.6 oz	160	2.5	33
Country Quick Oats, ½ c.,1.4 oz	150	3	27
Old Fashioned Oats, ½ cup, 1.4 oz	150	3	27
Oatmeal Express, avg. all flavors	200	2.5	42
Grits: Reg. all types, 1 pkg, avg.	130	0.5	29
Instant, all types, 1 pkg, 1 oz	100	0	22
Silver Palate Oatmeal, ⅓ c., 40g	160	3	26
Uncle Sam Oatmeal, 1.2 oz	130	3	24

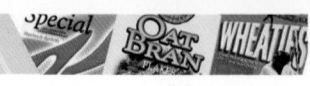

Quick Guide

Cold Cereals
Average All Brands

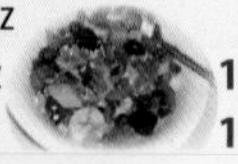

	C	**F**	**Cb**
Bran Flakes, ¾ c., 1 oz	95	0.5	24
Corn Flakes, 1 c., 1 oz	100	0	24
Granola, ¼ c., 1 oz	150	7.5	16
Oat Bran Cereal, ½ cup, 1½ oz	145	3	25
Puffed Rice, 1 cup, ½ oz	55	0	13
Puffed Wheat, 1 cup, ½ oz	45	0	10
Raisin Bran, ½ cup, 1 oz	90	0.5	22
Rice Crisps, 1 cup, 1 oz	105	0.5	24
Shredded Wheat, 1 bisc., 1 oz	85	0.5	20
Sugar-frosted Flakes, ¾ c, 1 oz	115	0	28
Wheat Flakes, ¾ cup, 1 oz	105	1	24

Breakfast/Cereal Bars/Pop Tarts: *See Page 33*

Ready-To-Eat Cereal

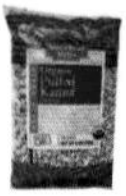

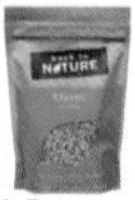

	C	**F**	**Cb**
Arrowhead Mills : *Per Cup*			
Flakes: Amaranth Flakes, 1.2 oz	140	2	26
Corn Flakes, 1.1 oz	120	0	27
Kamut Flakes, 1.1 oz	120	1	25
Multi Grain Flakes, 1½ oz	170	2	33
Oat Bran Flakes, 1.2 oz	140	2.5	24
Rice Flakes, 1.7 oz	180	1	40
Spelt Flakes, 1.1 oz	120	1	24
Puffs, Kamut, ½ oz	50	0	11
Shredded Wheat, 1.7 oz	190	1	38
Back to Nature: *Per ½ Cup, Unless Indicated*			
Energy Start:			
Cinnamon Crunch, 1 cup, 1.8 oz	200	2	43
Maple Nut Medley, 1 cup, 2.1 oz	250	5	45
Granola: Apple Blueberry, 1.7 oz	200	2.5	39
Cherry Vanilla, 1.7 oz	200	4	38
Chocolate Delight, 1.8 oz	210	6	37
Classic Granola, 1.7 oz	200	3	39
Cranberry Pecan, 1.7 oz	220	3	35
Ginger Rstd Alm., 1.5 oz	190	7	29
Honey Almond w. Flax, 1.5 oz	190	7	29
Sunflower & Pumpkin Seed, 1.7 oz	210	8	30
Wild Blueb. Walnut w. Flax, 1.5 oz	190	6	30

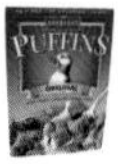

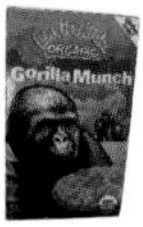

	C	**F**	**Cb**
Barbara's Bakery			
Brown Rice Crisps, sweetened, 1.1 oz	120	1	25
Corn Flakes, sweetened, 1 cup, 1.1 oz	110	1	25
Crispy Wheats, ¾ c., 1.1 oz	110	0.5	25
Honey Crunch 'n Oats. ⅔ cup, 1.1 oz	210	3	48
Organic B'fast O's, avg., ¾ cup, 1 oz	120	2	24
Wild Puffs, avg. all flavors, ¾ c., 1.1 oz	120	1	25
Puffins: Original, ¾ cup, 1 oz	90	1	23
Cinnamon, ⅔ cup, 1 oz	100	1	26
Honey Rice, ¾ c., 1 oz	120	1.5	25
Peanut Butter, ¾ c., 1 oz	110	2	23
Shredded Oats:			
Cinnamon Crunch, 1 cup, 2 oz	230	3	43
Bite Size, 1¼ cup, 2.1 oz	220	2.5	46
Vanilla Almond, 1 cup, 2 oz	220	3	42
Ultima Organic:			
Flax & Granola, 1 cup, 2 oz	210	3	43
High Fiber, 1 cup, 2 oz	180	2	48
Pomegranate, 1 cup, 2 oz	200	2	48
Breadshop Granola:			
Honey Gone Nuts, 1.85 oz	240	10	33
Other flavors, 1.8 oz, average	220	8	34
Cascadian Farms			
Honey Nut O's, 1 c., 1 oz	120	2	24
Multi-Grain Squares, ¾ c., 1 oz	110	1	25
Oats & Honey Granola, ⅔ c., 2 oz	230	6	42
Purely O's, 1 cup, 1.1 oz	110	2	22
Hearty Morning, ¾ cup, 1.9 oz	200	3	43
Raisin Bran, 1 cup, 1.9 oz	180	1	43
Dr McDougall's			
Big Cups: Cranberry Muesli	320	4	62
Organic Apple Cinn. Oatmeal	250	3	50
Organic Maple 4 Grain	260	3	52
Peach Raspb. Oatmeal & Barley	300	4	62
Oatmeal: Orig., no added sug., 1 oz	120	2	21
Light (50% less sugar):			
Apple Cinnamon, 1 Packet	120	1.5	24
Maple Brown Sugar, 1 Packet	150	2	28
Ener-G, Rice Bran, ½ cup, 2.4 oz	220	14	34
EnviroKidz: *Per ¾ Cup, 1 oz*			
Amazon Flakes	120	0	27
Gorilla Munch	120	0	27
Koala Crisp	110	1	25
Leapin Lemur	120	1.5	25
Panda Puffs	130	2.5	34

Ready-To-Eat (Cont)   **C F Cb**

Erewhon

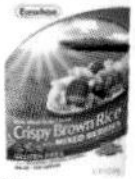

	C	F	Cb
Aztec, 1 cup, 1 oz	110	0	26
Corn Flakes, 1¼ cups, 2 oz	210	2.5	45
Crispy Brown Rice: 1 cup	110	0	25
w. Mixed Berries, 1 cup	120	0.5	27
Gluten Free, 1 cup, 1 oz	110	0.5	25
Kamut Flakes, ⅔ cup, 1.2 oz	110	0	25
Raisin Bran, 1 cup, 1.8 oz	170	1	40
Rice Twice, ¾ cup, 1 oz	120	0	26

Ezekiel 4.9 Flourless Cereals

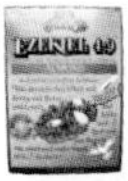

	C	F	Cb
Almond ½ cup, 2 oz	200	3	38
Golden Flax, ½ cup, 2 oz	180	2.5	37
Original, ½ cup, 2 oz	190	1	40

General Mills

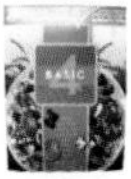

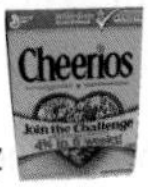

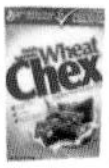

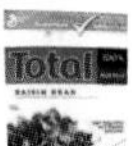

	C	F	Cb
Basic 4, 1 cup, 1.9 oz	200	2	43
Boo Berry, 1 cup, 1.2 oz	130	1	28
Cheerios: *Per ¾ Cup*			
Apple Cinnamon, 1 oz	120	1.5	25
Berry Burst, Triple Berry, 1 oz	100	1	22
Frosted, 1 oz	110	1	23
Fruity, 1 oz	100	1	23
Honey Nut, 1 oz	110	1.5	22
Multi Grain, 1 oz	110	1	24
Oat Cluster Crunch, 1.1 oz	100	1	22
Original, 1 cup, 1 oz	100	2	20
Yogurt Burst, all flavors, 1 oz	120	1.5	24
Chex: Corn, 1 cup, 1 oz	120	0.5	26
Chocolate, ¾ cup, 1.1 oz	130	2.5	26
Honey Nut, ¾ cup, 1.1 oz	120	0.5	28
Multi-Bran, ¾ cup, 1.6 oz	160	1.5	39
Rice, 1 cup, 1 oz	100	0.5	23
Wheat, ¾ cup, 1.6 oz	160	1	38
Cinnamon Tst Crunch, ¾ c., 1 oz	130	3	25
Cocoa Puffs, ¾ cup, 1.1 oz	110	1.5	23
Count Chocula, ¾ cup, 1 oz	110	1	23
Country Corn Flakes, 1 cup, 1.1 oz	120	0.5	28
Fiber One, ½ cup, 1 oz	60	1	25
Fiber One Honey Clusters, 1¼ cup	160	1.5	42
Golden Grahams, ¾ cup, 1 oz	120	1	26
Honey Nut Clusters, 1 cup, 2 oz	210	1	49
Kix: 1¼ cup, 1.1 oz	110	1	25
Berry Berry, ¾ cup, 0.9 oz	100	1.5	22
Lucky Charms, avg., ¾ cup, 1 oz	110	1	22
Oatmeal Crisp, Almond, 1 c., 2 oz	240	4.5	47
Raisin Nut Bran, ¾ cup, 1.75 oz	180	3	38
Reese's Puffs, ¾ cup, 1 oz	120	3	22
Total: Honey Clusters, ¾ c.	170	1	38
Raisin Bran, 1 cup, 1.9	160	1	40
Wheaties, ¾ cup, 1 oz	100	0.5	22

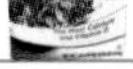

Glucerna 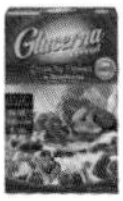   **C F Cb**

	C	F	Cb
Crunchy Flakes:			
'n Strawb., ¾ c., 1.1 oz	100	0.5	25
'n Almonds, ¾ c., 1.1 oz	100	1	24
'n Raisins, ¾ c., 1.2 oz	110	0.5	28

Health Valley
Organic Flakes:

	C	F	Cb
Amaranth Flakes, 1 cup, 1 oz	100	1	23
Blue Corn Flakes, ¾ cup, 1.1 oz	100	0	24
Cranberry Crunch, ¾ cup, 1.8 oz	190	4	38
Fiber 7, Multigrain Flakes, 1 c., 1.7 oz	160	1	37
Golden Flax, 1 cup, 1.75 oz	190	3.5	37
Oat Bran Flakes: 1 c., 1.75 oz	190	1.5	39
w. Raisins, 1 cup, 1.9 oz	200	1.5	43
Crunch-Ems!, avg., 1 c., 1 oz	110	0	27
Heart Wise, 1 cup, 2 oz	200	3	37

Heartland

	C	F	Cb
Granola: Original, ½ cup, 2.25 oz	290	11	41
Low-Fat Raisin, ⅔ cup, 2 oz	230	3	40

Kashi

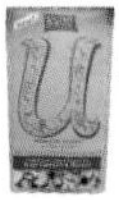

	C	F	Cb
7 Whole Grain: Flakes, 1 cup, 1.8 oz	180	1	41
Honey Puff, 1 cup, 1.1 oz	120	1	25
Nuggets, ½ cup, 2 oz	210	1.5	47
Puffs, 1 cup, 0.67 oz	70	0.5	15
Biscuit Cereals:			
Autumn Wheat, 1 cup, 1.9 oz	190	1	45
Cinnamon Harvest, 1 cup, 1.9 oz	190	1	44
Strawberry Fields, 1 cup, 1.1 oz	120	0	28
Kashi U, 1 cup, 2 oz	200	3.5	42
GoLEAN, 1 cup, 1.8 oz	140	1	30
GoLean Crunch! Orig., 1 c., 1.9 oz	190	3	36
Honey Almond Flax, 1 c., 1.9 oz	200	5	34
Good Friends: 1 cup, 1.9 oz	170	2	43
Cinna-Raisin Crunch, 1 c., 1.8 oz	170	1.5	41
Granola: Apple Orchard ½ c. , 1.9 oz	220	7	37
Cocoa Beach, ½ c., 1.9 oz	230	9	36
Mountain Medley, ½ cup, 1.9 oz	220	7	37
Summer Berry, ½ cup, 1.9 oz	210	6	37
Heart to Heart:			
Honey Toasted Oat, ¾ cup, 1.2 oz	110	1.5	25
Oat Flakes & Blueb. Clusters, 1 c	200	2.5	42
Oatmeal, avg. all flav., 1.5 oz pkg	160	2	33
Mighty Bites, Honey Cr., 1 c., 1.2 oz	110	1.5	23
Vive Probiotic, 1¼ cup, 1.9 oz	170	2.5	43

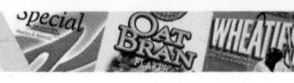

B — Breakfast Cereals

Ready-To-Eat (Cont)

	C	F	Cb
Kellogg's			
All-Bran: Bran Buds, ⅓ cup, 1.1 oz	70	1	24
Complete Wheat Flakes, ¾ c., 1.1 oz	90	0.5	23
Original, ½ cup, 1.1 oz	80	1	23
Strawberry Medley, 1 cup, 1.9 oz	170	1.5	44
Yogurt Bites, 1¼ c., 2 oz	190	3	44
Apple Jacks, 1 cup, 1 oz	110	0.5	25
Cereal Straws, all flav. (3), 1.1 oz	140	3.5	24
Cocoa Krispies, ¾ cup, 1.1 oz	120	0.5	27
Corn Flakes, Original, 1 cup, 1 oz	100	0	24
Corn Pops, 1 cup, 1 oz	110	0	26
Cracklin' Oat Bran, ¾ cup, 1.8 oz	200	7	35
Crispix, Original, 1 c., 1 oz	110	0.5	25
Crunch: Raisin Bran, 1 cup, 1.9 oz	190	1	45
Disney: Hannah Montana, 1 c., 1.1 oz	110	1	25
High Schol Musical, 1 cup, 1.1 oz	110	1	24
Froot Loops: Original, 1 cup, 1 oz	110	1	25
Reduced Sugar, 1¼ c., 1.1 oz	120	1	28
Grab'N Go Pack, 1 pouch	90	0.5	20
Marshmallow, 1 cup, 1.1 oz	120	1	27
Frosted Flakes, ¾ cup, 1.1 oz	110	1	27
Grab'N Go Pack, 1 pouch	80	0	21
Gold, ¾ cup, 1.1 oz	110	0.5	27
Red. Sugar, 1 c., 1.1 oz	120	1	28
Fruit Harvest, Straw./Blueb., ¾ cup	110	0	25
Granola, Low-Fat:			
with Raisins, ⅔ cup, 2.1 oz	230	3	49
without Raisins, ½ cup, 1.7 oz	190	2.5	40
Honey Smacks, ¾ cup, 1 oz	100	0.5	24
Jumbo Multi Grain Krispies, 1 c.	90	0	24
Mini Swirlz Cinnamon Bun, 1 cup	120	2	25
Mini-Wheats: Frosted Big Bite (5)	180	1	41
Frosted: Bite Size (24), 2.1 oz	200	1	48
Blueb. Muffins (24)	180	1	43
Unfrosted (30), 2.1 oz	200	1.5	46
Mueslix, ⅔ cup, 2 oz	200	3	40
Nutri-Grain Bars: *See Page 33*			
Product 19, 1 cup, 1.1 oz	100	0	25
Raisin Bran: Regular, 1 c., 2.1 oz	190	1.5	45
Extra, 1 cup, 1.9 oz	190	3	44

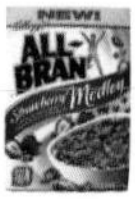

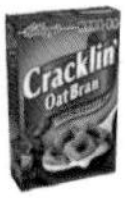

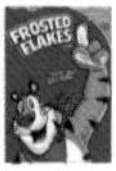

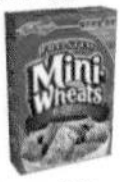

	C	F	Cb
Kellogg's (Cont)			
Rice Krispies: Orig. 1¼ cup, 1.2 oz	130	0	29
Berry, 1 cup, 1.1 oz	120	0	27
Frosted, ¾ cup, 1.1 oz	110	0	27
Cocoa, ¾ cup, 1.1 oz	120	1	27
Treats, ¾ cup, 1.1 oz	120	1.5	26
Smart Start:			
Antioxidants, 1 c., 1.8 oz	190	0.5	43
Smorz, 1 cup, 1.1 oz	120	2	25
Special K: Original 1 cup, 1.1 oz	120	0.5	23
Blueberry, ½ cup, 0.9 oz	100	0	23
Fruit & Yogurt, ¾ c., 1.1 oz	120	1	27
Red Berries, 1 c. 1.1 oz	120	0	26
Vanilla Almond, ¾ c.	110	1.5	25
Grab'N Go, avg., 1 pouch	100	1	22
Kozy Shak			
Ready Grains: *Per 7 oz Pkg*			
Apple & Cinnamon; Strawberry	210	2	38
Maple Brown Sugar	190	2	33
Original	180	2	30
Malt-O-Meal			
Apple Zings, 1 cup, 1.1 oz	130	1	30
Blueb. Muffin Tops, ⅔ cup	130	3.5	24
Cocoa Dyno-Bites, ¾ c., 1 oz	120	1	26
Coco Roos, ¾ cup, 1 oz	120	1.5	26
Colossal Crunch, ¾ cup, 1.1 oz	120	1.5	26
Frosted Flakes, ¾ cup, 1.1 oz	120	0	28
Frosted Mini Spooners, 1 c., 1.9 oz	190	1	45
Golden Puffs, ¾ cup, 1 oz	110	0	24
Honey Nut Scooters, 1 cup, 1 oz	110	1.5	24
Raisin Bran, 1 cup, 1.7 oz	220	1.5	49
Nature's Path			
Heritage, all types, ¾ cup, 1 oz	120	1	24
Honey'd Cornflakes, ¾ cup, 1 oz	120	0	26
Multigr. Oatbran Flakes, ¾ c., 1 oz	110	1	24
Flax Plus Granola: Ginger Zing, 1.9 oz	250	10	37
Hemp, 1.9 oz	260	10	37
Multibran ¾ cup, 1 oz	110	1.5	23
Pumpkin, 1.9 oz	260	10	37
Raisin Bran, ¾ c., 2 oz	190	2.5	41
Kamut Puffs, 1 cup, ½ oz	50	0	11
Optimum: Blueberry Cinn. 1 c. 2 oz	200	3	38
New England Natural Bakers			
Muesli, ½ cup, 2.1 oz	220	5	40
Granola: Almond Raisin Crisp, ½ c.	220	9	36
Apple Sunrise, ½ cup, 1.75 oz	210	7	34
Berry Good, ⅔ cup, 2.1 oz	250	6	44
Grateful Date, ½ cup, 1.7 oz	210	7	33
Honey Crunch; Pecan, ½ cup	285	13	37
Low-Fat Cranberry, ½ cup, 1.7 oz	200	2.5	41

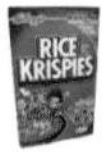

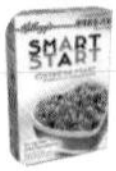

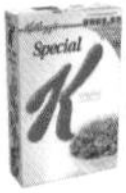

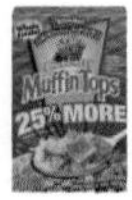

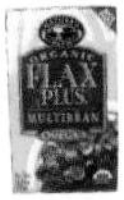

Ready-To-Eat (Cont) — C | F | Cb

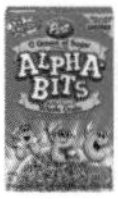

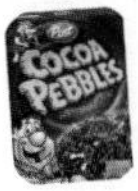

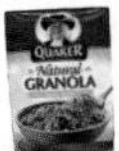

New Morning

	C	F	Cb
Cocoa Crispy Rice, ¾ cup, 1 oz	120	0.5	26
Fruit-e-O's, Organic, 1 cup, 1 oz	120	1.5	25
Oatios: Original, 1 cup, 1 oz	110	2	22
Apple Cinnamon, 1 oz	120	1	18

NutriSystem: *Per Package*

	C	F	Cb
Granola, Low-Fat	160	2.5	31
NutriCinnamon Squares	120	1	22
NutriFlakes (40% Bran Flakes)	110	1	23
NutriFrosted Crunch	110	1	19
Oatmeal, Apple Cinnamon	150	1.5	28

Peace

	C	F	Cb
Banana Nut Rainforest, 1 c., 1.95 oz	240	6	42
Essential 10, 1 cup, 1.95 oz	170	3	35
Granola, avg. all flavors, 2/3 cup	240	6	40
Hearty Raisin Bran, 1 cp, 1.95 oz	190	2	43
Crisps, Maple Pec.; Van. Alm., 1 c.	210	5	39

Post

	C	F	Cb
Alpha Bits, No Sugar, 1 c.	110	2	22
Bran Flakes, 1 oz	100	0.5	24
Grape-Nuts: 2 oz	200	1	48
Trail Mix Crunch, avg., 1.7 oz	180	3	37
Grape-Nuts Flakes, ½ cup	110	1	24
Honey Bunches of Oats, ¾ c. 1 oz	120	1.5	25
Just Bunches: Caramel, ⅔ cup, 2 oz	250	7	43
Honey, Rstd, ⅔ cup	250	7	43
Live Active Crunch:			
Mixed Berry, 1 c. 2 oz	190	1.5	43
Nut Harvest, 2 oz	210	7	38
Pebbles: Cocoa, ¾ cup, 1.1 oz	110	1.5	26
Fruity, ¾ cup, 1.1 oz	110	1	26
Raisin Bran, 1 cup, 2.1 oz	190	1	46
Selects: Banana Nut Crunch 2.1 oz	240	6	44
Cranberry Almd Crunch, ¾ cup	200	3.5	39
Shredded Wheat: Orig., 2 biscuits	160	1	37
Frosted, 1 cup, 1.8 oz	180	1	43

Quaker

	C	F	Cb
100% Natural Granola: ½ cup, 1.8 oz	210	6.5	37
w. Raisins, ½ c., 1.8 oz	215	6	38
Low-Fat: ⅔ cup	215	3	45
Oat Bran, 1¼ cup, 2 oz	210	3	43
Oatmeal Squares, Brown Sugar, 1 c.	210	2.5	44
Captain Crunch: Regular, ¾ cup, 1 oz	110	1.5	23
Crunch Berries, ¾ cup, 1 oz	100	1.5	22
Peanut Butter, ¾ oz, 1 oz	110	2.5	21

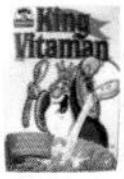

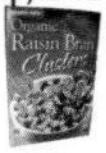

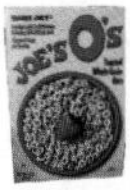

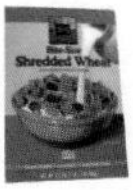

Quaker (Cont) — C | F | Cb

	C	F	Cb
Crunchy Corn Bran, 1 c., 1 oz	90	2.5	23
Honey Graham Oh's, ¾ c.	110	2	23
King Vitaman, 1½ c., 1.1 oz	120	1	26
Life, all types, ¾ c., 1.1 oz	120	1.5	26
Toasted Oatmeal: 1 cup, 1.7 oz	190	2	40
Brown Sugar Bliss, 1 cup, 1.7 oz	190	2	40
Honey Nut Heaven, 1 cup, 1.7 oz	190	2	40

Instant Oatmeal: *See Page 59*

Bars: *See Page 33*

Sweet Home Farm

	C	F	Cb
Honey Nut Granola, ½ cup, 1.9 oz	200	7	34
Low-Fat Granola, ½ cup, 1.9 oz	180	3	38

Trader Joe's

	C	F	Cb
Clusters: Raisin Bran, 1 cup, 2 oz	190	3	40
Super Nutty Toffee, ¾ cup, 2 oz	250	9	38
Avg. all other flavors			
⅔ cup, 1.3 oz	145	3.5	26
1 cup, 2 oz	220	5	39
Chocolate Decadence, ¾ cup, 2 oz	250	8	38
Cornflakes, 1 cup, 1.1 oz	110	0	26
Golden Flax Cereal, ¾ cup, 1.7 oz	200	3.5	37
Granola: Mango Passion, 2 oz	240	8	37
Gluten Free, ¾ cup, 2 oz	260	12	35
Trek Mix, ⅔ cup, 2 oz	240	8	37
Honey Nut O's, ¾ cup, 1 oz	120	1.5	24
Joe's O's, 1 cup, 1 oz	110	1.5	22
Morning Lite, 1 c., 1.85 oz	170	2.5	40
Shredded Wheats, Bite Size, 1 c., 1.7 oz	180	1	38
Soy Flax Clusters, 1 cup, 2 oz	190	3	38
Triple Berry O's, ¾ c. 1 oz	110	1	25
Toasted Oatmeal Flakes, ¾ c., 1.1 oz	110	1	23
Wheats, avg., 1 cup, 2 oz	200	1	42
Twigs, Flakes & Clusters, 1 c., 1.9 oz	170	1.5	41
Udi's, Granola, Au Naturel, ½ c., 2 oz	240	8	38

Uncle Sam

	C	F	Cb
Cereal w. Real Mixed Berries, 1 cup	190	4.5	39
Original, ¾ cup, 1.95 oz	190	5	38
Weetabix: 2 biscuits, 1.3 oz	120	1	28
Crispy Flakes: ¾ cup, 1.1 oz	110	0.5	24
& Fiber, 1¼ cup, 2 oz	170	1.5	44

Whole Foods (365)

	C	F	Cb
Corn Flakes, 1 cup, 1 oz	100	0	24
Honey Puffed Wheat, 1 oz	110	0	24
Frosted Flakes, ¾ c., 1 oz	110	0	26
Oat Bran Flakes, 1 c., 2 oz	220	3	45
Raisin Bran, 1 cup, 2 oz	200	0.5	44
Shredded Wheat, 1 cup, 1.7 oz	180	1	38
Frosted, 1 cup, 2 oz	210	1	45

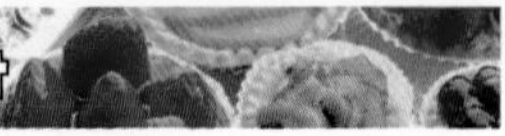

Ready-to-Eat

	C	F	Cb
Angel Food: Plain, no oil, 2 oz	145	0	33
Plain with oil, 2 oz	145	1	27
w. Cream Frosting	255	7	45
Almond Croissant, 5 oz	620	35	67
Apple Danish, 5 oz	450	18	67
Apple Pie: *See Pies/Tarts Page 136*			
Baklava, 1½" square, 1.75 oz	200	10	27
Banana w. Butter Cream, 2 oz	230	9	37
Banana Walnut, 3 oz	270	11	40
Bear Claw, 4½ oz	540	24	71
Black Forest, 3 oz (1/12)	345	11	59
Brownie: Small, 2" Square, 1 oz	130	8	14
Large, 3 oz	390	24	42
Bundt, average all types			
1 slice 3 oz (1/10)	300	13	42
Mini-Bundt, 5 oz	500	22	70
Cannoli	375	17	44
Carrot Cake: Plain, 3 oz	300	16	37
w. Cream Cheese Frosting	400	22	48
Cheesecake: Small serving, 3 oz	235	13	26
Large serving, 5 oz	395	21	44
w. Low-Fat Cheese/Fruit, 3 oz	170	4	28
Cheesecake Factory: 1 slice	630	45	53
Denny's Cheesecake, 1 slice	580	38	51
Chocolate Cake:			
Plain, no frosting, 1/12 of 9", 3½ oz	340	14	51
with chocolate frosting, 4 oz	415	18	62
Chocolate Croissant, 4¼ oz	470	26	54
Chocolate Eclair w. Custard, 3½ oz	260	16	24
Chocolate Fudge Cake, 3 oz	270	12	40
Chocolate Meringue, 1/6 pie	320	13	48
Churros, 1 stick, 1½ oz	125	5	18
Cinnamon Crumb Cake, 2½ oz	260	9	40
Cinnamon Roll: Small, 2 oz	220	8	34
Regular, 4 oz	440	16	68
Large, 6 oz	660	24	102
Brands ~ *See Page 69*			
Coffee Cake, 2 oz	180	6	30
Concha: Small, 2 oz	240	9	33
Large (5" diameter), 5½ oz	615	23	85
Cream Puff (custard fill), 4.6 oz	335	20	30
Creme Horns, each, 3 oz	210	5	36
Crumble Coffee Cake, 4½ oz	500	25	65
Danish Pastry:			
Small, 2½ oz	250	14	25
Large, 5 oz	500	28	50
Donuts: *See Page 68*			
Eclair, Choc., Cust. fill, 3½ oz	260	16	24
Fig Bars, average, each	160	3	31

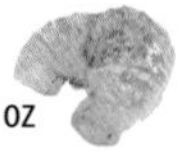

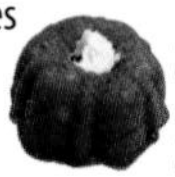

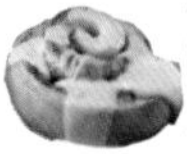

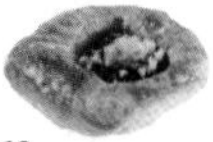

Ready-to-Eat (Cont)

	C	F	Cb
Fruit Cake, Dark/Light, 2 oz	185	5	34
Fudge Nut Brownie, each, 3½ oz	380	18	54
Gingerbread: From mix, 3" sq.	210	4	41
Honey Bun, each, 2.7 oz	310	15	39
Jelly Roll, 1/12 roll, 1.8 oz	150	2	32
Key Lime Pie, 4.3 oz	400	25	41
Kolacky, Apricot/Rasp., ½ oz (1)	60	3.5	8
Lady Fingers, 3 oz	310	4.5	59
Lemon Cake, 4 oz	440	24	49
Lemon Poppy Seed Creme, 1.6 oz	180	9	23
Marble Cake, 1 slice, 4 oz	430	23	50
Mississippi Mud Pie, 4 oz	480	22	67
Mud Cake, 1 piece, 4½ oz	380	20	44
Muffins: *See Page 69*			
Palmier Cookie, large, 4½ oz	490	25	62
Pineapple Upside Down, 2½ oz	230	9	36
Peach Melba, 3½ oz	300	8	52
Pecan Sticky Roll, 6½ oz	690	22	91
Pecan Twirls, 1 piece, 1.3 oz	170	7	26
Pies & Tarts: *See Page 136*			
Pound Cake, 3 oz	330	17	40
Raspberry Rugulah,			
1 pce, 1.2 oz	110	9	7
Scone, fruit, 2 oz	200	9	30
Sponge: Plain, 2½ oz	220	10	33
w. Cream & Strawberry Jam	390	12	69
w. Chocolate Frosting	290	12	45
Strawberry Creme, 4.7 oz	400	27	33
Strudel Bites, ¾ oz	60	2.5	9
Strudel, fruit, avg., 4.4 oz	300	17	32
Sweet Roll, avg., 1½ oz	150	6	23
Swiss Rolls, (2)	270	12	38
Tiramisu, 4.4 oz	440	22	34
Turnovers, fruit, avg., 3 oz	290	15	35

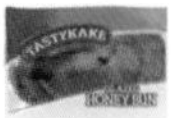

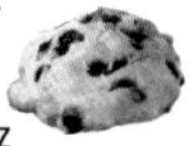

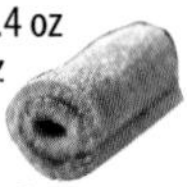

Cupcakes

	C	F	Cb
Average all Varieties			
Regular:			
Cake only, 1½ oz	140	5.5	20
Cake + Icing, 2½ oz	260	13	34
Large *(Muffin Size):*			
Cake only, 2½ oz	235	9	34
Cake + Icing, 5 oz	520	27	67
Mini (2-Bite):			
Cake only, 0.4 oz	40	1.5	5.5
Cake + Icing, 1 oz	110	5.5	13
Icing Only: Per 1 oz	115	7	13
Thick/Tall amount, 2½ oz	290	17	32
Starbucks Cupcakes:			
Triple Chocolate, 3¼ oz	360	20	46
Vanilla, 3 oz	320	16	43

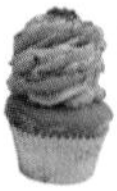

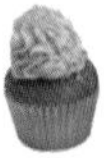

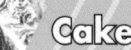

Cakes ~ Brands

	C	F	Cb
Albertson's Bakery			
Chocolate Ring Cake, ⅛, 3 oz	300	14	38
Lemon Ring Cake, ⅛, 3 oz	320	15	42
Sock it to me Ring Cake, ⅛, 3 oz	290	12	42
Cake Slices: *Per 1.6 oz Slice*			
Banana Nut Creme Cake	140	9	19
Blueberry Creme Cake	120	8	18
Butter Creme Cake	110	6	20
Cinnamon Butter Streusel Creme	140	9	20
Bimbo			
Concha, avg., 2.1 oz	240	9	33
Homestyle Pound Cake, 2.6 oz	300	15	37
Pecan Pound Cake, 2.9 oz	330	16	41
Raisin Pound Cake, 2.9 oz	340	16	43
Bon Appetite			
Banana Bread	440	25	49
Cheese Coffee Cake, 2.2 oz	270	15	31
Walnut Brownie, 3.5 oz	380	18	54
Sliced: Cheesecake, 4 oz	430	24	49
Lemon Cake, 4 oz	430	24	49
Marble Cake, 4 oz	430	24	50
Danish: Apple (1), 5 oz	420	22	50
Bear Claw (1), 5 oz	480	26	54
Cheese & Berries (1), 5 oz	500	28	52
Vienna Cream (1), 5 oz	480	28	54
Claim Jumper: Carrot Cake, 4.6 oz	450	24	54
Choc. Motherload Cake, 5.3 oz	520	27	73
Cheesecake Factory: *See Fast-Foods Section*			
Entenmann's			
Cheese-Filled Crumb Coffee, 2 oz	200	9	25
Chocolate Fudge, ⅙ cake, 2.75 oz	290	14	41
Coffee Cake, Cheese Topped, ⅑, 2 oz	200	9	26
Gourmet Cinn. Rolls, ½ roll	220	8	34
Louisiana Crunch, ⅑	330	15	47
Pecan Danish Ring, ⅙	250	15	26
Raspb. Danish Twist, ⅛	220	11	28
Enten-Minis:			
Butterscotch Cakes (2), 2 oz	250	10	37
Carrot Cakes (2), 2.8 oz	330	15	46
Choc. Creme Cupcakes (2), 2.8 oz	310	11	50
Sponge Creme Cupcakes (2), 2.3 oz	260	12	36
Muffins/Sweet Rolls: *See Page 69*			
Glenny's			
100 Calorie Brownie: *Per Brownie*			
Regular, 1.4 oz	100	4	12
Blondie, 1.4 oz	100	3	12
Peanut Butter, 1.4 oz	100	4	13

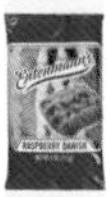

Great American Cookies

	C	F	Cb
Brownies: *Per Brownie*			
Cheesecake, 3.3 oz	430	23	54
Choc. Swirl Cheesecake, 3.3 oz	450	24	57
German Chocolate, 3.6 oz	420	22	55
Iced Fudge, 4.1 oz	500	23	71
Strawb. Swirl Cheesecake, 3.3 oz	430	23	55
Cookie Cakes: *Per Slice*			
By the Slice, 4.6 oz	580	27	83
Heart Shaped, 3.5 oz	440	21	64
Cookie Cakes (16"): 1 slice, 3.6 oz	460	22	67
M&M, 1 slice, 4 oz	500	24	73
Hostess			
100 Calorie Packs,			
Coffee Cakes, Cinn. (3)	100	3	21
Cinnamon Streusel Cake (1)	170	5	29
Chocodiles	230	11	36
Cup Cake: Choc. (1), 1.76 oz	180	6	31
Golden (1), 1.95 oz	200	7	33
Ding Dongs (2), 2.82	360	19	47
Ho Ho's (3), 3 oz	370	17	54
Snoballs (1), 1.7 oz	180	5	30
Suzy Q , 2 cakes, 4 oz	440	16	70
Twinkies, 1 cake, 1.5 oz	150	4.5	27
Fried Twinkie *(Page 175)*			
Zingers:			
Chocolate (1)	150	5	25
Devils Food, 4.2 oz	440	15	74
Raspberry (1)	160	7	24
Vanilla (1)	160	5	27
Little Debbie			
100 Calories: Choc. Cake (1), 1 oz	100	3	17
Yellow Cake w. Icing (1), 1 oz	100	3	18
Boston Crème Rolls (1), 2.2 oz	270	12	40
Brownies, Fudge (1), 2.15	290	13	40
Choc Chip Snack Cake (2), 2.4 oz	300	14	42
Chocolate Cup Cake	190	9	26
Coffee Cakes (1)	200	6	35
Devil Cremes (1) 1.65 oz	200	9	29
Devil Squares, 2 cakes, 2.2 oz	270	12	38
Fancy Cakes (2)	310	15	43
Frosted Fudge , 1.5 oz cake	190	9	26
Orange Cup Cake (1)	205	7	34
Star Crunch (1)	150	6	22
Smores (1)	190	7	30
Strawberry Shortcake Rolls, 2.1 oz	240	9	39
Swiss Cake Rolls (2), 2.15 oz	270	12	38
Zebra Cakes, 2 cakes, 2.6 oz	320	14	48
Nemo's			
Banana Cake, 3 oz	300	12	45
Chocolate Cake, 3 oz	300	12	44
Carrot Cake, 3.6 oz	390	21	47
Nilla, Cakesters,			
Vanilla /Strawb.(2), 1.76 oz	220	10	32

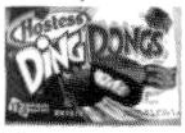

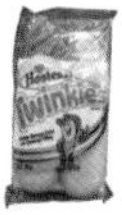

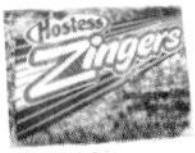

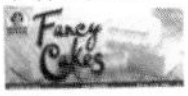

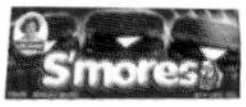

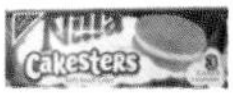

Cakes ~ Brands (Cont)

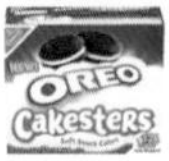

	C	F	Cb
Oreo			
Cakesters			
2 cake pkg, 2 oz	250	12	36
Pepperidge Farm			
Turnovers (Frozen): Apple, 3.15 oz	270	15	31
Raspberry, 3.15 oz	280	15	34
3-Layer Cakes:			
Coconut, ⅛, 2.5 oz	240	10	35
Chocolate Fudge, ⅛ cake, 2.5 oz	230	10	33
Golden, ⅛ cake, 2.5 oz	230	9	34
Apple Dumpling	230	11	29
Peach Dumpling	250	11	34
Rich's: Mini Eclairs (7)	300	16	36
Bavarian Creme (4), 2 oz	240	13	28
Safeway Select			
Molten Chocolate Lava Cake, 4½ oz	440	26	50
Sara Lee (Frozen)			
Cheesecake: *Per Slice*			
French Classic, ⅕ cake	400	24	38
French Strawberry, ⅙	320	18	37
New York Style Classic, ⅙ cake	480	30	47
Original Cream Cherry, ¼ cake	320	11	50
Original Cream, ¼ cake	330	17	35
Original Cream Strawberry, ¼ cake	310	11	48
Coffee Cakes: *Per Slice*			
Butter Streusel, ⅙ cake	190	10	22
Crumb Cake, ⅛ cake	190	8	30
Deluxe Cinnamon Rolls w. Icing (1)	320	15	41
Pecan Cake, ⅙ cake, 1.9 oz	310	10	22
Layer Cakes: *Per ⅛ Whole*			
Layer Coconut, ⅛ cake	260	14	33
Layer Double Chocolate, ⅛ cake	260	13	33
Layer Fudge Golden, ⅛ cake	260	13	34
Layer Vanilla, ⅛ cake	260	14	32
Pound Cakes: *Per ¼ of Cake, Unless Otherwise Staed*			
All Butter	300	16	35
Free & Light	200	4	39
Strawberry Swirl	290	11	44
Bites: *Per Serving*			
Original: (1)	20	1	3
(24)	440	27	43
Choc. Dipped Orig. Cheesecake	100	7	8
Choc. Dipped Praline Pecan (5)	90	6	8
Triple Choc. Fudge Brownie (1)	90	4	1

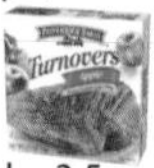

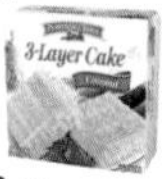

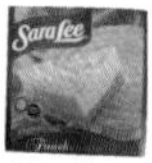

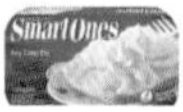

	C	F	Cb
Smart Ones (Weight Watchers)			
Brownie à la Mode	200	4	36
Chocolate Mousse	180	4	28
Chocolate Eclair	140	4	24
Choc. Chip Cookie Dough Sundae	170	3	32
Double Fudge Cake	220	7	35
Key Lime Pie, 3.3 oz	190	4.5	33
Mint Choc Chip Sundae, 2½ oz	150	3	28
Mocha Fudge Sundae, 2½ oz	160	4	27
Strawberry Shortcake, 3½ oz	170	6	25
Tastykake: Chocolate Jnr, 3.3 oz	340	12	55
Creme Filled Koffee Kakes, 3.15 oz	350	16	50
Koffee Kake Junior, 2.53 oz	280	10	44
Trader Joe's			
Bakery: Almond Ring Cake, ⅛, 1.8 oz	250	13	30
Carrot Cake, ⅛, 3.25 oz	480	33	42
Cheesecake Brownie Bites (1)	110	7	9
Danish Tea Cake, 1/13, 1.9 oz	200	9	28
Flourless Choc. Cake, 1 pce, 2 oz	260	17	23
Lemon Cake, ⅛, 3.25 oz	350	19	43
Mini Carrot Cake, 5 oz	450	19	68
Cupcakes: Chocolate, 3.2 oz	430	23	54
Vanilla, 3 oz	400	20	52
Frozen Dessert:			
Cappuccino Craving Cake, 1 pce	140	9	11
Chsecake Assortment: Plain, 3.5 oz	320	19	30
Choc Chip, 3.5 oz	350	20	36
Triple Choc, 3.5 oz	340	19	34
Tuxedo, 3.5 oz	320	17	34
Chocolate Cloud Cake, ⅛, 1.8 oz	160	10	15
Chocolate Ganache, ⅛, 3.5 oz	420	26	50
Choc Lava Cake (1), 3.8 oz	360	23	40
Ice Cream Cake, ⅑, 5 oz	370	18	48
Karat Cake, ⅛, 2.9 oz	320	19	37
Lemon Tarts (1), 3.3 oz	300	13	40
Mango Passion Torta Cotta, 1 pce	170	12	16
N.Y. Style Cheesecake, ⅐, 4.5 oz	400	28	32
Tiramisu Torte, ⅐, 3.2 oz	230	12	24
Tarts: Apricot Almond, ⅙, 4 oz	450	24	56
Lemon, ⅙, 2.7 oz	280	14	38
Linza, ⅙, 2 oz	200	7	32
Pear, ⅛, 3 oz	230	10	34

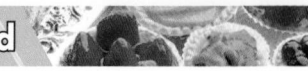

Cakes ~ Mixes

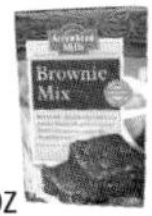

Made As Directed	C	F	Cb
Arrowhead Mills			
Cookie (1), avg. all types	**100**	4	16
Oatmeal Raisin (1), 0.7 oz	**80**	0	16
Gluten Free: Brownie, 1⁄20 pkg	**110**	2	21
Choc Chip (1), 0.7 oz	**70**	1	17
Betty Crocker			
Cakes (Super Moist): *Per 1⁄12 Cake*			
Butter Recipe Yellow	**250**	12	35
Cherry Chip	**290**	13	40
Chocolate varieties	**270**	13	34
Devil's Food	**270**	15	33
White	**230**	10	33
Other flavors, average	**270**	13	35
Per 1⁄10 Cake (Prepared): Carrot	**320**	14	41
If using No-Cholesterol Recipe, deduct 40 cals and 4g fat.			
Other Cakes: Pound Cake, 1⁄8	**260**	8	45
Gingerbread Cake, 1⁄8	**220**	6	39
Pineapple Upside Down, 1⁄6	**390**	13	65
Sunkist Lemon Bar (1)	**140**	4	24
Brownie Mix: *Per 1⁄20 Pkg*			
Chocolate Chunk	**180**	8	25
Dark Chocolate Fudge	**160**	10	24
Fudge	**170**	6.5	23
Low-Fat Fudge Brownie, 1⁄18 pkg	**140**	3	28
Original Supreme	**160**	7	26
Peanut Butter; Walnut, avg.	**180**	9	23
Triple Chunk	**180**	8	25
Cookie Mix: *Per 2 Cookies*			
Chocolate Chip	**170**	8	21
Double Chocolate Chunk	**150**	6	21
Oatmeal	**160**	7	22
Oatmeal Chocolate Chip	**160**	8	21
Peanut Butter	**150**	8	20
Rainbow Chocolate Candy	**160**	7	22
Sugar Cookie	**170**	8	22
Walnut Chocolate Chip	**170**	9	21
Warm Delights: *Per Bowl*			
Cinnamon Swirl Cake, 3.3 oz	**390**	10	72
Lemon Swirl Cake, 3.6 oz	**380**	9	72
Molten Caramel Cake, 3.4 oz	**360**	10	64
Molten Chocolate Cake, 3.4 oz	**370**	12	61

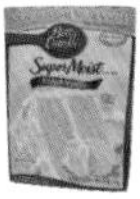
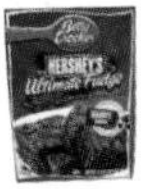
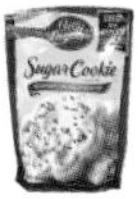

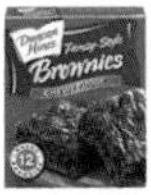
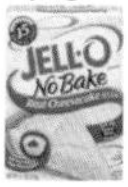
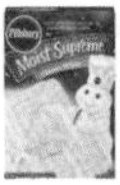

Duncan Hines	C	F	Cb
Brownie Mix: *Per 1 oz Brownie, Prepared*			
Candy Shop Peanut Butter Cup, 1 oz	**170**	8	23
Chewy Fudge	**170**	8	23
Double Fudge	**180**	8	26
Turtle	**160**	7	23
Cake Mix: *Per 1⁄12 Cake*			
Moist Deluxe Cake:			
Ban. Supreme/Yellow Cake, 1½ oz	**270**	12	36
Classic White, 1½ oz	**210**	6	36
Dark Choc./Devil's Food, 1½ oz	**290**	15	35
French Vanilla, 1½ oz	**250**	12	34
Jell-O No Bake Cheesecakes: *Prep'd As Directed*			
Chocolate Silk Dessert, 1⁄6 pkg	**290**	14	36
Homestyle Cheesecake, 1⁄6 pkg	**370**	17	50
Oreo, 1⁄6 pkg	**370**	17	51
Peanut Butter Cup, 1⁄8 pkg	**360**	20	42
Pumpkin Pie, 1⁄8 pkg	**250**	10	36
Real Cheesecake, 1⁄6 pkg	**350**	14	48
Krusteaz: Cinn. Crumb Cake, 1"	**230**	7	38
Lemon/Key Lime Bar, 2" bar	**160**	4.5	29
Pillsbury			
Moist Supreme: *Per 1⁄12 Cake*			
Devils Food	**260**	13	35
Classic White	**250**	8.5	35
Classic Yellow	**250**	11	35
Brownie Mix: Choc. Extreme, 1⁄16	**160**	8	22
Chocolate Fudge; Funfetti, 1⁄20	**170**	8	23
Fudge Supreme, 1⁄18	**150**	7	19
Mint Chocolate, 1⁄15	**160**	8	22

Cake Frostings

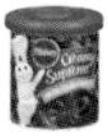

Betty Crocker	C	F	Cb
Drizzlers, 2½ Tbsp	**220**	13	26
Rich & Creamy, average, 2 Tbsp	**140**	5	23
Whipped, all flavors, 2 Tbsp	**100**	4.5	15
Easy Flow Icing, 1 Tbsp	**75**	3	12
Duncan Hines: *Per 2 Tbsp (1.2 oz)*			
Creamy Homestyle, avg all flavors	**140**	6	23
Homestyle Fat-Free, 6 tbsp	**100**	0	24
Whipped, avg., 3 Tbsp	**160**	9	20
Pillsbury: *Per 2 Tbsp (approx. 1⁄12 Tub)*			
Creamy Supreme: Choc Fudge	**140**	6	21
Classic White	**140**	5	22
Milk Choc	**140**	6	21
Vanilla; Vanilla Funfetti	**150**	6	25
Reduced Sugar: Choc., 2 Tbsp	**120**	8	16
Vanilla, 2 Tbsp	**120**	7	18
Whipped Supreme, avg all flavors	**100**	5	14

Quick Guide

Donuts
Average All Brands

	C	F	Cb
Plain, 1¾ oz	210	12	25
Sugared, 1¾ oz	220	11	27
Glazed, 2 oz	250	12	34
Chocolate Iced, 2 oz	260	14	29

Donuts ~ Brands

	C	F	Cb
Albertson's			
Donut Holes: Assorted	150	8	18
Powdered Sugar (4) 1.7 oz	210	12	24
Gem Donuts: Plain Cake (3) 1.6 oz	190	12	20
Chocolate (3)	260	16	25
Glazed (4), 1.9 oz	260	16	26
Sticky Donuts, 2.2 oz	230	10	32
Bon Appetite			
Cherry Donuts (1) 2 oz	260	15	30
Mini Donuts: Chocolate (4)	270	16	29
Powdered; Crumb, avg. (4)	240	12	32
Dolly Madison			
Regular, 1¾ oz	270	12	40
Donut Gems, Powdered Mini's (4), 2 oz	230	11	30
Coffee Cake, Cinnamon (1), 1.6 oz	170	6	29
Sweet Rolls, Cinnamon (1), 2 oz	230	10	31
Zingers (1), 1.5 oz	160	7	24
Dunkin' Donuts			
Apple N' Spice Donut	240	11	32
Blueberry Cake Donut	330	18	38
Boston Kreme Donut	280	12	38
Chocolate Frosted Cake Donut	340	19	38
Chocolate Glazed Cake Donut	280	15	33
Cinnamon Cake Donut	290	18	30
Glazed Cake Donut	320	18	37
Jelly Filled Donut	260	11	36
Old Fashioned Cake Donut	280	18	27
Powdered Cake Donut	300	18	30
Sugar Raised Donut	190	9	22
Vanilla Kreme Filled Donut	320	17	37

Donuts ~ Brands (Cont)

	C	F	Cb
Entenmann's			
Dark Choc. Frosted	280	19	28
Frosted Devil's Food	320	19	35
Glazed Buttermilk, 2¼ oz	270	14	34
Milk Chocolate Frosted, 2.4 oz	310	19	35
Powdered, 1¾ oz	230	14	25
Pop'ems (bite size): *Per 4 pieces*			
Glazed (4) 2 oz	240	12	31
Glazed Devil's Food (4) 2 oz	240	11	33
Popettes (bite size), 3 pcs, 1.8 oz	240	15	24
Hostess			
Dunkin Stix (3)	490	25	63
Donut Bites, 1 pouch, 2.3 oz	300	15	38
Regular: Plain, 1.4 oz	160	9	18
Choc. Frosted, 2 oz	230	13	26
Powdered, 1.7 oz	190	9	25
Old Fashioned Glazed, 2.1 oz	240	11	33
Donettes: Frosted (3) 1.76 oz	220	13	23
Crumb (4) 2 oz	220	9	32
Crunch (3), 2 oz	180	8	31
Powdered (4) 2.1 oz	240	12	31
Krispy Kreme			
Chocolate Glazed Cruller	290	15	37
Chocolate Iced Glazed	250	12	33
Chocolate Iced Kreme Filled	350	20	39
Chocolate Iced w. Sprinkles	270	12	38
Cinnamon Twist	240	15	23
Glazed Cruller	240	14	26
Glazed Kreme Filled	340	20	39
Maple Iced Glazed	240	12	32
New York Cheesecake	340	20	34
Original Glazed	200	12	22
Powdered Cake	280	14	37
Traditional Cake Doughnut	230	13	25
Doughnut Holes, Glazed (5)	200	11	25
Little Debbie			
Donut Sticks, 1.65 oz pkg	230	14	25
Mini Donuts: Frosted (4), 2.1 oz	290	17	32
Powdered (4)	210	10	29
Tastykake			
Cinnamon, 1.8 oz	210	11	26
Mini: Coated, 3 oz	380	22	42
Powdered Sugar (6) 2½ oz	280	13	37

Quick Guide **C F Cb**

Muffins: Ready-To-Eat
Average All Types:

	C	F	Cb
Small, 1 oz	80	3	12
Medium, 2 oz	160	6	24
Large, 3 oz	240	9	36
Extra Large, 4 oz	320	12	48
Giant, 6 oz	480	18	72
Super Size, 8 oz	640	24	96

Brands ~ Ready-To-Eat

	C	F	Cb
Albertsons: *Mini Muffins, Per 1.76 oz*			
Banana Nut (2)	160	11	20
Blueberry (2)	150	10	19
Honey Raisin Bran (2)	180	8	25
Awrey's: Blueberry, 2.5 oz	240	12	31
Raisin Bran, 1.5 oz muffin	160	8	23
Controlled Carb Gourmet			
Almond Blueberry Muffins, 3 oz	210	15	27
Entenmann's: Golden, 2.4 oz	240	12	29
Little Bites, Blueberry, 1 pouch	190	9	27
Hostess: Mini, 1 pouch, avg.	260	15	30
Fruit Pie/Tart, avg., 4.5 oz	475	20	68
Hearty Muffin: Blueberry, 6 oz	690	42	72
Banana Nut, 6 oz	750	48	72
Muffin Loaf: Blueberry, 3.8 oz	420	19	58
Banana Nut, 3.8 oz	460	24	56
100 Calorie Packs:			
Banana Streusel (3)	100	3.5	19
Blueb. Streusel (3)	100	3	20
Little Debbie: Banana Nut (1), 1.9 oz	210	9	30
Blueberry (1), 1.9 oz	190	8	27
Chocolate Chip (1), 1.9 oz	210	9	28
My Favorite Muffin:			
Chocolate Chip, 6 oz	630	33	81
Fat-Free, Blueberry; Cherry Pie, 6 oz	330	0	78
Otis Spunkmeyer: *Per Whole Muffin (4 oz)*			
Banana Nut, 4 oz	420	20	54
Chocolate Chip	420	22	52
Wild Blueberry	360	16	52
Starbucks: *See Fast-Foods Section*			
Trader Joe's:			
Banana Chocolate Chip, 4 oz	400	18	57
Triple Berry (1), 4 oz	310	11	49
Mini: Blueberry, 0.8 oz	110	6	12
Bran w. Raisin, 0.8 oz	80	3	13
Weight Watchers: Blueb., 2.5 oz	190	2.5	42
Double Chocolate, 2.5 oz	180	3	41
Fast-Food Restaurants: *See Page 183*			

Muffin Mixes **C F Cb**

Prepared: Per Muffin

	C	F	Cb
Betty Crocker: Apple Streusel (1)	230	8	37
Banana Nut (1)	210	10	27
Choc Chip; Cinnamon Streusel (1)	220	8	30
Wild Blueberry (1)	180	8	26
Water Muffins: Choc Chip (1)	160	5	26
Blueb.; Lemon Poppyseed, avg.	130	3.5	24
Cornbread (1)	180	6	24
Krusteaz: Banana Nut (1)	220	11	32
Choc Chip (1)	230	10	34
Lem. Poppyseed (1)	170	4.5	30
Oatbran (1)	180	4.5	31
Pillsbury: Hot Roll Mix	130	3	21
Just Add Milk Blueb. Muffin (1)	170	5	30
Ultimate: Blueberry Streusel (1)	190	12	35
Choc Fudge Choc Chip (1)	270	13	34
Sunmaid: Honey Raisin Bran (1)	210	7.5	33
Trader Joe's: Ban. Muffin Mix (1)	180	11	22

Sweet Rolls & Buns **C F Cb**

Note: It is best to weigh for accuracy as actual weight can be 10-50% higher than label weight·

	C	F	Cb
Bon Appetite: Cinn. Roll, 5 oz	580	34	64
Mammoth Cinnamon Roll, 5 oz	560	28	70
Cinnabon: Classic	815	32	117
Caramel Pecanbon	1100	56	141
Minibon, 1 roll	340	13	49
CinnaPretzel	750	6	156
Cinnabon Stix (5) no frosting	380	21	41
Cloverhill Bakery			
Jumbo Honey Bun, 4.75 oz	540	26	70
Entenmann's: Cinn. Bun (1), 4.5 oz	500	22	72
Hostess:			
Cinnamon Sweet Roll (1)	200	6	34
Honey Bun, Glazed:			
Net weight, 3.75 oz	440	25	51
Actual weight, 4.65 oz	550	31	63
Iced/Frosted, 3.5 oz	395	5.5	50
Little Debbie:			
Honey Buns, 1.76 oz	220	12	26
Pecan Spinwheels, 1 oz	100	4	16
McDonald's: Cinnamon Melts, 4 oz	460	19	66
Pillsbury: Cinnamon Roll, w. Icing	150	5	23
Reduced Fat (1) 1.5 oz	140	3.5	24
Ralph's, Cinnamon Roll, 2.5 oz	290	11	44
7-Eleven, Iced Honey Bun, 4.75 oz	520	24	71
Trader Joe's: Cinn. Roll, 2.35 oz	250	7	41
Low-Fat Cinn. Roll, 2.35 oz	180	2	36
Frosted Cinnamon Bun, 4 oz	380	9	66
Zen Bakery: Cinn. Raisin Roll (1), 3.2 oz	230	2	48

Quick Guide

Chocolate
Average All Brands

	C	F	Cb
Milk Chocolate, regular:			
Plain/Nuts/Fruit, average, 1 oz	155	10	16
1½ oz Bar	225	15	24
2 oz Bar	310	20	32
4 oz Block	620	40	64
8 oz Block	1240	80	128
1 Pound, 16 oz	2480	160	256
Dark/White Chocolate, 1 oz	155	9	17
Sugar Free *(Hershey's)* 1 pce, 0.3 oz	40	2	5
Chocolate-coated:			
Almonds, 5-6, 1 oz	155	9	16
Clusters, Nut, 3 pcs, 1.2 oz	210	14	20
Coffee Beans, 1.4 oz	220	13	22
Creme/Cordial Centers, 1.26 oz	170	6	28
Fudge, 1.5 oz	220	13	27
Macadamias, 10 pcs, 1.4 oz	220	16	21
Mints, 1 med., ½ oz	55	1	11
Nougat & Caramel, 1 oz	150	9	15
Peanuts, 12 med., 1 oz	150	10	15
Raisins, 28 med., 1 oz	110	4	19
Cooking Chocolate:			
Sweet/Semi-sweet, 1 oz	140	9	16
4 oz Bar *(Baker's)*	480	28	64
Chips: 1 Tbsp, ½ oz	70	4	9
½ cup, 3 oz	420	24	54
Unsweetened, 1 oz	140	14	8
Carob: Plain, 1 oz	150	9	16

Brands & Generic

Per Piece/Serving

	C	F	Cb
100 Grand: 1.5 oz bar	190	8	30
Super Size, 2.8 oz	360	14	58
Snack Size (1), .75 oz	95	4	15
Abba Zabba, 2 oz bar	240	5	48
After Dinner Mints, 1 small	25	1.5	3
After Eight Mint *(Nestlé),* each	35	1.5	4
Air Head, 1 bar, 15.6g	60	1	14
Allen Wertz: Simply Sugar Free			
Coffee Time (decaf), 4	45	1.5	8
Coffee Toffee, 6	120	3	23
Other types, 4	120	2.5	24
Almond Joy: 2 bars, 1.6 oz	220	13	26
King Size, 4 bars, 3.22 oz	440	26	52
Snack, 0.6 oz bar	80	4.5	10
Cookies (2), 1 oz	140	8	17
Almond Roca, 3 pcs, 1.27 oz	200	15	17
Almonds, sugar-coated (15), 40g	190	7	27

Brands & Generic (Cont)

Per Piece/Serving,

	C	F	Cb
Almond Clusters *(Trader Joe's),*			
2 pce, 1.2 oz	210	14	5
Altoids *(C & B),* 3 pcs	10	0	2
Andes, Thins, avg. all flav. (8), 1.4 oz	200	13	22
Anthon Berg: Cognac, each	180	8	25
Creamy Mint (4), 1.4 oz	180	6	31
Marzipan w. Madeira, 1.4 oz	175	7.5	26
Marzipan Brod	120	7	13
Atomic Fireball, 1 piece 0.3 oz	35	0	9
Baby Ruth: King Size, 3.7 oz bar	500	24	66
2.1 oz bar	280	14	39
Fun size, 2 bars	170	8	24
Minis, 4 bars	210	9	30
Baci *(Perugino):* 1 pce, ½ oz	75	6	7
3 pcs, 1.5 oz	230	18	21
Baskin-Robbins: 3 pce, 0.5 oz	60	1	12
Sugar Free, 4 pcs	40	1	15
Big Hunk, 2 oz	230	3	47
Bit-O-Honey, 1.7 oz	180	3.5	39
Chews, 6 pcs, 1.4 oz	150	3	32
Bliss *(Hershey's),* avg., 1 piece	35	2.5	4
Blow Pops, each, 0.6 oz	60	0	17
Bon Bons, 3 pieces	65	0	15
Boston Baked Beans, 11 pcs, 15g	70	2	11
Brach's: Almond Supremes (11)	210	13	21
Bridge Mix, 16 pcs, 1.4 oz	180	9	26
Chocolate Peanut Cluster, 3 pcs	210	14	19
Double Dippers (15), 1.4 oz	210	14	19
Maple Nut Goodies (8)	190	9	27
Milk Maid Caramel (4), 1.37 oz	160	4.5	27
Orange Slices (3), 45g	150	0	37
Special Treasure Butter Toffee (3)	80	2	15
Star Brites, Peppermint (3), 0.5 oz	60	0	15
Wild 'N Fruity (14), 1.4 oz	140	0	32
Breath Savers, all types, each	5	0	2
Brite Crackers, 1 bag, 1.5 oz	140	0	32
Bubble Gum: *See 'Gum' Page 77*			
Bulls Eyes, 3 pcs, 34g	130	3	23
Buncha Crunch: ⅓ cup, 1.4 oz	180	8	26
Movie Box, 3.2 oz	450	20	65
Burnt Peanuts, 31 pcs, 40g	170	6	29
Butterfinger: 2.1 oz bar	270	11	43
King Size (3), 3.7 oz	460	18	76
Fun Size, 1.3 oz	200	8	30
Giant (5 oz pkg), pieces in choc.,			
½ pkg, 2½ oz	340	16	48
Miniatures: 1 pce, 10g	45	2	7.5
4 pieces, 40g	180	8	29
Stix, 1 stick, 17g	90	4	12

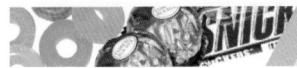

Brands & Generic (Cont)

Per Piece/Serving   **C** **F** **Cb**

	C	F	Cb
Butterfinger (Cont):			
Crisp Bar: 1.76 oz bar	250	14	32
King Size, 5 oz	680	32	96
Fun Size (2), 1.4 oz	210	11	25
Minis, 4 bars	180	8	29
Butter Mints, 7 pcs, 0.46 oz	50	0	12
Butterscotch: 3 pcs	60	0	15
Chips (Hershey's), 1 Tbsp	80	4	10
Dics (Walgreens), 3 pcs, 18g	70	0	17
Cadbury: Caramello Bar, 1.4 oz	200	9	28
Dairy Milk Bar, 7 pcs, 1.4 oz	200	11	23
Mini Eggs, 12 pcs,1.4 oz	190	8	28
Candy Apple, medium, 6.5 oz	280	0	60
Candy Cane, medium, 5", ½ oz	40	0	10
Candy Corn, 16 pcs, 1 oz	100	0	26
Candy Jar Mix (Jewel) (3), 0.6 oz	60	0	14
Candy Necklaces, 20g each	80	0	20
Caramels: each, 0.35 oz	40	1	8
Chocolate, each, 6.6g	25	0.3	6
Creams: 3 pcs, 1¼ oz	130	3	23
Caramel Nips: 2 pcs	60	1.5	11
Chocolate Parfait, 2 pcs	60	2	11
Peanut Butter, 2 pcs	60	2	11
Sugar Free Caramel, 2 pcs	60	1.5	12
Caramel Popcorn, ⅔ cup	150	6	23
Caramello Bar (Cadbury), 1.6 oz	220	10	29
Cella's Cherries, 3 pcs, 43g	160	6	27
Certs, Breath Mints, 1 pce	5	0	2
Charleston Chew: 1 bar, 40g	160	4.5	30
Mini (13), 1.4 oz	180	6	33
Charms: Blow Pop	60	0	17
Flat Pop, 15g	50	0	14
Chew-ets Peanut Chews:			
Original, 4 pcs, 47g	230	12	29
Chewz, 1 roll, 30g	120	1	28
Chick O Stick, 2 oz	240	9	42
Chocolate Mints (Hershey's), 3 mints	15	0	3
Chocolate Parfait Nips, 2 pcs	60	2	11
Chunky Bar (Nestlé),			
King Size, 2½ oz	340	19	43
Chupa Chups, 1 Pop	50	0	12
Cinn. Buttons (Walgreens), 3 pce	60	0	18

Per Piece/Serving   **C** **F** **Cb**

	C	F	Cb
Cinnamon Disks (Walmart), 3 pcs	70	0	18
Circus Peanuts, Marshmallow (Spangler),			
4 pieces, 1.5 oz	150	0	38
CocoaVia, Original Bars, 0.8 oz	100	6	12
Coconut Stacks, 8 pieces	290	13	37
Coffee Go Coffee/Cappuccino, ea.	18	0.5	4
Coffee Rio-Gold, each	15	0.5	3
Conversation Hearts (Necco), 1 lge	10	0	3
Cookie Dough Bites, 1.4 oz	200	10	27
Cote d'Or: Dark 86% Coca, 3.5 oz	605	55	19
Dark 70%, Orange, 3.5 oz	575	46	34
Dark Raspberry, 3.5 oz	580	46	34
Milk Intense, 3.5 oz	575	40	45
Cotton Candy, 1 oz	110	0	28
Cough Drops: See Page 77			
Cracker Jack, ½ cup, 1 oz	120	2	23
Creme Savers: See Lifesaves			
Crisped Rice, Choc Chip, 1 bar. 1 oz	115	4	20
Crows, 11 pieces, 1.4 oz	130	0	33
Crunch: Original, 1.55 oz bar	220	11	30
Fun Size, 1.34 oz	180	9	26
Miniatures: 6 pce	180	9	25
Dark, 1 pce	50	3	6
Buncha Crunch, 3.2 oz box	450	20	65
Crunch Crisp, 1.34 oz bar	190	11	24
Dots, 11 dots, 1.4 oz	130	0	33
Double Dip Stick, 1 stick	16	0.5	3
Dove			
Milk Choc: Singles Bar	200	12	22
Large Tablet Bar, 3.53 oz	540	33	60
Dark Choc: Singles Bar, 1.3 oz	190	12	22
Large Tablet Bar, 3.53 oz	510	33	60
Miniatures: Milk Choc, 1 pc, 0.3 oz	45	2.5	5
with Caramel, 1 piece, 0.3 oz	40	2	5
Choc Covered Almonds:			
Dark, 13 pieces	210	15	19
Milk, 13 pieces	220	15	19
Silky Smooth, Choc. w/ P'nut Butter			
5 pieces, 1.38 oz	220	14	20
Sugar Free: Dark (3.4 oz bag),			
All flavors, 1 piece	40	3	4
Tiramisu, Mint Caramel, 1 pc, 0.3 oz	40	2	5
Dum Dum Pops (Spangler), 1 pop	25	0	6.5

Brands & Generic (Cont)

Per Piece/Serving	**C**	**F**	**Cb**
English Toffee, 1 pce, 12g	70	4	6
Eda's Sugar Free, all flav., 5, ½ oz	40	0	15
5th Avenue: 2 oz bar	260	14	35
King Size bar	480	24	60
Fannie May: Single Wrapped Pieces			
Mint Milk, 1.55 oz	190	6	32
Pixie, 2 pcs, 1.6 oz	240	14	26
Trinidad, 1 pce, 1.15 oz	160	9	18
Fast Break *(Reese's):* 2 oz bar	260	12	35
3.5 oz bar	460	22	62
Ferrero Rocher: each	75	5	5
3 pcs, 1.3 oz	220	16	16
Rondnoir (4), 1.4 oz	220	14	21
Fifty 50 Snack Bars:			
Peanut Butter, 1.2 oz	190	14	17
Almond, 7 pce, 1.4 oz	150	17	18
Crunch Bar, 7 pce, 1.1 oz	110	12	16
Dark Choc, 7 pce, 1.4 oz	130	14	21
Milk Choc., 7 pce, 1.4 oz	150	16	19
Fluffy Stuff *(Charms),* 1.4 oz	150	0	40
Fondant: Choc-coated, 1.2 oz	125	3	27
Mint, 1 oz	105	0	25
Fran's: Gold Bar, 45g	250	14	17
Gold Bites (Almonds), 23g	120	7	13
Frooties, 12 pcs, 1.4 oz	160	3.5	32
Fruit Crystals *(Wonka),* 3 pcs	70	0	17
Fruit Drops, each, 4.25g	20	0	4
Fruit Gems *(Sunkist),* 4, 1.4 oz	130	0	33
Fruit Leathers, average, 0.5 oz	50	0.5	12
Fruit Pastilles *(Rowntree),* 1 roll	185	0	45
Fruit Rolls, 1 roll	80	1	17
Fruit Roll-Ups, ½ oz	50	1	12
Fruit Runts *(Walgreens),* 12 pcs	60	0	14
Fudge: Chocolate/Vanilla (1), 1 oz	120	4	20
with Nuts (1), 1 oz	145	9	115
Choco. Marshmallow, 1 oz	130	5	20
w. Nuts, 1 oz	135	6	19
Peanut Butter, 1 oz	115	3	19
Ghirardelli:			
Squares: Dark Choc. (4), 1.6 oz	220	17	23
Caramel (3), 1.6 oz	220	12	28
3.5 oz Bar: Dark Choc., 7.5 oz	500	43	43
Other varieties avg., 12 pcs	440	28	52
Intense Dark: Twilight, 3 pcs	200	17	17
Evening Dream, 3 pcs	190	15	20

Per Piece/Serving	**C**	**F**	**Cb**
Godiva: Hearts, 7 pieces, 1.4 oz	210	13	23
Bars: Milk/Dark, avg., 1½ oz	230	14	26
Extra Dark 72%, 1½ oz	230	17	18
Assorted Chocs: 2 pieces, 31g	160	10	17
Sugar Free, 3 pieces	200	15	23
Chocoiste: *Per 1.4 oz*			
Dark Choc: Amonds	210	17	16
Cherries (10)	160	7	28
Praline Pecans (7)	210	41	21
Whole Cashews (14)	220	15	19
Go Lightly: Choc Lovers Asst. (2)	220	16	28
Bags: Assorted Taffy, 5 pieces	130	3	36
Vanilla Caramels, 5 pieces	150	6	31
Sugar Free Creme Crunch (4)	150	5	33
Hard Candy (4), 16g	45	0	15
Goobers Peanuts, 1 pkg, 1.4 oz	210	14	22
Good & Plenty *(Hershey's)* (33), 1.16 oz	130	0	33
GooGoo Cluster, 1 bar, 1.75 oz	240	11	32
Gum Drops: 1 small, 0.1 oz	15	0	3
5 pcs, 0.63 oz	75	0	15
Gummi: Bears, 16 bears, 40g	140	0	34
Chewy Sweet Tarts (4), 1.5 oz	160	0	36
Novelties (Walgreens), 7	140	0	34
Savers, 10 pieces	130	0	30
Worms (1), 13 pcs, 39g	130	0	31
Guylian: Milk Choc., 8 squares, 1 oz	150	9	16
Dark Choc., 8 squares, 1 oz	140	9	13
Guylian Twists, 1 pc, 7g	45	3.5	3
Seashell Bar, 40g	210	13	21
Hard Candy: All flavors (3), 18g	60	0	16
1 regular piece	20	0	5
Heath: Original (1), 1.38 oz	210	13	24
Bites, 15 pcs, 1.38 oz	210	12	25
King Size, 2.8 oz	410	26	49
Snack Size, 3 pcs, 1.4 oz	230	14	27
Hershey's:			
Milk Chocolate: 1.55 oz bar	210	13	26
Cookies 'n' Creme, 2 bars, 1.2 oz	170	9	21
King Size, 2.6 oz bar	370	42	44
7 oz bar, 3 pcs	180	11	22
w. Almonds, 1.45 oz bar	230	14	22
Cacao Reserve:			
Milk Choc. (35% cacao), 4 blocks, 1.4 oz	220	15	21
Dark Choc. (65% cacao), 1.3 oz	160	13	19
Extra Dark (60% cacoa):			
Raspberry, 4 pcs, 1.4 oz	180	14	21
Pomegranate, 4 pcs, 1.4 oz	170	12	23
Candy-Coated Eggs:			
Milk Choc (4), 0.6 oz	90	4	12
w. Almonds (4) 0.6 oz	100	6	9

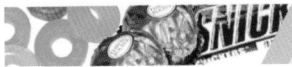

Brands & Generic (Cont)

Per Piece/Serving **C F Cb**

Hershey's (Cont):
Pot of Gold Chocolate:
Nut Assortment, 4 pcs 1.4 oz | **210** | 13 | 23
Caramel Assort., 4 pcs, 1.4 oz | **190** | 10 | 25
Chocolate Assortment, 1.4 oz | **200** | 12 | 24
Truffle Assortment, 1.5 oz | **200** | 9 | 27
Special Dark Choc.: 1.45 oz bar | **180** | 12 | 25
King Size, 2.6 oz | **330** | 22 | 45
Lge, 3 pcs, 1.27 oz | **170** | 11 | 22
Snack Size, 0.5 oz | **220** | 13 | 26
Snacksters, 1 pkg, 20g | **100** | 3.5 | 15
Sugar Free: Milk Choc. 5 pcs, 1.4 oz | **160** | 13 | 24
Peanut Butter Cups Minis (5) | **180** | 13 | 27
Special Dark Choc. (5), 1.4 oz | **190** | 15 | 23
York Peppermint Patties, 3 pcs | **80** | 3.5 | 28
Honeycomb: Plain, 1 oz | **115** | 0 | 27
Choc-coated, 2 pcs | **180** | 7 | 31
Hot Tamales, 20 pcs, 1.4 oz | **150** | 0 | 36
Hugs ~ *See Kisses*
Jawbreakers *(Sathers)*, 15, 17g | **60** | 0 | 16
Jellies, 3 medium, 1 oz | **130** | 0 | 33
Jells Raspberry *(Joyva)*, 3 pcs, 44g | **160** | 0 | 38
Jelly Beans: Small, 37 beans, 1.4 oz | **120** | 0 | 35
Regular, 13 beans, 40g | **150** | 0 | 37
1 bean | **10** | 0 | 3
Sugar Free, 35 beans | **80** | 0 | 37
Jumbo, 1 bean | **20** | 0 | 5
Jewel, 13 beans, 1.4 oz | **140** | 0 | 36
Sathers/Walgreens, 13 pcs | **150** | 0 | 38
Wonderbeans, 33 beans | **100** | 0 | 24
Jelly Bellys: each | **4** | 0 | 1
35 pcs, 1.4 oz | **140** | 0 | 37
Sugar Free Beans/Sours (35), 1.4 oz | **80** | 0 | 37
Jelly Rings *(Jewel)*, 5 pcs, 39g | **110** | 0 | 26
Jolly Rancher:
Blow Pop, 0.6 oz | **60** | 0 | 16
Gummies, 10 pcs, 1.38 oz | **120** | 0 | 29
Hard Candy (3), 0.63 oz | **70** | 0 | 17
Screaming Sours 3 pcs, 2 oz | **200** | 0 | 49
Jujubees, all types (52), 40g | **110** | 0 | 28
Juju Bears, | **130** | 0 | 34
Juju Mix *(Sathers)*, 11 pce, 1½ oz | **150** | 0 | 36
Jujyfruits, 16 pcs, 1.4 oz | **120** | 0 | 32

Per Piece/Serving **C F Cb**

Junior Caramels: 13 pcs, 1.48 oz | **190** | 6 | 33
Mini, 2 boxes, 0.85 oz | **110** | 3 | 19
Junior Mints: 1.83 oz | **220** | 4 | 45
16 pcs, 1.4 oz | **170** | 3 | 35
Kissables, 39 pcs, 1.4 oz | **180** | 9 | 28
Kisses, avg. all flavors:
1 piece, 0.16 oz | **25** | 1.5 | 2.5
6 pieces, 1 oz | **145** | 9 | 16
Kit Kat: 4-piece bar, 1.5 oz | **200** | 11 | 27
King Size, 8 pce, 3 oz bar | **400** | 22 | 54
Snack Size, 3 pc, 1.48 oz | **200** | 11 | 27
Extra Krispy Bar (1) | **220** | 12 | 29
White Choc, 4 piece, 1½ oz | **220** | 12 | 26
Kraft: Caramels (5), 1.4 oz | **160** | 3.5 | 31
Kudos: *See Page 139*
Lance: Peanut Bar, 2.3 oz pkg | **340** | 19 | 29
Lemon Drops (4) 0.6 oz | **60** | 0 | 16
Sugar Free *(Walgreens)* (3), 0.6 oz | **50** | 0 | 17
Lemonhead, 20, 1 oz | **100** | 0 | 28
Licorice: Average all types, 1oz | **100** | 0 | 25
Bites *(Switzer)*, each | **10** | 0 | 3
Chews *(Panda)*, each | **10** | 0 | 3
Tid Bits, each | **10** | 0 | 1.5
Twists: Black/Red, avg. 1 pce | **35** | 0 | 8
Sugar Free, 1 pce | **13** | 0 | 2.5
American Licorice Co.: Extinguisher (1) | **160** | 1.5 | 37
Red Vines, 7 pcs, 1.4 oz | **140** | 0 | 33
Sip-n-Chew, 1 pkg, 1 oz | **100** | 1 | 23
Snaps, 4 pcs, 1.4 oz | **140** | 0 | 34
Sour Punch, 6 pcs, 1.4 oz | **150** | 0.5 | 34
Super Ropes (1), 2 oz | **200** | 0 | 46
Superstring, 1⅓ pcs | **140** | 0 | 34
Sugar Free Red Twists (7) | **90** | 0 | 25
Lifesavers: Large size, 1 candy | **15** | 0 | 3
Regular, all flavors, 1 candy | **10** | 0 | 2.5
1 Roll (14 candies), 1.14 oz | **140** | 0 | 35
Creme Savers: 3 pcs, 0.5 oz | **60** | 1 | 11
Sugar Free, 4 pcs | **45** | 1.5 | 13
Gummies (10), 1.48 oz | **130** | 0 | 30
Pep-o-mint (4), 16g | **60** | 0 | 16
Fruit Splosion, 10 pcs, 1.4 oz | **130** | 0 | 30
Sugar-Free Delites: *Per Candy*
Orchard Fruits; Summer Blend | **7** | 0 | 2.5
Butter Toffee; European Collect. | **10** | 1 | 2.5

Brands & Generic (Cont)

Per Piece/Serving	C	F	Cb
Lik-m-aid *(Nestlé)*, Wonka Fun Dip, 1 pkg	50	0	13
Lindt: Lindor, Truffles avg. (1)	75	6	5
Milk Chocolate Bars: Raspb. (5)	200	10	25
Truffles, 7 pieces	240	18	18
Classic Recipe, Hazelnut (10)	230	16	20
70% Cocoa, 4 pcs	220	17	13
Lollipops: Mini, ¼ oz	25	0	6
Small, ½ oz	50	0	12
Medium, 1 oz	100	0	25
Giant (4" diam), 7 oz	790	0	198
M & M's:			
Milk Chocolate, 1 pce	5	0.1	0.5
20 pcs, 0.6 oz	70	3	10
1.7 oz pkg	240	10	34
¼ cup, 1.5 oz	210	9	30
Dark Choc.: 1.7 oz pkg	240	11	33
Fun Size, 18g pkg	90	4	13
Almond Choc., 1.3 oz pkg	200	11	21
Minis, Mega Tube, 1.1 oz tube	150	7	21
Peanut: 1.74 oz pkg	250	13	30
Fun Size, 18g pkg	90	4.5	11
Peanut Butter, 1.6 oz pkg	240	14	26
Premiums: Choc. Raspb. Almond			
¼ cup, 1½ oz	240	16	20
Dark; Triple, avg., 1½ oz	230	14	25
Mamba, 9 pcs, 1½ oz	170	2.5	36
Marshmallow Egg, 1 egg, 1 oz	120	3	22
Mary Jane, 5 pcs, 1.4 oz	160	4	32
Marshmallows: Firm/Soft, 1 oz	90	0	23
Regular size, 4 pcs, 30g	100	0	24
Mini-Marshmallow, ⅔ c., 1 oz	95	0	24
Choc-coat. Twists (Joyva), each	95	2	10
Fluff, 2 Tbsp, 0.63 oz	60	0	15
Kraft: Mini, ½ cup, 1 oz	100	0	24
Creme, 2 Tbsp	45	0	11
Jet-Puffed, 5 pcs, 1 oz	100	0	24
Funmallows, ⅔ cup, 30g	100	0	24
Marzipan, 2 Tbsp, 39g	160	4	29
Mauna Loa (10), 1.3 oz	220	16	21
Mexican Hats (7), 1.34 oz	120	0	30
Mentos: Regular (1)	10	0	3
Sugar Free (1)	5	0	2.5
Mike & Ike:			
Orig.: 1 pkg, 2.1 oz	220	0	55
23 pcs, 40g	140	0	36
Milkfulls *(Storck)*, 6 pcs, 1.4 oz	170	3	35
Milk Chocolate: *See Hershey's*			
Milk Duds, 13 pcs, 1.4 oz	170	6	28

Per Piece/Serving	C	F	Cb
Milky Way: Midnight Bar, 1.76 oz	230	8	36
Regular Bar, 58g	260	10	41
Fun size, 2 bars, 34g	150	6	24
Milky Way To Go, 51g	230	9	36
Miniatures: (5) 43g	190	8	30
Midnight Minis (5), 1.45 oz	190	7	29
Mints: Uncoated, 3 pcs	70	0	17
1 mint (¾" diam.)	7	0	1
1 large mint (1½" diam.)	15	0	3
Mon Cheri *(Ferrero)*, 4 pcs, 1.59 oz	260	18	20
Mounds: 1.7 oz bar	230	13	29
Snack, 0.6 oz	80	4.5	10
King Size, 3½ oz	460	26	58
Minis, 3 pcs, 1.45 oz	190	11	24
Mr Goodbar: 1.7 oz bar	260	17	26
King Size, 2.6 oz bar	380	26	38
Snack, 1.48 oz	220	15	22
Mrs Fields Choc, 2 pieces, 33g	160	8	22
Munch Bar, 1.42 oz	220	15	18
Necco Candy Wafers (40) 57g	220	0	56
Newman's Own:			
Caramel Cups: Milk Choc. (3)	160	8	21
Dark Chocolate (3)	160	9	20
P'Nut B. Cups, Milk Choc.. (3)	160	8	21
Nibs, all types, 1 pouch, 2.25 oz	220	2	50
Nips, all flavors, 2 pcs, 14g	60	2	11
Nougat: 3 pcs, 42 g	170	1	39
Choc. Covered, 1 oz	125	4	22
Nutrageous Bar *(Reese's)*, 1.8 oz	260	16	28
Oh Henry! 2.2 oz bar	300	17	26
Orange Slices: Jewel, 3, 1½ oz	140	0	35
Walgreens, 4 pcs, 1.6 oz	160	0	39
Pastel Mints *(Walgreens)*, 20 pcs	60	0	14
Patteez *(Sweet n' Low)*, 4 pcs	100	2	29
PayDay Bar: 1.85 oz bar	240	13	27
King Size, 3.4 oz bar	440	24	50
Snack Size, 0.7 oz	90	5	10
Avalanche, 1.8 oz bar	250	13	29
Peanut Bar, 1.6 oz bar	235	15	21
Peanut Butter Cups: *See Reese's; Newman's Own*			
Peanut Brittle: 1 piece, 1½ oz	190	5	32
Sugar Free *(Russell Stover)*			
4 pcs, 1.3 oz	140	10	24
Peanuts, choc-covered, 14 pcs	230	14	23
Pearson's Mint Patties, (5), 38g	150	2.5	31
Pecan Roll, ⅓ bar, 40g	190	10	24
Peppermints, 7 small, 0.5 oz	60	0	15
Brach's, 3 pcs	60	0	16

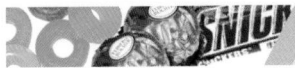

Candy ~ Chocolate (C)

Brands & Generic (Cont)

Per Piece/Serving

	C	F	Cb
Pez, 1 roll	35	0	9
Planters: Choc. Peanuts (25) 7 oz	220	15	20
Orig. Peanut Bar, 1.6 oz	230	14	22
Hersheys, 2½ oz	390	24	34
Pops ~ See Lollipops			
Pop Rocks, 0.34 oz pkg	35	0	9
Pretzels: Choc-covered, Mini (6), 38g	200	9	25
White Choc Bites (23), 40g	200	9	25
Pretzel Flipz (Nestlé), 8 pcs, 1 oz	130	5	20
Raisinets: Milk Choc: 1 pkg, 1.6 oz	190	8	30
King Size, 2.8 oz	330	13	56
Movie Pack, 3.5 oz	380	16	64
Dark Choc., ¼ c., 1.6 oz	180	8	32
Reese's			
Peanut Butter Cups: 2 cups, 1.5 oz	220	13	24
King Size (1), 2.8 oz	420	24	44
Mini, 5 pcs, 1.55 oz	220	13	25
8-Pack, 1 pce, ½ oz	80	4.5	9
Snack Size, 1 pce, 0.74 oz	110	6.5	12
Sugar Free: 5 pcs, avg., 1.38 oz	180	13	27
Caramel Filled (2),1.4 oz	150	11	27
Big Cup: Regular, 1.4 oz	200	12	22
King Size (2), 2.8 oz	400	22	24
White Chocolate (2), 1.5 oz	220	13	22
Reese's Pieces: 50 pcs, 1.3 oz	200	9	24
King Size, 51 pcs, 1.4 oz	190	9	24
Reese's Sticks: 1.5 oz	210	13	23
King Size (1), 3 oz	440	26	46
Snack Size (1), 0.6 oz	90	5	9
Reese's Whipps: (40% less fat),1.5 oz	230	9	36
Minis, 3 pcs, 1.48 oz	190	7	29
Clusters, 3 pcs, 1½ oz	220	13	24
Crispy Crunchy Bar: 1.7 oz	260	15	24
2 pcs, 1.2 oz	190	11	18
King Size, 3.1 oz bar	460	26	52
Fast Break, 2 oz bar	260	12	35
Snacksters, 1 pkg, ¾ oz	100	4	14
Peanut Butter Chips, 1 Tbsp, 15g	80	4	8
Chocolate Layered Cookies (4), 2 oz	280	14	36
Rice Krispies Treats (Kellogg's):			
1 bar, average all varieties	90	2.5	17
Rice Crunchy Bars, 1.4 oz bar	200	11	23
Riesen Choc. Chew, 4 pcs, 1.26 oz	170	6	28
Rocky Road, 2 oz bar	240	11	34
Roca Thins, all flavors, 4 pcs	210	16	22
Rolo: All types, per roll, 1.7 oz	220	10	33
Bites, 7 pieces, 1.4 oz	200	9	29
Root Beer Barrels (3) 0.63 oz	60	0	17

Per Piece/Serving

C F Cb

Russell Stover Candy:

Boxed Chocolates: Chocolate Coated

	C	F	Cb
Assorted (2), 1.13 oz	150	6	23
Cherry Cordials (3), 1.34 oz	150	5	25
Dairy Cream Caramels (2), 1.16 oz	150	7	22
Elegant Assortment, 3, 1.59 oz	210	10	28
French Choc. Mints, 4, 1.34 oz	220	13	22
Nut, Chewy & Crisp Centers, 2	160	8	21
Pecan Delights, 2, 1.83 oz	270	16	32
Sugar Free: Assort. Candies, 3, 1.55 oz	180	13	26
Pecan Delights, 2, 1.66 oz	210	17	27
Bags: Assorted Fruit, 3, 0.6 oz	40	0	17
Butter Cream Caramels, 3, 1.52 oz	150	10	25
Chocolate Peanuts, 25, 1.4 oz	190	14	20
Chocolate Truffles, 3, 1.52 oz	180	13	23
Peanut Butter Cups, 2, 1.2 oz	160	12	17
Salt Water Taffy (Brach's), 5	170	2.5	36
Seashells (Guylian), 1 shell, 1.4 oz	210	13	21
See's Candies:			
Almond Royal, 5 pieces, 1.3 oz	190	13	18
Butterscotch Chews (5), 1.5 oz	210	12	27
Krispy's: Caffe Latte, 5 pcs 1.3 oz	180	8	27
Mint, 5 pieces, 1.3 oz	170	8	27
Little Pops:			
Butterscotch (4), 0.5 oz	70	2	13
Cafe Latte (4), 0.5 oz	70	2	12
Chocolate (4), 0.5 oz	70	3	11
Vanilla (4), 0.5 oz	50	2	9
Lollypops, average, 20g	90	3	17
Milk Molasses Chips, 6 pieces, 1.4 oz	180	8	27
Milk Peppermints, 2 pieces, 1.23 oz	150	4	28
Peanut Butter Bar, 1 oz	150	10	15
Peppermint Twists (3), 0.53 oz	60	0	15
Raisins, Dark/Light (28), 1.4 oz	170	7	29
Toffee-ettes, 3 pieces, 1.6 oz	270	21	18
Sugar Free: Dark Bar, 1.5 oz	180	16	24
Dark Walnut Clusters, 1.5 oz	220	20	18
Peanut Brittle, 1.5 oz	170	14	17
Skittles: Sour, 2 oz bag	230	2.5	51
Tropical/Wild Berry, 2.17 oz	250	2.5	56
Fun Size, 1 bag, 0.5 oz	60	1	14
Tear & Share, 4 oz bag	420	4.5	93
Smarties:			
Candy Rolls (1), 7g	25	0	6
Giant, 2 pcs, 7g	25	0	6

Brands & Generic (Cont)

Per Piece/Serving	C	F	Cb
Snack Barz (Hershey's), 25g	120	5	16
Snickers: 2.07 oz bar	280	14	35
King Size, 3.29 oz	440	22	56
Fun Size, 2 bars, 34g	160	8	21
Adventure Bar, 1.87 oz	250	12	32
Amond Bar, 1.76 oz	230	11	32
Creme Egg (1), 1.2 oz	170	10	20
Cruncher, 1.56 oz	220	11	28
Cruncher To Go, 2.54	350	18	45
Fudge, 1.78 oz	250	13	31
Marathon Bar, avg., 1.9 oz bar	210	8	26
Miniatures, 4 pieces, 1.27 oz	170	8	22
Munch Bar, 1.4 oz bar	220	15	18
Sno Caps, ¼ cup, 40g	180	8	30
Soft 'N Chewy Butter Toffee, ea.	30	0.5	5
Sorbee: Choc., ½ bar, 1.4 oz	180	12	25
Crystal Light Hard Candy, 4 pcs	25	0	13
(Note: Carb figures include Isomalt which has fewer calories than sugar.)			
Sour Patch: All types, 1.5 oz	140	0	32
1 straw	20	0	5
Spearmint Leaves: Jewel, 5, 40g	140	0	35
Walgreens, 4 pieces, 46g	160	0	39
Spree Candies: Original, 15 pcs	50	0	13
Chewy Spree, 8 pcs	60	0	13
Starburst: Candy Canes, 0.5 oz	70	0	18
Fruit Chews, each	20	0.4	4
2 oz pkg	240	5	48
Jellybeans, 1.5 oz	150	0	37
Jellybean Egg, 2 oz	200	0	51
Tropical Fruit, 2.07 oz pack	240	5	49
Starlight Mints, 3 pcs, 0.56 oz	60	0	15
Suckers (Walgreens) (1), 0.39 oz	45	0	11
Sugar Babies, 30 pcs, 1.55 oz	180	1.5	41
Sugar Coated Peanuts, 1 oz	120	8	10
Sunbursts Sunflowers (Kimmie):			
Candy Bar Bag, 1.7 oz	190	9	27
Coffee Break Tube, 1.41 oz	200	11	22
Swedish Fish (7), 1.48 oz	150	0	38
Sweet 'N Low: Chews, each	20	0.5	5
Coffee Cremes (1)	40	3	6
Wafer Bars, avg., 3 pcs	140	7	23
Mint Cremes, 3½ pcs	120	9	22
Mint Patteez, 4 pcs	100	2	29
Sweet Escapes: See Hershey's			
Symphony: 1.5 oz bar	220	14	23
Large, 5 pcs	200	13	21
Snack: Chocolate (1), 0.6 oz	90	5	10
w. Almds & Toffee (1), .5 oz	230	14	23

Per Piece/Serving	C	F	Cb
Taffy, 1 pce, 1 oz	60	0	17
Take 5 (Hershey's): 1.5 oz	200	11	25
King Size, 2.25 oz	300	16	37
Snack Size, 2 pces	210	11	26
Marshmallow, 1.3 oz	180	9	22
3 Musketeers: Original, 2.13 oz	260	8	46
Fun Size, 3 pieces, 1.66 oz	190	6	34
Minis, 7 pce, 1.4 oz	180	6	30
Mint Bar, 2 pieces, 1.24 oz	150	5	26
Pop'ables (15)	180	6	31
Tang-a-Roos, 1 roll	25	0	6
Terry's Choc Orange, (5), 1.5 oz	230	12	27
Tic Tac, all varieties, each	2	0	0
Toblerone: 1.8 oz bar	260	13	32
1 bar: 3.5 oz	510	30	63
1.23 oz bar	180	9	23
Toffees, Regular, 1 oz	160	9	18
Toll House Milk Choc. Morsels, 1Tbsp	70	4	9
Tootsie Pops (1), 0.6 oz	60	0	15
Tootsie Roll: 2.25 oz roll	245	2	50
Midgees, 6 pieces, 1.4 oz	140	3	28
Truffles: Regular, 12g	60	4	6
Large (Godiva), 0.75 oz	110	6.5	12
Extra Large (J.Schmidt), 1½ oz	220	13	24
Turtles (Nestlé): Avg., each	80	4.5	10
Sugar Free, 3 pieces, 38g	150	11	20
Twists (Sugar Free): Licorice; Strawberry,			
7 twists, 40g	90	0	25
Twix: 2 cookies, 2 oz	280	14	37
Fun Size, 0.5 oz	80	4	10
Twix 4 To Go	480	24	64
Minis, 3 pcs, 1 oz	150	8	20
Caramel, 0.85 oz	130	6	16
Peanut Butter 4 To Go	480	28	48
Peanut Butter, 1.8 oz	280	17	28
Twizzlers: Bites (17), 1.4 oz	140	0.5	32
Cherry Nibs, 2.3 oz pkg	220	2	50
Pull 'n' Peel Cherry, 1.16 oz	100	0	25
Sourz Assorted, 1.8 oz	180	1.5	40
Twists Strawberry, 1.6 oz	150	1	35
U-No Bar 1.5 oz	250	17	22
Weight Watchers (Whitman's):			
Butter Cream Caramel (3)	150	8	23
Caramel Medallions (3)	160	9	24
English Toffee Squares (3)	150	9	21
Mint Patties (3)	150	9	23
Peanut Butter Cups (4)	180	8	31
Pecan Crowns (3)	160	10	24

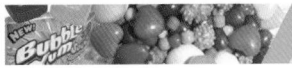

Brands & Generic (Cont)

Per Piece/Serving	C	F	Cb
Werther's: Original, 3 pce, 0.56 oz	70	1.5	14
Chewy Caramel (6), 1.31 oz	170	5	30
Caramelts (8), 1.4 oz	250	18	18
Sugar-Free, 5 pieces	40	1	14
Whatchamacallit Bar, 1.6 oz	230	12	28
King Size, 2.6 oz	370	20	45
Whitman's: Sampler (4), 1.75 oz	240	11	33
12 oz Box, 4 pieces, 1.59 oz	220	12	27
Sugar Free, 10 oz Box, 3 pcs, 1.42 oz	180	12	25
Reserve, 7 oz Box, 2 pcs, 1.16 oz	160	9	21
Whoppers, 18 pcs, 1.4 oz	190	8	28
Wonka: Wonka Bar (1), 2.6 oz	360	19	49
Laffy Taffy: Orig., 5 bars, 1.5 oz	160	2	36
Stretchy & Tangy, 1½ oz	165	4	33
Nerds, 0.5 oz	60	0	14
Gobstopper, 9 pcs, 0.5 oz	60	0	14
Runts Fruit Box, 1.8 oz	210	0	49
Yogurt Candy,			
Coated Raisins, 27 pcs, 40g	180	8	28
York Peppermint Pattie:			
Regular, 1.4 oz	140	2.5	31
Fun Size, 0.6 oz	60	1	14
King Size, 1.45 oz	150	3	33
York Mints, 3	10	0	3
Zachary Choc. Peanuts, 1.48 oz	240	15	21
Zagnut, 1.52 oz bar	200	8	31
Zero Bar: 1.8 oz bar	230	8	37
King Size, 3.4 oz	400	14	68
Zingos, 3 pce, 2g	5	0	2

Gum ~ Per Piece

	C	F	Cb
Bazooka, each	15	0	4
Beechies	6	0	2
Big League Chew	10	0	2
Double Bubble Ball	20	0	5
Bubble Yum	25	0	6
Sugarless	10	0	3
Candilicious	30	0	2
Carefree (Sugarless/Regular)	5	0	2
Chiclets, 1 piece	5	0	1
Clorets, 1 stick	10	0	2
Dentyne	5	0	0.5
Estee, bubble/regular	5	0	2
Extra (Wrigley's),			
Sugar-Free	5	0	2
Freshen-Up	10	0	3
Hubba Bubba: Regular	20	0	5
Sugar-free, average	14	0	0.5
Ice Breakers	5	0	2
Jolt Gum, 2 pcs	10	0	3
Super Bubble	15	0	4
Trident, Original; White	5	0	1
Wrigley's, all flavors	10	0	2

Carob Candy

Per Piece/Serving	C	F	Cb
Carob: Plain/Natural, 1 oz	155	9	15
Carob Coated: Raisins, 1 oz	130	8	15
Almonds/Peanuts, 1 oz	150	10	14
Malt Balls, 1 oz	135	8	15
Caramels, 1 oz	110	4	18
Dates, 1 oz	125	5	20
Soybeans	145	9	16
Trail/Party Mix, 1 oz	150	9	15
Carob Chips, unsweetened, 1 oz	155	9	15

Cough Drops

	C	F	Cb
Beech Nut, 1 drop	10	0	2
CVS, Sour Lemon Throat Drops			
Diabetic Tussin, 1 drop	0	0	0
Halls Defense Vit. C, 1 drop	15	0	4
Sugar Free, 1 drop	5	0	3
Halls Fruit Breezers, 1 drop	15	0	4
Halls Menthol Drops, 1 drop	15	0	4
Sugar Free, 1 drop	5	0	4
Halls Plus, 1 drop	20	0	5
Listerine Lozenge (Amer. Chicle)	10	0	2
Luden's Throat Drops, all flavors, 1	10	0	2
Sugar Free, 1 drop	0	0	0
Pine Bros, 1 cough drop	10	0	2
Ricola: Cough Drops (1)	10	0	3
Sugar-Free Lemon Mint (2)	0	0	1
Rite Aid, Menthol Cough (1)	10	0	3
Robitussin: Regular, 1 drop	15	0	3
Honey Cough, 1 drop	40	0	10
Sugar Free Throat, 1 drop	10	0	3
Sunny Orange Vit. C, 1 drop	10	0	3
Rolaids Sodium Free, 1	5	0	1
Sathers Peppermint Lozenges, 1	15	0	3
Squibb Cough/Throat Loz.'s, 1	15	0	4
Sucrets (Beecham) Lozenges, 1	10	0	2
Wintergreen Loz. (Walgreens), 1	15	0	3

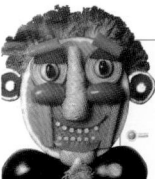

Eat at least 5 servings of fruit and vegetables every day . . . and Enjoy Better Health!

Quick Guide C F Cb

Firm/Hard Cheeses
(American, Cheddar, Colby, Swiss)
Regular Cheese:

	C	F	Cb
Thin Deli slice, ¾ oz	90	7	0
1 oz slice/piece	115	9	0.5
8 oz package	915	75	3
16 oz (1lb) package	1830	150	6
Cubes: 1" cube, ¾ oz	85	7	0.5
1¼" cube, 1 oz slice	115	9	0.5
Diced: 1 cup, 4½ oz	530	40	2
Grated: 1 Tbsp, ¼ oz	30	2.5	0
Shredded: Cheddar, ¼ cup, 1 oz	115	9	0.5
1 cup, 4 oz	455	37	1.5
Cheddar, Red.-Fat, ¼ cup, 1 oz	80	6	1
Mozzarella: ¼ cup, 1 oz	85	6.5	0.5
Part-Skim, ¼ cup, 1 oz	70	5	1
Sliced: 1 thin (3½" sq.), ¾ oz	85	7	0.5
Rectangular (7"x 4"x ⅛ "), 1½ oz	170	14	0.5
Round (3¼" diam. x ⅛ "), ¾ oz	85	7	0.5
Semi-circular, 1¼ oz			
(5½" long, 3½" radius, ⅛" thick)	140	12	0.5
Fat-Free: Average all brands, 1 oz	40	0	2
Low-Fat: Average all brands, 1 oz	50	2	0.5
Reduced Fat: Avg. all brands, 1 oz	80	5	0.5

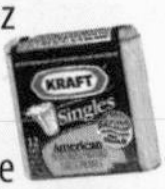

Cheese C F Cb

Per 1 oz Unless Indicated
American:

	C	F	Cb
Regular: 1 slice, 1 oz	105	9	0.5
Alpine Lace, 1 oz	90	7	2
Kraft, 0.7 oz slice	70	5	2
Shedded, ¼ cup, 1 oz	115	9	0.5
Land O'Lakes, 0.7 oz slice	70	5	2
Light: *Kraft* (2% Milk), 0.7 oz slice	50	3	1
Fat-Free: *Kraft,* 0.7 oz slice	30	0	2
Borden, Singles, 0.8 oz slice	80	0	2
Babybel *(Laughing Cow),* 21g	70	6	0
Light Original, 21g pce	50	3	0
Blue/Bleu, 1 oz	100	8	0.5
Bonbel *(Laughing Cow),* 1 pce	70	6	0
Brick *(Land O'Lakes),* 1" cube, 1 oz	110	8	1
Brie, 1 oz	95	8	0
Camembert, 1 oz	85	7	0
Caraway, 1 oz	105	8	1
Castello *(Wegman's),* avg., 1 oz	120	12	0

Cheddar: (Also see 'Quick Guide') C F Cb

	C	F	Cb
Regular: 1 oz	115	9	0.5
Alpine Lace, 1 oz	90	7	0
Reduced-Fat/Low-Fat:			
Borden, Shredded, ¼ cup, 1 oz	80	6	1
Cabot Vermont, 50% Light, 1 oz	70	4.5	0.5
Lifetime, 1oz	45	1.5	3
Fat-Free, *Kraft,* 0.7 oz slice	30	0	2
Cheese Balls *(Kaukauna),* 1 oz, avg.	100	7	0.5
Cheese Curds: Fresh, ¼ cup, 1 oz	110	9	0
Breaded & Fried ~ *See Page 80*			
Cheese Logs *(Kaukauna),* avg., 1 oz	100	7	0.5
Cheshire, 1 oz	110	9	1.5
Colby: Regular, 1 oz	110	9	0.5
Reduced-Fat *(Kraft),* 1 oz	80	6	0
Colby-Jack, regular, 1 oz	110	9	1

Cottage Cheese: *Average All Brands*

	C	F	Cb
Creamed (4% milk fat): 2 Tbsp, 1 oz	30	1	1.5
½ cup, 4 oz	120	5	6
w. fruit, ½ cup, 4 oz	130	4	15
Reduced-Fat (2%): 2 T., 1 oz	25	0.5	1
½ cup, 4 oz	100	2	4
Low-Fat (1%): 2 Tbsp, 1 oz	20	.5	1
½ cup, 4 oz	80	1	3
Fat-Free/Non-Fat: 2 Tbsp, 1 oz	20	0	1
(Jewel), ½ cup, 4 oz	80	0	5
Friendship: Low-Fat P'apple, 4 oz	120	1	16
Non-Fat w. Peach, ½ cup, 4 oz	110	0	15
Pot Style, ½ cup, 4 oz	90	2.5	3
Hood w. Chive/Onion, 4 oz	90	1	5
Knudsen:			
Free: Non-Fat, ½ c., 4.oz	80	0	7
2% Milk Fat, ½ c., 4 oz	100	2.5	6
Cottage Doubles, avg, 5.5 oz ctn	150	2.5	18
On the Go! Free, 4 oz ctn	70	0	7
Low-Fat, 4 oz ctn	90	2.5	6
Lactaid: Low-Fat, ½ cup, 4 oz	80	1	7
Light N' Lively: Fat-Free, 4.4 oz	80	0	8
Low-Fat, ½ cup, 4.4 oz	80	1.5	6
Live Active (Low-Fat 2%):			
Plain, 1/2 cup, 4 oz	90	2	10
Mixed Berry; Pineapple, avg., 4 oz	120	1.5	18

Cream Cheese: *See Page 81*

	C	F	Cb
Edam, Regular, 1 oz	100	8	0.5
Farmer *(Friendship),* 2 Tbs	50	2.5	0
Feta: Regular, 1 oz	75	6	1
Crumbled, ½ cup, 2½ oz	190	15	3
Red.-Fat *(Athenos),* 1 oz	60	4	1
Fontina, 1 oz	110	9	0.5
Gjetost (Goat's Milk, fresh), 1 oz	130	8	12

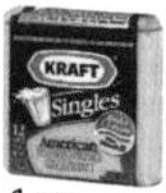

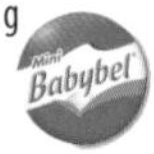

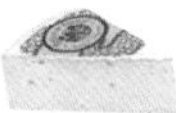

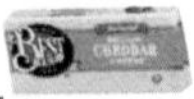

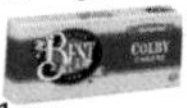

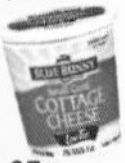

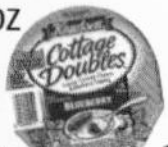

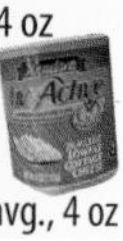

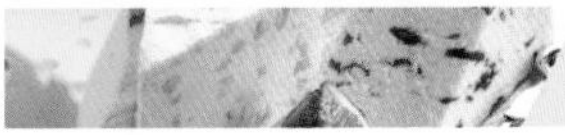

Goat's Milk Cheese:	C	F	Cb
Chevre, Soft, 1 oz	80	6	1
Chavril: 3 Tbsp, 1 oz	60	4.5	0.5
Semi-Soft, 1 oz	100	8.5	1
Hard, 1 oz	130	10	0.5
Gorgonzola, 1 oz	100	8	0.5
Galbani Dolcelatte, 1 oz	95	8	1
Gouda, 1 oz	100	8	0.5
Gruyere, 1 oz	115	9	1
Havarti *(Land O'Lakes)*, 1 oz	110	8	1
Italian Blend *(Sargento)*, 1 oz	90	7	1
Jarlsberg *(Wegman's)*, 1 oz	100	8	0
Jarlsberg Red. Fat, shredded, 1 oz	70	4	0
Kefir *(Alta Dena)*, 2 Tbsp, 1 oz	70	6	2
Labneh (Lebanese cream chse), 1.8 oz	70	4	4
Lactose Free Cheese *(Lifetime)*, 1 oz	40	0	1
Limburger, 1 oz	95	8	0
Mascarpone *(Wegman's)*, 1 oz	130	13	1
Mexican:			
Cacique: Cotija, 1 oz	110	9	0
Queso Fresco, 1 oz	80	6	0
Queso Quesadilla, 1 oz	70	5	2
Ranchero, 1 oz	80	6	0
Chi-Chi's: Con Quéso, 2 Tbsp	90	7	4
Hot/Medium/Mild/Acante, 2 T.	10	0	2
Kraft, Taco, shredded, ¼ cup, 1 oz	100	8	2
Sargento, Shredded, ¼ cup, 1 oz	110	9	0.5
Supremo Chihuahua: Quéso Bianco	100	8	0
Quéso Fresco; Rancherito	80	6	0
Monterey, 1 oz	105	8.5	0
Monterey Jack: Regular, 1 oz	110	9	0
Kraft 2% Milk Red. Fat, 1 oz	80	6	1
Alpine Lace, Co-Jack, 1 oz	90	7	0
Weight Watchers, 1 oz	90	6	1
Mozzarella:			
Regular: 1 oz	85	6.5	0.5
Land O'Lakes/Polly-O, 1 oz, avg.	90	6	1
Shredded, ¼ cup, 1 oz	90	7	1
Light: *Polly-O Lite,* Shred., 1 oz	60	2.5	1
Kraft 2% Milk Fat, Red. Fat, 1 oz	70	4	1
Sargento Reduced Fat, ¼ c., 1 oz	80	4.5	1
Part Skim: *Alpine Lace,* 1 oz	70	5	1
Borden/Kraft, Shred., ¼ c., 1 oz	80	5	1
Polly-O, String (2% milk), 1 stick	70	4.5	0.5
Fat-Free: *Polly-O,* 1 oz	35	0	1
Kraft, shredded, ¼ cup, 1 oz	45	0	2
Muenster: Regular, 1 oz	105	9	0.5
Low-Fat, 1 oz	85	5	1
Myzithra, grated, 4 T. 1 oz	80	4	2
Neufchatel: 1 oz	75	6	1
Philadelphia, 1 oz	70	6	1
Flavored: Fruit/Herbs	80	7	1
Chocolate *(Hickory Farms)*, 1 oz	110	8	1

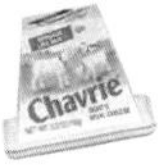

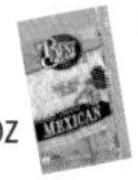

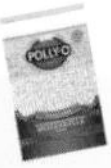

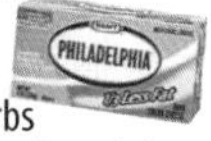

	C	F	Cb
Parmesan: Fresh/Block, 1 oz	110	7.5	1
Grated (Packaged): 1 Tbsp	20	1.5	0
1 oz quantity	120	8	1
½ cup, 1¾ oz	215	14	2
w. Romano *(Frigo)*, grated, 1 oz	110	7	0
Kraft Reduced-Fat Topping, 1 T.	20	1	2
Pizza Cheese, shredded:			
Regular *(Kraft)* ¼ cup, 1 oz	90	7	1
Port de Salut, 1 oz	100	8	0
Port Wine *(Kaukauna)*, 1 oz	90	6	4
Pot *(Sargento)*, 1 oz	25	0	1
Provolone: Regular, 1 oz	100	7.5	0.5
Reduced-Fat: *Alpine Lace,* 1 oz	80	5	1
Sargento, 1 slice, ⅔ oz	50	3.5	0
Pub *(Rondele)*, 1 oz, avg.	95	7	1
Quark: 40% fat, 1 oz	47	3	1
20% fat, 1 oz	32	1.5	1
Skim/Non-Fat, 1 oz	22	0	1.5
Queso: Anejo/Asadero/Blanco, 1 oz	105	9	1
Chichuahua/De Papa, 1 oz	110	9	2
Ricotta Cheese:			
Whole Milk, 2 Tbsp, 1 oz	50	3.5	1
½ cup, 4½ oz	215	16	4
Part Skim, 2 Tbsp, 1 oz	40	2	1.5
½ cup, 4½ oz	170	10	6
Light/Low-Fat, 2 Tbsp, 1 oz	25	1	1.5
½ cup, 4½ oz	125	5	6
Fat-Free, ½ cup, 4½ oz	100	0	10
Baked Ricotta, 2 oz portion	130	9	3
Romano: Block/Loaf, 1 oz	110	8	1
Grated (Pkg): 1 oz	120	9	1
1 Tbsp, 5g	20	1.5	0
Roquefort, 1 oz	105	9	0.5
Sheep's Milk, 1 oz	45	3	1
Smoked: *Wegman's,* 1 oz	100	8	0
Tillamook, Smoked Cheddar, 1 oz	110	9	0
Stilton *(Wegman's)*, 1 oz	110	10	0
String *(Frigo/Kraft/Sargento)*, 1 oz	80	6	0.5
Light String-Ums *(Kraft)*, 1 oz	80	4.5	1
String Lite *(Frigo)*, 1 oz	60	2.5	0.5
Light *(Sargento)*, 1 stick, 0.7 oz	50	2.5	0.5
Swiss: Regular, 1 oz	110	8	1.5
Reduced-Fat: *Alpine Lace,* 1.2 oz	110	7	1
Kraft, 2% Milk, 0.7 oz slice	50	2.5	2
Taco Cheese *(Kraft)* shredded, ¼ cup	120	10	1
Tilsit, 1 oz	100	7.5	0.5
Tybo, 1 oz	100	7	0.5
Vermont *(Cabot)*, 1 oz	110	9	0
Wensleydale, 1 oz	100	8	0.5
Whey Cheese, 1 oz	125	8	9

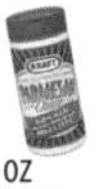

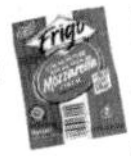

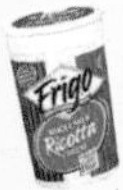

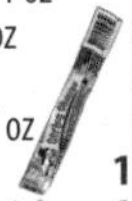

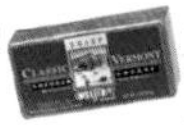

C Cheese

Cheese Products

	C	F	Cb
Cheese Food:			
Average all flavors: ¾ oz slice	70	5	2
1 oz slice	95	7	2.5
Alouette: *Per 2 Tbsp., 0.8 oz*			
Berries & Cream	80	6	4
Light Garlic & Herbs	50	4	2
Peppercorn Parmesan	80	8	1
Sundr. Tomato & Basil	80	7	1
Cabot, Jalapeno, 50% Red-Fat, 1 oz	70	4.5	0
Cracker Barrel, Extra Sharp Ched., 1 oz	120	10	0
Handi-Snacks: *(Kraft)*			
Breadsticks 'n Cheez, 1.1 oz	110	4.5	13
Ritz Crackers 'n Cheez, 1 oz pkg	100	6	10
Polly-O Stringcheese Stick, each	80	6	0.5
Kraft: American Shred., 1Tbsp	25	2	0.5
Singles: 1 slice, ¾ oz	60	4.5	1
Fat-Free, 1 sl., 0.7 oz	25	0	2
Snack Pack, 1½ oz	160	13	1
Cubes: Regular, avg, 7 cubes, 1 oz	120	10	1
2% Milk, 7 cubes, 1 oz	90	6	1
Kraft Natural:			
Cheese Sticks: Cheddar (1), 1 oz	120	10	0
Mozzarella, 1 stick, 1 oz	80	5	0
Colby Jack, Red. Fat (1), 1 oz	90	6	0.5
Lifetime Cholesterol Reducing,			
Slices, 1 Slice, 19g	30	1	1
Block, 1"cube, 1 oz	45	1.5	1
Lifeway Farmers Kefir, 2 Tbsp, 1 oz	25	1.5	4
Precious Cheddar Chse Sticksters, 1 oz	110	9	1
Rondele: Spreadable., 2 T., 1 oz	70	7	1
Light, 2 Tbsp, 1 oz	50	4	2
Sargento Chef Style,			
Cheddar, shred., ¼ c., 1 oz	110	9	1
Mozzarella, shrd., ¼ cup	80	6	1
Smart Balance:			
Creamy cheddar-flavor, 1 slice, ⅔ oz	40	2	2
Cheese Product Shreds, 1 oz	80	5	0
Cream Cheese Spreads ~ *See Next Page*			
Smart Beat, Fat-Free, 0.6 oz slice	40	2	2
Velveeta: Regular, ⅜" slice, 1 oz	60	4.5	2
Extra Thick, 1.2 oz	100	7	3
Shredded, ¼ c., 1.3 oz	130	9	3
WisPride: Port Wine,			
Ball/Cup, 2 T., 1.1 oz	90	7	4
Light, 2 T., 1.1 oz	70	3.5	5

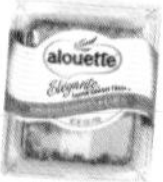

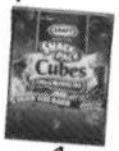

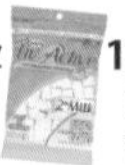

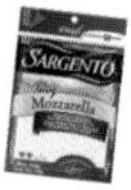

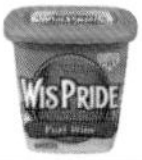

Cheese Whiz (Sauce/Dip)

	C	F	Cb
Original, 2 Tbsp, 1.1 oz	90	7	4
Light, 2 Tbsp, 1.1 oz	80	3.5	6
Salsa Con Queso, 2 T., 1.1 oz	90	7	4

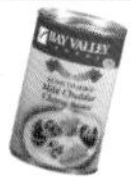

Cheese Curds

	C	F	Cb
Fresh: ¼ cup, 1 oz	110	9	0
1 cup, 4 oz	440	36	0
Breaded & Fried:			
A&W, 5 oz	570	40	27
Culver's, 6.7 oz	670	38	54

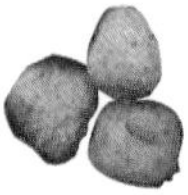

Cheese Substitutes

	C	F	Cb
Galaxy:			
Grated Parmesan, 2 tsp, 0.18 oz	15	0.5	0
Oat/Rice Slices, 1 slice, 0.7 oz	40	2	1
Veggie Yellow American, 1 sl., ½ oz	40	2.5	0.5
Veggie Mozz. Singles, 1 sl., ½ oz	40	2.5	0.5
Lifetime Rice Cheese, 1" cube, 1 oz	95	7	2
Mori Nu Tofu: Mozzarella, 1 oz	70	4	2
Fat-Free Mozz./Ched./Jack, 1 oz	40	0	2
Soya Kaas: Cheddar, 1 oz	60	4	0
Fat-Free, all varieties, 1 oz	40	0	2
Soy-Sation Shredded Cheese, 1 oz	70	4	2
Tofu Rella, avg. all varieties, 1 oz	60	4	0
Tofutti Better Than Cream Chse, 1 oz	85	5	9
Trader Joe's: *Per Slice*			
Soy Cheese:			
Cheddar Flavor, 0.7 oz	45	2	3
Mozzarella Flavor, 1 oz	70	4	3
Sliced Yogurt Cheese, 1 oz	100	8	0

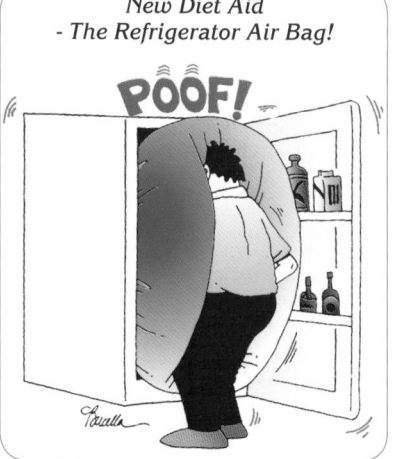

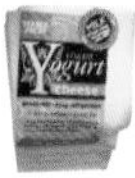

*New Diet Aid
- The Refrigerator Air Bag!*

POOF!

Cream Cheese C F Cb

Regular/Soft, average all brands:

	C	F	Cb
2 Tbsp, 1 oz	90	9	2
8 oz pkg	720	72	13
w. Chives/Herbs/Pimento, 1 oz	75	2.5	10
w. Fruit/Strawb./P'apple, 1 oz	90	8	4

Philadelphia *(Kraft): Per 2 Tbsp*

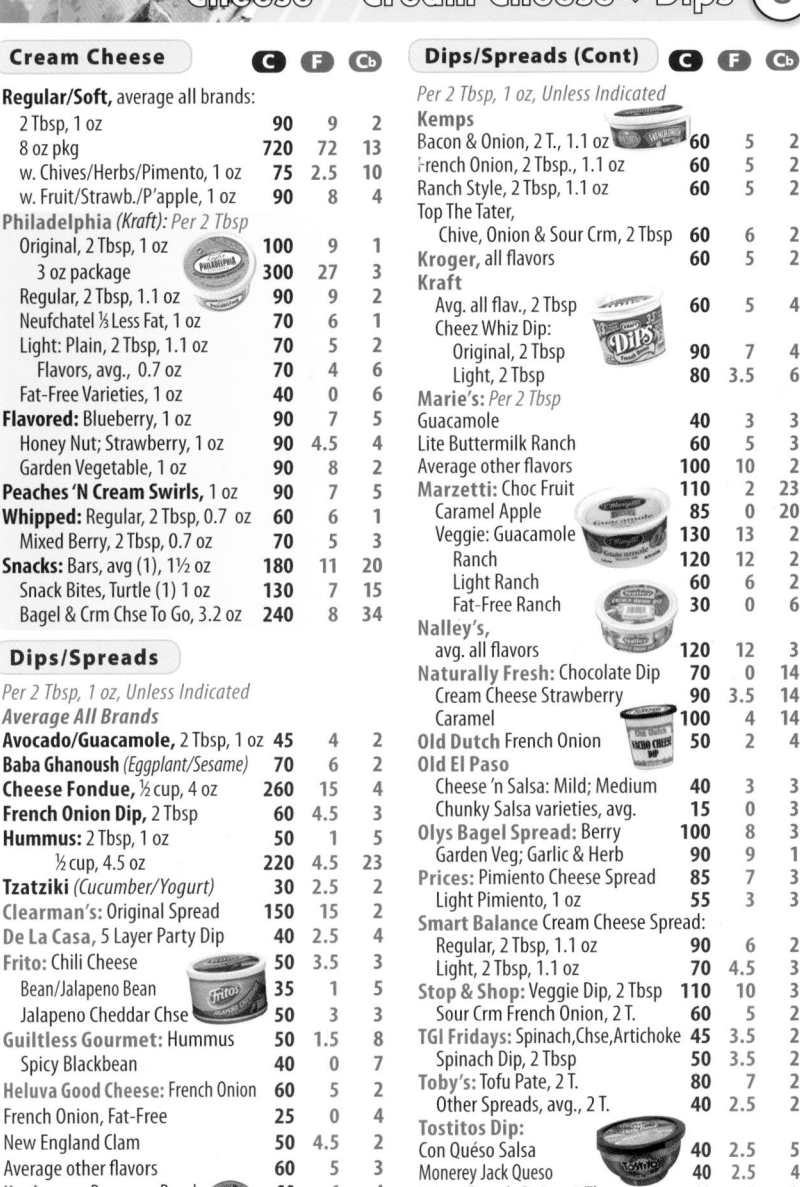

	C	F	Cb
Original, 2 Tbsp, 1 oz	100	9	1
3 oz package	300	27	3
Regular, 2 Tbsp, 1.1 oz	90	9	2
Neufchatel ⅓ Less Fat, 1 oz	70	6	1
Light: Plain, 2 Tbsp, 1.1 oz	70	5	2
Flavors, avg., 0.7 oz	70	4	6
Fat-Free Varieties, 1 oz	40	0	6
Flavored: Blueberry, 1 oz	90	7	5
Honey Nut; Strawberry, 1 oz	90	4.5	4
Garden Vegetable, 1 oz	90	8	2
Peaches 'N Cream Swirls, 1 oz	90	7	5
Whipped: Regular, 2 Tbsp, 0.7 oz	60	6	1
Mixed Berry, 2 Tbsp, 0.7 oz	70	5	3
Snacks: Bars, avg (1), 1½ oz	180	11	20
Snack Bites, Turtle (1) 1 oz	130	7	15
Bagel & Crm Chse To Go, 3.2 oz	240	8	34

Dips/Spreads

Per 2 Tbsp, 1 oz, Unless Indicated
Average All Brands

	C	F	Cb
Avocado/Guacamole, 2 Tbsp, 1 oz	45	4	2
Baba Ghanoush *(Eggplant/Sesame)*	70	6	2
Cheese Fondue, ½ cup, 4 oz	260	15	4
French Onion Dip, 2 Tbsp	60	4.5	3
Hummus: 2 Tbsp, 1 oz	50	1	5
½ cup, 4.5 oz	220	4.5	23
Tzatziki *(Cucumber/Yogurt)*	30	2.5	2
Clearman's: Original Spread	150	15	2
De La Casa, 5 Layer Party Dip	40	2.5	4
Frito: Chili Cheese	50	3.5	3
Bean/Jalapeno Bean	35	1	5
Jalapeno Cheddar Chse	50	3	3
Guiltless Gourmet: Hummus	50	1.5	8
Spicy Blackbean	40	0	7
Heluva Good Cheese: French Onion	60	5	2
French Onion, Fat-Free	25	0	4
New England Clam	50	4.5	2
Average other flavors	60	5	3
Kaukauna: Parmesan Ranch	90	6	4
Smokey Cheddar	90	7	3

Dips/Spreads (Cont) C F Cb

Per 2 Tbsp, 1 oz, Unless Indicated

	C	F	Cb
Kemps			
Bacon & Onion, 2 T., 1.1 oz	60	5	2
French Onion, 2 Tbsp., 1.1 oz	60	5	2
Ranch Style, 2 Tbsp, 1.1 oz	60	5	2
Top The Tater,			
Chive, Onion & Sour Crm, 2 Tbsp	60	6	2
Kroger, all flavors	60	5	2
Kraft			
Avg. all flav., 2 Tbsp	60	5	4
Cheez Whiz Dip:			
Original, 2 Tbsp	90	7	4
Light, 2 Tbsp	80	3.5	6
Marie's: *Per 2 Tbsp*			
Guacamole	40	3	3
Lite Buttermilk Ranch	60	5	3
Average other flavors	100	10	2
Marzetti: Choc Fruit	110	2	23
Caramel Apple	85	0	20
Veggie: Guacamole	130	13	2
Ranch	120	12	2
Light Ranch	60	6	2
Fat-Free Ranch	30	0	6
Nalley's,			
avg. all flavors	120	12	3
Naturally Fresh: Chocolate Dip	70	0	14
Cream Cheese Strawberry	90	3.5	14
Caramel	100	4	14
Old Dutch French Onion	50	2	4
Old El Paso			
Cheese 'n Salsa: Mild; Medium	40	3	3
Chunky Salsa varieties, avg.	15	0	3
Olys Bagel Spread: Berry	100	8	3
Garden Veg; Garlic & Herb	90	9	1
Prices: Pimiento Cheese Spread	85	7	3
Light Pimiento, 1 oz	55	3	3
Smart Balance Cream Cheese Spread:			
Regular, 2 Tbsp, 1.1 oz	90	6	2
Light, 2 Tbsp, 1.1 oz	70	4.5	3
Stop & Shop: Veggie Dip, 2 Tbsp	110	10	3
Sour Crm French Onion, 2 T.	60	5	2
TGI Fridays: Spinach,Chse,Artichoke	45	3.5	2
Spinach Dip, 2 Tbsp	50	3.5	2
Toby's: Tofu Pate, 2 T.	80	7	2
Other Spreads, avg., 2 T.	40	2.5	2
Tostitos Dip:			
Con Quéso Salsa	40	2.5	5
Monerey Jack Queso	40	2.5	4
Wise: French Onion, 2 Tbsp	60	5	3
Nacho Cheese	50	4.5	3

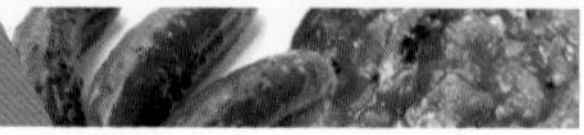

Condiments, Sauces

Average of Brands & Homemade

	C	F	Cb
Apple Sauce: *Also see Page 104*			
Sweetened, ¼ cup, 2½ oz	55	0	13
Unsweetened, ¼ cup, 2 oz	25	0	7
Barbecue Sauce: Avg., 2 Tbsp, 1 oz	40	0	10
Bull's Eye, Original, 1 Tbsp, ½ oz	30	0	7
Bearnaise Sauce, ¼ cup, 2½ oz	190	19	5
Buffalo Wing Sce: Honey Mustard, 1 T.	40	3	3
Average other varieties, 1 Tbsp	25	2	2
Catsup (Ketchup), regular, 1 Tbsp	15	0	4
Cheese, h/made, ¼ cup, 2½ oz	150	10	12
Chef-Mate, Hot Dog, ¼ cup	70	2.5	9
Chili Sauce: *Heinz,* 1 T, ½ oz	20	0	4.5
Del Monte, 1 Tbsp, ½ oz	20	0	5
Cocktail Sauce, ¼ cup	110	0	15
Fat-Free *(Walden Farms)* 1 Tbsp	0	0	0
Cranberry, all types, ¼ c., 2½ oz	110	0	27
Demi Glaze Gold, 2 tsp	30	0.5	3
Honey Mustard *(French's)* 1 tsp	5	0	1
Horseradish: 1 tsp	2	0	0
Kraft, 1 tsp	20	1.5	1
Ketchup: Regular, 1 T., ½ oz	15	0	4
Heinz One-Carb, 1 Tbsp	5	0	1
Mole: *Doñg Maria,* 2 Tbsp, 1 oz	200	13	10
Rogelio Bueno 2 Tbsp, 1 oz	160	11	12
Mushroom Sauce, ½ cup, 2 oz	50	2	5
Mustard, average, 1 tsp	5	0	0.5
Pesto Sauce, ¼ cup, 2 oz	90	5	8
Pizza Sauce, cnd., ¼ cup, 2 oz	30	0	6
Seafood Cocktail Sce, ¼ c.	60	0	15
Soy Sauce: Avg., 1 Tbsp	10	0	1
Kikkoman Lite Soy, 1 Tbsp	10	0	1
Sour Cream Sce, ½ cup	250	15	22
Spaghetti Sce, ½ cup, 4½ oz	135	6	19
Steak Sauce: A1, 1 Tbsp, ½ oz	15	0	3
Lea & Perrins, 1 Tbsp, ½ oz	25	0	5
Carb Well *(A1)* 1 Tbsp, ½ oz	5	0	1
Strawb. Puree Sce, Unsweet., 2 T.	10	0	2
Sweet & Sour Sauce:			
Contadina, 1 Tbsp	40	1	8
Kraft, 1 Tbsp	60	0	13
La Choy, 2 Tbsp, 34g	60	0	14
Tabasco Sauce, 1 tsp	2	0	0
Taco Sauce, average, 2 Tbsp, 1 oz	10	0	1
Tartar Sauce: Heinz, 2 Tbsp, 1 oz	120	11	4
America's Choice, 2 Tbsp, 1 oz	160	17	1
Hellmann's, Regular, 2 Tbsp, 1 oz	80	7	4
McCormick, Fat-Free, 2 Tbsp, 1 oz	35	0	6
Teriyaki Sauce *(Kikkoman)* 1 T., ½ oz	15	0	3
Vinegar, White or Wine, 2 Tbsp	4	0	1
White Sauce, ½ cup, 5 oz	130	7	10
Worcestershire Sauce, 1 tsp	5	0	1

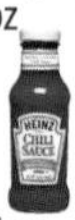

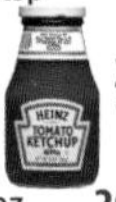

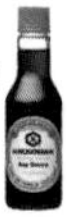

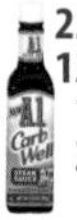

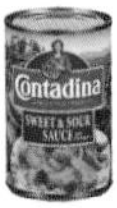

Pickles & Relish

Average All Brands

	C	F	Cb
Bread & Butter Pickles, 4 sl., 1 oz	25	0	6
Chutney, 2 Tbsp, 1¼ oz	50	0	11
Dill Pickle:			
Slices, 4 slices, 1 oz	4	0	1
1 large,			
(3¾"x 1¼" diam.), 2¼ oz	12	0	3
Extra lrg (4"x 1¾" diam.), 5 oz	30	0	6
Halves: Small, 1 oz	3	0	0.5
Large, 2½ oz	8	0	2
Sweet, small, ½ oz	22	0	6
Gherkins, sweet, 1 med., 1 oz	30	0	7
Green Chiles, chopped, 2 Tbsp	5	0	1
Horseradish, 1 Tbsp	10	0	2
Jalapenos, pickled (2), 2 oz	10	0.5	2
Jalapeno Relish, 1 Tbsp, ½ oz	5	0	1
Mustard, avg. all brands, 1 tsp	5	0	0.5
Peppers, Hot/Mild (1), 1.6 oz	20	0	4
Pickled: Beets, ½ cup, 4 oz	75	0	19
Onions, 1 medium, ¾ oz	10	0	2
Cocktail Onion, 1 onion	2	0	0
Red Cabbage, ½ cup, 3 oz	65	0	15
Pickles: Sweet, 2 Tbsp, 1 oz	35	0	0
Large (3" x ¾ diam.), 1¼ oz	40	0	10
Pickle in a Pouch, 1 large	12	0	3
Relishes: Sandwich Spread, 1 tsp	20	1	5
Cranberry-Orange, 1 Tbsp	30	0	7
Hot Dog *(Heinz),* 1 Tbsp, ½ oz	17	0	3
Sweet Pickle, 1 Tbsp, ½ oz	20	0	5
Sweet Cauliflower, 1 oz	35	0	8
Sauerkraut, Drained, 1 cup, 5 oz	25	0	6

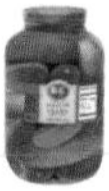

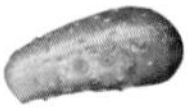

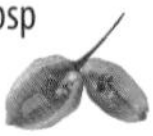

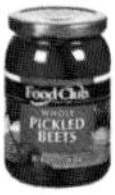

Salsa

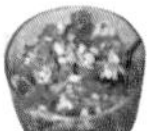

	C	F	Cb
Average all Types:			
Regular, no oil, 2 Tbsp, 1 oz	15	0	3.5
Made with oil, 2 Tbsp, 1 oz	40	3	8
Kaukauna, 2 Tbsp, 1 oz	15	0	3
La Victoria, 2 Tbsp, 1 oz	10	0	2
Old El Paso, 1 Tbsp, 1 oz	10	0	3
TGI Friday's, 1.2 oz	15	0	4

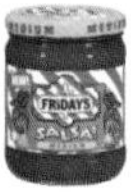

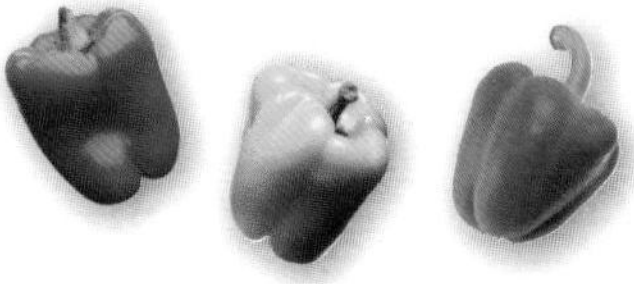

Quick Guide   C F Cb

Cookies

Average All Brands: Per Cookie

	C	F	Cb
Biscotti: Small, 0.5 oz	70	3	10
Regular, 1 oz	140	6.5	18
Chocolate Chip Cookies:			
Small/Thin 0.5 oz	70	3.5	9
Regular, 1 oz	140	7	18
Large, 2.5 oz *(Mrs Fields)*	330	16	46
Extra Large, 4 oz	555	28	73
Oatmeal/Oatmeal Raisin:			
Small/Thin 0.5 oz	65	2.5	10
Regular, 1 oz	130	5	20
Large, 2.5 oz *(Mrs Fields)*	330	14	44
Extra Large, 4 oz	510	20	78
Peanut Butter:			
Small/Thin 0.5 oz	70	3.5	9
Regular, 1 oz	135	7	17
Large, 2.5 oz *(Mrs Fields)*	330	17	41
Extra Large, 4 oz	540	27	67
Low-Fat Cookies			
Choc Chip (Low-Fat), ½ oz (1)	65	2	10
Oatmeal Raisin (Fat-Free), 1 oz (1)	95	0.5	22
Peanut Butter (Low-Fat), 1 oz (1)	105	5	15

Quick Guide   C F Cb

Crackers

Average All Brands: Per Cracker

	C	F	Cb
Cheese Crackers: Plain, 1" square	5	0	0.5
Small, octagonal	10	0	1
Round (2" diam.)	15	0	1.5
Sandwich (Peanut Butter)	35	1.5	4
Graham, 2½" square,1 cracker	30	0.5	5
Melba Toast, plain, 1 piece	20	0	4
Oyster & Soup Crackers, ½ oz	60	2	10
(40 small oysters/20 lge hexagons)			
Rice Crackers: 1 small	9	0	1.5
Rice Snacks, Oriental-Style, 1 oz	130	2.5	23
Saltines, 5 crackers	65	2	11
Snack-type, 1 round cracker	15	0	2
Soda Crackers *(Saltine)*, 2	25	1	4.5
Water Cracker *(Carr's)*: Regular, 1	30	0	7
Small, 1 piece	15	0	3
Wheat, thin, 1 cracker	9	0.5	1.5
Zweiback Toast, 1 piece	35	1	6

Brands   C F Cb

Albertsons

	C	F	Cb
Animal Crackers (6), 1 oz	130	3.5	22
Chocolate Chip:			
Original (3), 1 oz	150	7	20
Chewy (2), 1 oz	130	6	18
Chunky (1), 0.6 oz	80	3.5	10
Chocolate Sandwich Cremes (3) 1.1oz	150	6	23
Double Filled (2) 1 oz	130	6	20
Fudge Graham (3), 1 oz	140	7	19
Fudge Wafer (3), 1 oz	140	8	18
Graham Crackers: Cinnamon (2)	130	3	25
Honey (2), 1 oz	140	3	24
Low-Fat Honey (2), 1 oz	110	1	22
Marshmallow Ring (1), 1 oz	130	6	20
Milk Chocolate Chip (1), 2.5 oz	310	14	30
Striped Shortbread (3), 1.1 oz	160	7	21
Sugar (1), 2.5 oz	270	9	22
Triple Chocolate (1), 2.8 oz	310	12	33
White Chocolate Chip (1), 2.5 oz	280	11	37
Vanilla Wafers (9), 1.1 oz	160	4.5	24

Annie's

Cheddar Bunnies

	C	F	Cb
Regular: 1 oz Snack Pack	150	7	19
7½ oz Box	1125	52	140
Sour Cream & On., 1 oz	140	6	18
White Cheddar, 1 oz	140	6	18
Whole Wheat, 1 oz	130	6	17
Bunny Classics: Buttery Rich, 1 oz	140	5	20
Cheddar, 1 oz	140	7	18
Saltine, 1 oz	140	3	22
Bunny Grahams: Friends, 1 oz	130	4.5	22
Chocolate, 1 oz	130	3.5	22

Austin

Crackers: *Per Package*

	C	F	Cb
Cheese w. Cheddar Cheese, 1.38 oz	190	10	23
Cheese w. Cheddar Jack Cheese	200	11	23
Cheese & Peanut Butter	190	10	23
Mega Stuffed P'nut Butter, 1.68 oz	240	13	26
Sandwich: Chocolatey P'nut Butter	190	8	26
Grilled Cheese Flavored, 1.38 oz	190	9	24
PB & J Flavored, 1.38 oz	190	8	26
Toasty Crackers w. P'nut Butter, 1.3 oz	190	9	23
Wheat Crackers w. Cheddar Cheese	190	10	24
Zoo Animal Crackers, 1 oz	120	1.5	23
Sandwich Cremes: *Per Package*			
Lemon OHs!; Vanilla Cremes, 1.2 oz	170	7	24

Baker's (Erin)	C	F	Cb
Original Breakfast Cookies: *Per 3 oz*			
Peanut Butter	330	11	49
Peanut Butter & Jelly	320	9	52
Vegan Peanut But. Choc. Chunk	320	10	48
Other varieties, average	300	6	54
Minis: *Per 1 oz Cookie*			
Peanut Butter	110	3	16
Other flavors, avg.	100	2	18
Brownie Bites, average, 1 oz	100	2	18
Barbara's Bakery			
Cookies: Fig Bars, avg. (1)	60	0	14
Snackimals (10), average	120	4	19
Crackers: Rite Lite Rounds (5), avg.	60	2	11
Wheatines (4), average	60	1	11
Blue Diamond			
Nut Thins:			
Almond: (16)	130	3.5	23
Cheddar (16)	130	4	23
Smokehouse (16)	130	3	23
Hazelnut (16)	130	3	23
Pecan (16)	130	3.5	23
Brent & Sam's			
Chocolate Chip Pecan (2)	110	6	13
Key Lime White Chocolate (2)	110	5	14
Oatmeal Raisin with Pecans (2)	110	5	14
Triple Chocolate Bliss (2)	110	5	14
White Chocolate Macadamia (2)	110	6	14
Carr's			
Crackers:			
Poppy & Sesame Seed (4)	80	5	9
Table Water (5)	70	1.5	13
Whole Wheat (2)	80	4	10
Cookies, Ginger Lemon Cremes (2)	130	5	20
Cheez·It ~ *See Sunshine (Page 89)*			
Chips Ahoy! ~ *See Nabisco (Page 87)*			
Country Choice			
Ginger Snaps (5)	140	5	22
Sandwich Cremes (2), avg.	130	5	19
Soft Baked, avg. all varieties (1)	100	4	16
Vanilla Wafers (7)	140	5	22
Dr. Kracker			
Crackers, Flatbread, avg., all flav., 1 oz	100	4	11
Snacker: Klassic 3-Seed (8), 1 oz	120	5	13
Seeded Spelt (8), 1 oz	120	6	12
Spelt Sunflower Cheese (8), 1 oz	100	6	12
Avg., other flavors (8), 1 oz	120	5	15

Per Cookie/Cracker, Unless Indicated

Famous Amos	C	F	Cb
(Bite Size Cookies)			
Chocolate Chip: 4 cookies, 1 oz	150	7	20
1.4 oz Snack bag	210	10	28
3 oz (99cents) bag	450	21	60
12 oz bag	1800	84	240
15 oz box	2250	105	300
Sandwich Creme: Choc. (3), 1 oz	170	7	25
Oatmeal Macaroon (3), 1.2 oz	140	6	20
Peanut Butter (3)	160	7	22
Vanilla (3), 1.2 oz	170	7	25
Chocolate: 3 cookies, 1.2 oz	170	7	25
2.2 oz bag	310	9	33
14 oz pkg	1980	82	290
Fig Newtons ~ *See Nabisco, Page 87*			
Girl Scouts			
Cookies: Caramel DeLites (2)	140	7	19
Peanut Butter Sandwich (3)	160	6	26
Goldfish ~ *See Pepperidge Farm, Page 88*			
Grandma's			
Peanut Butter Sandwich Creme (5)	210	10	28
Rich 'N Chewy, Choc Chip, pkg.	270	12	38
Vanilla Sandwich Creme (5)	210	9	30
Vanilla Creme Mini Cookie Bites (9)	150	7	22
Homestyle: Chocolate Chip (1)	190	9	25
Fudge Choc. Chip (1)	170	7	27
Oatmeal Raisin (1)	180	6	30
Peanut Butter (1)	200	10	24
Great American Cookies			
Cookies: Original; Pecan (1)	230	12	31
Chewy Pecan Supreme (1)	230	12	31
Chewy Choc. Supreme/Sugar (1)	200	9	29
Double Fudge/Reese's (1), avg	235	11	32
Oatmeal (1)	230	10	33
Original M&M/Reese's (1)	240	12	32
Peanut Butter M&M (1)	250	13	28
Snickerdoodles (1)	240	11	33
White Chunk Macadamia (1)	250	14	30
Double Doozies: Original (1)	690	34	94
M&M Big Bite (1)	340	17	46
Brownies: Cheesecake (1)	430	23	54
German Chocolate (1)	420	22	55
Iced Fudge (1)	500	23	71
Iced Fudge Nut (1)	500	27	64
Strawberry Swirl Cheesecake (1)	430	23	55
Cookie Cakes: 16" Cookie (1)	460	22	67
16" M&M Cookie (1)	500	24	73
Heart Shaped (1)	440	21	64
Sliced Cookie Cake, 1 slice	580	27	83

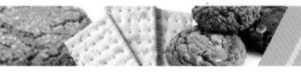

Cookies ◇ Crackers C

Per Cookie/Cracker, Unless Indicated

Health Valley | C | F | Cb

Cookies

	C	F	Cb
Cookie Cremes Sandwich (2) avg.	125	5	19
Oatmeal Raisin Cookie (1)	90	3.5	14
Mini: Choc. Chocolate Chip (4)	130	7	16
Other varieties (4)	120	5	16

Crackers

	C	F	Cb
Original: Amaranth Bran Graham (6)	120	3	22
Oat Bran Graham (6)	120	3	22
Rice Bran (6)	110	3	19
Cracked Pepper; Sesame (4)	70	3	10
Stoned Wheat; Whole Wheat (4)	70	3	9

Hershey's

Brownies:

	C	F	Cb
Hershey's, 1 pkg	380	18	56
Reese's, 1 pkg	380	18	54
Cookies: York Cookies (2)	130	8	17
Almond Joy Cookies (2)	140	8	17
Hershey's Layered (2)	130	6	19
Reese's (2)	150	8	17
Reese's Layered (2)	140	7	18
Soft Baked (1)	340	16	50

Joseph's Cookies

	C	F	Cb
Brownies: Original, 1½ oz bag	150	7	26
Pecan Walnut (9)	100	5	15
Crispy Bite Size: *Per 4 Cookies*			
Almond; Chocolate Peanut Butter	95	5	13
Choc. Walnut; Pecan Chocolate Chip	95	5	13
Chocolate Chip	100	5	13
Lemon; Peanut Butter, avg.	95	4	15
Oatmeal Choc Chip w. Pecans	100	6	14
Oatmeal; Pecan Shortbread, avg.	100	5	15

Kashi TLC

	C	F	Cb
Cookies: *Per Cookie*			
Happy Trail Mix	130	5	21
Oatmeal: Dark Choc.	130	5	21
Raisin Flax	130	5	20
Crackers:			
Mini: Fire Roasted Vegetable (15)	130	3.5	21
Honey Sesame (15)	130	3	22
Party: Mediterranean Bruschetta (4)	120	4	18
Roasted Garlic & Thyme (4)	130	4.5	18
Stoneground 7 Grain (4)	130	5	17

Per Cookie/Cracker (Unless indicated)

Keebler Crackers | C | F | Cb

	C	F	Cb
Club: Original (4)	70	3	9
Reduced Fat (5)	70	2	12
Grahams: Original (8), 1 oz	120	3.5	22
Low-Fat varieties (8), 1 oz	110	1.5	23
Town House: Original (5)	80	4.5	10
Reduced Fat (6)	60	1.5	11
Wheatables: Reduced Fat (19)	140	4	22
Other varieties, average (17)	140	6	20

Keebler Cookies:

Chips Deluxe:

	C	F	Cb
Chocolate Lovers; Coconut (1)	80	4.5	10
Original (2)	170	9	19
Rainbow (1)	80	4	10
Rainbow Mini's 1.4 oz pkg	200	10	27
Soft & Chewy (1)	80	3.5	11
Country Style Oatmeal (2)	130	6	19
Danish Wedding (4)	130	6	18
E.L. Fudge: Original (1)	90	3.5	13
Double Stuffed (2)	180	9	24

Fudge Shoppe:

	C	F	Cb
Deluxe Grahams, regular (3)	140	7	17
Fudge Sticks (3), avg.	150	8	20
Fudge Stripes: Regular, avg. (3)	150	7	21
Mini's, 1 pkg	200	9	27
100 Calorie Pkg	100	3.5	16
Grasshopper (4)	140	7	19
Gripz, avg., 1 pouch	125	5	22
Iced Animal (6)	140	5	22

Sandies Cookies:

	C	F	Cb
Choc Chip Pecan (2)	170	10	18
Pecan Shortbread (2)	160	10	18
Reduced-Fat (2)	160	7	21
100 Calorie Pkg	100	3	17
Soft Batch, Choc Chip; P'nut Butter	160	7	22
Vienna Fingers: Regular (2)	150	6	23
Reduced Fat (2)	140	4.5	24
Wafers: Vanilla (8)	150	6	21
Mini Vanilla (18)	140	6	21

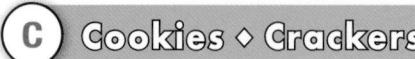

C · Cookies ◇ Crackers

Per Cookie/Cracker, Unless Indicated

Kroger	C	F	Cb
Cookies: Chip Mates			
Original (2), 1 oz	120	6	16
Chewy (2), 1 oz	130	6	17
Chunky (2), 1 oz	150	7	20
Olde Southern Pecan Shortbread, 1 oz	150	9	15
Sugar Wafer (3), 1.1 oz	160	9	20
Vanilla Wafers (7), 1.1 oz	130	3.5	23
Crackers:			
Grahams, Original /Honey (4)	120	3	20
Saltines, Original, 5 crackers, 0.5 oz	60	1.5	10
Kid-O's			
Mint (2) 1 oz	130	6	19
Choc. Lovers Dbl Filled Choc, (2) 1 oz	130	5	19
Double Filled Sandwich (2) 1 oz	130	6	20
Chocolate Sandwich (3) 1.15 oz	150	6	23
Lance			
Nekot, Peanut Butter, 1 pkg	240	11	30
Strawberry Cookies (5)	190	8	27
Crackers: Toasty, 1 pkg	180	9	16
Nipchee, 1 pkg	190	9	23
Toastchee: Original, 1 pkg	220	11	23
Reduced-Fat, 1 pkg	190	8	23
Malt Crackers, 1 pkg	190	10	18
Little Debbie			
Fig Bars (1)	160	3	31
Marshmallow Pies, avg. (1)	180	7	28
Marshmallow Treats (1)	160	4	31
Oatmeal Creme Pies (1)	170	7	26
Nutty Bars (2), 2 oz	310	18	33
Crackers: Cheese w. P'nut Butter (4)	140	7	15
Toasty w. P'nut Butter (4)	140	7	15
Lu			
Le Petit Beurre (4)	140	4	24
Le Petit Ecolier, avg. (2)	130	6	17
Pim's, Orange (2)	100	3	16
Macaroni & Cheese			
Original Cheddar, 1 serving, 1.1 oz	150	7	18
Mild Cheddar, 1 serving, 1.1 oz	150	7	18
White Cheddar, 1 serving, 1.1 oz	150	7	19
Manischewitz			
Matzo Boards: *See Page 105*			
Chocolate Macaroons, each	45	2	8
Matzo Cracker, Miniatures (10)	110	0	25
Tam Tam Crackers: Everything (10)	130	5	19
Onion (10)	140	5	21

Per Cookie/Cracker, Unless Indicated

Miss Meringue	C	F	Cb
Chocolettes			
Mint, (10), 1.1 oz	130	3.5	24
Van.; Strawberry Van. (10), 1.1 oz	130	3.5	24
Macaroons			
Traditional Recipe (1), 1.3 oz	180	10	20
Madeleines			
Chocolate (2), 1.2 oz	160	9	18
Traditional Recipe (2), 1.2 oz	160	9	19
Meringue Classiques			
Cappuccino (4), 1.1 oz	110	0	26
Mint Chocolate Chip (4), 1.1 oz	120	1.5	25
Triple Choc. (4), 1.1 oz	120	1.5	25
Vanilla Rainbow/Van. (4), 1.1 oz	110	0	27
Meringue Minis			
Chocolate (13), 1.1 oz	110	0	26
Chocolate Chip (12), 1.1 oz	130	1.5	27
Mint Choc. Chip (12), 1.1 oz	120	1.5	26
Orange Creamsicle (13), 1.1 oz	110	0	27
Van.; Rainbow Van. (13), 1.1 oz	110	0	27
Sugar-Free Choc. (13), 0.5 oz	40	0	8
Sugar-Free Vanilla (13), 0.5 oz	35	0	9
Mother's			
Chocolate Chip (4), 1 oz	150	7	20
Circus Animals (6), 1 oz	150	7	20
Coconut Cicadas (5), 1.2 oz	160	8	21
Double Fudge (2), 1.3 oz	170	7	27
English Tea (2), 1.3 oz	180	7	27
Macaroons (2), 1 oz	170	11	17
Oatmeal (2), 1 oz	130	5	19
Taffy (2), 1.3 oz	180	8	27
Vanilla Creme (2), 1.3 oz	180	7	26
Iced: Lemonade (4), 1 oz	140	7	19
Oatmeal (4), 1.2 oz	130	5	20
Mrs Fields Cookies: *See Fast-Foods Section*			
Murray Sugar Free Cookies			
Double Fudge (3)	160	9	23
Fudge-Dipped: Grahams (4)	150	8	19
Mint Cookies (4)	130	7	16
Shortbread (5)	130	5	21
Vanilla Wafers (4)	150	10	19
Gingersnaps (7)	130	5	23
Lemon/Choc/Creme Sandwich (3)	130	6	20
Lemon Wafers (4)	130	8	19
Oatmeal (3)	140	7	21
Peanut Butter (3)	150	9	16
Shortbread (8)	130	5	21
Shortbread Pecan (3)	170	11	18
Vanilla Wafers (9)	130	5	24

Nabisco Cookies: C F Cb

Per Cookie/Cracker (Unless Indicated)

Chips Ahoy!

	C	F	Cb
Big & Soft: Choc Chunk (1)	170	7	27
Oatmeal Choc Chunk (1)	180	8	26
Chewy Oatmeal (2)	120	5	17
Choc. Chip (3)	160	8	22
Reduced-Fat (3)	140	5	23
Mini Choc. Chips Bite-Size (14)	150	7	20
Snak Saks (5)	150	8	21
Peanut Butter Chunky (1)	90	5	10
White Fudge Chunky (2)	80	4.5	11
Ginger Snaps (4)	120	2.5	23
Lorna Doone (1)	140	7	20
Mallomars (1)	120	5	18
Newtons: Fig Newtons (2)	110	2	22
Fig/Strawb. Minis, 1 pkg, 1.34 oz	130	3	27
100% Whole Grain (2)	110	2	21
Fat-Free (2)	90	0	22
Fruit Crisps, avg. (2)	100	2	20
Raspberry/Strawberry (2)	100	1.5	21
Nilla Wafers: (8), 1 oz	140	6	21
Reduced-Fat (8), 1 oz	110	2	24
Nutter Butter:			
Sandwich Cookies (2), 1 oz	130	5	20
Bites: Minis, 1 pkt, 1 oz	130	6	19
Go-Paks (10), 1 oz	140	6	21
Snak-Saks (10), 1 oz	140	6	21
Wafers, Peanut Butter (5)	160	9	18
Oreo:			
Sandwich Cookies: Chocolate (3)	160	7	25
Reduced-Fat (3), 1.2 oz	150	4.5	27
Sugar Free (2), 0.8 oz	100	5	16
Golden: Original (3), 1.2 oz	170	7	25
Chocolate (3), 1.2 oz	170	7	25
Double Stuff: Original (2), 1 oz	140	7	21
Chocolate (2), 1 oz	150	7	21
Cool Mint (2), 1 oz	140	7	20
Peanut Butter (2), 1 oz	140	6	20
Fudge Covered (1), 0.7 oz	100	5	13
Fudge Rings (3), 1 oz	120	4.5	19
Fun Stix, Chocolate; Golden 1 pkt	90	3.5	13
Go-Pak, Bite Size Choc (9), 1 oz	130	6	21
Snak-Saks: Bite Size Choc (9) 1 oz	130	6	21
Mini Golden Vanilla (9), 1 oz	140	6	21
Cakesters: Original (2), 2 oz	250	12	36
Choc Creme (2), 2 oz	250	12	36
Teddy Grahams:			
Honey; Cinn. Snacks (24)	130	4	23
Chocolate (24)	130	4.5	22
Snak Saks,			
Mini Choc Chip/Honey (47)	130	4	22

Nabisco Cookies (Cont): C F Cb

100 Calorie Packs: *Per Pack*

	C	F	Cb
Chips Ahoy! Thin Crisps	100	3	18
Barnum's Animals			
Choco Crackers	100	3	17
Honey Maid Thin Crisps	100	3	16
Lorna Doone Crisps	100	3	16
Milk Choc. Pretzels	100	3.5	16
Oreo Thin Crisps	100	3	16
Ritz Toasted Chips, Minis, 0.8 oz	100	3	17
Ritz Snack Mix Toasted, 0.8 oz	100	3	16

Nabisco Crackers: *Per Serving*

	C	F	Cb
Barnum's Animals (8)	120	3.5	22
Cheese Nips:			
Baked Cheddar, 1 oz	150	6	19
Cheddar; Packs-2-Go!, 1.2 oz	170	7	22
Four Cheese, 1 oz bag	150	7	18
Mini Go-Pak (53), 1 oz	150	6	19
Flavor Originals:			
Better Cheddars (22)	160	8	18
Chicken in a Biskit (12)	160	8	19
Sociables Baked Savory (7)	70	3.5	9
Vegetable Thins (11)	150	7	20
Honey Maid:			
Grahams: Avg. (8)	130	3.5	24
Low-Fat (8), avg.	120	2	25
Mini S'Mores (9)	140	6	21
Premium Saltine: Fat-Free (5)	60	0	13
Hint of Salt (5)	60	1.5	12
Multigrain (5)	60	1.5	10
Original (5)	70	1.5	11
Unsalted Tops (5)	70	1.5	11
Premium, Soup & Oyster (22)	60	1.5	11
Minis, Original (21)	70	2	11
Wheat Thins: Big (11)	150	6	21
Multi-Grain (17)	130	4.5	22
Original (16), 1.1 oz	150	6	21
Parmesan Basil (15) 1 oz	140	5	21
Ranch (14), 1 oz	140	6	19
Reduced-Fat (16), 1 oz	140	4	21
Sundried Tomato & Basil (15) 1 oz	140	6	20
Toasted Chip, Multi-Grain (15)	140	4.5	22
Wheatsworth, Stone Ground Wheat (5)	80	3.5	10
Zwieback, 8g	35	1	6

Newman's Own Organics	C	F	Cb
Alphabet Cookies (10) avg.	120	3	22
Champion Chip: Chocolate Chip (4)	160	7	21
Expresso Chocolate Chip (4)	150	7	21
Wheat-Free & Dairy-Free (4)	160	8	21
Other varieties, avg.	160	8	21
Fig Newman's: Fat-Free, 2 bars	120	0	28
Low-Fat, 2 bars	140	2	28
Wheat/Dairy-Free, 2 bars	120	1.5	26
Newman-O's: Original (2)	130	4.5	20
Choc. Creme (2); Mint Creme (2)	130	4.5	20
Ginger-O's (2)	120	4.5	19
Wheat-Free & Dairy-Free (2)	130	4.5	21

Oreo Cookies ~ *See Nabisco, Page 87*

Peek Freans			
Assorted Creme (2)	140	6	19
Nice Biscuits (2)	160	6	25
Shortcake (2)	140	7	18

Pepperidge Farm			
Cookies			
Brussels (3)	150	7	20
Brussels Mint (3)	190	10	22
Chessmen (3)	120	5	18
Choc Chunk: Double (1)	140	7	18
Dark Choc. Chunk Nantucket (1)	140	7	16
Dark Choc. Pecan Chesapeake (1)	140	8	15
Milk Chocolate, Macadamia Nut Sausalito (1)	140	8	16
White Choc. Macadamia (1)	130	6	17
Other varieties, avg. (1)	140	7	18
Collection: Ginger Family (4)	160	5	26
Golden Orchard (3)	140	6	21
Geneva (3)	160	9	19
Homestyle: Ginger Man (4)	130	4	21
Shortbread (2)	140	7	16
Sugar (3)	140	6	20
Milano: Milk Choc. (3)	170	9	21
Other varieties, avg. (2)	130	7	16
Soft Baked Cookies: Oatmeal (1)	140	5	22
Milk Chocolate Chunk (1)	150	7	21
Molasses (1)	130	3.5	22
Snickerdoodle; Sugar (1)	140	5	22
100 Calorie Pouches: *Per Packet*			
Chessmen	100	3.5	15
Dark Choc. Chunk	100	3.5	15
Goldfish	100	3.5	14
Oatmeal Raisin	100	3	16

Pepperidge Farm (Cont)	C	F	Cb
Crackers			
Entertaining Quartet (4)	70	2.5	10
Golden Butter (4)	70	2.5	11
Harvest Wheat (3)	80	3.5	11
Wheat Crisps (17), 1 oz	140	5	21
Goldfish, avg. all flavors:			
1 oz (55)	140	5	20
1.5 oz Pouch	210	9	27
2 oz ctn	280	10	40
Pretzel Thins:			
Simply (11)	110	0	21
Savory Cheddar (11)	140	3	26
Snack Sticks:			
Artisan Cheese (11)	130	3.5	21
Toasted Sesame (12)	130	5	19

President's Choice			
Milk Choc Chunk Pecan (1), 0.8 oz	120	7	14
Peanut Butter (2), 1 oz	140	8	15
The Decadent: Choc Chip (2), 1.1 oz	160	8	21
Chocolate Chunk (2), 1.1 oz	160	8	21
White Chocolate Chip (2), 1.1 oz	160	8	19

Ritz			
Crackers: Orig., ½ oz	80	4.5	10
Reduced-Fat, ½ oz	70	2	11
Honey Butter (5), 06 oz	80	4	10
Peanut Butter, 1.4 oz pkg	190	9	24
Real Cheese, 1.4 oz pkg	200	11	22
Whole Wheat, ½ oz	70	2.5	11
100 Calorie Snack Mix, 1 pkg, 0.8 oz	100	3	16
Ritz Bits Sandwiches: Cheese, 1 oz	150	9	17
Cheese Go-Pak (12) 1 oz	150	9	17
Cheese Packs 2 Go!, 1.5 oz	220	13	24
Peanut Butter Go-Pak, 1 oz	160	8	18
Peanut Butter Packs 2 Go!, 1.2 oz	170	10	20
Real Cheese, 1 oz	150	9	16
Ritz Chips: Toasted Original, 1 oz	130	4.5	21
Cheddar; Sour Crm & Onion, 1 oz	130	6	19

Safeway Select			
Homestyle: Choc. Chunk Brownie	120	5	19
Oatmeal Raisin, 1 oz	130	6	18
Indulgent: Double Choc Chunk, 1 oz	130	7	18
Milk Choc. Macadamia Nut, 1 oz	140	8	17
Pecan Choc Chunk, 1 oz	140	9	16
White Choc. Macadamia Nut, 1 oz	140	8	17
Tuxedos: Chocolate (3), 1.3 oz	180	7	26
Cinnamon Bun; Vanilla (3), 1.3 oz	180	8	26
Mint Creme (2), 1 oz	140	7	20
Vanilla Creme Wafers (4)	150	8	20

Snackwell's

	C	F	Cb
Creme S'wich (2) 1 oz	110	3	20
Creme Sandwich, Packs To Go!, 1 pkg	210	5	38
Devil's Food Cake, Fat-Free (1) ½ oz	50	0	12
Lemon Creme Sandwich Sugar Free (3)	130	6	23
Shortbread Sugar Free (3) 1 oz	130	6	21

South Beach Living

Cookies: Per Package

	C	F	Cb
Peanut Butter	100	5	15
Oatmeal Choc. Chip	100	5	16

Stella D'Oro

	C	F	Cb
Almond Toast (3)	115	2.5	21
Anginetti, 1 oz	130	3.5	22
Anisette Sponge Low-Fat (2)	95	1	19
Anisette Toast Low-Fat (3)	125	1	27
Biscotti, average, ¾ oz	95	4	13
Breakfast Treats: Chocolate Cookie (1)	90	3	15
Original (1)	90	3	15
Original Mini, 1 oz	120	3.5	21
Viennese Cinnamon (1)	90	2.5	16
Coffee Treats: Almond Toast, 1 oz	100	2	20
Angel Wings, 1 oz	170	12	14
Anisette Sponge (2)	90	1	18
Anisette Toast, 1.1 oz	130	1	27
Banana Walnut Toast, 1 oz	100	2	19
Blueberry; Cinnamon Toast, 1 oz	100	1	20
Roman Egg Biscuits, 1.1 oz	130	4	21
Continental Cookie Collection, 1 oz	130	4.5	20
Egg Jumbo, 1.1 oz	120	1.5	26
Lady Stella Assortment, 1 oz	130	4.5	20
Margherite (2)	130	4.5	20
Margherite Mini, 1.1 oz	150	5	24
Swiss Fudge (2) 1.1 oz	170	9	22

Streit's

Wafers: Chocolate (3)

	C	F	Cb
Wafers: Chocolate (3)	160	9	19
Vanilla (3)	170	11	18
Rolls, Chocolate (3)	105	6	12

Sunshine

	C	F	Cb
Krispy: Original; Whole Wheat (5)	60	1.5	11
Oyster & Soup, 16 crackers	60	1	11
Wheat (5)	60	1.5	11
Cheez-It: Original (27), 1 oz	150	8	17
Reduced-Fat (29), 1 oz	130	4.5	20

Also See Snacks ~ Page 154

Per Cookie/Cracker (Unless Indicated)

Trader Joe's

	C	F	Cb
100 Calorie Packs, avg	100	3	18
Cherry Granola (2), 1 oz	110	4	18
Chocolate Almond Lacey's (2)	170	12	16
Chocolate Chip: Small (4), 1.1 oz	140	7	18
Large, Singles (1), 1.7 oz	280	14	35
Caramel Cashew (3), 1 oz	140	7	16
Dark Choc Chunks w. Almonds (3)	140	7	17
Dunkers: Choc Chip (2), 1.2 oz	160	7	21
Choc Coated Choc. Chip (2), 1.3 oz	190	9	25
Ginger Snaps (5), 1 oz	140	6	21
Joe Joe's S'wich Cremes, Choc./Vanilla (2), 1 oz	130	6	19
Lemon Crisps (5)	120	4	19
Meringues: Low-Fat, Chocolate (4)	120	1.5	25
Fat-Free Vanilla (4)	110	0	27
Very Mini Meringues, Van. (100)	100	0	24
Oatmeal Raisin (1), 1.8 oz	270	12	35
Pecan Southern Style (4), 1 oz	150	9	15
Righteous Rounds Choc Chip (5), 1 oz	130	4	20
Thins: Meyer Lemon (9), 1 oz	160	5	25
Triple Ginger (9), 1 oz	140	4.5	24
Triple Choc Chunk (1), 1 oz	140	7	20
Ultimate Vanilla Wafers (5), 1 oz	120	6	15
Water Crackers (4)	60	1	12

Triscuit

Baked Whole Wheat Crackers: Per Serving

	C	F	Cb
Original (15) 1 oz	120	4.5	19
Thin Crisps, Orig. (15) 1 oz	130	5	21
Roasted Garlic (8)	120	4.5	20

Voortman

Shortbread Cookies (2), 1.3 oz — 180 | 10 | 22

Sugar Free Cookies:

	C	F	Cb
Shortbread Cookies (2), 1.3 oz	180	10	22
Chocolate Chip (2), 1.4 oz	160	9	26
Lemon Wafers (3), 1 oz	130	8	17
Peanut Butter Wafers (4), 1 oz	150	8	17
Vanilla Wafers: Regular (3), 1.1 oz	140	7	20
Sugar Free (3), 1 oz	130	8	17

Zesta

Crackers: Whole Grain Wheat (5)

	C	F	Cb
Crackers: Whole Grain Wheat (5)	60	1.5	11
Fat Free, 5 crackers	60	0	13
Original, 5 crackers	60	1.5	11
Export Sodas (3)	60	1.5	10

365 (Whole Foods):

	C	F	Cb
Choc Chip (5), 1 oz	130	6	19
Classic Fig Bars (2), 1.3 oz	140	2.5	27
Lady Fingers (5), 1.1 oz	120	1.5	25
Lemon Wafers (5), 0.9 oz	120	5	17
Oatmeal (6), 1 oz	130	4.5	20
Sandwich Cremes (2), average	130	5	20
Sugar (5), 1.1 oz	130	4	22

Thaw, Bake & Serve | C | F | Cb

Grands! Biscuits (Pillsbury): *Per Biscuit*

	C	F	Cb
Extra Rich	210	10	26
Butter Tastin'; Buttermilk, avg.	180	8	25
Reduced Fat	160	6	25
Flaky; Butter Tastin'; Buttermilk	190	9	24

Pillsbury Cookies: *Per 1 oz*

Refrigerated Cookie Dough

Big Deluxe Classics:

	C	F	Cb
Oatmeal Raisin (1)	150	6	24
Peanut Butter Cup (1)	170	8	22
White Chunk Macadamia Nut (1)	170	9	22
Other varieties (1)	170	9	22
Ready To Bake: Sugar Cookie (2)	170	8	22
Chocolate Chip w. Walnuts (2)	170	9	22
Chocolate Chunk Chip (2)	180	9	22
Peanut Butter w. Reese's Pces (2)	170	8	21
S'mores (1); Choc. Candy (2)	160	7	23
Create n Bake: Peanut Butter	130	6	16
Chocolate Chip	130	7	18
Oatmeal Choc. Chip; Sugar, avg.	130	6	17

Refrigerated Dough:

	C	F	Cb
Cinnamon Roll	150	5	23
Flaky Cinnamon Twists w/ Icing (1)	180	9	22
Flaky Supreme w/ Icing (1)	370	19	48
Grands Cinnamon Rolls w/ Icing (1)	310	9	54

Simply Bake Bars:

	C	F	Cb
P.B. Choc.; Turtle Supreme, 1/10 pkg	180	9	23

Spread & Bake Brownies:

	C	F	Cb
Choc. Fudge, 1/12 pkg	150	6	24
Triple Choc Chunk, 1/12 pkg	160	6	24

Toll House *(Nestlé)*

Refrigerated Dough

	C	F	Cb
Chocolate Chunk (2)	180	9	23
Fudgy Brownie w/ Filling (1)	150	7	20
Jumbo Chocolate Chip (1)	180	9	23
Mini Chocolate Chip (3)	160	8	21
Walnut Chocolate Chip (2)	180	9	22

Ultimates Refrigerated Dough

	C	F	Cb
Chocolate Chip Lovers (1)	180	9	23
Choc. Chips & Chunks w. Pecans (1)	190	10	22
P. Butter Chips & Choc Chunks (1)	180	9	23
Triple Chocolate Decadence (1)	170	8	23
Turtle (1)	180	9	23
White Choc. Macadamia Nut (1)	190	10	22

Crispbreads | C | F | Cb

Per Serving

	C	F	Cb
Finn Crisp: Original, rye (1)	40	0	10
Other types (1)	19	0	3
Kavli Norwegian: Crispy Thin (3)	50	0	11
Hearty Thick (2)	60	0	12
Malsovit Meal Wafers (1)	75	4	7
New York Flatbread Crisps (1)	35	0	7
Ry-Krisp: Natural (2)	50	0	11
Seasoned (2)	60	1	11
Sesame (2)	60	2	10
Ryvita: Dark/Light (2)	70	0	16
WASA: Crisp'n Light 7 Grain (3)	60	0	13
Fiber (1)	30	1	5
Hearty (1), 0.5 oz	45	0	11
Light Rye (2), 0.5 oz	60	0	14
Multi Grain (1), 0.5 oz	45	0	10
Whole Wheat (1), 0.5 oz	50	1	10

Matzos

Manischewitz

	C	F	Cb
Egg 'n Onion Matzo, 1 oz	100	1	23
Mandelin (9)	35	2	4
Matzo Meal, 1/4 cup	130	0	28
Matzo Farfel, 1 cup, 2.7 oz	180	0.5	60
Passover Egg Matzos, 1.1 oz	120	0	28
Tam Tam Crackers, Onion (10)	140	5	21
Thin Salted; Thin Tea Matzos, 0.9 oz	100	0	22
Unsalted, 1 oz	90	0	20
Whole Wheat, 1 oz	110	0.5	23
Crackers: Miniatures (10)	110	0	25
Passover Egg Matzo (11)	110	0	20

Streit's

	C	F	Cb
Mediterranean Matzos, 1 Matzo, 1 oz	90	0.5	18
Unsalted Matzos, 1 Matzo, 1 oz	100	0	23

There are 1440 minutes in every day...

Schedule 30 of them for exercise!

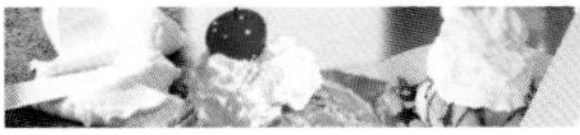

Quick Guide

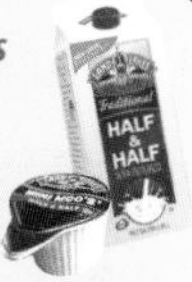

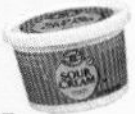

Cream
(C) (F) (Cb)

Average All Brands

Half & Half Cream:

	C	F	Cb
1 Tbsp, 0.5 oz	20	1.5	0.5
2 Tbsp, 1 oz	40	3	1
¼ cup, 2 oz	80	6	2
Single Serve Cup, ⅜ fl.oz	15	1.5	0.5
Light: Coffee/table (20% fat): 1 T.	30	3	0.5
2 Tbsp, 1 oz	60	6	1

Sour Cream:

	C	F	Cb
Regular: 1 Tbsp, 0.5 oz	25	2.5	1
1 cup, 8 oz	490	48	10
Low-Fat/Light: 1 Tbsp, 0.5 oz	20	1.5	1
2 Tbsp, 1 oz	40	3	2
Fat-Free: Average, 2 Tbsp, 1 oz	25	0	4
Hood, 2 Tbsp, 1 oz	25	0	4
Kroger, 2 Tbsp, 1 oz	20	0	3
Naturally Yours; Oak Farm, 2 T.	20	0	3
Knudsen, 2 Tbsp, 1 oz	30	0	5

Sour Cream Substitute:

	C	F	Cb
Albertson's, 2 Tbsp, 1 oz	60	5	2
Tofutti Sour Supreme, 2 T., 1 oz	85	7	9

Whipping Cream:

Heavy (37% fat):

	C	F	Cb
1 T. fluid/2 T. whipped	50	5.5	0.5
¼ cup whipped	100	11	1
½ cup fluid/1 c. whipped	400	44	3.5

Light (30% fat):

	C	F	Cb
1 Tbsp fluid/2 Tbsp whipped	45	4.5	0.5
½ cup fluid/1 cup whipped	350	37	4

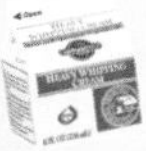

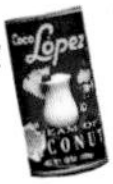

Coconut Cream/Milk
(C) (F) (Cb)

	C	F	Cb
Coconut Cream (Canned),			
Plain/unsweetened: 2 Tbsp, 1 oz	75	6.5	3
½ cup, 4 oz	285	26	12
Sweetened: *Coco Lopez,* 1 oz	130	5	21
½ cup, 4 oz	520	20	84
Coconut Milk (Canned):			
Natural Value: Reg., ¼ c., 2 fl.oz	120	11	5
Lite, ¼ cup, 2 fl.oz	55	5	1
Thai Kitchen: Lite, ¼ cup, 2 fl.oz	45	4	1
Premium, 2 fl.oz	120	10	4
Coconut Water (Center), 1 cup	45	0.5	9

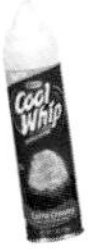

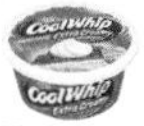

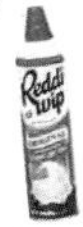

Whipped Toppings
(C) (F) (Cb)

Average All Brands

	C	F	Cb
Cream (Pressurized): 2 T.	20	1	1
¼ cup	45	4	2
½ cup	90	8	4
Cream Topping: Lite, 2 Tbsp	20	1	3
Cool Whip: Extra Creamy, 2 T.	25	2	2
Lite, 2 Tbsp, 7g	15	1	2
Free, 2 Tbsp, 9g	15	0	3
Kraft: Dream Whip, 2 Tbsp	10	0	2
Reddi-Wip: Original, 2 T., 8g	15	1	0.5
Chocolate, 2 Tbsp, 8g	15	1	1
Extra Creamy, 2 Tbsp, 8g	20	1.5	0.5
Fat-Free, 2 Tbsp, 8g	5	0	1

Creamers (Non-Dairy)

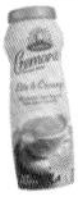

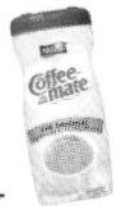

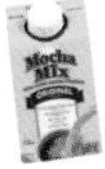

Powder:

Coffee-Mate/Cremora/N-Rich

	C	F	Cb
Original, 1 tsp	10	0.5	1
1 heaping tsp	25	2	2
Lite, 1 tsp	10	1.5	2
Flavors: 4 tsp	60	3	8
Fat-Free: Average, 4 tsp	50	0	11

Liquid/Refrigerated: *Per Tablespoon*

Coffee-Mate

	C	F	Cb
Unflavored: Original, 1 Tbsp	20	1	2
Fat-Free, 1 Tbsp	10	0	2
Low-Fat, 1 Tbsp	10	0.5	1
Flavors: French Vanilla, 1 T.	35	1.5	5
Avg., other flavors, 1 Tbsp	35	1.5	5
Fat-Free, all flavors, 1 Tbsp	25	0	5
Hood, Country Creamer, 1 Tbsp	20	1.5	2
International Delight:			
Average all flavors, 1 Tbsp	40	1.5	7
Fat-Free French Vanilla, 1 Tbsp	30	0	7
Kroger			
Coffee, Fat-Free & Lactose Free:			
French Vanilla, 1 Tbsp	30	0	6
Hazelnut, 1 Tbsp	35	1.5	6
Mocha Mix: Original, 1 Tbsp	20	1.5	2
Fat-Free, 1 Tbsp	10	0	1
Lite, 1 Tbsp	10	0.5	1
Silk: Original, 1Tbsp	15	1	1
French Vanilla; Hazelnut, 1 Tbsp	20	1	3

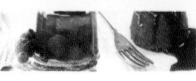

Ready-To-Serve | C | F | Cb
	C	F	Cb
Instant Pudding, Reg., ½ cup	170	4	30
Reduced Calorie: *Estee*	70	0	12
Jell-O Snacks, sugar-free, ½ cup	60	1	13
Royal Flan,Van. sugar-free, ½ c.	80	0	21
Hunt's Snack Pack: *Per 3.5oz Cup*			
Puddings, average all flavors	120	3.5	22
Jell-O Puddings			
Pudding & Pie Filling: *Per ¼ Pkg*			
Cook & Serve, avg, prep.	100	0	22
Instant, regular, avg.	100	0	25
Fat & Sugar Free, avg.	30	0	8
Pudding Snacks: Fat-Free, 4 oz	100	0	23
Cheesecake Snack, Strawb. 3½ oz	130	2	26
Smoothie Snacks, 4 oz	100	2.5	18
Kozy Shack Puddings			
Regular Puddings:			
Chocolate, ½ cup, 4 oz	140	3.5	24
Key Lime, ½ cup	110	0	25
Low-Fat (1% Milk), 6-Pack,			
Avg., 1 pudding cup	110	1	20
No Sugar Added, 4-Pack:			
Apple Pie A-la-Mode	70	3	10
Chocolate, 1 pudding cup	90	3	11
Other flavors, avg., 1 cup	70	3	10
Flans: Creme Caramel, 1 cup	150	3.5	27
Restaurant Style, 1 cup	190	6	28
Rice Pudding: Orig., ½ cup, 4 oz	130	3	22
Cinnamon Raisin, ½ cup, 4 oz	140	3	24
European Style, ½ cup, 4 oz	130	3.5	22
No Sugar Added, 1 pudding cup	90	3	14
Rice, Country Peaches, ½ cup	140	4.5	23
Soy Puddings, avg., 1 cup	115	2	22
Tapioca: All Natural, 1 pudding cup	130	3	23
No Sugar Added, 1 pudding cup	90	3	11
Frozen Desserts: Cream Puffs (6)	260	20	15
Choc. Truffle Rolls (8)	240	13	27
Mini Eclairs (5)	250	16	23
Mini Napoleons (5)	280	14	35
Tiramisu, 1 cup	220	10	29
Kraft Handi Snacks: *Per Cup (3.5 oz)*			
"Doubles", avg. all flavors	100	1	22
Chocolate Pudding Fat-Free	90	0	21
Rice Pudding	140	6	19
Vanilla Pudding	90	1	20
Kroger: *Per Container*			
Butterscotch, 3½ oz	110	2	22
Chocolate, 3½ oz	110	2.5	21
President's Choice			
Key Lime Pie (36 oz), ⅛ pie, 4.5 oz	440	22	59
Mississippi Mud Pie (36 oz), ⅑, 4 oz	405	22	49

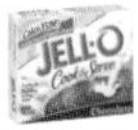

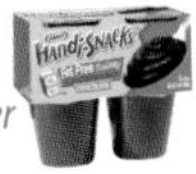

Ready-To-Serve (Cont) | C | F | Cb
	C	F	Cb
Swiss Miss Pudding Snacks: *Per 4 oz Cup*			
Chocolate, Low-Fat	130	2	26
Chocolate Vanilla Swirl	140	3.5	27
Creamy Vanilla	140	3.5	24
Milk/Dark Chocolate	150	3.5	27
Old Fashioned Tapioca	140	3.5	24

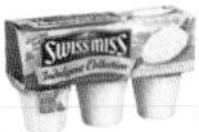

Homemade Puddings
	C	F	Cb
Apple Tapioca, ½ cup	150	0	32
Bread Pudding, ½ cup	250	8	40
Blancmange, ½ cup	140	5	19
Chocolate, ½ cup	190	6	30
Crème Brûlée, ½ cup	400	35	16
Plum Pudding, 2 oz	170	3	32
Rice with Raisins, ½ cup	200	4	38
Sponge Pudding, 3½ oz	340	16	45
Tapioca Cream, ½ cup	110	4	15
Trifle, ½ cup	180	7	26

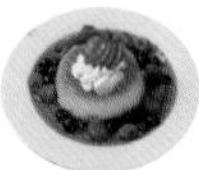

Custards
	C	F	Cb
Custard Mix: Dry, ⅙ pkg	85	1	17
Prep. w. 2% milk, ½ cup	140	3.5	21
Jello Flan, w. 2% milk, ½ cup	140	2.5	20
Royal-Flan: Prep. w. 2% milk, ½ c.	130	2.5	18
Homemade Custard			
Baked: Plain, ½ cup, 4½ oz	150	7	16
w. skim milk, artif. sweetened	70	3	4
Boiled, ½ cup	165	7	18

Meringues
	C	F	Cb
Meringue Swirl, ½ oz	50	0	8
Meringue Shell, 1 oz shell	100	0	16

Gelatin • Parfait • Jell-O
	C	F	Cb
Gelatin Mix: *Jell-O, Royal ~ Made Up*			
Regular, all flavors, ½ cup	80	0	18
Sugar Free/Low Calorie, ½ cup	10	0	0
Creme Gelatin/Parfait: *Per ½ Cup*			
Ida Mae, ½ cup	60	2	10
Reser's, Dessert Parfait (110g)	100	2	19
Gel Snacks *(Jell-O):* Regular, 3.5 oz	90	0	22
X-Treme Snacks:			
Cherry/Raspb., 3½ oz	70	0	17
Watermelon/Apple, 3½ oz	100	0	24

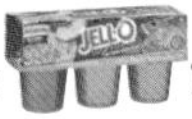

Chicken Eggs

Fresh Eggs

Raw (weight with shell):	C	F	Cb
Small, 40g	65	4	0
Medium, 44g	70	4	0
Large, 50g	75	4.5	0
Extra Large, 56g	80	5	0
Jumbo, 63g	90	5.5	0
Egg Yolk, 1 extra large	63	5	0
Egg White, 1 extra large	16	0	0

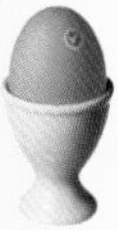

Dried Egg Powder

	C	F	Cb
Whole Egg, ¼ cup, 1 oz	170	12	0
1 Tbsp	30	2	0
Egg White, ¼ cup, 1 oz	105	0	0
Egg Yolk, ¼ cup, 1 oz	195	18	0

Egg Substitutes

¼ Cup (Equivalent to 1 Egg) ~ Zero Cholesterol.

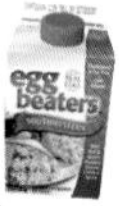

	C	F	Cb
Better 'n Eggs (*Papetti*), ¼ cup, 2 oz	30	0	1
Egg Beaters (*Fleischmann's*) Frozen/Liquid, Regular/Flavors, ¼ c., 2.2 oz	30	0	1
Ener-G, Egg Replacer, 1½ tsp, 4 g	15	0	4
Egg Substitute (*Albertson's*), ¼ c.	30	0	1
Egg Whites, 4 Tbsp, ¼ cup, 2 oz	30	0	0
Nature Egg, Simply Egg White, ¼ c., 2 oz	25	0	0
Second Nature, Fat-Free, ¼ c., 2 fl.oz	35	0	1

Other Eggs

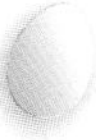

	C	F	Cb
Duck, 1 large, 2½ oz	130	9.5	0
Goose, 1 large, 5 oz	280	19	0
Quail, 3 eggs, 1 oz	42	3	0
Turkey, 1 large, 3 oz	135	9.5	0
Turtle, 1 egg, 1¾ oz	75	5	0

Omega-3 Fat Enriched

	C	F	Cb
Eggland's Best, 1 large	70	4	0
Eggs Plus (*Pilgrim's Pride*), 1 large	70	4.5	1

Note: Cholesterol content same as regular eggs, but Omega-3 fats inhibit blood cholesterol increase. (Extra Notes ~ See Page 271)

Updated Nutrition Data ~ www.CalorieKing.com
Persons with Diabetes ~ See Disclaimer (Page 24)

Cooked Eggs   C F Cb

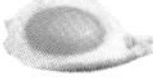

	C	F	Cb
Boiled Egg: Same as raw egg			
Hard-Cooked (*Egg·Lands*), Peeled	60	3.5	0
Fried Egg:			
With fat: 1 large egg	105	9	0.5
2 small eggs	175	13	1
No fat/nonstick pan, 1 large	75	5	0.5
Deviled Egg, 2 halves	145	13	0.5
Eggs Benedict (2) on toast or English muffin	860	56	25
Eggs Florentine (2) on toast or English Muffin	890	59	25
Pickled Egg, 1 large	80	5.5	0
Poached Egg, 1 large	65	4	0
Quiche (Homemade, average):			
Egg & Bacon, 1 slice, 5.3 oz	580	43	27
Ham & Cheese, 1 slice, 5.3 oz	475	33	29
Scotch Egg, 1 egg	300	21	16
Scrambled Eggs: 1 large egg:			
w. 1 Tbsp milk + 1 tsp fat	120	9	1
w. 1 Tbsp skim milk/no fat	85	5.5	1
2 large eggs:			
w. 2 Tbsp milk + 2 tsp fat	260	20	2
w. 2 Tbsp skim milk/no fat	180	11	2

Omelets

	C	F	Cb
1 Egg: Plain (w. 1 tsp fat)	125	10	0.5
with ½ oz cheese	175	15	0.5
w. ½ oz cheese + ½ oz ham	200	16	0.5
2 Eggs: Plain (w. 2 tsp fat)	250	20	1
with 1 oz cheese	360	29	2
w. 1 oz cheese+1 oz ham	410	32	2
3 Eggs: Plain (w. 1 Tbsp fat)	360	29	1.5
w. 2 oz cheese	580	47	2.5
w. 2 oz cheese+2 oz ham	680	53	2.5
Extras: Tomato/Onion/Veggies	20	0	4.5
Egg Substitute (*EggBeaters*):			
2 eggs (½ cup) + 1 tsp fat	100	4	2
3 eggs (¾ cup) + 2 tsp fat	160	8	3
Extras: 1 oz cheese	110	9	1
1 oz ham	50	3	1
Tom./Onion/Veggies	20	0	4.5

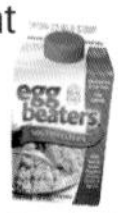

Egg Nog   ~ Per ½ Cup (4 fl.oz)

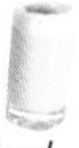

	C	F	Cb
Average all Brands, ½ cup	170	9.5	17
Regular: *Borden*	160	9	17
Hood (Golden)	180	9	22
Light/Low-Fat: *Horizon; Hood*	140	4	22

Breakfast Sides

	C	F	Cb
Toast: Plain, 1 thick slice	85	1	13
with 2 tsp butter/marg.	155	9	13
with 3 tsp/1 Tbsp fat	190	13	13
English Muffin: Plain, 2 oz	130	1	26
with 3 tsp fat	230	12	26
Bacon, 2 strips	70	5	0
Ham, Lean, 2 oz	100	3	0
Hash Browns:			
½ cup, 3 oz	125	6.5	14
1 cup serving, 6 oz	250	13	28
Sausages, 2 links (1 oz ea.)	180	16	1.5

Frozen Egg Breakfasts

	C	F	Cb
Aunt Jemima Great Starts: *Per Package*			
Griddle Cake w. Ham, Egg, Cheese	240	8	33
Sausage, Egg & Cheese Biscuit	340	21	27
Sausage, Egg & Cheese Croissant	350	23	22
Jimmy Dean			
Biscuit, Sausage, Egg & Cheese (1)	440	31	27
Croissant: Ham & Cheese (1)	280	13	29
Sausage, Egg & Cheese (1)	430	29	30
Muffin, Sausage, Egg & Cheese	350	21	28
Omelet: 3 Cheese (1)	290	23	4
Ham & Cheese (1)	250	19	4
Pillsbury: Toaster Scrambles,			
Cheese Sauce, Egg & Bacon	180	12	16
Cheese Sauce, Egg & Sausage	180	11	16
Red Baron			
Scrambles: Bacon (1), 5 oz	390	19	37
Sausage (1), 5 oz	360	17	37
Western (1), 5 oz	370	17	37
Swanson Great Starts			
Frozen Pancake/Waffles: *See Page 122*			

Frozen Egg Rolls

	C	F	Cb
Chun King/La Choy: *Average All Brands*			
Chicken Egg Rolls, Mini, 6 rolls	210	9	25
Pork & Shrimp Egg Rolls:			
Mini, 6 rolls, 3 oz	210	9	27
Shrimp Egg Rolls, Mini, 6 rolls	190	6	28
Lotus: Pork, 3.8 oz	180	7	18
Vegetable, 3.8 oz	70	1.5	13
Kahiki: Pork, 3 oz	140	3.5	20
Chicken, 3 oz	160	6	19
Vegetable Egg Roll, 3 oz	130	3.5	21

Fast-Foods/Restaurants

	C	F	Cb
Arby's: Bacon & Egg Croissant	335	22	23
Au Bon Pain: Scrambled Eggs, 6 oz	210	18	6
Bob Evans:			
Farmers Market Omelette	620	43	14
Ham & Cheddar Omelette	475	33	4
Three Cheese Omelette	490	37	4
Western Omelette	485	32	7
Bojangles: Egg Biscuit	400	30	26
Bacon, Egg & Cheese Biscuit	550	42	27
Bruegger's Bagels:			
Breakfast Sandwiches:			
Egg & Cheese	420	18	71
Egg, Cheese & Sausage	460	23	65
Burger King: Croissan'wich			
Bacon Egg & Cheese	350	19	27
Ham Egg & Cheese	340	17	28
Sausage & Cheese	380	24	26
Carl's Jr, Bacon & Egg Burrito	550	32	37
Chick-Fil-A			
Chicken, Egg & Cheese Bagel	500	20	49
Denny's: Sirloin Steak & Eggs	420	31	1
Omelette: Ham & Cheddar	590	44	4
Ultimate with Hash Browns	870	66	28
Veg.-Cheese w. Hash Browns	700	49	30
Del Taco, Egg & Cheese Burrito	450	24	39
Dunkin Donuts			
Bacon, Egg & Cheese Croissant	510	31	39
Ham, Egg & Cheese Bagel S/wich	520	17	75
Eat 'N Park: Cheese Omelette	390	30	2
Western Omelette	345	21	7
Hardee's: Big Country Bacon Platter	980	56	90
Loaded Omelet Biscuit	640	44	37
IHOP: T-Bone Steak & Eggs	1310	86	63
Colorado Omelette	790	68	5
Jack in the Box			
Bacon, Egg & Cheese Biscuit	440	25	37
McDonald's: Egg McMuffin	300	12	30
Bacon, Egg & Cheese Bisc., Reg.	420	23	37
Scrambled Eggs (2)	170	11	1
Whataburger			
Breakfast Platter w. Bacon (2 sl.)	740	45	53

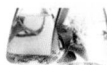

Fats ◇ Spreads & Oils (F)

Quick Guide **C F Cb**

Butter & Margarine
Average All Brands

	C	F	Cb
Regular: 1 tsp (5g)	35	4	0
1 Pat/Single Portion, 5g	35	4	0
1 Tbsp, approx. ½ oz	100	11	0
2 Tbsp, 1 oz	205	23	0
1 Stick, ½ cup, 4 oz	815	92	0
1 Pound, 2 cups, 16 oz	3260	368	0
Light (Regular) 40% Fat:			
1 tsp (5g)	25	3	0
1 Tbsp, ½ oz	75	8.5	0
2 Tbsp, 1 oz	150	16	0
Whipped Butter (Regular):			
1 tsp (4 g)	30	3	0
1 Tbsp (10g)	70	7.5	0
1 Stick, ½ cup, 2 ⅔ oz	545	62	0
Whipped Light Butter (40% Fat):			
1 tsp, 5g	25	3	0.5
1 Tbsp, 9g	45	5	1
2 Tbsp, 18g	90	10	2
Unsalted: Same as Regular			

Flavored Butter/Spreads
Average All Brands

	C	F	Cb
Honey Butter (60% Fat):			
1 Tbsp, ½ oz	90	8	4
Downey's, 1 Tbsp, ½ oz	60	1	11
Garlic Butter (80% Fat):			
1 Tbsp, ½ oz	100	11	0
Sweet Cream Butter:			
Regular, 1 Tbsp	100	11	0
Stick *(Parkay),* 70% Fat, 1 Tbsp	90	10	0
Tub *(Land O'Lakes),* 60% Fat, 1 T.	80	8	0

Ghee (Clarified Butter)

(Example: *Purity Farms*)
Note: Ghee is 100% fat compared to regular butter (80% fat + 20% water)

	C	F	Cb
1 tsp (5g)	45	5	0
1 Tbsp, ½ oz	120	14	0
2¼ Tbsp, 1 oz	250	28	0

Light & Reduced Fat Spreads
Per 1 Tbsp, ½ oz (Unless Stated) **C F Cb**

	C	F	Cb
Albertson's: Country (48%), 1 T.	60	7	0
Butter Blend, 1 Tbsp	80	9	0
Benecol: Spread, 1 T., 14g	70	8	0
Light, Spread, 1 T., 14g	50	5	0
Blue Bonnet, Homestyle (48% Veg Oil)	60	7	0
Brummel & Brown, Spread, 1 T.	45	5	0
Country Crock *(Shedd's):* Regular	60	7	0
Light; Calcium & Vitamins	50	5	0
Spreadable Butter, 1 Tbsp	80	9	0
Downey's, Honey Butter, 1 Tbsp	60	1	11
Fleischmann's: Soft Spread	70	8	0
Original Stick, 1 Tbsp	100	11	0
Light Spread, 1 Tbsp	40	4.5	0
'I Can't Believe It's Not Butter': Reg.	80	8	0
Light Soft Spread	50	5	0
Imperial: Stick, 1 Tbsp	80	8	0
Tub, 1 Tbsp	50	5	0
Land O'Lakes: Butter in Half, 1 T.	100	11	0
Honey Butter, 1 Tbsp	90	8	4
Light Butter Whipped	50	6	0
Light Butter, 1 Tbsp	50	6	0
Parkay: Squeeze, 1 Tbsp	70	8	0
Light Spread, 1 Tbsp	50	5	0
Original Stick, 1 Tbsp	80	9	0
Original Spread, 1 Tbsp	60	7	0
Promise: Buttery, 1 Tbsp	80	8	0
Fat-Free, 1 Tbsp	5	0	0
Light, 1 Tbsp	45	5	0
Smart Balance: 67% Buttery, 1 T.	80	9	0
Heart Right, 1 Tbsp	80	8	0
Light (37%), 1 Tbsp	45	5	0
Omega Plus, 1 Tbsp	80	9	0
Smart Beat, Fat-Free, 1 Tbsp	50	0	1
Smart Squeeze, 1 Tbsp	5	0	1

Butter Substitutes

	C	F	Cb
Butter Buds: 1 serving, ½ tsp	5	0	2
Sprinkles, 1 tsp	5	0	0
Earth Balance, Non GMO,1 Tbsp	100	11	0
Molly McButter, ½ tsp	5	0	1
Shedd's Willow Run, Soy, 1 T.	100	11	0
Sunsweet, Lighter Bake, 1Tbsp, 19g (Butter/Oil Replacement)	35	0	9

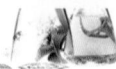

Spreads Comparison · C · F · Cb

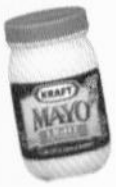

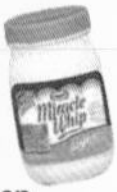

	C	F	Cb
Mayonnaise: Regular, 1 T.	90	10	0
Light, average, 1 Tbsp	45	0	2
Fat-Free, 1 Tbsp	10	0	2
Miracle Whip (Kraft):			
Regular, 1 Tbsp	40	3	2
Light, 1 Tbsp	25	1.5	3
Free, 1 Tbsp	15	0	3
Smart Beat Dressing: 1 Tbsp	10	0	3

Extra Listings for Mayonnaise & Dressings
~ See Page 89 ~

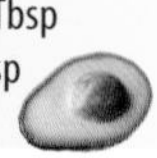

	C	F	Cb
Avocado, mashed, 1 Tbsp	45	4	2.5
Peanut Butter, 1 Tbsp	100	8	3.5
Nutella, 1 Tbsp	95	5.5	11

Animal Fats/Lards · C · F · Cb

Average All Types
Beef Tallow/Drippings, Lard (Pork), Chicken, Duck, Goose, Turkey.

	C	F	Cb
1 Tbsp (13g)	115	13	0
2¼ Tbsp, 1 oz	255	28	0
1 cup, 7¼ oz	1850	205	0
½ pound, 8 oz	2040	227	0
Ghee/Butter Oil: 1 Tbsp, ½ oz	120	14	0
2¼ Tbsp, 1 oz	250	28	0

Vegetable Shortening

Average All Types (example: Crisco)

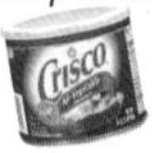

	C	F	Cb
1 Tbsp, 13g	115	13	0
2¼ Tbsp, 1 oz	250	28	0
1 cup, 7¼ oz	1810	205	0

Vegetable Oils

Includes almond, avocado, canola, corn, coconut, flaxseed, grapeseed, linseed, mustard, olive, palm, peanut, rice bran, safflower, sesame, sunflower, soybean, wheat germ. Note: Oil is 100% fat.

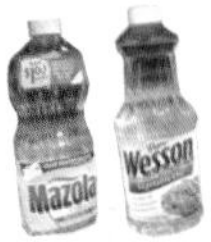

	C	F	Cb
1 tsp, 5g	45	5	0
1 Tbsp, ½ oz	120	14	0
2 Tbsp, 1 oz	250	28	0
1 cup, 7¾ oz	1930	205	0

Fish Oils

Average All Types (Includes cod liver, herring, salmon, sardine): 1 Tbsp, ½ oz **125 14 0**

Cooking Sprays/Squeezes

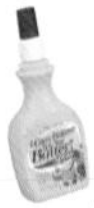

Cooking Sprays *(PAM, Mazola, I Can't Believe It's Not Butter, Weight Watchers, Wesson):*

Per serving	2	0	0
1-3 second spray	6	1	0
I Can't Believe It's Not Butter			
Parkay Buttery Spray	0	0	0
Squeeze (Parkay), 1 Tbsp, ½ oz	70	8	0

Olestra (Olean)

Olestra *(Olean)*	0	0	0

Note: *Olean is Proctor & Gamble's* brand name for olestra – a no-calorie cooking oil that gives snacks (like potato chips, tortilla chips and crackers) taste and texture without adding fat or calories.

Examples:
- *Frito-Lay* Light Products
  (Lays, Ruffles, Tostitos, Doritos)
- *Pringles* Fat-Free Potato Crisps

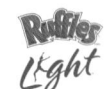

Quick Guide

Mayonnaise

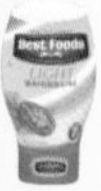

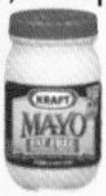

	C	F	Cb
Regular			
Average All Brands, 1 Tbsp	90	10	0
Best Foods, Kraft, 1 Tbsp	90	10	0
½ cup, 4 oz	720	80	0
Light/Reduced Fat			
Kraft, 1 Tbsp	45	4	2
Best Foods, 1 Tbsp	35	3.5	1
Hain, Safflower Oil, 1 Tbsp	100	11	0
Hellman's, 1 Tbsp	90	10	0
Smart Balance, Omega, 1 Tbsp	50	4.5	2
Spectrum: Canola Mayo, 1 Tbsp	100	11	0
Light Canola Mayo Eggless, 1 Tbsp	35	3.5	0
Fat Free			
Kraft: 1 Tbsp	10	0	2
½ cup, 4 oz	80	0	16
Smart Beat, 1 Tbsp	10	0	3
Sugar Free: Dukes Mayo, 1 Tbsp	100	12	0

Mayonnaise Style Dressing

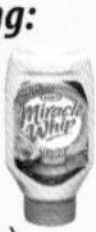

	C	F	Cb
Best Foods Sandwich Spread, 1 T.	60	5	2
Miracle Whip Salad Dressing:			
Regular, 1 Tbsp, ½ oz	35	3	2
Light, 1 Tbsp, ½ oz	25	1.5	3
Free, 1 Tbsp, ½ oz	15	0	3
Nayonaise (Nasoya)			
(Tofu Base/Dairy Free/Eggless)			
Regular, 1 Tbsp, ½ oz	35	3.5	1
Fat-Free, 1 Tbsp, ½ oz	10	0	2

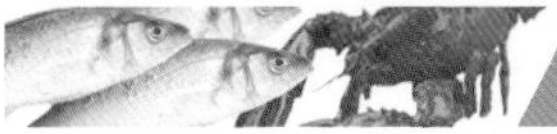

Quick Guide

Fresh Fish   🅒 🅕 🅒ᵇ

Low Oil (Less than 2.5% fat)
White/Lightly-colored flesh. Examples:
Cod, Flounder, Haddock, Halibut, Mahi Mahi,
Perch, Pike, Pollock, Snapper, Sole, Whiting.

Per 4 oz Edible Portion

	C	F	Cb
Raw, 4 oz (no bones)	90	1	0
Steamed, Broiled, Baked	130	1	0
Fried: Lightly Floured	210	8	3.5
Breaded	260	12	8
In Batter	320	16	27

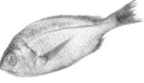

Medium Oil (2.5-5% fat)
Lightly-colored flesh. Examples: 🅒 🅕 🅒ᵇ
Bluefin Tuna, Catfish, Kingfish, Orange Roughy,
Salmon (Pink), Swordfish, Rainbow Trout, Yellowtail.

Raw, 4 oz (no bones)	140	5	0
Baked, Broiled, 4 oz	175	6	0
Fried, 4 oz	230	11	8

High Oil (Over 5% fat) 🅒 🅕 🅒ᵇ
Darker-colored flesh. Examples:
Albacore Tuna, Bluefish, Herring, Mackerel,
Salmon (Atl./Chinook/Sockeye), Sardines, Trout,
Whitefish.

Raw, 4 oz (no bones)	230	16	0
Baked, Broiled, 4 oz	275	17	0
Fried, 4 oz	340	23	12

Cooking Yields (Fin Fish):
4 oz Raw wt. = 3½ oz Cooked wt.
4 oz Cooked wt. = 5 oz Raw wt.

Calorie & Fat Variations
The amount of fat/oil in fish varies with the species,
season and locality. Within the same fish, fat/oil content
is generally higher towards the head.

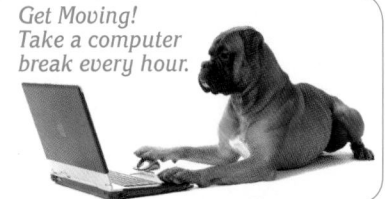

Get Moving!
Take a computer
break every hour.

Fish & Shellfish   🅒 🅕 🅒ᵇ

Edible Weights: (no bones/shell)

	C	F	Cb
Abalone, Raw, 3 oz	90	0.5	5
Ahi Tuna, grilled, 6 oz fillet (no fat)	235	2	0
Anchovy: Paste, 1 Tbsp, ¼ oz	15	1	0.5
Cnd. in oil, drnd., 5 only, ¾ oz	40	2	0
Pickled, 1 oz	50	3	0
Barracuda (Pacific), raw, 4 oz	130	3	0
Bass: Sea, raw, 4.6 oz fillet	125	2.5	0
Striped: Raw, 1 fillet, 5½ oz	150	3.5	0
Baked, 3 oz	105	3	0
Blue Fish: Raw, 1 fillet, 5¼ oz	185	6.5	0
Baked, 3 oz	130	5	0
Butterfish, raw, 3 oz	125	7	0
Cajun & Creole Dishes: *See Page 176*			
Calamari, breaded/fried, 7 oz	350	15	16
Carp, raw, 3 oz	110	5	0
Catfish (Wild): Raw, 4 oz	110	3	0
Fried, breaded, 1 fillet, 3 oz	200	12	7
Baked, 3 oz	90	2.5	0
Caviar, black/red, 1 Tbsp, 16g	40	3	0.5
Clams: Raw, 3 oz (4 lge/9 small)	65	1	2
Fried, breaded, 6.6 oz (20 small)	380	21	20
Canned, drained, ½ cup, 2½ oz	120	1.5	4
Minced, ¼ cup, 2 oz	25	0	2
Clam Juice: (*Snow's*) 1 Tbsp	0	0	0
Cod, Atlantic/Pacific: Raw, 4 oz	95	1	0
Baked/Broiled, 1 fillet, 6¼ oz	190	2	0
Canned, 3 oz	90	1	0
Minced, ¼ cup, 2 oz	25	0	0
Smoked/Dry Heat, 3 oz	90	1	0
Crab: Alaska King, raw, 1 leg, 6 oz	145	1	0
1 leg, cooked, 4¾ oz	130	2	0
Blue: Raw, 1 crab			
(⅓ lb whole crab, ¾ oz flesh)	20	0.2	0
Steamed, 3 oz	85	1	0
Canned, drained, ½ cup, 2½ oz	65	1	0
Dungeness, 1 crab, 5¾ oz edible			
(from 1½ lb whole crab)	180	2	2
Imitation Crab Legs/Stix, 3oz	80	0.5	13
Crab Cakes (Low-fat), (1), 2 oz	95	4.5	0.5
Regular (1), 3 oz	130	6.5	0.5
Crab Legs, restaurant (*Red Lobster*)	260	4.5	0
Crayfish, raw, 4 oz (edible)	90	1	0
Croaker, raw, 3 oz	90	3	0
Cuttlefish, raw, 3 oz	70	1	1
Dolphinfish, raw, 1 fillet, 7 oz	175	1.5	0
Eel: Raw, 3 oz	155	10	0
Smoked/Dry Heat, 3 oz	200	13	0
Fish & Chips: *Arthur Treacher*	1540	101	132
Denny's, no condiments	960	54	83
Fish S'wich w. Tartar Sce, 5½ oz	430	23	41
Fish Sticks (1), frozen, breaded, 1 oz	70	3.5	6

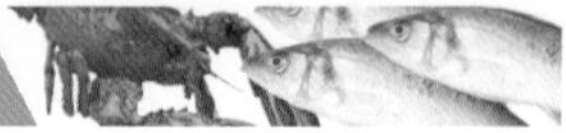

Fish & Shellfish (Cont)

Edible Weights: (no bones/shell)	C	F	Cb
Fish Oil, 1 Tbsp, ½ oz	125	14	0
Flounder/Sole: Raw, 4 oz	105	1.5	0
Baked, 1 fillet, 4½ oz	150	2	0
Frozen Fish & Entrees: *See Page 113-124*			
Gefilte Fish: *See Kosher/Deli Foods, Page 178*			
Grouper, raw, 4 oz	105	1	0
Haddock: Raw, 4 oz	100	1	0
Broiled, 1 fillet, 5¼ oz	170	1.5	0
Smoked, 3 oz	100	1	0
Baked, 3 oz	95	1	0
Halibut: Raw, 4 oz	125	3	0
Baked, ½ fillet, 2¾ oz	225	5	0
Herring: Atlantic, raw, 4 oz	180	10	0
Pickled, 2 pieces, 1 oz	80	5	3
In Sour Cream, 1 oz	55	3	5
Party Snacks, ¼ cup, dr., 2 oz	120	5	0
Rollmops, 1½ oz	110	8	6
Canned: Plain, drained, 3 oz	130	8	0
in Tomato Sauce, 3.5 oz	140	8	2
Smoked, kippered, 4 oz	245	14	0
Jellyfish: Raw, 4 oz	30	0	0
Dried, Salted, 1 cup, 2 oz	20	1	0
King Fish, raw, 4 oz	120	2.5	0
Ling, raw, 4 oz	100	0.5	0
Lobster, Northern: Raw, 4 oz	105	1	0.5
1 Lobster, 6¼ oz			
(from 1½ lb whole lobster)	160	1.5	1
Cooked, 1 cup, 5 oz	140	1	2
Lobster Newberg, avg. ¾ cup	360	20	9
Lobster Thermidor, avg. 1 serving	370	22	15
Lobster Salads, avg. ½ cup	220	13	5
Lobster Tail, restaurant *(Red Lobster)*	260	3	0
Lomi Salmon, ¼ cup, 4 oz	20	1	3
Lox, Regular/Nova, 2 oz	65	2.5	0
Mackerel: Atlantic, raw, 4 oz	230	16	0
Broiled, 3 oz fillet	230	16	0
Jack, canned, ½ c., 3⅓ oz	150	6	0
King, raw, 4 oz	120	2	0
Pacific/Jack: Raw, 4 oz	180	9	0
Broiled, 3 oz	170	9	0
Spanish, raw, 4 oz	160	7	0
Mahi-Mahi, raw, 4 oz	125	1	0
Milkfish, raw, 4 oz	170	7.5	0
Monkfish: Raw, 4 oz	85	1.5	0
Baked, 3 oz	80	2	0
Mullet, striped, raw, 4 oz	135	4.5	0
Mussels: Raw, 4 oz (edible wt.)	100	2.5	4
1 cup, 5¼ oz (edible wt.)	130	3.5	5
Cooked, moist heat, 3 oz	150	4	6

	C	F	Cb
Ocean Perch: Raw, 4 oz	105	2	0
Baked, 3 oz	105	2	0
Octopus, common, raw, 4 oz	95	1	2.5
Orange Roughy, raw, 4 oz	85	1	0
Oysters: Common, raw, 4 oz	70	2	4
Eastern raw: 6 medium, 3 oz	50	1.5	4.5
1 cup, 8¾ oz	150	4	14
Fried/breaded, 6 med., 3 oz	170	11	10
Pacific, raw, 1 med., 1¾ oz	40	1	2
Oysters Rockefeller, 3 oysters	220	13	12
Perch, average, raw, 4 oz	105	1	0
Pike: Northern, raw, 4 oz	100	1	0
Walleye, raw, 4 oz	105	1.5	0
Pollock, raw, 4 oz	105	1	0
Pout (Ocean), raw, 4 oz	90	1	0
Pompano, Florida, raw, 4 oz	185	11	0
Porgy/Scup, raw, 4 oz	150	4	0
Quahogs ~ See Clams			
Red-Snapper, raw, 4 oz	115	1.5	0
Rockfish, Pacific, raw, 4 oz	110	2	0
Roe, raw, 2 Tbsp, 1 oz	40	2	0.5
Sablefish: Raw, 4 oz	220	17	0
Smoked, 3 oz	220	17	0
Salmon:			
Raw: Chinook, 4 oz	205	12	0
Atlantic; Coho/Silver, 4 oz	210	12	0
Chum; Pink, 4 oz	135	4	0
Red/Sockeye, 4 oz	190	10	0
Baked: Atlantic/Coho, 3 oz	160	5	0
Smoked Salmon: Chinook, 3 oz	100	4	0
Pacific Supreme, 2 oz	100	4	0
Canned Salmon: *Average All Brands*			
Pink: 1 oz	40	2	0
¼ cup, 63g (2.2 oz)	90	5	0
3¾ oz can, whole	155	8.5	0
7½ oz can, whole	300	17	0
Skinless/boneless, ¼ c., 2 oz	70	2	0
Red Sockeye: 1 oz	50	3	0
¼ cup, 63g (2.2 oz)	110	7	0
3¾ oz can, whole	190	12	0
Atlantic, ½ cup, 3½ oz	230	14	0
Chinook/King, ½ cup	210	14	0
Chum, ½ cup, 3½ oz	140	5	0
Coho/Silver, ½ cup	155	5	0
Atlantic Steaks: Small, 8 oz	320	14	0
Medium, 12 oz	480	21	0
Large, 16 oz	640	28	0
Salmon Cake, take-out, 3 oz	240	15	6

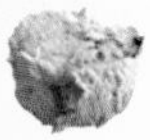

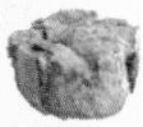

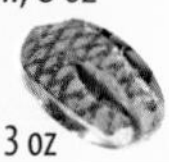

Fish (Cont)

	C	F	Cb
Sardines (Canned): *Average All Brands*			
In Oil, undrained, 1 oz	85	7	0
Drained of oil, 1 oz	60	3	0
3¾ oz can, drained, (3¼ oz)	190	11	0
1 lge/2 med. ⅗ " small, 0.8 oz	50	3	0
In Tom./ Mustard Sce, 1 oz	55	3	0
3¾ oz can (3 sardines)	210	12	1
Sashimi: *See Japanese Foods, Page 178*			
Scallop: Raw, 6 lge/15 small, 3 oz	80	0.5	2
Breaded/fried, 6 pces, 3½ oz	200	10	10
Sea Bass, raw, 4 oz	110	2	0
Seafood Salad, (Deli Style), ½ cup, 3.5 oz	250	21	11
Shark: Raw, 4 oz	150	5	0
Batter-dipped, fried, 4 oz	220	13	6
Baked, 4 oz	185	7	0
Shark Fin, dried, 1 oz	30	0	0
Shrimp: Raw, in shell, ½ lb	140	2	1.5
Raw, shelled, 3 oz (12 lge)	90	1.5	0.5
Breaded/fried, 3 oz (11 lge)	210	11	10
Canned, 1 oz (10 shrimp)	30	0.5	0
Tiger, cooked, 1 shrimp, ½ oz	15	0.5	0
Battered, fried, 1 shrimp	60	4	3
Shrimp Cocktail, restaurant-style	140	2	1
Smelt, Rainbow, raw, 4 oz	110	3	0
Snapper: Raw, 3 oz	85	1	0
Cooked, 1 fillet, 6 oz	220	3	0
Sole, Raw, 4 oz	105	1.5	0
Squid: Raw, 4 oz	105	1.5	3.5
Fried, 3 oz	150	6	7
Surimi (Imitation Crab), 4 oz	110	0.5	17
Sweet & Sour Fish, ½ dish, 10 oz	580	29	53
Swordfish raw:			
Small Steak, 4 oz	135	4.5	0
Medium Steak, 6 oz	205	7	0
Tilapia, Rain Forest Fillets, 4 oz	110	2	0
Trout, Rainbow: Raw, 4 oz	135	4	0
Broiled, 3 oz	125	5	0
Smoked, 2 oz	110	6	0
Tuna: *Average All Brands*			
Raw: Albacore, 4 oz	190	8	0
Bluefin, 4 oz	165	5.5	0
Skipjack, Yellowfin, 4 oz	125	1	0
Broiled, 3 oz	115	1	0
Canned:			
In Water, drained:			
Chunk/Solid: 2 oz can	75	1.5	0
3 oz can	110	2.5	0
6 oz can	220	5	0
In Oil, drained:			
Chunk Light: 2 oz	110	5	0
6 oz can, drained	315	14	0

Tuna (Cont)	C	F	Cb
Solid White, 2 oz	105	4.5	0
6.3 oz can, drained	330	14	0
Tuna Salad: Deli Style, ½ c., 4oz	300	24	15
Lower fat, 4 oz	210	10	11
Whitefish: Raw, 4 oz	150	6.5	0
Baked, 3 oz	145	6.5	1
Smoked, 3 oz	90	1	0
Whiting: Raw, 4 oz	100	1.5	0
Baked, 3 oz	100	1.5	0
Yellowtail: Raw, 4 oz	165	6	0
Grilled, 3 oz (from 4 oz raw)	160	6	0

Other Canned/Packaged Fish

	C	F	Cb
Bumble Bee:			
Tuna Salad Kit: Original	300	22	18
Fat-Free Kit	150	1.5	24
w. Mayonnaise Kit	420	23	24
Seafood Salad w. Crab Kit	180	5.5	27
Sensations Bowls: Spring Thai Chili	160	7	9
Other varieties, average	110	4	2
Lunch on the Run, Tuna Salad Kit	560	31	59
Chicken of the Sea			
Albacore Tuna in Water, 2.5 oz pouch	80	2	0
Light Tuna in Oil, 3 oz pouch	100	4	0
Prime Fillet Pink Salmon Steaks, 4 oz	150	4.5	2
Shrimp, Regular, Broken, 6 oz can	120	0	0
Starkist			
Pouch: *Per 3 oz Pouch, Drained*			
Tuna Chunk Light, in water, 2 oz	60	0.5	1
Albacore Tuna, in water, 2 oz	70	1.5	1
Lunch-To-Go Kit: Chunk Light Tuna w. Mayo/Crackers, 4.5 oz	240	9	20
Tuna Creations, all varieties, 2 oz	70	1	0

Frozen Fish Products

Gorton's: *Page 120*
Kroger: *Page 121*
Van De Kamp's: *Page 124*
Restaurant Chains: *Page 182*
Captain D's Seafood: *Page 94*
Long John Silver's: *Page 221*
Shoney's: *Page 249*
Southern Tsunami: *Page 253*
Wahoo's Fish Taco: *Page 265*

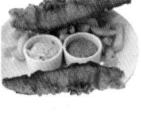

Flours & Grains

	C	F	Cb
Amaranth Flour, ½ cup, 3½ oz	365	6.5	65
Arrowroot Flour, ½ cup, 2¼ oz	230	0	56
Barley: Regular, ½ cup, 2.6 oz	255	1	55
Pearled, raw, 3½ oz	350	1	78
Buckwheat: Regular, ½ c., 3 oz	290	3	61
Groats: Roasted, dry, ½ c., 2.9 oz	285	2	62
Roasted, cooked, 3½ oz	80	0.5	17
Flour, whole-groat, ½ cup, 2 oz	200	2	42
Bulgur: Dry, ½ cup, 2½ oz	240	1	53
Cooked, ½ cup, 3.2 oz	75	0.5	17
Carob Flour, ½ cup, 1.8 oz	115	0.5	46
Corn Kernels avg., ckd, ½ c.	80	0.5	18
Corn Bran, ½ cup, 1.3 oz	85	1	33
Corn Flour/Masa, ½ cup, 2 oz	215	2.5	43
Corn Grits: Dry, ½ cup, 2¾ oz	290	1	62
Cooked, ½ cup, 4¼ oz	70	0.5	15
Corn Germ, toasted, ½ cup, 4 oz	100	1.5	22
Cornmeal: Average all Types,			
3 Tbsp, 1 oz	105	0.5	22
½ cup, 2½ oz	255	1	54
Mixes: same as above	230	1	48
Made Up, ½ cup, 4.8 oz	95	0.5	20
Cornstarch: 1 Tbsp, 8g	30	0	8
½ cup, 2¼ oz	245	0	58
Couscous: Dry, 1 oz (yield 3 oz ckd)	110	0	22
1 cup cooked, 5½ oz	175	0.5	37
Farina: Dry, ½ cup, 3.1 oz	325	0.5	69
Cooked, ½ cup, 4.1 oz	55	0	12
Flaxseed: Seeds, 1 Tbsp, 8g	45	3.5	2
Ground, 2 Tbsp, 8g	60	4.5	4
Garbanzo (Chick Pea), ½ c., 1.6 oz	180	3	27
Kuzu Root Starch, 1 Tbsp, 10g	35	0	9
Matzo Meal, ½ cup, 2.2 oz	230	0.5	48
Millet: Raw, ½ cup, 3½ oz	380	4	73
Cooked, ½ cup, 3 oz	105	1	21
Oat Bran: Raw, ⅓cup, 1.1 oz	75	2	21
Cooked, ½ cup, 3¾ oz	45	1	13
Oats, rolled/oatmeal:			
Dry/Groats, ½ cup, 1.5 oz	160	3	28
Cooked, ½ cup, 4.2 oz	75	1	13
Polenta: *See Cornmeal*			
Potato Flour, ½ cup, 2.8 oz	285	0.5	66
Psyllium Husks, 1 Tbsp (5g)	20	0	4
Quinoa: Dry ½ cup, 3 oz	320	5	59
Cooked, ½ cup, 3¾ oz	130	2	24
Rice Bran, ½ cup, 2 oz	180	12	28
Rice Flour, ½ cup, 2¾ oz	290	1	63

Flours & Grains (Cont)

	C	F	Cb
Rice Polish, ½ cup, 3½ oz	360	0.5	80
Rye Flour: Dark, ½ cup, 2.3 oz	210	2	44
Medium, ½ cup, 1.8 oz	180	1	40
Light, ½ cup, 1.8 oz	190	1	41
Rye Grain: ½ cup, 3 oz	280	2	59
Flakes, ¼ cup, 1 oz	100	0.5	21
Semolina, ½ cup, 3 oz	300	1	61
Sorghum, ½ cup, 3.4 oz	325	3	72
Soy Flour:			
Defatted, 1 cup, 3½ oz	330	1	38
Low-Fat, 1 cup, 3 oz	325	6	33
Full-Fat, 1 cup, 3 oz	365	17	29
Soy Meal, defatted, 1 cup, 4.3 oz	415	3	49
Spelt Flour, ½ cup, 2 oz	190	1	41
Tapioca, Pearl:			
Dry, ½ cup, 2.7 oz	270	0	67
3 Tbsp, 1 oz	100	0	25
Teff (Seed) Flour, 2 oz	215	2	42
Tortilla Flour Mix, ½ cup, 2 oz	220	6	37
Triticale: ½ cup, 3.4 oz	325	2	70
Flour, whole-grain, ½ c., 2.3 oz	220	1	48
Wheat Bran, unproc., ½ c., 1 oz	65	1	19
Wheat Flakes, ½ cup, 1½ oz	160	1	35
Wheat Germ: Raw, ¼ cup, 1 oz	105	3	15
Toasted, ¼ cup, 1 oz	110	3	14
Wheat Flour:			
White, All Purpose/Self-Rising,			
1 level Tbsp, 0.28 oz	30	0	6
½ cup, 2.2 oz	230	0.5	48
1 cup, 4.4 oz	455	1.5	95
Whole Wheat, 1 cup, 4.2 oz	405	2	87

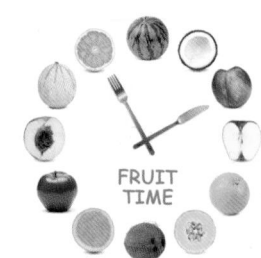

FRUIT TIME

not Quinoa Flakes

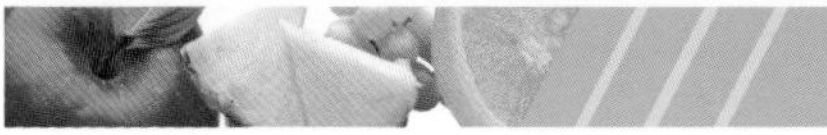

Weights As Purchased	C	F	Cb
Acerola, 1 cup, 20 pcs, 3½ oz	30	0	7.5
Apples: Whole, average all varieties,			
1 small (4 per lb), 4 oz	55	0	13
1 medium (3 per lb), 5½ oz	70	0	17
1 large (2 per lb), 8 oz	110	0	26
1 extra large, 11 oz	150	0	36
without skin: 1 medium, 4½ oz	60	0	14
1 cup slices, 4 oz	55	0	13
Candy/Caramel Apple, 1 med., 6½ oz	245	4	54
Nut Coated, 1 medium, 7 oz	325	11	56
Chiquita Apple Bites, 10 sl., 3½ oz	50	0	12
Apricots: 1 small (12 per lb)	17	0	4
1 medium (8 per lb), 2 oz	25	0	6
1 large (5-6 per lb), 3 oz	40	0	10
Asian Pear (Nashi Fruit), 1 med., 7 oz	85	0	21
Avocado (w/out seed/skin):			
Avg., ½ medium, 3½ oz	160	15	8
1 salad slice, ½ oz	25	2	1
Mashed/Puree, 2 Tbsp, 1 oz	50	4.5	2
¼ cup, 2 oz	90	9	5
Californian, ½ medium, 3 oz	160	14	8
Mashed/Puree, ½ c., 4 oz	190	18	10
Florida, ½ medium, 5½ oz	180	15	12
Mashed/Puree, ½ c., 4 oz	140	11	9
½ cup cubed, 3 oz	105	8	7
Banana, (weight with skin):			
1 small (6", 4 per lb), 4 oz	90	0	23
1 medium (7", 3 per lb), 5 oz	105	0	27
1 large (8"), 7 oz	120	0	30
1 extra large (9"), 9 oz	135	0	35
w/out skin, 1 oz	25	0	6
Black Raspberries, 1 cup, 5 oz	70	0	16
Blackberries, 1 Cup, 5 oz	60	0.5	14
Blueberries: Approx. 20, 1 oz	15	0	4
1 Cup, 5 oz	80	0.5	20
1 pint, 14 oz	225	1	57
Boysenberries, 1 cup, 4.5 oz	60	4.5	14
Breadfruit, ½ cup, 4 oz	115	0	30
Cactus Pear, 1 fruit, 3½ oz	40	0	9
Cantaloupe: Flesh (no rind), 1 oz	10	0	2
1 cup pieces/balls, 5.5 oz	55	0	13
½ Circle Slices (no rind):			
1 thin (¼"), 1 oz	10	0	2
1 medium (½"), 2 oz	20	0	5
1 thick (¾"), 3 oz	30	0	7
Wedges (Length cut, no rind):			
1 thin, 1/16 medium, 2 oz	20	0	5
1 thick, ⅛ medium, 4 oz	40	0	9
Whole (Weights with seeds and rind):			
½ small, 20 oz	195	1	46
½ medium, 28 oz	270	1.5	65
½ large, 2½ lb	370	2	90
Carambola (Starfruit), 1 med, 3 oz	30	0	6
Cassava, ⅓ cup, 2½ oz	115	0	27
Cherimoya, 1 cup, 5.5 oz	115	1	27

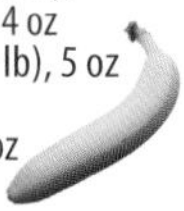

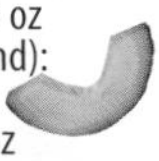

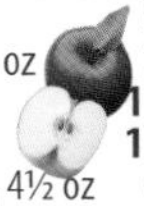

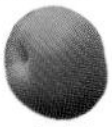

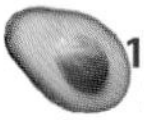

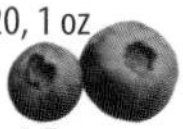

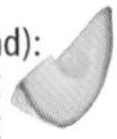

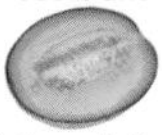

Weights As Purchased	C	F	Cb
Cherries: Sweet (Red/White), raw,			
8 cherries, 2 oz	30	0	8
1 cup, 4½ oz	75	0	19
½ lb (30 cherries)	130	0.5	32
Sour, red, raw, 1 cup, 4 oz	50	0	12
Clementine, 1 med., 2.6 oz	35	0	9
Coconut: Fresh,			
1 piece, 2"x2"x ½", 1 oz	100	10	4.5
Shredded, fresh, ½ cup, 1.4 oz	140	13	6
Sweetened, dried, ½ cup, 1.6 oz	235	16	22
Crabapples, ½ cup slices, 2 oz	40	0	11
Cranberries, ¼ cup, 1 oz	25	0	6.5
Currants, raw, ½ cup, 2 oz	35	0	8
Custard Apple, 4 oz, edible	115	1	28
(from 7 oz with skin/seeds)			
Dates: *See Dried Fruits*			
Dragon Fruit (Pitahaya),			
1 medium, 11½ oz	330	1.5	76
Durian, flesh, 4 oz	165	6	31
Elderberries, ½ cup, 2½ oz	55	0.5	13
Feijoa (Pineapple Guava),			
1 medium, 2 oz	30	0.5	5.5
Figs, green/black:			
1 medium, 2 oz	40	0	10
1 large, 3 oz	60	0	15
Gooseberries, raw, ½ c., 2½ oz	35	0	7
Grapefruit: Average all types,			
½ fruit, 10 oz (6 oz flesh)	55	0	13
1 cup sections w. juice, 8 oz	75	0	18
Grapes: Average, 1 cup, 5½ oz	105	0	28
1 small bunch, 4 oz	80	0	20
1 medium bunch, 7 oz	140	0	36
1 large bunch, 16 oz	315	0	82
Granadilla, flesh, 3½ oz	95	0	23
Guava: 1 medium, 4 oz	80	1	16
Honeydew: 1 slice, ¾" thick, 3 oz	30	0	7
1 wedge, ⅛ of 7" diam.),			
12 oz (with rind)	80	0	20
1 cup cubes/balls, 6 oz	60	0	14
½ small (4½ lb whole)	180	0.5	42
½ medium (6lb whole)	230	1	56
Honey Murcots, 1 only, 5 oz	45	0	11
Jaboticaba, flesh, 4 oz	75	2	15
Jackfruit, flesh, ⅛ average, 4 oz	105	0	27
Java-Plum, 4 plums, ½ oz	10	0	2
Jujube, 3 oz	65	0	17
Kiwifruit, 1 medium, 2.7 oz	45	0	11
1 large, 3.2 oz	55	0.5	13
Kumquats, 5 medium, 3½ oz	65	1	15
Kiwano, ½ medium, 5 oz	35	0	8
Langsat, Duku 1 medium, 2 oz	25	0	5
Lemon: 1 medium, 3 oz	25	0	8
1 wedge, 1 oz	5	0	1.5
Peel, grated, 1 Tbsp	5	0	1

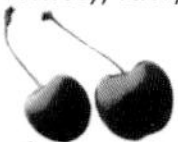

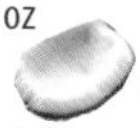

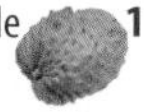

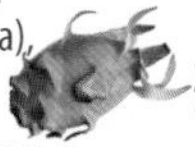

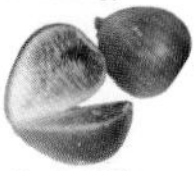

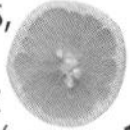

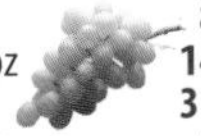

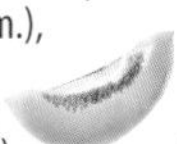

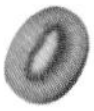

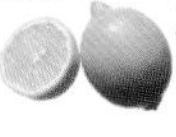

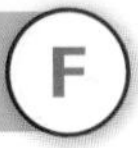

Handwritten notes:
- fresh cranberries 4 Grams/cup of sugar
- med banana 14g/sugar

Weights As Purchased	C	F	Cb
Limes, 1 med. (2" diam.), 2.4 oz	20	0	7
Loganberries, froz., ½ cup, 2½ oz	40	0	9
Longans, 5 fruit, ½ oz	10	0	2.5
Loquats, 4 fruit, 2¼ oz	30	0	8
Lychees, 4 fruit, 2¼ oz	30	0	7
Mamey Apple: ¼ fruit, 7 oz	100	1	25
Mandarin: 1 small, 3 oz	35	0	9
1 medium, 4 oz	45	0	11
1 large, 6 oz	50	0	13
Mango: Flesh, ½ cup slices, 3 oz	55	0	14
1 small mango, 7 oz	90	0.5	24
1 medium, 10 oz	130	0.5	34
1 cheek, 4 oz	60	0	14
1 large, 17 oz	220	1	58
1 extra large mango, 24 oz	310	1.5	82
Marionberries, 1 cup, 5 oz	75	1	15
Melon, avg, 1 cup, cubes/balls, 6 oz	60	0	14
Monstera Deliciosa (Taxonia), Edible part, 4 oz	50	0	11
Mulberries, 20 fruit, 1 oz	15	0	3
Nashi Fruit (Asian Pear), 1 med., 7 oz	85	0	21
Nectarines: 1 medium, 4 oz	50	0	12
1 large, 5½ oz	70	0	16
Oheloberries, ½ cup, 2½ oz	20	0	5
Olives (Pickled): Green, 10 lrg, 1½ oz	60	6.5	1.5
Ripe, Greek Style, 10 med., 1 oz	70	6	4
Ripe (Black) Californian:			
1 small/medium	5	0	0.2
1 large/extra large	6	0.5	0.5
1 jumbo	7	0.5	0.5
1 colossal	11	1	0.5
Oranges: Avg. all varieties (wts with skin)			
1 small, 5 oz	45	0	11
1 medium (3" diam.), 7 oz	85	0	21
1 large, 10 oz	130	0	33
Californian Valencia, 1 medium (2¾" diam.), 6 oz	60	0	14
Calif. Navels (3" diam.), 7 oz	70	0	17
Sunkist Navel, large, 14 oz	130	0	30
Florida Orange, 1 med, 7 oz	70	0	17
Flesh only, 1 cup, 6 oz	85	0	21
Peel, 1 Tbsp	0	0	0
Papaya: ½ cup, cubed, 2½ oz	30	0	7
1 medium, (5"x3" diam.), 16 oz	120	0	30
Green (unripe), ½ cup, 3½ oz	20	0	5
Passionfruit, 1 medium, 1¼ oz	35	0	8
PawPaw (see Papaya)			
Peaches: 1 small/donut, 3 oz	30	0	7.5
1 medium (4 per lb), 4 oz	45	0	11
1 large, 6 oz	65	0	16
1 extra large, 10 oz	110	0	27

Weights As Purchased	C	F	Cb
Pears, Average all types:			
1 mini, 2½ oz	35	0	8
1 small, 5 oz	75	0	18
1 medium, 7 oz	105	0	25
1 large, 9 oz	135	0	33
1 extra large, 12 oz	175	0	42
Pepino, ½ medium, 4 oz	20	0	4
Persimmons: Native, 1 oz	35	0	9
Japanese (2½"d. x 2½"h), 7 oz	120	0	30
Seedless (Maui), 1 med., 5 oz	100	0	25
Pineapple (wts without skin):			
1 thin slice (½"), 2 oz	25	0	6
1 thick slice (¾"), 3 oz	40	0	10
1 cup, diced, 5½ oz	75	0	19
1 medium, 1½ lb (peeled)	325	0	86
Wedges *(Del Monte)*, 12 oz pkg	195	0	47
Canned: *See Page 104*			
Pitanga, (Surinam-Cherry) (5), 1.2 oz	10	0	2
Plaintains, ½ cup slices, 2½ oz	90	0	22
Plums: Average all types,			
Mini/Damson, (1" diam.), ½ oz	7	0	1.5
Small (2" diam.), 2¼ oz	30	0	7
Med. (2½" diam.), 3½ oz	45	0	10
Large (3" diam.), 5 oz	60	0	14
Pluot (plum-apricot), 1 med., 5 oz	80	0	19
Pomegranate, 1 medium, 10 oz	105	0.5	25
Pummelo, flesh, ½ cup, 3½ oz	35	0	9
Prickly Pear, (Nopal):			
1 small, 2½ oz	20	0	5
1 medium, 5 oz	40	0	10
Quince, 1 medium, 3½ oz	55	0	14
Rambutan (Rambotang), Red/Yellow, 1 medium, 2 oz	15	0	4
Raspberries, ½ cup, 2 oz	30	0	7
10 Raspberries, ¾ oz	10	0	2
1 Cup, 4¼ oz	65	1	15
1 Pint, 11 oz	160	2	37
Sapodilla (Chico), 1 med., 7½ oz	140	2	34
Sapote, ½ medium, 8 oz	150	0.5	38
Satsuma Tangerine, 1 med., 3 oz	45	0	11
Soursop, 1 cup pulp, 8 oz	150	0.5	38
Starfruit, 1 medium, 3 oz	30	0	6
Strawberries: 1 cup, 5½ oz	50	0.5	12
6 medium/3 large, 2 oz	20	0	4
1 pint, 14 oz	115	1	27
Chocolate Dipped, 1 large	45	2.5	6
Sugar Apple (Custard Apple) ½ cup pulp, 4 oz	120	0	30
Tamarillo, 1 med., 3 oz	20	0	3
Tamarind: 1 fruit (3"x1")	5	0	1.5
Pulp, ½ cup, 2 oz	140	0.5	37

Weights as Purchased

	C	F	Cb
Tangelo, 1 small, 4 oz	55	0	13
1 medium, 5 oz	70	0	17
1 large, 7 oz	95	0	23
Tangerine, 1 medium, (2½" diam.), 4 oz	50	0	13
Tangor, 1 medium, 4 oz	35	0	7
Tomatillos (3), 3½ oz	35	1	6
Tomatoes:			
1 small (2¼" diam.), 3 oz	15	0	3
1 medium (2¾" diam.), 5 oz	25	0	5
1 large (3½" diam.), 8 oz	40	0.5	9
1 extra large (3" diam.), 12 oz	60	0.5	14
Grape, 5 medium, 2 oz	10	0	2
Yellow Tear Drop, 3 medium, 1 oz	5	0	2
Cherry: 4 medium, 2 oz	10	0	2
1 cup, 5 oz	25	0	6
Slices (Medium Tomato):			
2 thin slices, 1 oz	5	0	1
2 thick (⅜"), 2 oz	10	0	2
Wedge, ¼ medium tomato, 1¼ oz	6	0	1
Chopped, 1 cup, 6½ oz	35	0.5	7
Fried Green Tomato, 2 slices, 2½ oz	140	11	9
Canned Tomatoes/Products: See Page 168			
Tree Tomato (Tamarillo), 3 oz	20	0	5
Ugli Fruit, Tangelo type, 5 oz	40	0	8
Watermelon: Flesh only/no rind, 1 oz	8	0	2
1 thin slice, (¼ circle, ⅜"), 2 oz	15	0	4
1 Extra			
1 cup cubes or balls, 5½ oz	45	0	11
10 balls, 4.3 oz	35	0	9
Buffet Slice, thin, 1 oz	8	0	2
Regular (Long Shape):			
1 thick (1") slice (¼ circle, 4½" radius)			
9 oz w. skin (5½ oz no rind)	50	0	12
1 thin (½") slice (¼ circle)	25	0	6
1 thick (1") slice (½ circle)			
18 oz with rind	100	1	22
1 whole melon (15" long, 7½"diam.)			
20 lb w. rind, (10 lb no rind)	1360	7	330
Seedless (Round Shape):			
Medium size (13 lb, 8¼" diam.)			
1 whole, 8½ lb (no rind)	1160	5	280
Wedge (⅛ whole melon),			
26 oz (with rind)	145	1	35
Flesh only (no rind), 8 oz	70	0.5	17
Mini size (6 lb, 6½" diam.),			
1 whole, 3½ lb (no rind)	480	2.5	110
Wedge (⅛ whole),			
1½ lb (with rind)	60	0.5	14
Xoconostle: *see Prickly Pear*			

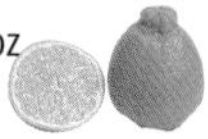

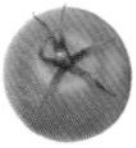

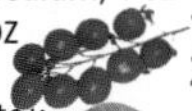

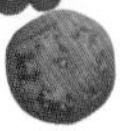

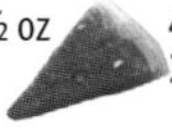

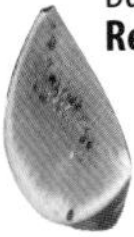

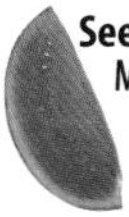

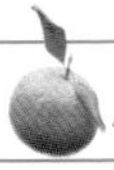

FRUIT & VEGETABLE JUICES
~ *See Beverages Page 41*

Dried Fruit	C	F	Cb
Apples, 5 rings, 1 oz	80	0	19
Apricots, 8 halves, 1 oz	65	0	16
Banana Chips, ½ cup, 1½ oz	220	14	25
Banana Flakes, 4 Tbsp, 1 oz	80	0	20
Cranberries *(Craisins):*			
Sweetened, ¼ cup, 1 oz	100	0	24
Unsweetened, ¼ cup, 1 oz	80	0	19
Choc-coated, 1 oz	135	7.5	18
Currants, ¼ cup, 1¼ oz	100	0	25
Dates: 5 medium dates, 1½ oz	120	0	29
Large Calif.: 1 date, 0.7 oz	55	0	13
3 dates, 2 oz	170	0	39
½ cup, chopped, 3 oz	240	0	58
Pecan Date Rolls, 1 oz	100	2.5	19
Date Crumbles *(Bob's Redmill),*			
1 oz, ¼ cup	90	0	22
Figs, 3 medium figs, 1 oz	90	0	23
Goji Berries, 3 Tbsp, 1 oz	100	1	20
Longans; Lychees, 1 oz	80	0	20
Mango Slices, 5 pieces, 1.4 oz	25	0	6
Papaya Spears, 2 pieces, 1.4 oz	120	0	30
Peaches, 2 halves, 1 oz	60	0	15
Pears, 3 halves, 2 oz	140	0.5	34
Plums *(Sunsweet)* (5), 1.4 oz	100	0	24
Prunes (dried Plums): w. pits, 1 oz	70	0	17
1 medium (60/lb)	16	0	4
1 large (50/lb)	22	0	5
1extra large (40/lb)	25	0	6
Without pits, 4 med., 1 oz	70	0	17
Cooked: w. sugar, ½ cup, 5 oz	155	0	38
w/out sugar, ½ cup, 4½ oz	135	0	33
Raisins: 2 Tbsp, 1 oz pkg	85	0	20
½ cup, 2.8 oz	220	0.5	56

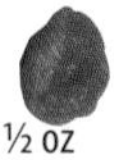

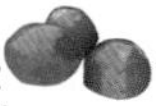

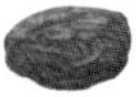

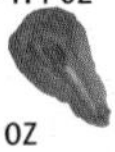

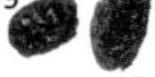

Candied/Glazed Fruit	C	F	Cb
Apricot, 1 medium, 1 oz	70	0	17
Cherry, (Maraschino) (1)	8	0	2
Citron/Fruit Peel, 1 oz	85	0	20
Ginger, 1 oz	90	0	21
Pineapple, 1 slice, 1¼ oz	120	0	29

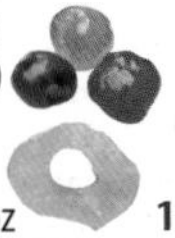

Fruit Leather/Rolls	C	F	Cb
Average All Brands, 1 oz	105	1	24
Fruit By The Foot, (Betty Crocker)			
1 roll, ¾ oz	80	0	17
Fruit Gushers, (Betty Crocker), 1 oz	90	1	20
Fruit Roll-Ups, (Betty Crocker) 1 roll	50	1	12
Stretch Island, Leathers, 2 pces, 1 oz	90	0	24

Canned/Bottled Fruit

Solids & Liquids:
Per ½ Cup (Approx. 4½ oz)

	C	F	Cb
Apricots: In water/diet	35	0	8
In juice/lite	60	0	15
In syrup	105	0	28
Black/Blueberries: Heavy syrup	120	0	30
In light syrup	110	0	26
Cherries, pitted: in water	55	0	15
In light syrup	85	0	22
In heavy syrup	105	0	27
In extra heavy syrup	135	0	34
Maraschino, 1 oz	50	0	12
Pie Cherries, ⅔ cup, 5 oz	90	0	23
Fruit Salad: In water/diet	35	0	10
In juice/Light	60	0	16
In heavy syrup	95	0	25
Gooseberries, Light syrup	90	0	24
Grapefruit: Juice pack	45	0	12
In light syrup	75	0	20
Lychees, ½ cup, 4.5 oz	105	0	26
Mixed Fruit: In water/diet	40	0	10
In fruit juices/light syrup	70	0	18
In heavy syrup	90	0	24
Peaches (halves/slices): In water/diet	30	0	7
In juice/light	55	0	14
In light syrup	70	0	18
drained, ½ peach	55	0	14
In heavy syrup	100	0	26
Pears: In water/diet	35	0	10
In juice/light	60	0	16
In heavy syrup	100	0	26
Pineapple: All types			
In own juice	75	0	20
In heavy syrup	100	0	26
1 slice (ring), drained, 1½ oz	15	0	4
Prunes: In heavy syrup	125	0	33
In Liqueur, ½ cup, 125g	280	0	70
Stewed in Water, ½ cup	135	0	35
Tropical Fruit Salad: In light syrup	80	0	21
In heavy syrup	110	0	29

Fruit Snack Cups

	C	F	Cb
Deli/Take-Out: Small, 6 oz	70	0	16
Large, 12 oz	140	0	32
Yogurt & Fruit Cup, 15 oz	380	4.5	75
Del Monte Fruit Cups			
Fruit Cups: *Per 4 oz Cup*			
Strawberry Banana	70	0	17
Mandarin Or. Segments	70	0	17
Pineapple Tidbits	70	0	18
Tropical Fruit	70	0	18
Fruit Naturals: *Per 8 oz Cup*			
Cherry Mixed Fruit	140	0	35
Peach Chunks	140	0	35
Pineapple Chunks	140	0	35
Red Grapefruit	120	0	30
Fruit-n-Gel Cups: *Per 4½ oz Cup*			
Mixed Fruit/Peaches in Fruit Gel	95	0	23
Lite varieties in Gel, avg.	60	0	14
Pull Top Cans: in 100% Juice, 4 oz	80	0	20
Lite varieties, 4 oz	50	0	13
Super Fruits: *Per ½ Cup*			
Mixed Fruit Chunks in Juice	70	0	17
Peach Chunks in Juice	60	0	15
Pear Chunks in Juice	70	0	18
Dole Fruit Bowls			
4 oz Bowls: Diced Peaches	80	0	20
Mixed Fruit; Tropical Fruit	80	0	19
Pineapple	60	0	16
Fruit-n-Gel Bowls (4.3 oz): Regular	90	0	23
Reduced Sugar	60	0	16
Mott's: Healthy Harvest, 4 oz cup	50	0	13
Vons: Fruit Cocktail,			
In heavy syrup, ½ cup, 4.5 oz	100	0	25
In lite syrup, ½ cup	60	0	14

Apple & Fruit Sauces

	C	F	Cb
Apple Sauce:			
Regular/sweetened, 2 Tbsp, 1 oz	20	0	6
4 oz package	85	0	22
¼ cup	50	0	13
Fruit Sauces & Purees:			
Average all fruit types, 2 Tbsp, 1 oz	25	0	6
½ cup, 4 oz	100	0	24
Mott's:			
Classics, avg. 4 oz	100	0	24
Apple Sauce: Original, 4 oz	100	0	24
Fruit Flavored, avg., 4 oz	90	0	23
No Sugar Added, 4 oz	50	0	12
Ocean Spray: *Per ¼ Cup*			
Jellied Cranberry Sauce	110	0	25
Whole Berry Cranberry Sce	110	0	27

Pie Fillings ~ See Page 136

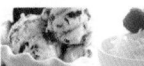 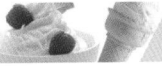

Ice Cream ◇ Frozen Yogurt

Quick Guide — **C** **F** **Cb**

Ice Cream
Vanilla: *Average All Brands*
Other flavors ~ See Brand Listings.

Regular Ice Cream (10% fat):
Examples: *Borden/Hood*

	C	F	Cb
3 fl.oz scoop	105	5	12
½ cup, 4 fl.oz	140	7	17
1 Pint, 16 fl.oz	560	28	68
½ Gallon (4 Pints)	2240	112	272

Rich (16% fat):
Example: *Hood (Red Sox)*

	C	F	Cb
3 fl.oz scoop	135	7.5	15
½ cup, 4 fl.oz	180	10	20
1 Pint	720	40	80

Super-Rich (20% fat): *Haagen-Dazs/Ben & Jerry's*

	C	F	Cb
3 fl.oz scoop	200	13	18
½ cup, 4 fl.oz	270	17	24
1 Pint	1080	68	96

Reduced-Fat/Light (6% fat):
Breyer's Light/Hood Light

	C	F	Cb
3 fl.oz scoop	95	3	15
½ cup, 4 fl.oz	125	4	20
1 Pint	500	16	80

Fat-Free: *Baskin-Robbins FF/Borden FF/ Breyers FF/Dreyers FF/Hood FF*

	C	F	Cb
3 fl.oz scoop	70	0	16
½ cup, 4 fl.oz	90	0	21
1 Pint	360	0	84

Soft Serve: Regular, ½ cup

	C	F	Cb
Regular, ½ cup	190	11	19
1 cup	380	22	38
Light, ½ cup	110	2	19
1 cup	220	4	38

Quick Guide

Frozen Yogurt
Average All Brands — **C** **F** **Cb**

		C	F	Cb
Hard:	Low-Fat, ½ cup	110	3	19
	Non-Fat, ½ cup	110	0	24
Soft:	Low-Fat, ½ cup	120	4	17
	Non-Fat, ½ cup	100	0	30

Brands: *See Ice Cream & Ices Section*

Quick Guide — **C** **F** **Cb**

Gelato/Ices/Frozen Custard
Gelato: *Per ½ Cup*

	C	F	Cb
Milk base: Vanilla	160	6	25
Choc. Hazelnut	230	15	21
Water base, ½ cup	100	0	26

Frozen Custard: *Per ½ Cup*

	C	F	Cb
Chocolate	140	6	18
Orange Sherbet	105	2	21
Vanilla	130	6	16

Ice (Milk base): Average all flavors

	C	F	Cb
Hard (4% fat), ½ cup	100	3	15
Soft Serve (3% fat), ½ cup	110	2	19
Shaved Ice: Average, 12 fl. oz	160	0	40
Sherbet: Avg., ½ cup	110	1.5	22
Sorbet: Fruit (no fat), ½ cup	70	0	19
Fruit Ice Pops	80	0	20

Tofu Frozen Desserts: *See Page 35*

Sundaes — **C** **F** **Cb**

Baskin Robbins:

	C	F	Cb
Banana Royale	620	28	87
Banana Split	1010	34	173
Brownie	920	47	119
Oreo	1290	57	188
Reeses Peanut Butter Cup	1220	80	109
Snickers	1000	46	139
Denny's: Banana Split	810	31	125
Oreo Blender Blaster	890	44	113
Oreo Sundae	760	37	103
Chocolate, Topping, 2 oz	140	0.5	36

Other Toppings ~ *See Page 203*

McDonald's:

	C	F	Cb
Hot Caramel Sundae	340	8	60
Hot Fudge Sundae	330	10	54
Strawberry Sundae	280	6	49
Toppings: Peanuts, ¼ oz	45	3.5	2

Ice Cream, Cones & Cups

Average All Brands — **C** **F** **Cb**

	C	F	Cb
Wafer Cone/Cup, average	20	0	4
Sugar Cone, average	50	0	14
Waffle Cone:			
Small	50	1	10
Large	90	0.5	19
Brands:			
Oreo Chocolate Cone	50	1	10
Comet Sugar Cone	50	0	11
Keebler Sugar Cone	50	0	10

Updated Nutrition Data ~ www.CalorieKing.com
Persons with Diabetes ~ See Disclaimer (Page 24)

Ice Cream & Frozen Yogurt

Brands

C **F** **Cb**

Baskin-Robbins: *See Fast-Foods Section*

Ben & Jerry's

Hand Scoop: *Per ½ Cup*

	C	F	Cb
Butter Pecan, 86g	260	20	17
Cake Batter, 92g	240	14	24
Cherry Garcia, 87g	200	11	23
Chocolate, 88g	200	12	21
Chocolate Chip Cookie Dough, 87g	220	12	26
Chocolate Therapy, 86g	210	12	25
Cinnamon Buns, 88g	240	12	30
Coconut Seven Layer Bar, 92g	275	17	25
Coffee, Coffee BuzzBuzzBuzz, 88g	230	14	23
Half Baked, 88g	230	11	28
Imagine Whirled Peace, 91g	250	15	26
Mint Chocolate Chunk, 88g	230	14	23
New York Super Fudge Chunk, 87g	250	17	24
One Cheesecake Brownie, 92g	235	14	23
Phish Food, 88g	230	11	32
Strawberry Cheesecake, 86g	210	11	24
Sweet Cream & Cookies, 88g	240	13	24
Triple Caramel Chunk, 88g	230	12	38
Vanilla, 88g	190	12	18

Original: *Per ¼ Tub*

	C	F	Cb
Banana Split, 110g	270	15	30
Cake Batter, 105g	280	17	28
Cherry Garcia, 105g	240	14	27
Chocolate Chip Cookie Dough, 104g	270	14	32
Chocolate Macadamia, 102g	270	18	25
Everything But The…, 109g	300	19	31
Imagine Whirled Peace	270	16	28
Karamel Sutra, 107g	270	14	32
Mission To Marzipan, 102g	260	13	32
New York Super Fudge Chunk, 106g	300	19	29
One Cheesecake Brownie, 103g	250	15	26
Peanut Butter Chocolate, 108g	350	19	40
Phish Food, 101g	270	12	37
Strawberry Banana, 95g	150	1.5	32
Triple Caramel Chunk, 107g	280	16	32
Turtle Soup, 104g	280	15	30
Vermonty Python, 106g	310	19	30
Vanilla Fudge Brownie, 108g	310	14	43

Frozen Yogurt: *Per ½ Cup*

	C	F	Cb
Fro Yo: Half Baked, 99g	180	3	35
Cherry Garcia, 100g	160	3	31
Chocolate Fudge Brownie	170	2.5	34
Strawberry Banana, 95g	150	1.5	32
Sorbet: Avg. all flavors	115	0	30

Blue Bunny: *Per ½ Cup*

C **F** **Cb**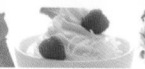

Fat-Free, No Added Sugar:

	C	F	Cb
Brownie Sundae, 74g	90	0	23
Caramel Toffee Crunch, 71g	90	0	24
Vanilla, 71g	80	0	20

Reduced-Fat, No Added Sugar:

	C	F	Cb
Banana Split, 71g	120	5	20
Butter Pecan, 71g	130	6	16
Rocky Road, 71g	130	6	21
Turtle Sundae, 71g	140	7	20
Hi Lite: Chocolate, 65g	110	3	17
Fudge Nut Sundae, 65g	120	4	19
Homemade Vanilla, 67g	110	3.5	18

Personals (Light):

	C	F	Cb
Bunny Tracks, 68g	130	5	20
Choc. Raspb. Cheesecake	100	2.5	18
Super Fudge Brownie, 67g	120	3	23

Frozen Yogurt:

	C	F	Cb
Brownie Fudge Fantasy, 74g	110	0	24
Homemade Vanilla, 74g	100	0	19
Strawberry Cheesecake	100	0	21

Bars/Pops: See Page 110

Breyers: *Per ½ Cup*

	C	F	Cb
CarbSmart: Butter Pecan	120	8	13
Chocolate	90	6	13
Rocky Road	110	7	14
Vanilla	90	6	13
All Natural: Butter Pecan, avg.	150	10	14
Cherry Vanilla	130	6	18
Cookies & Cream; Rocky Road	150	7	19
Vanilla, Chocolate	130	6	15
Double Churn:			
Fat-Free: Creamy Vanilla	90	0	21
Cappuccino Choc Chunk	100	0	25
Caramel Swirl	100	0	23
Light: Butter Pecan	120	5	16
Choc. Mocha Silk; Mint Choc. Chip	130	5	19
Rocky Road	130	4.5	22
Vanilla, Chocolate, Strawberry	100	3	17
No Sugar Added: Butter Pecan	110	6	14
Chocolate Fudge Brownie	90	1.5	20
Peanut Butter; Triple Choc., avg.	115	6	17
Fun & Indulgent: Brownie Mud Pie	130	3.5	23
Bubble Yum Original	120	3	21
M&M Cookie Dough	150	5	23
Oreo	160	8	20
Snickers	170	8	20

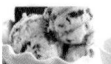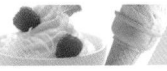

Brands (Cont)

	C	F	Cb
Brigham's: *Per ½ Cup, 4 fl.oz*			
Ice Cream: Big Dig	210	12	24
Chocolate	200	12	20
Coffee	190	12	17
Frozen Pudding	180	9	20
Just Jimmies	220	13	21
Mocha Almond; Pistachio	210	15	18
Vanilla	190	12	18
Elan Frozen Yogurt			
Average all flavors, ½ cup, 4 fl.oz	135	3	24
Bruster's			
Frozen Yogurt: *Per 3 fl.oz*			
Chocolate	150	4.5	24
Vanilla	150	4	24
Fat Free, No Added Sugar Ice Cream: *3 fl.oz*			
Chocolate	100	0	26
Choc. Caramel Swirl	120	0	31
Cinnamon	100	0	23
Coffee	100	0	24
Fudge Ripple	110	0	30
Vanilla	100	0	23
Other varieties, average	110	0	30
Carvel Ice Cream: *See Fast-Foods Section*			
Coldstone Creamery: *See Fast-Foods Section*			
CremaLita (Soft Serve)			
Calories will vary with density (air in product) and serving size. Best to weigh product and calculate on 25 cals per 1 oz weight.			
Vanilla: Small (4 fl.oz cup),			
If 4 oz weight*	100	0.5	23
If 6 oz weight*	150	1	35
(*) Most common weights			
Medium (8 fl.oz cup), 11 oz wt	275	1.5	63
Chocolate: Small, 6 oz weight	160	1	36
Dairy Queen/Brazier: *See Fast-Foods Section*			
Dippin' Dots			
Dots 'n Cream: *Per ½ Cup*			
Banana Split	220	14	22
Caramel Cappuccino	190	12	18
Mint Chocolate	230	14	25
Vanilla Over The Rainbow	210	12	23
Wild About Chocolate	240	14	26
Dove: *Per ½ Cup*			
Beyond Vanilla	240	15	23
Caramel Pecan Perfection	300	18	30
Chocolate & Brownie Affair	300	19	31
Chocolate & Cherry Courtship	270	16	27
Irresistibly Raspberry	240	12	30
Unconditional Chocolate	290	17	31
Vanilla with Chocolate Soul	300	18	30
Other varieties, avg.	300	19	30

	C	F	Cb
Dreyers/Edys: *Per ½ Cup, 4 fl.oz*			
Grand: Chocolate	150	8	17
Fudge Swirl	150	7	19
Mint Chocolate Chip	160	9	18
Neapolitan; Vanilla Bean, avg.	140	8	15
Real Strawberry	130	6	16
Vanilla	140	8	15
Other flavors, avg.	160	9	18
Loaded, Chocolate Fudge Brownie	120	4	19
Slow Churned: Light, Neapolitan	100	3	15
Cookie Dough	130	4.5	20
Cups ½ Fat ⅓ Calories:			
Chocolate, 1 cup	170	6	25
Mint Chocolate Chip, 1 cup	210	8	29
Yogurt Blends: Cookies & Cream	120	4	20
Other flavors, avg	100	2	17
Friendly's: *Per Single Scoop*			
Ice Cream: Butter Crunch	130	6	16
Chocolate	110	6	10
Chocolate Alm. Chip	120	7	11
Coffee	110	6	13
Hunka Chunka PB Fudge	180	11	17
Pistachio	130	7	15
Strawberry	110	5	14
Vanilla	120	6	14
Vienna Mocha Chunk	140	8	16
Frozen Yogurt: *Per ½ Cup*			
Raspberry Swirl, Non-Fat	90	0	19
Sundaes: *Per 3 Scoops*			
Royal Banana Split	880	35	132
Jim Dandy	1080	46	156
Reese's Peanut Butter Cup	870	51	90
Friend-Z's, Reese's P'nut Butter Cup	860	45	96
Gelati-da			
Gelato: *Per ½ Cup (4 oz)*			
Amaretto Chocolate	150	4.5	23
Choc Mint Milano	120	2.5	22
Coffee Fudge Latte	130	2	22
Limoncello	120	3	20
Red Raspberry	130	1.5	25
Vanilla Marsala	120	2	21
Haagen-Dazs			
Ice Cream, Sorbet, Frozen Yogurt: *See Fast-Foods Section*			
Bars: *See Page 111*			
Hola Fruta!: *Per ½ Cup, 95g*			
Pure Fruit Sherbet: Margarita	140	1	30
Peach	130	1	30
Pina Colada	140	1.5	31
Pomegranate; Raspberry	140	1	32
Pomegranate & Blueberry	150	1	31
Strawberry	130	1	31

Ice Cream & Frozen Yogurt

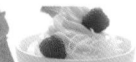

Brands (Cont)

	C	F	Cb

Hood: *Per ½ Cup*
Frozen Fat-Free Yogurt:

	C	F	Cb
Maine Blueberry & Sweet Cream	90	0	19
Mocha Fudge	100	0	22
Pomegranate Swirl	100	0	21
Strawberry	80	0	18
Strawberry Banana	90	0	20
Vanilla	90	0	19

Ice Cream: *Per 66g*

	C	F	Cb
Birthday Party	150	8	19
Chippedy Chocolaty	150	9	19
Chocolate	140	7	17
Classic trio	140	7	17
Cookie Dough Delight	160	8	20
Cookies 'N Cream	140	7	17
Creamy Coffee	140	7	16
Fudge Twister	150	7	20
Golden Vanilla	140	7	17
Maple Walnut	150	9	17
Natural Vanilla Bean	140	7	16
Patchwork	140	7	17

New England Creamery ~ www.CalorieKing.com

Bars: *See Page 111*

I Can't Believe It's Yogurt: *See Fast-Foods Section*
Jerseymaid (Vons): *Per ½ Cup*

	C	F	Cb
Cookies & Cream	160	8	18
Choc Chip; Mint Choc Chip	150	9	16
Heavenly Hash; Nut Chunky Choc.	170	10	17
Mocha Almd Fudge; Rocky Road	160	10	17
Neapolitan; Vanilla	140	8	15
Strawberry	130	6	17

Oberweis: *Per 6 oz Scoop*
Super Premium:

	C	F	Cb
Chocolate	480	31	43
Chocolate Peanut Butter	550	39	42
Cookie Dough	500	28	56
Vanilla	460	31	40

Purely Decadent: *Per ½ Cup*

	C	F	Cb
Belgian Chocolate, 3.5 oz	180	7	30
Blueberry Cheesecake, 3.5 oz	180	6	33
Gluten Free: Key Lime Pie, 3.5 oz	190	7	34
Peanut Butter Zig Zag, 3.5 oz	230	13	32
w. Coconut Milk: Choc., 3 oz	150	9	20
Coconut, 3 oz	170	10	19
Cookie Dough, 3 oz	190	9	24
Mint Chip, 3 oz	170	9	20
Vanilla Bean, 3 oz	150	8	19

Red Mango Frozen Yogurt:
No Toppings Included

	C	F	Cb
Original/Green Tea/Tangomonium:			
Small	110	0	24
Regular	190	0	42
Large	270	0	60
Pomegranate: Small	120	0	26
Regular	210	0	46
Large	300	0	66

Rice Dream (Non-Dairy):
Per ½ Cup, 70g, Unless otherwise specified

	C	F	Cb
All Natural: Carob Almond	190	9	27
Cocoa Marble Fudge	150	6	25
Cookies & Dream; Mint Carob Chip	170	8	25
Neapolitan; Sweet Peach Pie	150	6	23
Orange Vanilla Swirl	160	7	22
Strawberry, 80g	160	8	25
Vanilla	150	6	22
Van. Hazelnut Fudge	150	7	22
Supreme: Chocolate Caramel Chai	150	7	22
Sweet Peach Fudge	150	6	23

Bars: *See Page 112*

	C	F	Cb
So Delicious Organic: Butter Pecan	160	7	22
Chocolate Velvet, 81g	130	3.5	23
Cookies 'N Cream, 83g	150	4	26
Creamy Vanilla, 81g	130	3	24
Dulce de Leche, 83g	130	3	26
Mint marble Fudge, 84g	140	3	27
Mocha Fudge, 84g	130	3	26
Neapolitan; Strawberry, 81g	120	3	23

Soy Delicious: *Per ½ Cup*

	C	F	Cb
It's Soy Delicious: Choc Almond	140	4.5	23
Choc Peanut Butter	135	3.5	24
Pistachio Almond	130	4.5	23
Other flavors, avg.	110	1.5	25

Soy Dream (Non-Dairy): *Per ½ Cup, 70g*

	C	F	Cb
Butter Pecan	150	9	19
Chocolate	120	6	17
Chocolate Fudge Brownie	130	7	18
French Vanilla; Vanilla	140	8	17
Green Tea	140	8	18
Mocha Fudge	140	7	21

Starbucks: *Per ½ Cup*

	C	F	Cb
Caramel Macchiato	240	13	27
Coffee	210	13	21
Java Chip Frappuccino	250	15	25
Mocha Frappuccino	220	13	23

Stonyfield Farm (Organic)
Premium Ice Cream: *Per ½ Cup, 100g*

	C	F	Cb
Chocolate Raspberry Swirl	230	13	25
Cookies 'N Dream	270	16	27
Creme Caramel	250	14	29
Gotta Have Java	250	16	22
Gotta Have Vanilla	240	16	21
Vanilla Chai	240	16	21

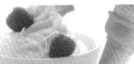

Brands (Cont)	C	F	Cb
Stop & Shop: *Per ½ Cup, 4 fl.oz*			
Butterscotch Ripple	140	7	19
Chocolate	140	8	18
Chocolate Chip (Reg./Chunky)	150	9	17
Country Club	130	6	19
Heavenly Hash	170	8	22
Neapolitan; Vanilla	140	8	16
Vanilla Fudge Swirl	150	8	18

Tasti D-Lite (Soft Serve): *Per ½ Cup, 4 fl.oz*
Calories will vary with density (air in product) and serving size
Best to weigh product and calculate on 25 cals per 1 oz weight.

	C	F	Cb
Banana	70	1.5	11
Blueberry Cheesecake	90	1.5	14
Brownie Batter	90	2	14
Buttercrunch	100	3	13
Chocolate Marshmallow	90	1.5	16
Vanilla Cream; Vanilla Marshmallow	80	1.5	13

TCBY

	C	F	Cb
Soft Serve Frozen Yogurt: *Average all Flavors*			
98% Fat-Free:			
Kids, 2.68 oz	90	1.5	18
½ Cup, 3.4 oz	110	2	23
Small, 6.7 oz	220	4	46
Regular, 8.7 oz	285	5	60
Large, 11 oz	365	6.5	76
Non-Fat: ½ Cup, 3.4 oz	110	0	24
Small, 6.7 oz	220	0	48
Regular, 8.7 oz	285	0	62
Large, 11 oz	365	0	79
No Sugar Added/Fat-Free: ½ c.	90	0	24
Small, 6.7 oz	190	0	50
Regular, 8.7 oz	230	0	62
Large, 11 oz	300	0	79
Hand Scooped Frozen Yogurt			
Chocolate Chocolate: Child, 2 oz	90	2.5	15
Small, 4 oz	190	5	30
Medium, 6 oz	280	8	45
Large, 8 oz	380	10	60
No Added Sugar:			
Chocolate Swirl: Child, 2 oz	70	0	16
Small, 4 oz	130	0.5	32
Medium, 6 oz	200	1	49
Large, 8 oz	270	1.5	65
Tofutti, Non-Dairy Dessert: *Per ½ Cup*			
Premium Pints: Better Pecan	210	13	21
Chocolate Cookie Crunch	210	11	26
Chocolate Supreme	180	11	18
Vanilla	210	13	21
Vanilla Almond Bark	240	15	24
Vanilla Fudge; Wildberry, avg.	190	9	25

Per Serving

	C	F	Cb
Turkey Hill: *Per ½ Cup, 4 fl.oz*			
Premium: Black Cherry	130	6	18
Butter Pecan	160	10	15
Choco Mint Chip	160	9	17
Choc. Peanut Butter	180	11	18
Cookies 'n Cream	150	8	19
French Vanilla	140	7	16
Rocky Road	170	8	23
Tin Roof Sundae	150	8	19
Lite: Moose Tracks	130	6	19
Peanut Butter Mania	130	5	19
Vanilla Bean	100	2.5	16
Other flavors, average	130	4	19
All Natural: Avg. all flavors	150	8	17
No Sugar Added: *Per ½ Cup*			
Cherry Fudge Ripple	80	0	22
Dutch Chocolate; Vanilla	70	0	20
Peanut Brittle	120	0	19
Frozen Yogurt:			
Choc. Chip Cookie Dough	120	2	23
Low-Fat, Mint Cookies 'n Cream	110	1.5	22
Fat-Free: Choc. Marshmallow	110	0	24
Other flavors, average	100	0	19
Sherbet	120	1	26

Walgreens

	C	F	Cb
Premium One Pint Container: *Per ½ Cup*			
Banana Split	130	5	20
Creme de Menthe	160	9	19
Homemade Vanilla	130	7	16
New York Cherry	130	6	17
Rocky Road	150	7	18
Strawberries 'n Cream	130	6	14
Toasted Butter Pecan	170	10	18
Waffle Cone	150	7	19
Scoops Orange Sherbert	120	1	26
Premium 1.75 Quarts Container: *Per ½ Cup*			
Banana Split	150	6	22
Homemade Vanilla	150	8	17
New York Cherry	150	7	20
Old Fashioned 1.75 Quarts (Square)			
Avg., all flavors, ½ cup	140	7	16
Whole Soy Frozen Yogurt			
Average all flavors,			
½ cup, 2½ oz	120	1	25

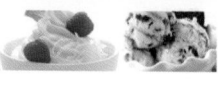

Ice Cream Bars & Pops

Bars & Pops

	C	F	Cb
Per Bar/Serving			
Barq's			
Root Beer &			
Ice Cream Float, 4 fl.oz cup	120	3	22
Ben & Jerry's			
Bars: Cherry Garcia (1)	270	19	28
Half Baked (1)	360	18	46
Vanilla (1)	310	21	26
The Cone: Cherry Garcia	310	16	41
Vanilla Almond (1)	440	27	47
Big Bear: *See Klondike*			
Blue Bunny:			
Pops: Banana, 1.87 oz	35	0	9
Bomb Pops, avg., 1.87 oz	60	0	16
Bars: Big Fudge, 2.72 oz	110	1.5	21
Big Star, 1.66 oz	130	8	13
Caramel Ice Cream Crunch, 1.69 oz	150	10	14
Choc. Ice Cream Sundae Crunch	170	9	21
Chocolate Raspberry, 2.82 oz	270	18	25
English Toffee, 1.38 oz	130	9	12
Milk Choc. with Almond, 3.14 oz	320	23	25
Orange Dream, 2.12 oz	80	1.5	16
Root Beer Float, 2 oz	80	2	14
King Size: Chocolate Eclair, 3 oz	240	12	30
Cookies 'n Cream, 2.89 oz	250	15	28
Crunch with Candy Center, 3.21 oz	370	29	28
Strawberry Shortcake, 3 oz	230	12	29
FrozFruit:			
Banana; Strawb. Cream, avg.	160	6	27
Creamy Pina Colada	180	10	21
Creamy Coconut	150	10	14
Champ Cones: Caramel Lovers, 3.75 oz	350	19	40
Caramel Nut (1)	320	19	34
Fudge Nut (1)	330	19	35
Vanilla, 3.53 oz	330	19	35
Sandwiches: Big Bopper, 5.01 oz	460	23	60
Big Double Strawberry, 3.84 oz	270	10	41
Big Mississippi Mud, 3.77 oz	280	12	39
Big Neapolitan, 3.67 oz	260	11	37
Chips Galore, 3.42 oz	310	16	40
Breyers			
Berry Swirls; Fruit Variety	40	0	10
Pomegranate Blends	40	0	10
Strawberry Tropical Raspb	25	0	5

Per Bar/Serving	C	F	Cb
Breyers (Cont)			
Ice Cream Poppers:			
Heath (27)	410	30	32
Hershey's Kisses:			
Chocolate (26)	470	31	31
Vanilla (26)	460	34	33
Oreo (27)	410	27	38
Reese's (27)	470	34	35
Double Churn Light Bars: Rocky Rd	180	9	23
Creamy Vanilla	160	8	21
Vanilla & Almond	170	9	21
No Sugar Added: Creamy Vanilla	150	9	18
Krunch	150	9	18
Butterfinger *(Nestle):* 54g Bar	210	15	17
Loaded Bar, 80g	270	17	28
California Natural: Mango Sorbet	130	0	33
Lemon & Strawberry Sorbet Cups	120	0	31
Chiquita: Swirls, all flavors	80	3	12
Cool Classics:			
Artic Blasters: Crispy Bar	160	11	15
Fudge Bar	80	0	20
Ice Cream Bar	150	10	13
Orange Cream	100	2.5	18
Icepix: Grape; Cherry; Orange	35	0	8
Honedew; Watermelon Cantelope	35	0	9
Sugar-Free Banana	15	0	3
Squeeze Freeze:			
Blue Raspberry; Cherry Cola	60	1	15
Sour Apple; Cherry	40	0	9
Creamsicle: Sugar-Free Pops (2)	40	0.5	12
Orange, 2.3 oz	100	2	20
Crunch *(Nestle):*			
Caramel	210	14	19
Vanilla Flavored	220	15	18
Reduced-Fat	140	8	15
Loaded, King Size, 2.68 oz	270	17	15
Dove: Milk Chocolate w. Vanilla	330	21	31
Milk Chocolate w. Almonds	340	23	28
Dark Chocolate with Vanilla	330	21	33
Dreyers/Edys			
Dibs: With Chocolaty Coating (26 Pieces)			
Chocolate	360	25	30
Crunch	340	24	30
Drumstick	350	25	30
Mint	340	24	30
Real Fruit Bars: Orange & Cream	80	1.5	16
Strawberry-Banana Smoothie	100	2	20

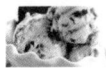
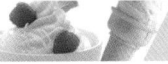

Bars & Pops (Cont)

Per Bar/Serving

	C	F	Cb
Drumstick *(Nestlé)*: Classic Van.	290	16	33
Vanilla Caramel	320	17	37
Vanilla Fudge	310	16	37
King Size, Triple Choc.	390	21	46
Simply Dipped: Vanilla	270	13	37
Cookies & Cream	300	14	39
Mint	290	14	38
Edy's, Fruit Bars:			
Creamy Coconut	120	3	21
Grape; Lemonade; Lime	80	0	20
Orange & Cream	80	1.5	16
Strawberry Banana Smoothie	100	2	20
Fat Boy			
Bars on a Stick Sundaes:			
Casco Vanilla Nut, 3 oz	290	22	22
Cherry Nut, 3 oz	300	22	26
Peppermint, 3 oz	280	20	26
Sandwiches: Chocolate, 3 oz	210	9	31
Cookies n' Crm 3 oz	240	10	36
Raspberry Cheesecake, 2.8 oz	210	7	34
Strawberry, 3 oz	220	10	30
Vanilla, 3 oz	220	10	31
Fruit A Freeze:			
All Natural Creamy: Cappuccino	140	5	20
Coconut	160	9	20
Mango Cream	110	3.5	18
Strawberry	120	4.5	20
Choc. Covered Creamy: Banana	190	11	22
Coconut	240	16	24
Strawberry	190	12	20
Fudge Bar *(Nestlé)*: Polar	90	2	16
Mini's	80	2	14
Fudgesicle: *(The Original Brand)*			
Fudge Bar	100	2	17
Fat-Free	60	0	13
No Added Sugar	40	1	10
Good Humor: Oreo Bar	250	15	28
Candy Center Crunch	310	23	24
Chocolate Eclair	220	10	30
Premium Vanilla	260	17	24
Reese's P'nut Butter Cups	310	21	27
Toasted Almond	240	12	30
Cones: King	250	13	30
Premium Sundae	260	15	29
Triple Choc. Brownie	420	19	58
Vanilla & Chocolate	390	21	44
Sandwiches: Chocolate Chip	270	10	44
Giant Neapolitan	250	9	38
Giant Vanilla	220	4	43
Snack Pops, average all flavors	210	13	23

Per Bar/Serving

	C	F	Cb
Haagen-Dazs:			
Chocolate & Dark Chocolate	290	20	24
Coffee & Alm. Crunch Snack Size	190	13	15
Vanilla & Almonds	310	22	22
Vanilla & Dark Choc.	300	21	23
Vanilla & Milk Choc.	290	21	22
Healthy Choice: Fudge Bar	80	1	13
Caramel Swirl S'wich	150	2	30
Mocha Swirl	90	1.5	17
Sorbet & Cream Bar	90	1	17
Vanilla Sandwich	130	2	25
Hood: Chocolate Eclair	150	10	14
Fudge Bar, Fudge Stix	90	0	20
Orange Cream	90	1.5	19
Rocket	120	5	16
Hoodsie Cups: Van./Choc.	100	5	12
Pops	60	0	16
Sundae	120	5	19
Sandwiches: Vanilla	180	6	29
Light	160	3	29
Ice Cream Sandwich *(Nestle)*: Mini	90	2.5	15
Super	260	11	39
Vanilla	160	4	29
Icee Freeze, 2.25 oz	70	0	17
Klondike			
Caramel Pretzel Bar	260	15	29
Choco Taco	290	15	36
Dark Chocolate Bar	250	14	29
Heath	230	15	24
Krunch	250	14	30
w. Crispy Pieces	260	17	24
Neapolitan	250	17	22
Oreo Bar	260	17	26
Original Vanilla, 3 oz	250	14	29
3.6 oz	330	23	28
Reese's Bar	260	16	26
Triple Chocolate	230	14	26
Whitehouse Cherry	250	14	31
Cones: Nascar; Vanilla	280	14	35
Vanilla Caramel; Vanilla Fudge	290	14	37
Sandwiches			
Oreo	230	10	34
Vanilla	260	5	50
Slim-a-Bear Sandwich			
100 Calorie, Vanilla	100	1.5	21

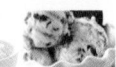

Bars & Pops (Cont)

	C	F	Cb
Per Bar/Serving			
Luigi's Real Italian Ice			
Squeeze Tubes (1)	70	0	18
M&M's			
Cookie Ice Cream Sandwich:			
Single, 3 oz	260	12	34
6 pack, 1 sandwich, 2.3 oz	220	10	29
Cone, Single, 2.8 oz	250	12	33
Treats	190	15	13
Minute Maid: Juice Bars	60	0	15
Soft Frozen Lemonade	70	0	19
Molli Coolz!: *Per 2.5 oz Cup*			
Cookies N' Cream	140	10	10
Rocks: Cherry & Blue Raz & Lemon	80	1.5	15
Strawberry	50	0.5	12
Nestlé: Push Up Pop, average	70	1	16
Crunch Vanilla, 2.2 oz bar	220	15	18
Mini Sandwiches	90	2.5	15
Rolo Chocolate Cone	260	14	30
Rolo King Size, 4 oz	300	19	30
Vanilla Sandwich	160	4	29
Drumstick: Chocolate	310	17	34
Vanilla Fudge	310	16	37
Oreo: Sandwich	260	11	38
Popsicles			
Regular: Big Stick	70	0	17
Dora The Explorer; Scribblers	30	0	8
Firecracker	35	0	9
Rainbow	45	0	11
SpongeBob Pop-Ups	80	1	16
Super Heros	40	0	11
Sugar Free: Orange Cherry Grape	15	0	4
Tropicals	15	0	4
Slow Melts: Ice Age	40	0	10
Mighty Minis	40	0	10
Creamsicle:			
Low Fat, Orange & Raspberry	70	1	13
No Added Sugar, Orange; Cherry; Berry	25	0	5
Sugar-Free, Orange; Cherry; Berry	40	2	10
Reese's Peanut Butter Ice Cream	270	18	24
Rice Dream Vanilla Nutty Bar, 95g	320	24	27
Safeway Select Coffee Almd Bar	270	17	26
Skinny Cow			
Ice Cream Cones, avg.	150	3	29
Fudge Bars, Low-Fat	100	1	22
Minis Fudge Pops (2)	100	2	19
Sandwiches, average	140	2	30

	C	F	Cb
Slim A Bear ~ *See Klondike*			
Per Bar/Serving			
Snickers: Ice Cream Bar, 50g	180	11	18
Snack Size (1)	90	6	9
Cone, 2.9 oz	280	15	33
Snow Cone *(Wonder):* 7 fl.oz Cone	60	0	15
So Delicious Sugar Free: Fudge Bar	80	5	12
Vanilla Bar	150	14	15
Soy Dream (Non-Dairy):			
Lil' Dreamers, all flavors	100	4	15
Sweet Nothings: Fudge Bar	100	0	23
Mango Raspberry	100	0	23
Tofutti (Non-Dairy):			
Cuties: Cookies 'N Cream	130	6	11
Peanut Butter	130	8	20
Vanilla	130	6	17
Sticks: Choc. Fudge Treats	30	1.5	6
Hooray! Hooray!	150	9	10
Marry Me Bar	170	8	22
Mint By Mintz	170	7	7
Totally Fudge Pops	95	1.5	19
Trader Joe's Fruit Floes: Cafe Latte	130	0	26
Caribbean	80	0	21
Lime Juice	60	0	16
Mango	120	0	30
Strawberry	100	0	24
Bars: Ice Cream Sandwich	480	21	60
Mini Mint Sandwich	170	6	27
Raspberry & Vanilla Cream	80	3.5	10
Turkey Hill: Double Decker	190	7	30
Vanilla Bean	190	7	29
Light S'wich, Van. Bean	160	3	32
Sundae Cone	320	18	33
Twix Bar, 2.65 oz	280	16	31
Walgreens			
Choc Nut Sundae Cones	200	11	24
Ice Cream S'wiches, 2.2 oz	170	5	28
Turbo Tubes, 2.26 fl.oz	90	1	20
Weight Watchers			
Bars: Candy Bar	150	9	16
English Toffee Crunch	110	6	13
Giant: Chocolate Cookies & Crm	130	5	24
Choc. Fudge Brownie	140	1.5	35
Cookies & Cream	130	5	23
Latte Bar	90	1	21
Cones: Avg. all flavors	140	4	30
Cups: Choc. Chip Cookie Dough	140	2.5	31
Giant Choc./Van. Fudge Sundae	160	1	37
Mint Chocolate Chip	140	3.5	29
Sandwiches: Choc./Van. Round	140	1.5	31
Vanilla Ice Cream	120	2	28

Canned & Packaged Meals

B & M: *Per ½ Cup (4½ oz)*

	C	F	Cb
Baked Beans: Original	180	3	31
Barbeque	190	0.5	39
Vegetarian	160	1	31
Raisin Brown Bread, ½" slice, 2 oz	130	0.5	29

Banquet

Homestyle Bakes: *Per Serving, Prepared*

	C	F	Cb
Asian Style Fried Rice	250	1.5	49
Beef Stew & Biscuits	270	6	42
Chicken & Dumplings	230	4.5	33
Creamy Chsy Chkn Alfredo	400	22	36
Creamy Chicken & Biscuits	350	18	39
Lasagna	290	11	36
Pasta & Meatballs	310	10	41

Betty Crocker

Complete Meals: *Per Serving, ⅕ Package*

	C	F	Cb
Cheesy Beef Taco	240	4.5	42
Chkn & Buttermilk Biscuits	280	11	37
Chkn Fettuccini Alfredo	230	6	34
Stroganoff	200	4.5	30
Three Cheese Chicken	240	7	36

Hamburger Helper: *Per Cup, Prepared*

	C	F	Cb
Beef Fried Rice	300	12	22
Beef Pasta	280	9	24
Cheeseburger Macaroni	310	10	26
Cheesy Hashbrown	400	19	39
Cheesy Ital. Sausage	290	9	29
Cheesy Jambalaya	320	13	28
Chili Macaroni	270	16	26
Crunchy Taco	340	13	33
Salisbury	280	9	24

Tuna Helper: *Per Serving*

	C	F	Cb
Creamy Parmesan	290	7	36
Other varieties, average	310	12	37

Chicken Helper: *Per Cup, Prepared*

	C	F	Cb
Cheesy Chicken Enchilada	330	10	40
Chicken Fried Rice	250	7	22
Italian Fettuccini Alfredo	330	9	29

Side Dishes/Casseroles: *Per Serving, Prepared*

	C	F	Cb
Au Gratin, ⅔ cup	150	4	23
Cheddar & Bacon; Cheesy Scallops	140	4	25
Roasted Garlic	120	5	20
Scalloped Potatoes, ½ cup	130	5	25
Sour Cream and Chives, ⅔ cup	120	2.5	21

Deluxe Potatoes: *Per ½ Cup, Prepared*

	C	F	Cb
Cheesy Cheddar Au Gratin	180	8	25
Loaded Au Gratin	140	4	25
Three Cheese Mashed Pot. Bake	190	9	24

Betty Crocker (Cont)

	C	F	Cb

Seasoned Skillets: *Prepared*

	C	F	Cb
Hash Brown, ½ cup	120	3	18
Roasted Garlic & Herb, ⅔ cup	170	7	21
Traditional, ½ cup	180	7	22

Bowl Appetit: *Per Bowl*

	C	F	Cb
Cheddar Broccoli Rice	290	6	52
Homestyle Chicken Pasta	250	5	44
Pasta Alfredo	350	9	55
Teriyaki Rice	250	1	57
Three-Cheese Rotini	340	7	59

Bush's Best: *Per ½ Cup*

	C	F	Cb
Black Beans	110	0.5	23
Chili Beans	120	1	20
Dark Red Kidney Beans	105	0	22
Garbanzo Beans	105	2	20
Refried Beans: Traditional	150	3	24
Fat Free	130	0	24
Baked Beans: Vegetarian	130	0	29
Other flavors, average	150	1	32

Campbell's

Beans: *Per ½ Cup*

	C	F	Cb
Baked Beans	160	2.5	30
Pork & Beans	140	1.5	25

Chunky Microwavable Bowls: *Per Cup*

	C	F	Cb
Firehouse; Roadhouse	230	8	25

Spaghetti O's: *Per Cup*

	C	F	Cb
Original	180	1	36
in Meat Sauce	180	2	32
with Meatballs	240	8	32

Supper Bakes: *Per ⅙ Box, Dry Mix*

	C	F	Cb
Cheesy Chicken with Pasta	150	3	24
Garlic Chicken with Pasta	190	1.5	36
Herb Chicken with Rice	160	1.5	33
Lemon Chicken with Rice	160	1.5	43

Chef Boyardee: *Per Cup*

	C	F	Cb
Beefaroni in Tomato Sauce	260	10	33
Beef Ravioli in Tomato & Meat Sce	240	8	35
Cheesy Burger Macaroni	200	5	30
Cheesy Burger Ravioli	250	6	38
Pepperoni Pizzaroli	250	7	38
Spaghetti & Meatballs in Sce	270	10	32
99% Fat-Free: Beef Ravioli in Sce	170	1.5	33
Cheese Ravioli in Tomato Sce	240	2.5	45

Forkables, Sports; Sealife:

	C	F	Cb
Pasta in Sauce with Meat	250	7	37

Microwaveable Big Bowls: *Per ½ Bowl*

	C	F	Cb
Beefaroni in Tomato Sauce	250	9	31
Lasagna	250	7	33
Mini Beef Ravioli in Sauce	240	8	33

Chef Boyardee (Cont)	C	F	Cb
Microwaveable Cups: *Per Cup*			
Beefaroni	210	8	27
Beef Ravioli	190	5	29
Macaroni & Cheese	190	8	23
Spaghetti & Meatballs	200	8	23
Mini Bites: *Per Cup*			
Beef Ravioli w. Meatballs	280	12	33
Pasta Shells w. Meatballs	250	10	29
Spaghetti w. Meatballs	250	10	30
Overstuffed: Beef Ravioli in Sauce	270	6	44
Italian Sausage Ravioli in Sauce	240	4.5	40
Twistaroni: Cheesy Nacho	220	7	32
Tomato & Beef	230	5	38
Dinner Kits: *Per Serving*			
Cheese Pizza	260	4.5	45
Lasagna	210	4	35
Dennison's Chili: *Per Cup*			
Chili Con Carne w/Beans:			
Original	350	15	31
Chunky	300	10	32
99% Fat Free: Beef Chili w. Beans	210	2	29
Turkey Chili w. Beans	210	3	29
Dinty Moore *(Hormel Foods)*			
7½ oz Can: Beef Stew, 1 can	190	10	15
24 oz Can: Beef Stew, 1 cup	210	10	19
Microwave Cup: Beef Stew, 7.5 oz	150	6	15
Chicken & Dumplings, 7.5 oz	200	6	26
Noodles & Chicken, 7.5 oz	190	9	20
Other varieties, average	180	8	17
Dr. McDougall's: *Per 10 oz*			
Ramen Noodles, Chicken flavor	200	1	40
Rice Pilaf, average	260	2	52
Eden Organics: *Per ½ Cup (4½ oz)*			
Baked Beans w. Sorghum, Mustard	150	0	27
Black Eyed Peas	90	1	16
Black Soybeans	120	6	8
Refried: Black Beans	110	1.5	18
Pinto; Kidney Beans, avg.	85	1	17
Farmhouse			
Pasta: *Per ¾ Cup*			
Chicken Pasta	370	15	49
Creamy Garlic	420	20	49
Herb & Butter	430	20	48
White Cheddar Pasta	380	14	50
Rice: *Per ⅓ Cup (Prepared as Directed)*			
Chicken Rice	230	4	43
Long Grain & Wild Herb Butter	250	7	43
Other varieties, average	230	5	41

French's Fried Onions	C	F	Cb
Regular: 2 Tbsp, ¼ oz	45	3.5	3
¼ cup, ½ oz	90	7	6
1 cup, 2 oz	360	28	24
Cheddar: 2 Tbsp, ¼ oz	45	3.5	3
¼ cup, ½ oz	90	7	6
1 cup, 2 oz	360	28	24
Health Valley			
Chili, average all varieties, 1 cup	150	1	31
Microwavable Chili: *Per Cup*			
Vegetarian Spicy	120	1	25
Vegetarian Spicy 3 Bean	140	1	28
Heinz			
Vegetarian Beans, ½ cup	140	0.5	27
Hormel: *Per Cup*			
Compleats: *Per 10 oz Serving*			
Beef & Beans in BBQ Sauce	390	11	43
Beef Pot Roast	270	6	29
Beef Steak Tips	270	9	29
Chicken & Dumplings	260	8	34
Chicken & Noodles	240	8	27
Chicken & Rice	280	11	34
Chicken Alfredo	360	20	28
Chicken Breast w. Mash Potatoes	200	3	24
Chicken Breast w. Dressing	290	6	35
Homestyle Beef w. Pot. & Gravy	220	6	30
Lasagne with Meat Sauce	280	7	42
Meatloaf w. Pot & Gravy	310	11	34
Salisbury Steak	280	11	30
Santa Fe Style Chicken	280	4	41
Sesame Chicken	320	8	41
Spaghetti w. Sauce	280	8	36
Teriyaki Chicken w. Rice	270	1.5	51
Turkey & Hearty Vegetables	180	3.5	24
Turkey & Dress. w. Gravy	280	8	31
Kid's Kitchen: Beans & Wieners	310	13	37
Cheesy Mac 'N Cheese	270	14	24
Mini Beef Ravioli	240	6	38
Noodle Rings & Chicken	140	4	18
Chili (15 oz Can): *Per ½ Can*			
With Beans:			
Reg./Hot/Chunky, average	260	7	33
Turkey (99% Fat Free)	210	3	28
Vegetarian (99% Fat Free)	190	1	35
Less Sodium Without Beans:			
Hot/Chili, 1 cup	220	9	18
Chunky No Beans	220	9	18
Turkey No Beans	190	3	16

	C	F	Cb
Hungry Jack Potatoes			
Instant Potato Flakes, ⅓ cup	80	0	19
Hunt's			
Manwich Sloppy Joe, Original, ¼ cup	30	0	7
Knorr Lipton:			
Sides: Dry Mix Only			
Note: Figures are only for package contents and not for extra ingredients added in preparation.			
Asian: Chicken Fr. Rice, ½ c., 2.3 oz	220	1.5	47
Teriyaki Noodles, ¾ cup, 2.3 oz	240	2	48
Teriyaki Rice, ½ cup, 2.1 oz	240	1.5	51
Cajun: Garlic Butter Rice, ½ c., 2.4 oz	240	4	46
Red Beans & Rice, ½ cup, 2.8 oz	290	1	52
Fiesta: Mexican Rice, ½ cup, 2.4 oz	240	1	52
Spanish Rice, ½ cup, 2.3 oz	240	1	52
Taco Rice, ½ cup, 2.4 oz	230	1	48
Pasta: Alfredo, ⅔ cup, 2.2 oz	240	4.5	40
Alfredo Broccoli, ⅔ cup, 2.2 oz	240	4.5	41
Butter, ⅔ cup, 2.2 oz	240	4	43
Butter & Herb, ⅔ cup, 2 oz	230	3.5	44
Cheesy Cheddar, ¾ cup, 2.1 oz	220	2	41
Parmesan, ⅔ cup, 2.1 oz	220	4.5	37
Stroganoff, ⅔ cup, 2 oz	210	2	39
Rice: Cheddar Broccoli, ½ c., 2.4 oz	230	1.5	48
Chkn Flav. Broccoli, ½ c., 2.3 oz	210	1	46
Chicken Flav. Rice & Pasta, ½ cup	230	2.5	47
Sides Plus Veggies:			
Butter & Herb Rotini, 1 c., 2.5 oz	260	3.5	49
Cheddar Chse Rice, ¾ c., 2.2 oz	220	2	42
Sth Western Style Rice, ⅔ c. 2.5 oz	250	1.5	52
Vegetable Fr. Rice, ½ c., 2.3 oz	240	1.5	50
Kraft			
Dinners: *Per Serving, Prepared*			
Macaroni & Cheese: Chsy Alfredo	380	14	50
Pasta & Sauce	310	9	49
Scooby-Doo	290	6	50
Spirals	290	6.5	48
Thick 'N Creamy	380	15	50
Bistro Deluxe:			
Creamy Portobello Mushroom	310	11	40
Sundried Tomato Parmesan	300	11	40
Deluxe: Orig.; Sharp Cheddar	320	9	47
Easy Mac, avg. all varieties	230	4	42
Velveeta Shells & Cheese, Orig.	360	12	49
Velveeta Potatoes: *Per ½ Cup, Prepared*			
Cheesy: Au Gratin	180	6	26
Bacon Scalloped	200	7	26
Mashed Potatoes	200	12	21

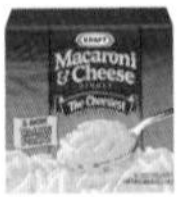

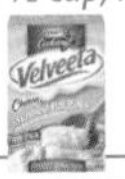

	C	F	Cb
Kroger: *Prepared as Directed*			
Kitchen Creation Skillet Dinners: *Per Cup Prep'd*			
Cheeseburger	300	10	22
Creamy Broccoli	300	14	33
Lasagna	280	9	26
Salisbury	280	10	24
Three Cheese	340	16	30
Noodles & Sauce: *Per Cup, Prepared*			
Alfredo	310	9	44
Butter	290	11	39
Chicken Flavor	250	3	42
Stroganoff	290	10	42
La Choy			
Beef Chow Mein, 1 cup	90	2	11
Chicken Chow Mein, 1 cup	100	3	10
Chop Suey Vegetables, ½ c.	15	0	3
Chow Mein Noodles, ½ cup	130	5	19
Lightlife			
Smart Deli: Baked Ham, 4 sl. 2 oz	70	1	3
Pepperoni Slices, 13 slices, 1 oz	50	1	2
Roast Turkey Style, 4 slices, 2 oz	80	0	6
Santa Fe Chicken, 4 slices, 2 oz	80	0	4
Smart Sausages:			
Chorizo Style, 1 link, 3 oz	140	8	5
Italian Style, 1 link, 3 oz	140	7	7
Smart Stuffers: *Per 4 oz*			
Chick'n Cordon Melt (1)	210	8	15
Chick'n Parmesan (1)	200	8	14
Turkey w. Cranberry (1)	220	7	22
Smart Tenders:			
Lemon Pepper (3)	140	6	8
Savory chick'n (3), 3 oz	150	7	7
Tempeh: BBQ; Ginger Teriyaki, 3 oz	160	6	16
Flax; Soy, avg., 4 oz	225	9	16
Garden Veggie, 4 oz	250	10	17
Three Grain; Wild Rice, 4 oz	230	9	21
Zesty Lemon, 3 oz	160	8	10
Lunchables (Oscar Mayer): *Per Package*			
Cracker Stackers Ham & Cheddar	410	21	39
Mini Beef Taco Wrapz, 5.7 oz	400	10	61
Nachos Chse & Salsa, 4¾ oz	500	18	66
Maxed Out: Combo Ham & Ched.	660	22	101
Combo Turkey & Cheddar, 5.4 oz	680	22	106
Pizza: Pepperoni, 7.1 oz	530	17	75
Extra Cheesy, 7.3 oz	510	12	77
Ultimate Nachos w. Dip & Salsa	580	27	75
Lunchmakers (Armour)			
Loco Nachos	400	14	69
Cheese Pizza	360	9	53

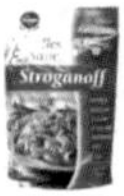

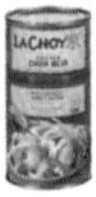

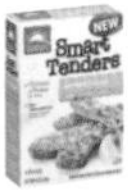

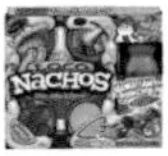

Maruchan

	C	F	Cb
Ramen Noodles: Beef/Chicken/Shrimp Flavors, ½ block, 1½ oz	190	7	26
Noodles: Instant Lunch,			
Roast Beef Flavor	290	12	38
Roast Chicken Flavor	290	12	37
With Shrimp Flavor	290	12	38
Yakisoka: *Per ½ Package*			
Cheddar Cheese Flavor	280	14	31
Chicken Flavor	260	11	35
Teriyaki	260	10	36

Minute Rice: *1 Cup, Prepared*

	C	F	Cb
Ready To Serve:			
Brown Rice	170	4.5	28
Chicken Rice Mix	190	4	35
White Rice	190	4	34

Nissin

	C	F	Cb
Choice Ramen: *Per Cup*			
All flavors	140	1	28
Top Ramen: *Per ½ Dry Noodle Block, w. Seasoning*			
Beef/Chicken Flavor	190	7	27
Chow Mein: *Per ½ Pkg, 56.7g*			
w. Shrimp	280	14	32
Chicken Flavor	240	9	34
Spicy Chicken Flavor	260	11	36
Teriyaki Beef/Thai Peanut	270	12	36
Noodle Cups: *Per Cup*			
Beef/Shrimp Flavor	300	13	38
Beef Flavor Minestrone	270	11	37
Chicken Flavor	300	13	38

Old El Paso

	C	F	Cb
Dinner Kits: *Prepared*			
Chicken Soft Taco (2)	320	10	32
Enchilada Bake (2)	520	23	36
Fajita w/o meat (2)	320	11	33
Hard Taco w. Beef (2)	290	19	19
Soft Taco w. Chicken (2)	320	10	21
Side Dishes: *Prepared*			
Spanish Rice, ⅓ pkt	270	7	54
Cheesy Mexican Rice, ⅓ pkt	280	7	55
Refried Beans: Traditional, ½ cup	90	0.5	16
w. Green Chili, ½ cup, 4.3 oz	90	0.5	16
Vegetarian, ½ cup, 4.16 oz	90	0.5	16
Fat-Free varieties, ½ cup, 4.37 oz	100	0	18

Pasta Roni: *Per Cup (Prepared)*

	C	F	Cb
Angel Hair Pasta varieties, avg.	310	14	39
Asian Garlic Chicken	280	11	39
Butter Herb Italiano	300	11	41
Chicken & Broccoli	360	15	49
Chicken Flavor	300	12	39
Shells & Cheddar	290	12	39

Pasta Roni (Cont): *Per Cup, Prep'd*

	C	F	Cb
Chicken Quesadilla	310	13	40
Fettuccine Alfredo	450	24	48
Four Cheese Corkscrew	370	15	49
Tomato Parmesan	270	9	40
Nature's Way: Creamy Parmesano	270	7	43
Mushroom in Cream Sauce	280	9	41
Olive Oil & Italian Herb	250	8	38

Rice-A-Roni

Classic Favorites: *Per Cup, Prepared*

	C	F	Cb
Beef; Herb & Butter; Rice Pilaf, avg.	310	9	51
Broccoli Au Gratin	360	17	46
Chicken	310	9	51
Lower Sodium	270	5	51
Chicken & Broccoli	230	5	40
Chicken & Garlic	260	8	41
Fried Rice	310	10	51
Spanish Rice	260	7	44

(Reduced Fat Recipe: If only 1 Tbsp fat is used instead of 2 Tbsp, deduct 35 calories and 4g fat.)

	C	F	Cb
Nature's Way: Parmesan & Romano	280	9	42
Italian Cheese & Herb	340	12	52
Long Grain & Wild Rice	250	7	43
Savory Whole Grains:			
Chicken & Herb Classico	260	8	41
Roasted Garlic Italiano	270	9	41
Spanish	250	8	42

Ronzoni Bistro: *Per 8 oz*

	C	F	Cb
Penne with Chicken & Broccoli	210	7	23
Rotini with Tomato & Basil	260	10	34
Spaghetti Meatballs	260	9	32

Rosarita

Refried Beans: *Per ½ Cup*

	C	F	Cb
Traditional	120	2	18
Vegetarian; Spicy	120	2	19
No-Fat: Black Bean	110	0	19
Traditional	100	0	19

S & W: *Per ½ Cup*

	C	F	Cb
Baked Beans, avg. all types	140	0.5	28
Black Beans, 4.48 oz	70	0	18
Chili Beans w. Santa Fe Sce	90	0	21
Kidney Beans, 4.66 oz	100	0.5	23
White Beans, 4.48 oz	80	0.5	19

Shedd's

	C	F	Cb
Country Crock Side Dishes			
Garlic Mashed Pot., ⅔ cup, 5 oz	160	7	22
Homestyle Mashed Pot., ⅔ cup	180	9	23
Deluxe: Cheddar Broccoli Rice, 1 cup	270	11	35
Elbow Macaroni & Cheese, 1 cup	370	17	40
Four Cheese Pasta, 1 cup, 8.11 oz	380	17	41
Loaded Mashed Potatoes, ⅔ cup	200	11	23

Simply Asia

	C	F	Cb
Noodle Bowls: *Per 8.5oz Bowl*			
Roasted Peanut	510	14	78
Sesame Teriyaki	410	3.5	79
Soy Ginger	420	5	78
Spicy Kung Pao	420	5	78
Quick Noodles: *Per 8.8 oz Tray*			
Pad Thai	460	3	93
Szechwan Garlic Chow Mein	460	7	83
Other varieties, average	430	3	86
Stir-Fry Meals: *Per ½ Cup*			
Honey Teriyaki	240	2	47
Mandarin Orange	230	1	49
Spicy Kung Pao	230	3	43
Take Out Noodle Boxes: *Per ½ Box*			
Honey Teriyaki	380	3	73
Pad Thai	390	3	79
Sweet & Sour	370	2	75
Other varieties, average	400	5	71

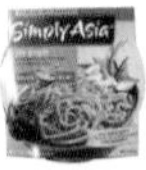
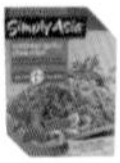
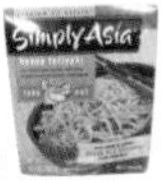

South Beach Living *(Kraft)*

	C	F	Cb
Wraps/S'wiches: *Per Package*			
Deli Ham & Turkey	220	10	23
Grilled Chicken Caesar	230	11	22
Southwestern Style Chicken	240	11	26
Turkey & Bacon Club	240	12	24

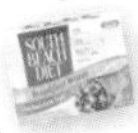

Stagg Chili

	C	F	Cb
14.3 oz Box: *Per Cup*			
Chili w. Beans: Classic/Dynamite	335	17	29
Country/Laredo	320	16	29
Ranch House Chicken	240	8	26
Silverado	250	7	30
White Chili	260	12	20
No Beans: Steakhouse/Dble	320	22	14
Low-Fat: Veg. Garden 4 Bean	200	1	37
Turkey Ranchero	240	3	31

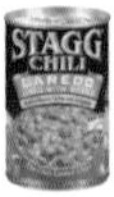

Taco Bell

	C	F	Cb
Home Originals: *Per Serving*			
Dinner Kits: Taco, ⅙ pkg	250	11	20
Cheesy Dbl Decker Taco, ⅙ pkg	350	16	30
Soft Taco, ⅕ pkg	370	13	40
Ultimate Nachos, ¼ pkg	280	14	31
Refried Bean: *Per ½ Cup Serving*			
Fat-Free, w. Green Chilies, 4.6 oz	100	0	18
Vegetarian Blend, 4.6 oz	120	1	20

Tasty Bite

	C	F	Cb
Vegetarian Entrees: *Per ½ Package, 5 oz*			
Agra Peas & Greens	140	10	9
Bengal Lentils	160	8	16
Bombay Potatoes	100	4	13
Jaipur Vegetables	170	11	10
Jodhpur Lentils	100	4	12
Madras Lentils	120	5	14
Punjab Eggplant	140	9	13

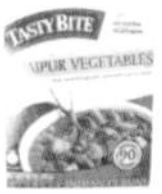

Thai Kitchen

	C	F	Cb
Microwaveable Take-Out Meals: *Per ½ Package*			
Original Pad Thai	240	2	52
Thai Basil & Chili	230	5	43
Thai Peanut	220	4.5	42
Noodle Carts: *Per 2¼ oz Tray*			
Pad Thai	230	2.5	49
Thai Peanut	280	6	51
Rice Noodle Soup Bowls, avg. all flavors, 2.4 oz	250	3	49
Stir-Fry Rice Noodles: *Per ½ Package*			
Thai Curry	290	2	63
Thai Peanut	310	6	54

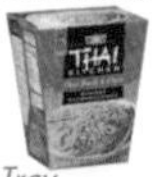
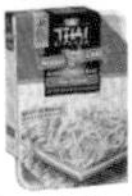

The Spice Hunter: *Per Cup Meal*

	C	F	Cb
Stuffed Potato: Creamy Butter	140	3.5	25
Broccoli & Cheddar	170	3	31
Sour Cream & Chives	160	2	31
Risotto: 3 Cheese	260	3	47
Spinach & Garlic	180	2.5	32
Wild Mushroom	230	0.5	47

Tofurky

	C	F	Cb
Deli Slices, avg., 5 pces, 1.83 oz	100	3	6
Holiday: Dumplings (2), 4 oz	210	1	45
Tofurky Roast, ⅕ pkg, 5.19 oz	250	6	13
Jurky, 4 pieces	100	2	9
Sausages: Beer Brats (1), 3.5 oz	280	16	8
Kielbasa (1), 3.5 oz	240	12	12
Sweet Italian Sausage (1), 3.5 oz	270	13	12

Trader Joe's

	C	F	Cb
Turkey Chili w. Beans, 1 cup	230	3	30
Chicken Chili w. Beans, 1 cup	290	9	32
Pasta, Shells & White Cheddar, 1 cup	280	6	48
Refried Beans, avg., ½ cup	115	0.5	21
Organic Baked Beans, avg., ½ cup	140	0	29
Black Beans: Regular, ½ cup	110	0	19
Cuban Style, ½ cup	100	0.5	19
Pasta Bowls: *Per 5 oz Bowl*			
Penne w. Crmy Vodka Marinara Sce	400	8	72
Fusilli with Tomato Basil Sauce	380	5	72
Potatoes: Garlic Mashed, ½ cup	150	7	19
Cheddar Cheese Au Gratin, ½ cup	140	5	21

Uncle Ben's	**C**	**F**	**Cb**
Country Inn: *Per Cup, Prepared w/o Margarine*			
Broccoli Rice Au Gratin	200	2	43
Other varieties, avg.	200	1	43
Ready Rice: *Per 1 Cup, Prepared*			
Butter & Garlic Flavored Rice	220	4	41
Roasted Chicken	220	3.5	41
Teriyaki	220	3	42
Whole Grain Brown	240	3	39
Valley Fresh			
Chicken: *Per 2 oz*			
White & Dark Chunk	80	3.5	0
Premium Chunk White	70	2	0
Turkey, Premium Chunk White	80	3	0
Van Camps			
Pork & Beans, ½ cup	110	1	23
Orig. Baked Beans, ½ cup	140	1	30
Beanee Weenee Original, 10½ oz	340	11	39
White Wave			
Seitan: Chicken w. Broth, 5 oz	110	2	4
Traditional, 3 oz	90	1	3
Soy Milks & Yogurts: *See Pages 48, 170*			
Tofu: *See Page 162*			
Worthington/Loma Linda			
Big Franks: 1 link, 1.8 oz	110	6	3
Low-fat, 1 link, 1.8 oz	80	2.5	3
Chili, 1 cup, 8.10 oz	280	10	25
Choplets, 2 slices, 3.2 oz	90	1	4
Diced Chik, 2 oz	50	0	2
Linketts, (1), 1¼ oz	70	4	1
Little Links, 2 links, 1.6 oz	90	5	3
Low-Fat Veja-Links (1), 1 oz	45	1.5	3
Multigrain Cutlets, 2 sl., 3¼ oz	100	1	5
Prime Stakes (1) 3¼ oz	120	6	7
Redi-Burger, ⅝" slice, 3 oz	120	2.5	7
Saucettes, 1 link, 1 oz	90	6	1
Super Links (1) 1.7 oz	110	8	2
Tender Bits (6), 2.8 oz	120	4	7
Tender Rounds (6), 2.8 oz	120	4.5	6
Veja-Links (1), 1 oz	50	3	1
Vege-Burger, ¼ cup, 2 oz	60	0.5	2
Vegetable Skallops, ½ cup, 3 oz	90	1	4
Vegetarian Burger, ¼ cup, 1.9 oz	70	1.5	3

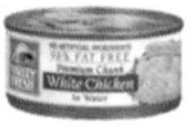

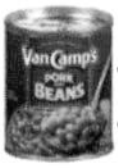

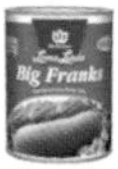

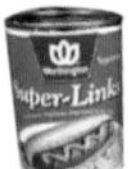

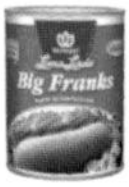

Yves Veggie Cuisine	**C**	**F**	**Cb**
Breakfast: Patties (2) 1.8 oz	80	2	4
Canadian Veg. Bacon, 3 slices	80	0.5	2
Burgers: Meatless Beef Burger (1)	110	4	8
Lentil & Veggie Burger (1) 2.6 oz	130	3.5	19
Deli: Bologna, 4 slices	80	2.5	2
Ham, 4 slices	100	2	5
Pepperoni, 6 slices	60	1	4
Roast Beef, 4 slices	110	2.5	4
Salami, 4 slices	80	0	4
Smoked Chicken, 4 slices	100	1.5	5
Turkey, 4 slices	100	1.5	5
Hot Dogs & Brats:			
Jumbo Dog (1) 2.7 oz	110	3	5
Good Dog (1) 2 oz	70	3.5	2
Hot Dog (1), 1.6 oz	50	0.5	2
Tofu Dog, avg. (1), 1.3 oz	45	1	2
Brats: Veggie Classic (1), 3.3 oz	160	5	9
Zesty Italian (1), 3.3 oz	150	5	9
Entree: Chili, 10.5 oz	240	1	37
Lasagne, 10.5 oz	300	3	51
Mac n Soy Cheese, 10½ oz	340	9	52
Santa Fe Beef, 10½ oz	360	9	57
Thai Lemongrass Veggie Chicken	330	9	49
Skewers:			
Lemon Herb Chicken, 2.8 oz	100	1	7
Meatless:			
Ground: Turkey, ⅓ cup, 1.95 oz	60	1	4
Taco Stuffers, ⅓ cup, 1.95 oz	90	2.5	5
Rounds: Original, ⅓ c., 1.95 oz	60	0.5	5
Asian Lettuce Wrap, ⅓ c. 1.95 oz	60	0.5	8
Strips: Beef, 3 oz	120	1	4
Chicken, 3 oz	110	1	3
Zatarain's			
Beans & Rice Mix: *Per 1 Cup Prepared*			
Black Beans	230	0.5	37
Blackeyed Peas	220	0.5	46
Caribbean Rice	320	6	61
Chicken Creole	130	0.5	28
Chicken Flavor	210	1	44
Fire Roasted Vegetables	170	0	38
Garlic & Herb	160	1.5	34
Gravy & Rice	200	0.5	45
Rice Pilaf	210	1	45
Smothered Chicken Rice	130	0	28
Yellow Rice	220	0	46
Ready-to-Serve Complete Meals: *Per Packet*			
Blackened Chicken & Yellow Rice	300	4.5	52
Dirty Rice with Pork, 8.8 oz	375	6	72
Jambalaya with Sausage, 6.5 oz	350	12	48
Red Beans with Rice & Ssg, 6.5 oz	350	7	57
Southern Chicken Rice, 8.8 oz	400	6	77

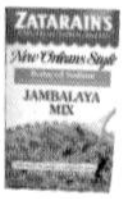

Amy's (Vegetarian) C F Cb

Per Serving

	C	F	Cb
Asian Meals: Thai Stir Fry, 9.5 oz	310	11	45
Asian Noodle Stir Fry, 10 oz	290	7	50
Bowls: Brown Rice & Vegs, 10 oz	260	9	36
Santa Fe Enchilada, 10 oz	350	11	47
(Other Varieties ~ www.CalorieKing.com)			
Burritos: Bean & Rice, 6 oz	280	6	48
Bean & Cheese, 6 oz	300	9	43
Breakfast Burrito, 6 oz	250	7	38
Entrees: Cheese Enchilada, 4.9 oz	240	14	18
Cheese Lasagna, 10.3 oz	380	14	44
Macaroni & Cheese, 9 oz	400	16	47
Macaroni & Soy Cheeze, 9 oz	370	15	42
Roasted Vege Lasagna 9.8 oz	350	11	47
Tofu, 9.5 oz	310	11	41
Whole Meals: Chse Enchilada, 9 oz	350	15	38
Black Bean Enchilada	330	8	53
Black Bean Tamale Verde	330	10	55
Veggie Loaf, 10 oz	290	8	47
Pot Pies: Broccoli	430	22	46
Mex. Tamale; Shepherd's Pie,	155	4	27
Vegetable, 7½ oz	420	19	54
Snacks: Nacho, 5-6 pcs	210	8	26
Chse Pizza, 5-6 pcs	190	7	22
Veggie Burgers:			
Californian Veggie (1), 2½ oz	140	5	19

Extra Product Listings ~ www.CalorieKing.com

Bagel Bites

Three Cheese, 4 pieces, 3 oz	210	6	30
Cheese Sausage & Pepperoni, 4 pcs	210	7	30

Banquet

	C	F	Cb
Chicken, Breaded: Brst Patties (1)	160	9	11
Chicken Breast Nuggets (6), 3 oz	240	16	12
Crispy Chicken, Skinless, 4.2 oz	360	23	13
Popcorn Chicken, 11 pieces	180	9	18
Wings: Hot & Spicy, 3 oz	260	17	8
Honey Barbecue, 3 oz	270	17	12
Crock Pot Classics			
Chicken & Dumplings, ⅔ cup	200	8	21
Hearty Beef & Veggies, ⅔ cup	140	6	15
Meatballs in Stroganoff Sauce, ⅔ c.	300	14	29

Banquet (Cont) C F Cb

	C	F	Cb
Dinners:			
Boneless Pork Rib, 10 oz	370	17	47
Chicken Fingers, 7.1 oz	460	15	69
Fettuccine Alfredo, 8 oz	290	12	34
Lasagna w. Meat Sauce, 8 oz	270	8	35
Mac & Cheese, 8 oz	260	6	40
Macaroni & Beef, 8 oz	200	4	32
Meatloaf Meal, 9.5 oz	280	13	28
Pepperoni Pizza, 5.75	350	13	46
Salisbury Steak Meal, 9.5 oz	290	16	25
Spaghetti & Meatballs, 9 oz	380	16	42
Swedish Meatballs, 10.25 oz	440	18	51
Turkey , 9.25 oz	280	7	41
Hearty One Dinners:			
Chicken Fried Beef Steak	750	42	66
Chicken Fried Chicken	660	40	48
Select Recipe: Chicken Parmesan	360	16	37
Corn Dog Meal, 7.5 oz	460	16	68
Fried Chicken Meal, 9 oz	440	26	30
Slow Cooked Beef Meal	220	6	27
Pot Pies: Beef, 7 oz	450	27	36
Chicken/Turkey, avg., 7 oz	385	21	35

Birds Eye – Voila!

Per 1 Cup, Cooked

Voila!: Beef & Broccoli Stir Fry	210	6	27
Chicken Parmesan	240	8	31
Creamy Tomato Penne w. Chkn	210	4.5	29
Garlic Chicken	240	8	21
Garlic Shrimp	220	8	27
Shrimp Scampi	190	2.5	31
Sweet & Sour Chicken	200	1	38
Family Skillets: Alfredo C	250	6	35
Cheesy Chicken	250	6	35
Cheesy Macaroni Beef	370	15	44

Boca (Vegetarian)

	C	F	Cb
Burger: Cheeseburger, 2.5 oz	100	4.5	6
All American Flame Grilled, 2.5 oz	120	5	6
Vegan, Original, 2.5 oz	70	0.5	6
Organic Burgers: Vegan, Orig.	100	2.5	9
Roasted Garlic/Onion	130	3	10
Chik'n: Nuggets (4), 3 oz	180	7	17
Patties (1), 2.5 oz	160	6	15
Sausages: Italian, 2.5 oz	130	6	6
Vegie Patties, Bruschetta	70	1.5	9

Boston Market

	C	F	Cb
Dinners: Beef Sirloin & Ndles, 14 oz	460	12	58
Chicken Parmesan	620	24	69
Salisbury Steak	710	40	53
Swedish Meatballs	760	43	57
Turkey Breast Medallions w. Pot.	360	14	35
Entrees: Chicken Pot Pie, 8 oz	560	36	43
Honey Roasted Chicken, 9.2 oz	410	17	46

Claim Jumper

	C	F	Cb
Beef Pot Roast, 8 oz	220	10	22
Chicken & Noodles, 8 oz	300	15	24
Chicken Alfredo, 8 oz	300	12	32
Chicken Fried Beef Steak, 16¼ oz	720	39	71
Country Fried Chicken, 17¼ oz	700	34	75
Lasagna w. Meat Sauce, 8 oz	310	14	30
Meatloaf Dinner, 15¼ oz	520	31	36
Rst Turkey Brest w. Broccoli, 14 oz	430	17	47
Salisbury Steak, 16 oz	640	35	48
Pot Pies: Beef, 1 cup, 8 oz	580	41	39
Chicken & Broccoli, 1 cup	550	37	39

Contessa

	C	F	Cb
Green Cuisine Meals: *Per Serving, Unprepared*			
Beef Goulash, 9 oz	250	5	34
Burgundy Beef Stew, 9 oz	240	11	22
Chicken Cacciatore, 9 oz	240	7	28
Chicken Tandoori w/ Sauce, 8 oz	200	3.5	27
Kung Pao Shrimp w/ sauce, 8 oz	200	3.5	30
Shrimp Mediterranean w/ sauce, 10 oz	400	5	63
Microsteam: *Per 1 Cup Prepared*			
Chicken Alfredo	270	13	27
Italian Sausage Rigatoni	310	11	43
Spaghetti Bolognese	250	11	27

Croissant Pockets

	C	F	Cb
Five Cheese Pizza	350	17	35
Ham & Cheddar	320	16	33
Pepperoni Pizza	370	21	33
Philly Steak & Chse	340	18	34

GardenBurger

	C	F	Cb
Veggie Burgers: *Per Patty*			
Potabella	90	2.5	16
Sun-Dried Tomato Basil	100	2.5	17
The Original	100	3	18
Garden Steaks: Gourmet Tuscany	210	8	36
Gourmet Hula	250	8	48
Garden Variety: Breaded Chik'n	160	9	13
Breakfast Sausage	60	3.5	4
Herb Crusted Cutlet	140	7	13

Gorton's

	C	F	Cb
Fish Fillets:			
Battered:			
Beer Battered (2), 3.63 oz	250	17	17
Crisp Battered (2), 3.81	230	12	22
Lemon Peppered Battered (2), 2.7 oz	270	18	20
Breaded: Classic Crunchy Golden (2)	240	12	23
Crunch Tilapia (2), 3.8 oz	240	12	23
Garlic & Herbs (2)	230	12	21
Lemon Herb (2)	240	13	22
Potato Crunch (2)	240	14	20
Grilled: Garlic/Lem. Butter (1)	100	3	1
Salmon (1), 3.15 oz	100	3	1
Tilapia (1), 3.15 oz	80	2.5	1
Shrimp:			
Crunchy Butterfly (5)	250	11	27
Shrimp Scampi, 4 oz	120	6	8
Grilled: Classic, 4 oz	110	1.5	5
Shrimp Scampi, 4oz	130	4.5	3

Healthy Choice

	C	F	Cb
Cafe Steamers:			
Chicken Margherita, 10 oz	320	7	45
Chicken Pesto Classico	320	9	39
Chicken Red Pepper Alfredo, 10.3 oz	250	5	30
Grilled Basil Chicken	290	6	39
Grilled Whiskey Steak	250	4	34
Rstd Beef Merlot, 10.6 oz	230	8	21
Roasted Chicken Fresca, 10.6 oz	230	5	29
Roasted Chicken Marsala, 10.4 oz	250	6	30
Complete Meals:			
Beef Pot Roast, 11 oz	260	5	40
Chkn Parmigiana, 11.6 oz	340	9	49
Grilled Chicken Teriyaki, 11 oz	280	4	44
Homestyle Salisbury Steak, 12.5	290	6	42
Lemon Pepper Fish	310	4.5	53
Oven Roasted Chicken	260	5	37
Sweet & Sour Chicken	400	10	61
Select Entrees:			
Bacon & Smokey Cheddar Chicken	260	6	32
Chicken Alfredo, 8.5 oz	230	3.5	31
Honey Ginger Chicken, 8.5 oz	310	4.5	53
Salisbury Steak, 8 oz	190	6	18

Hot Pockets

C F Cb

Calzones: Per ½ Calzone, 4.2 oz

	C	F	Cb
4 Meat & 4 Cheese	290	12	33
Pepperoni & 3 Cheese	310	15	33
Supreme	280	12	32

Paninis: Per ½ Panini

	C	F	Cb
Bruschetta Chicken	190	6	25
Deli Style Ham & Swiss	220	8	26
Steak & Cheddar	230	8	27

Stuffed Sandwiches: Per 4 oz Sandwich

	C	F	Cb
Barbecue Sauce w. Beef Steak	340	14	44
Beef Taco	320	13	37
Cheeseburger	310	13	37
Four Cheese Pizza	320	13	27
Meatballs & Mozzarella	340	16	36
Philly Steak & Cheese	310	13	37
Sausage & Pepperoni Pizza	340	16	36

Soft Baked Subs: Ham 'N Cheese

	C	F	Cb
Soft Baked Subs: Ham 'N Cheese	260	9	34
Meatballs & Mozzarella	320	15	34
Philly Steak & Cheese	300	13	34
Spicy Peperoni Pizza	360	19	34
Twisted Stix, average, 1 pce	130	4.5	18

Hungry-Man

Hungry-Man Dinners:

	C	F	Cb
Boneless Fried Chkn	860	44	86
Boneless Pork Rib	840	36	105
Buffalo Chicken Strips	970	46	103
Classic Fried Chicken	1040	59	64
Meatloaf	690	29	74
Mexican Style Fiesta	600	23	87
Roasted Carved Turkey	560	18	78
Rotisserie Chicken	460	36	31
Salisbury Steak	580	31	50

Hungry-Man XXL Dinners: Per ½ Package

	C	F	Cb
Backyard BBQ, 12 oz	570	28	52
Carved Turkey Breast	430	18	47
Gr. Beef Steak Strips	620	14	94
Meatloaf	690	27	86
Roasted Carved Turkey Dinner	1360	70	114
Southern Fried Boneless Chicken	500	26	44

XXL Sandwiches: Per 8 oz Sandwich

	C	F	Cb
Angus Beef Charbroil	700	41	55
Buffalo Fried Chicken	660	27	70
BBQ Pork Ribs	750	45	60
Country Fried Pork	660	33	70
Chili Cheese Dogs	300	15	31
Crispy Fried Chicken	670	30	68

José Olé

C F Cb

Breakfast Burrito

	C	F	Cb
Egg & Bacon, 4 oz	250	9	32
Egg & Ham, 4 oz	250	8	34
Egg & Sausage, 4 oz	270	10	34
Premium: Chicken Monterey, 5 oz	270	7	41
Steak & Cheese (1), 5 oz	310	10	40

Burrito: Steak & Cheese

	C	F	Cb
Burrito: Steak & Cheese	310	10	40
Chicken Monterey (1)	270	7	41

Chimichangs:

	C	F	Cb
Mini Steak & Cheddar (3), 3.85 oz	340	17	38
Premium: Chicken & Cheese (1), 5 oz	330	12	44
Steak & Cheese (1), 5 oz	350	15	40

	C	F	Cb
Empanadas, Chkn & Cheddar (2)	320	15	34

Snacks: Beef & Chse Tacos (4)

	C	F	Cb
Snacks: Beef & Chse Tacos (4)	200	11	19
Chimichangas, 3 pces	340	17	38
Taquitos, 4 pces	200	10	24
Quesadillas, 3 pces	240	8	32

Tacos: Beef & Cheese, Soft (1), 5 oz

	C	F	Cb
Tacos: Beef & Cheese, Soft (1), 5 oz	270	10	31
Mini Beef & Cheese (4), 3 oz	200	11	19

Taquitos, Corn, average, 3 pieces

	C	F	Cb
Taquitos, Corn, average, 3 pieces	200	9	26
Flour, average 2 pieces	235	12	28

Kid Cuisine

	C	F	Cb
All American Fried Chicken	480	20	47
All Star Chicken Breast Nuggets	440	17	53
Chse Blaster Mac & Cheese Meal	390	9	64
Magical Cheese Stuffed Crust Pizza	420	11	62
Popstar Popcorn Chicken	430	13	64
Twist & Twirl Spaghetti w. Meatballs	420	12	60

Kroger

Meals Made Simple

	C	F	Cb
Chicken Alfredo, 1¾ cups, 7.4 oz	410	16	47
Chicken Parmesan, 1¾ cups, 6.4 oz	270	8	34
Shrimp Asparagus, 2¼ cups, 6.9 oz	220	6	30
Shrimp Fried Rice, 1¼ cups, 8 oz	190	0.5	36
Shrimp Linguini, 1⅓ cups, 8 oz	340	8	51

Oven Ready

	C	F	Cb
Breaded Calamari Rings (15), 3 oz	200	11	19
Coconut Shrimp with Dipping Sce	350	21	27
Shrimp Scampi (7), 4 oz	320	29	4

Pot Pies: Beef, (1), 7 oz

	C	F	Cb
Pot Pies: Beef, (1), 7 oz	450	27	36
Chicken (1), 7 oz	390	22	36
Turkey (1), 7 oz	370	20	36

Lean Cuisine

	C	F	Cb
Cafe Classics Entrees: *Per Meal*			
Beef & Broccoli	260	5	39
Beef Chow Fun	320	5	54
Beef Portabello	220	6	25
Chicken with Almonds	250	4	38
Sun Dried Tomato Pesto Chicken	290	9	34
Thai Style Chicken	290	7	39
Cafe Classic Bowls:			
Chicken Teriyaki	250	2	44
Grilled Chicken Caesar	240	7	25
Three Chse Stuffed Rigatoni	240	6	35
One Dish Favorites: Mac. & Chse	290	7	41
Angel Hair Pomodoro	250	5	42
Chicken Enchilada Suizo	270	4	47
Lasagna w/ Meat Sce	320	7	43
Linguini Carbonara	300	8	43
Pasta Romano w/ Bacon	280	7	43
Spaghetti with Meatballs	270	5	38
Paninis, average all flavors	340	8	42
Flatbread Melts, average (1)	330	9	42
Pizzas ~ *See Page 138*			

Lean Pockets

Per Single Pocket

	C	F	Cb
Cheeseburger	290	8	41
Four Cheese Pizza	300	7	45
Meatballs & Mozzarella	290	9	40
Pepperoni Pizza	280	8	40
Philly Steak & Cheese	270	7	39
Stuffed Quesadilla, avg.	360	9	48
Whole Grain: Chkn Broccoli & Cheddar	250	6	39
Garlic Chkn White Pizza, 4.48 oz	270	8	38
Grilled Chicken Mushr. & Spinach	250	6	37
Ham & Cheddar	270	8	40
Meatball & Mozzarella	230	7	33
Supreme Pizza	220	6	33
Turkey, Broccoli & Cheese	260	8	39
Mexican Style, average all flavors	250	7	36
Soft Baked Subs, average	250	7	36
Breakfast, average	140	4.5	18

Marie Callender's

	C	F	Cb
Complete Dinners: *Per Meal*			
Country Fried Chicken & Gravy	560	26	61
Golden Battered Fish Fillet	410	12	60
Grilled Chicken Breast	400	17	32
Honey Roasted Chicken	340	12	37
Honey Roasted Turkey	320	10	31
Meatloaf & Gravy w. Pot.	460	19	40
Old Fashioned Beef Pot Roast	310	9	34
Salisbury Steak & Gravy	390	15	38
Spaghetti w. Meat Sauce	620	19	88
Swedish Meatballs	450	21	44
Pasta Al Dente:			
Cavatappi Genovese, 11 oz	400	16	40
Fettuccine Chkn Balsamico, 10.5 oz	420	17	44
Penne Chicken Modesto, 11 oz	400	18	39
Rigatoni: Con Pesce, 10.5 oz	340	12	44
Marinara Classico, 10.5 oz	460	24	41
Tortellini Romano, 10 oz	460	15	62
Pot Pies: Grilled Chicken Alfredo	680	39	58
Savory Herb Turkey, 10 oz	660	36	64

Michael Angelo's *Per Single Serve Package*

	C	F	Cb
Baked Ziti & Meatballs, 12 oz Tray	480	15	60
Chicken Alfredo, 12 oz	470	14	57
Chicken Cacciatore, 10 oz	260	8	26
Chicken w/ Creamy Garlic, 10 oz	310	9	31
Chicken Piccata, 10 oz	510	24	52
Chicken Toscana, 12 oz	490	15	58
Eggplant & Chkn, 12 oz	360	16	28
Eggplant Parmesan, 12 oz	480	28	16
Four Cheese Lasagna, 12 oz	600	33	42
Lasagna with Meat Sauce, 12 oz	450	16	45
Manicotti with Sauce, 12 oz	460	24	11
Shrimp Scampi, 10 oz	570	30	53
Vegetable Lasagna, 12 oz	345	11	35

Morningstar Farms

	C	F	Cb
Burgers: *Made with Organic Soy*			
Classic	150	6	9
Mushroom Lovers	110	6	8
Spicy Black Bean	120	4	13
Tex Mex Burger	110	1	17
Thai Burger	100	3.5	7
Patties: Breakfast Pattie (1)	80	3	4
Chik Patties, Original (1)	140	5	16
Garden Veggie Pattie (1)	110	3.5	9
Italian Herb Chik Pattie (1)	170	5	22

Morningstar (Cont)

	C	F	Cb
Grillers: Original Veggie Burger	130	6	5
Prime Veggie Burger	170	9	4
Vegan	100	2.5	7
Chik'n: Buffalo Wings (5)	200	8	20
Chik'n Nuggets (4)	190	9	1

Safeway Select

	C	F	Cb
Beef Salisbury Steak, 9.35 oz	400	25	23
Bow Tie Pasta Pepperoni, 9.5 oz	340	14	36
Chicken Parmesan, 9.25 oz	350	11	48
Classic Lasagna, 11 oz	280	9	35
Fettucini Alfredo, 11.5 oz	480	15	75
Five Vegetable Lasagna, 10.6 oz	330	7	58
Orange Chicken, 9 oz	450	15	64
Pasta Primavera, 9 oz	300	11	41
Pot Roast, 9 oz	280	14	26
Spaghetti w. Meat Sauce, 12 oz	450	16	61
Swedish Meat Balls, 11.5 oz	470	24	43
Triple Rich Mac. & Cheese, 7.95 oz	360	18	37

South Beach Living

	C	F	Cb
Caprese Style Chicken	240	8	10
Garlic Parmesan Chicken	270	10	22
Orange Beef Slices	220	7	23
Roasted Turkey	240	9	27
Savory: Beef	220	8	16
Pork	230	9	13

Stouffer's

	C	F	Cb
Entrees, Homestyle: *Per Serving*			
Beef Stroganoff, 9.75 oz	380	17	34
Breaded Boneless Pork Cutlet, 10oz	370	21	31
Chicken a la King, 11.5 oz	360	12	44
Lasagna Bake w. Meat Sce, 11½ oz	350	10	49
Macaroni & Cheese, 6 oz	340	16	33
Meatloaf w. Pot. & Glaze, 16 oz	600	31	4
Roast Turkey Breast, 16 oz	460	19	51
Salisbury Steak w. Mac & Cheese	710	39	48
Spag. w. Meat Sce, 12 oz	350	12	44
Stuffed Pepper, 10 oz	210	9	23
Swedish Meatballs, 11.5 oz	560	27	47
Turkey Tetrazzini, 12 oz	450	23	38
Corner Bistro:			
Flatbread Melts:			
Chicken Quesadilla, 6 oz	370	15	41
Steak, Mushr. & Cheddar	390	17	40
Stromboli: Italian-Style Supreme	430	19	45
Chicken, Broccoli & Cheddar, 6 oz	360	11	45
Pepperoni & Provolone, 6 oz	430	17	45

Stouffer's (Cont)

	C	F	Cb
Easy Express: *Per Serving*			
Cheesy Garlic Lasagna, 7.8 oz	330	13	36
Cheese Manicotti, 9.8 oz	340	16	33
Rigatoni with Chicken, 4.7 oz	260	10	29
Easy Express Skillets: *Per Bowl*			
Broccoli & Beef; Garlic Chkn, avg.	350	6	57
Chicken Alfredo, 12.5 oz	410	10	48
Teriyaki Chicken, 12.5 oz	310	4.5	44
Yankee Pot Roast, 8 oz	300	8	38
Side Dish: Cheddar Pot. Bake, 5 oz	270	17	21

Swanson

	C	F	Cb
Classics:			
Breaded Fish Fillet, 7.3 oz	370	14	45
Boneless Fried Chicken, 7.5 oz	240	13	21
Chicken Strips w. Fries, 6¾ oz	300	10	39
Macaroni & Cheese, 10.25oz	430	16	62
Meatloaf, 9.5 oz	270	13	22
Mexican Style Fiesta	380	15	51
Roasted Carved Turkey	310	11	39
Salisbury Steak, 9.5 oz	330	15	32
Pot Pies: Beef (1), 7 oz	390	24	33
Chicken/Turkey (1), 7 oz	380	22	34

TGI Friday's

	C	F	Cb
Beer Battered Onion Rings (3)	180	8	26
Buffalo Wings (3)	180	11	4
Chicken Quesadilla	290	13	26
Honey BBQ Wings (3)	150	9	6
Mozzarella Sticks & Sce, 1 oz	80	4.5	7
Popcorn Chicken, 3 pces, 2.6 oz	250	8	29
Potato Skins, Ched. & Bacon, 3 pces	210	12	20

Trader Joe's

	C	F	Cb
Meals: *Per Serving*			
Asian Style Chkn Stir Fry w. Sce, 8 oz	190	1	30
Chicken Chow Mein, ⅓ pkg, 6.35 oz	220	2	37
Chicken Fried Rice, 1 cup, 5 oz	200	3.5	33
Chicken Quesadilla (1), 6 oz	320	16	26
Citrus Glazed Chicken w/ rice, 8 oz	270	5	40
Macaroni & cheese, 1 cup, 6.98 oz	360	15	42
Rice Bowls, average, 11 oz bowl	390	3.5	55
Shrimp Stir Fry, 6.4 oz	70	0.5	6
Sweet & Sour Shrimp w. Rice, ⅓ pkg	190	0	39
Turkey Saus. Stromboli, ¼ loaf, 4.5 oz	250	7	31
Pies: Chicken Pot Pie, ½ Pie, 8 oz	360	22	28
Spinach Pie, ¼ pie, 6 oz	240	4	37

Tyson

	C	F	Cb
Any'tizers:			
Buffalo Style: Chicken Wyngs, 3 pces	150	7	8
Hot Wings (Bagged), 3 pces	230	15	1
Chicken Peperoni Minis (3)	200	11	10
Chicken Cordon Bleu Minis (3)	180	10	9
Popcorn Chicken (Boxed), 6 pces	220	10	19
Popcorn Chicken Bites (Bag), 7 pces	180	9	11
Fully Cooked Chicken: *Per Serving*			
Buffalo Style Chicken Strips (2)	230	10	21
Fajita Chicken Strips, 3 oz	110	4	1
Grilled Chicken Breast Strips, 3 oz	100	1.5	3
Honey BBQ Chicken Strips (1)	180	8	18
Southwestern Style Chkn Brst Strips	120	3	3
Spicy Chicken Breast Fillets (1)	320	17	25
100% All Natural Breaded Chicken			
Breast: Fillets (1), 4.5 oz	240	9	20
Patties (1), 2.57 oz	180	11	12
Sthn Style Tenderloins (1)	150	7	9
Tenders (5)	240	14	15
Crispy Strips (2)	200	10	13
Nuggets (5), 3.2 oz	270	17	15
Skillet Creations: *Per Serving*			
Asian Style Orange Chicken, ½ pkg	340	5	50
Chicken Tuscany & Penne, ½ pkg	320	6	44
Grilled Chicken Fajitas (2)	250	7	32

Van De Kamp's

	C	F	Cb
Crispy Battered Halibut (3), 4 oz	230	11	22
Crunchy Fish Sticks (6), 4 oz	260	13	26
Fish Shaped Nuggets (4), 4.25 oz	260	12	29
Baked: Fish Fillet (2), 3.67 oz	150	1.5	25
Fried: Battered Fillets (2)	190	9	20
Breaded: Butterfly Shrimp, 7 pces	250	11	27
Popcorn Shrimp, 20 pces, 4 oz	260	11	30

Weight Watchers

	C	F	Cb
Smart Ones Bistro Selections: *Per Meal*			
Chicken Carbonara	250	4.5	32
Chicken Fettucini	340	6	47
Chicken Parmesan	290	5	35
Meatloaf w. Mashed Pot.	250	8	23
Picante Chicken & Pasta	260	4	32
Roasted Chicken w/ Potato	180	4	20
Sirloin Beef Asian Veg.	220	5	27
Stuffed Turkey Breast	290	6	42
Sweet & Sour Chicken	210	2	31
Teriyaki Chicken & Veg.	230	2.5	39
Thai Style Chicken & Rice Noodles	260	4	43

Weight Watchers (Cont)

	C	F	Cb
Smart Ones Anytime Selections: *Per Meal*			
Calzone Italiano, 10 oz	290	6	47
Chicken & Cheese Quesadilla, 8 oz	220	7	26
Classic Favorites: *Per Meal*			
Angel Hair Marinara	230	4	40
Broccoli & Cheddar Roasted Potato	240	7	35
Chkn Enchiladas Suiza	290	5	49
Lasagna Bake w/ Meat Sauce	270	4	43
Lemon Herb Chkn Piccata	230	1.5	31
Macaroni & Cheese	270	2	52
Pasta Primavera	280	6	44
Rst Turkey Medallions	220	1.5	38
Salisbury Steak	260	7	26
Shrimp Marinara	180	1.5	31
Spaghetti w/ Meat Sauce	310	6	48
Spicy Szechuan Style Vege & Chkn	240	5	36
Swedish Meatballs	270	5	35
Three Cheese Macaroni	300	6	48
Traditional Lasagna w. Meat Sce	300	6	43
Tuna Noodle Gratin	240	4.5	37
Fruit Inspirations: *Per Meal*			
Cranberry Turkey Medallions	250	2	43
Honey Mango BBQ Chkn	240	3.5	34
Orange Sesame Chicken	320	8	48
Pineapple Beef Teriyaki	260	4.5	38
Morning Express, Breakfast: *Per Meal*			
Breakfast Quesadilla	220	6	28
Canadian Style Bacon Eng. Muffin	210	6	27
English Muffin Sandwich, 4 oz	210	5	27
Stuffed Breakfast Sandwich, 4 oz	240	7	28

Worthington/Loma Linda

	C	F	Cb
Chic-ketts, 2 slices	110	5	2
Dinner Roast, ¾" slice	180	11	6
Fried Chik'n w. Gravy, 2 pieces	150	10	5
FriPats, 1 pattie, 2¼ oz	130	6	5
Leanies, 1 link, 1.4 oz	100	7	2
Meatless: Chicken Style Roll, ⅜" sl.	90	4.5	2
Smoked Turkey Roll, ⅜" slice	130	8	4
Prosage, Links, 2 links, 1.6 oz	80	3	3
Stakelets, 2.5 oz pce	150	7	7
Stripples, 2 slices	60	4.5	2
Swiss Stake, 1 piece	130	6	9

Zatarains

Per 12oz Package Unless Indicated

	C	F	Cb
Blackened Chicken Alfredo, 10.5 oz	500	25	46
Jambalaya seasoned with Chicken	400	5	69
Jambalaya seasoned with Sausage	480	14	77
Red Beans & Rice with Sausage	510	20	68

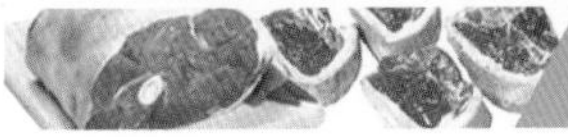

Note: Cooking reduces weight of meat by 20-45% due to water and fat losses. Average weight loss is 30%. Actual loss depends on cooking method and cooking time. Examples:

 4 oz raw wt. = approx. 3 oz cooked wt.
 4 oz cooked wt. = approx. 5½ oz raw wt.

What 3 oz Cooked Meat Looks Like
- Half the size of this book (4¼" x 3" x ⅜" thick)
- Rectangular piece (4" x 2½" x ½" thick)
- Deck of cards (3½" x 2½" x ⅝" thick)

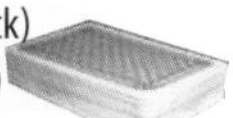

STEAK QUICK GUIDE

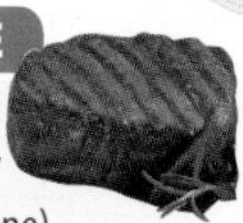

Sirloin (Choice Grade)
External fat trimmed to ¼"
Broiled, Edible Portion (no bone)

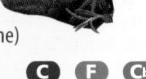

	C	F	Cb
Small/Regular Serving, 3 oz (cooked)			
(from 4-4½ oz raw)			
Lean + external fat (¼"), 3 oz	225	13	0
Lean + marbling, 3 oz	195	10	0
Lean only, 3 oz	160	6	0
(No external fat or marbling)			
Medium Serving, 5 oz (cooked wt)			
(from approx. 7 oz raw)			
Lean + external fat (¼"), 5 oz	350	21	0
Lean + marbling, 5 oz	325	17	0
Lean only, 5 oz	265	10	0
Large Serving, 8 oz (cooked wt)			
(from 11-12 oz raw)			
Lean + external fat, 8 oz	600	36	0
Lean + marbling, 8 oz	520	27	0
Lean only, 8 oz	425	15	0
Extra Large Serving, 12 oz (cooked wt)			
(from approx. 16-17 oz raw)			
Lean + external fat (¼"), 12 oz	900	52	0
Lean + marbling, 12 oz	740	40	0
Lean only, 12 oz	640	23	0
Pan Fried			
Sirloin (choice), medium serving:			
Lean + external fat (¼"), 5 oz	460	33	0
Lean only, 5 oz	340	16	0

Other Steaks

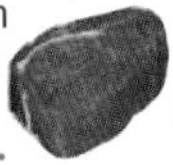

C F Cb

	C	F	Cb
Filet Mignon (Tenderloin):			
1 Medium steak (6 oz raw wt.)			
Broiled, with ¼" fat trim			
Lean + fat (¼"), 4 oz	360	27	0
Lean only, 3½ oz	230	12	0
New York/Club Steak:			
Top Loin/Short Loin			
1 steak, regular (9¼ oz raw, ¼" fat)			
Broiled: Lean + fat (¼"), 6¼ oz	580	43	0
Lean + marbling, 5½ oz	400	25	0
Lean only, 5¼ oz	360	20	0
Porterhouse Steak:			
1 Medium, (6 oz raw wt. no bone), broiled			
Lean + fat (¼"), 4¼ oz	410	33	0
Lean only, 3½ oz	210	11	0
1 Large (12 oz raw wt. no bone), broiled			
Lean + fat (¼") 8½ oz cooked	820	66	0
Lean only, 7 oz cooked	420	22	0
T-Bone Steak: *Broiled or Grilled*			
Medium Size: *8 oz raw weight*			
(Approx. 6 oz cooked)			
Lean + Fat (¼"), 5 oz, no bone	400	28	0
Lean only, 4 oz (no bone)	265	12	0
Large Size: *12 oz raw weight*			
(Approx. 9 oz cooked)			
Lean + fat (¼"), 7 oz (no bone)	560	39	0
Lean only, 6 oz (no bone)	400	18	0
Extra Large Size: *20 oz raw weight*			
(Approx. 16 oz cooked)			
Lean + Fat (¼"), 12 oz (no bone)	960	66	0
Lean Only, 10 oz (no bone)	660	30	0

Also See Fast-Foods & Restaurants Section ~
Lone Star Steakhouse
Outback Steakhouse

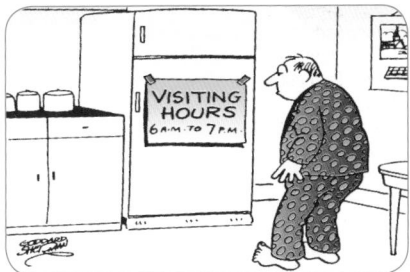

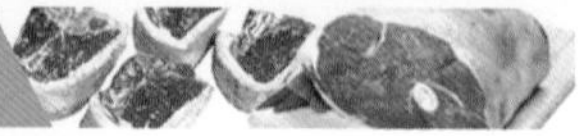

Beef – Individual Cuts

Average All Grades	C	F	Cb
Edible Weight (no bone)			
Brisket, whole, braised:			
Lean + fat (¼" trim), 3 oz	330	27	0
Lean + marbling, 3 oz	250	17	0
Lean only, 3 oz	185	9	0
Chuck blade, braised:			
Lean + fat (¼"), 3 oz	310	24	0
Lean + marbling, 3 oz	295	22	0
Lean only, 3 oz	245	13	0
Flank: Raw, 4 oz	175	8	0
Braised, 3 oz	225	14	0
Broiled, 3 oz	155	6	0
Round, bottom, braised:			
Lean + marbling, 3 oz	190	7.5	0
Lean only, 3 oz	185	6.5	0
Round, eye/tip, roasted:			
Lean + fat (¼"), 3 oz	205	11	0
Lean (with marbling), 3 oz	150	5	0
Round, top: Per 3 oz (cooked wt)			
Braised, Lean + fat	210	10	0
Lean only	170	4	0
Broiled, Lean + fat	180	8	0
Lean only	160	5	0
Pan-fried, Lean + fat	235	13	0
Lean only	195	7	0

Beef Ribs

	C	F	Cb
Back Ribs (7" long, visible fat trimmed to ¼")			
10.3 oz raw (with bone) or 3½ oz cooked (braised, no bone)			
1 average rib	410	34	0
3 ribs	1230	102	0
Short Ribs (2½" long, visible fat trimmed to ¼")			
6 oz raw (with bone) or 2½ oz cooked (braised, no bone)			
1 average rib	320	28	0
3 ribs	960	85	0

Ground Beef

	C	F	Cb
Ground Beef, Raw: Per 4 oz			
70% lean (30% fat)	380	34	0
75% lean (25% fat)	335	29	0
80% lean (20% fat)	290	23	0
85% lean (15% fat)	245	17	0
90% lean (10% fat)	200	12	0
95% lean (5% fat)	155	6	0
Baked/Broiled: Reg. (70%), 3 oz	230	16	0
Lean (80%), 3 oz	215	14	0
Extra lean (90%), 3 oz	185	10	0
Pan-Broiled: Reg. (70%), 3 oz	230	15	0
Lean (80%), 3 oz	210	14	0
Extra lean (90%), 3 oz	195	10	0
Ground Beef Patties: Average (23% Fat)			
Raw, 4 oz	330	25	0
Broiled, 3 oz (from 4 oz raw)	250	19	0

Quick Guide

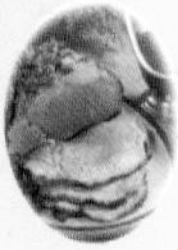

Roast Beef (Roasted)	C	F	Cb
Round (Eye/Tip, average) Average All Cuts			
Small/Regular Serving, 3 oz			
(2 thin slices/1 thick slice)			
Lean + fat (¼"), 3 oz	200	11	0
Lean only, 3 oz	150	5	0
Medium Serving, 5 oz			
(3-4 thin slices)			
Lean + fat, 5 oz	330	19	0
Lean only, 5 oz	245	9	0
Large Serving, 8 oz (3 thick slices)			
Lean + fat, 8 oz	525	30	0
Lean only, 8 oz	390	14	0

Roast Dinner Extras

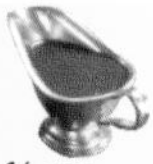

	C	F	Cb
Gravy: Thin, 2 Tbsp	20	0.5	3.5
Thick, 2 Tbsp	50	2	0.5
1 Ladle/4 Tbsp	100	4	1
Veggies: Beans, green, ½ cup	20	0	5
Cauliflower w. cheese sce, 4 oz	135	9	15
Corn, kernels, ¼ cup	35	0	9
Carrots, ¼ cup	20	0	3
Peas, ¼ cup	35	0	6
Potato: Roasted w. fat, 1 small	155	8	30
Baked in Jacket, 1 large	280	0	63
with 1 Tbsp whipped butter	350	8	63
with Sour Cream, 2 Tbsp	270	5	64
Sweet Potato/Yam, 1 medium	105	1	24
Beef Kebob (Cooked):			
Beef & Veggies, 2 oz	160	10	4
If very lean meat	100	4	4

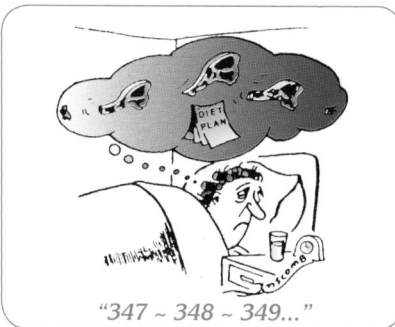

"347 ~ 348 ~ 349..."

Updated Nutrition Data ~ www.CalorieKing.com
Persons with Diabetes ~ See Disclaimer (Page 24)

Lamb   Ⓒ Ⓕ Ⓒᵇ

Choice Grade

Leg (Whole), roasted:

	C	F	Cb
Lean + fat, 3 oz	220	14	0
Lean only, 3 oz	160	7	0

Leg (Sirloin Half), roasted:

Lean + fat, 3 oz	250	18	0
Lean only, 3 oz	175	8	0

Leg (Shank Half), roasted:

Lean + fat, 3 oz	190	11	0
Lean only, 3 oz	155	6	0

Loin Chop, broiled:

1 chop (raw wt., 4¼ oz):

Lean + fat (2¼ oz edible)	180	12	0
Lean only (1.6 oz edible)	85	3.5	0

Rib Chop, broiled/roasted:

1 chop (raw wt., 3½ oz)

Lean + fat (2½ oz edible)	255	21	0
Lean only (1¾ oz edible)	105	6	0

Shoulder (Arm/Blade):

Braised: Lean + fat, 3 oz	295	21	0
Lean only, 3 oz	240	12	0
Broiled: Lean + fat, 3 oz	240	17	0
Lean only, 3 oz	170	8	0
Roasted: Similar to Broiled			

Cubed Lamb (Leg/Shoulder):

For stew or kabob

Braised, lean only, 3 oz	190	8	0
Broiled, lean only, 3 oz	160	6	0

Veal   Ⓒ Ⓕ Ⓒᵇ

Edible Weights

Leg (Top Round):

	C	F	Cb
Braised: Lean + fat, 3 oz	180	6	0
Lean only, 3 oz	175	5	0
Pan-fried, breaded:			
Lean + fat, 3 oz	195	8	9
Lean only, 3 oz	185	6	9
Pan-fried, not breaded:			
Lean + fat, 3 oz	180	7	0
Lean only, 3 oz	155	4	0
Roasted: Lean + fat, 3 oz	135	4	0
Lean only, 3 oz	130	3	0

Veal (Cont)   Ⓒ Ⓕ Ⓒᵇ

Loin Chop: 1 chop, 7 oz raw wt.

	C	F	Cb
Braised: Lean + fat, 3 oz	240	15	0
Lean only, 3 oz	190	8	0
Roasted: Lean + fat, 3 oz	185	11	0
Lean only, 3 oz	150	6	0

Rib, roasted: Lean + fat, 3 oz

Lean + fat, 3 oz	195	12	0
Lean only, 3 oz	150	7	0

Shoulder, Arm/Blade, roasted:

Lean + fat, 3 oz	155	7	0
Lean only, 3 oz	140	5	0

Sirloin, roasted:

Lean + fat, 3 oz	170	9	0
Lean only, 3 oz	145	6	0

Cubed for Stew, braised:

Leg/Shoulder, lean only, 3 oz	160	4	0

(1 lb raw yields approx. 9¼ oz cooked)

Pork

Fresh Pork (Cooked Wt., no bone)
(4 oz raw wt. = approx. 3 oz cooked wt.)

Blade Steak, broiled:

	C	F	Cb
Lean + fat, 3 oz	220	15	0
Lean only, 3 oz	190	11	0

Country Style Ribs, broiled/roasted:

Lean + fat, 3 oz	280	22	0
Lean only, 3 oz	210	13	0

Spareribs, braised: lean & fat, 6 oz

(from 1 lb raw wt)	675	52	0

Leg (Ham), whole, roasted:

Lean + fat, 3 oz	230	15	0
Lean only, 3 oz	180	8	0

(Ham, cured ~ See Cold Meats)

Loin Chops, broiled: Average
(From 1 chop: 5 oz raw wt. w. bone
or 4 oz raw wt., no bone)

Lean + fat, 3 oz	200	11	0
Lean only, 3 oz	165	7	0

Loin Roast, roasted:

Lean + fat, 3 oz	210	13	0
Lean only, 3 oz	180	8	0

Rib Chops, (Boneless), broiled:

Lean + fat, 3 oz	220	14	0
Lean only, 3 oz	185	9	0

Rib Roast, roasted:

Lean + fat, 3 oz	215	13	0
Lean only, 3 oz	180	9	0

Pork (Cont)

	C	F	Cb
Sirloin Chop, broiled:			
Lean + fat, 3 oz	180	8	0
Lean only, 3 oz	165	6	0
Sirloin Roast, roasted:			
Lean + fat, 3 oz	175	8	0
Lean only, 3 oz	170	7	0
Tenderloin (Boneless), roasted:			
Lean + fat, 3 oz	125	4	0
Lean only, 3 oz	120	3	0
Ground Pork			
Raw: Average, ¼ lb, 4 oz	300	24	0
Broiled, 3 oz	250	18	0
Pan-fried, drained, 3 oz	260	19	0

Bacon

	C	F	Cb
Raw: 1 med. slice (20 lb), ¾ oz	95	9	0
1 thick slice (12 lb), 1⅓ oz	175	17	0
(1 lb raw yields approx. 5 oz cooked)			
Broiled/Pan-Fried: 1 med. sl., 8g	40	3	0
3 medium slices, 24g	125	10	0
2 thin slices, ½ oz	75	6	0
1 thick slice, 12g	65	5	0
Canadian Bacon: Cooked, 1 slice, 1 oz	45	2	0.5
Packaged, 3 slices, 2 oz	90	4	1
Bacon Bits, 1 Tbsp, ¼ oz	35	2	0
Breakfast Strips, Broil., 1 sl., 12 g	50	4	0

Ham

	C	F	Cb
Boneless Ham, cooked:			
Regular, (approx. 13% fat):			
Roasted, 3 oz	150	8	0
Extra Lean (5% fat):			
Roasted, 3 oz	125	5	0
Whole Ham, cooked:			
Lean + fat (as purchased)			
Roasted, 3 oz	210	15	0
Lean only, Roasted, 3 oz	135	5	0
Canned Ham: Similar to boneless ham			
Chopped, canned, 3 oz	200	16	0
Ham Patties, cooked, 1 patty, 2¼ oz	220	20	1
Ham Steak, extra lean, 2 oz	70	2.5	0
Lunch Slices: See Deli Meats, Page 131			

Game & Other Meats

	C	F	Cb
Bison Steak,			
lean, 6 oz (raw)	205	4	0
Boar (wild), roasted, 3 oz	140	4	0
Buffalo Steak: New West Foods, 4 oz	70	3	0
Trader Joe's, 1 patty	430	30	1
Caribou, roasted, 3 oz	140	4	0
Deer/Venison, roasted 3 oz	135	3	0
Goat (Capretto): Raw, 3 oz	95	2	0
Roasted, 3 oz	120	2.5	0
Ostrich: Blackwing Ostrich Meats,			
Sport Jerky, ½ oz pce	25	0	0
Sausage Patties (2) 2 oz	60	0.5	0
New West Foods:			
Ground Ostrich, 4 oz	165	7	0
Ostrich Steak, 4 oz steak	130	2.5	0
Rabbit: Roasted, 3 oz	165	7	0
Stewed, 1 cup, diced, 5 oz	290	12	0

Variety & Organ Meats

	C	F	Cb
Brain (Lamb): Braised, 3 oz	125	9	0
Pan-fried, 3 oz	230	19	0
Chitterlings, pork, simmered, 3 oz	260	25	0
Ears, pork, simmered, 1 ear, 4 oz	185	12	0
Feet, pork: Simmered, 3 oz	200	14	0
Cured, pickled, 3 oz	170	14	0
Hormel, 2 oz	80	6	0
Head Cheese (Pork Snouts/Ears/Vinegar/Spices):			
1 oz slice	50	4	0
Heart, Beef, braised, 3 oz	140	4	24
Jowl, pork, raw, 4 oz	750	80	0
Kidneys, braised, 3 oz	140	5	0
Liver (beef): Raw, 4 oz	150	4	4
Braised, 3 oz	140	4	3
Pan-fried, 3 oz	185	7	7
Pancreas, pork, braised, 3 oz	185	8	0
Pork Cracklins, 0.5 oz	80	6	0
Pork Hocks, 1 piece, 6 oz	340	23	0
Scrapple, pork, 2 oz	120	8	8
Spleen, pork, braised, 3 oz	130	3	0
Stomach, pork, raw, 4 oz	185	12	0
Sweetbreads: Beef, ckd., 3 oz	125	9	0
Lamb, cooked, 3 oz	125	9	0
Tail, pork, simmered, 3 oz	340	31	0
Tongue, braised: Veal, 3 oz	170	9	0
Beef/Lamb/Pork, average, 3 oz	235	17	0
Tripe, beef, raw, 3 oz	85	3.5	0

Updated Nutrition Data ~ www.CalorieKing.com
Persons with Diabetes ~ See Disclaimer (Page 24)

Quick Guide

Franks & Weiners

Average All Brands

	C	F	Cb
Regular/Smoked: *Per Frank*			
Regular, 1.5oz (10/16 oz pkg)	140	13	1
Jumbo, 2 oz (8/16 oz pkg)	170	16	0
Bun Length, 2 oz	180	17	2
Extra Long, 2.75 oz	240	21	2
Small/Cocktail (50/lb) each	30	3	0.5
Beef Franks: *Per Frank*			
Regular, 1.6 oz (10/16 oz pkg)	140	13	2
Jumbo, 2 oz (8/16 oz pkg)	170	15	2
Bun Length, 2 oz	180	16	2
¼ lb Dog, 4 oz	300	24	4

Franks & Weiners

	C	F	Cb
Ball Park			
Franks & Wieners: *Per Frank*			
Angus Beef Franks	170	15	3
Cheese	190	16	3
Turkey Franks	120	7	6
GrillMaster: Deli Style Beef; Beef	250	21	3
Hot 'N Spicy; Smokehouse	255	24	4
Lite: Franks; Beef	100	7	3
Foster Farms			
Chicken/Turkey Franks (1), 2 oz	140	12	1
Hebrew National			
Beef: 1.72 oz link	150	14	1
Dinner Frank, 4 oz	350	32	1
Jumbo, 3 oz link	270	26	1
97% Fat-Free, 1.72 oz link	45	1.5	3
Jennie-O			
Turkey Franks:			
1.2 oz link	70	5	1
Jumbo, 2 oz link	120	10	2
Oscar Mayer			
Reg./Smoked, 98% Fat-Free, 1.76 oz	40	0.5	3
Beef, Light, 1.6 oz	90	7	2
Cheese Frank, 1.6 oz	140	13	1
Turkey Frank: 1.6 oz	100	8	2
Bun Length, 2 oz link	120	10	3
Shelton's			
Chicken Franks, 1.2 oz link	70	6	0
Turkey Franks, 1.2 oz link	60	4.5	1
Zacky Farms			
Turkey Franks, 2 oz link	160	12	1

Quick Guide

Fresh Sausages

Pork/Beef: *Average All Types*

	C	F	Cb
Small: Raw, 4" link, 1 oz	85	7.5	0
Broiled/Pan-fried	80	7	0
Medium: Raw, 2 oz	170	15	0
Broiled/Pan-fried	165	14	0
Large: Raw, 3 oz	255	22	0
Broiled/Pan-fried	245	21	0
Italian: Raw, 3.2 oz	315	28	0.5
Cooked, 2.4 oz	230	18	3
Chorizo: Beef Chorizo, 2.5 oz pce	250	23	5
Pork Chorizo, 2 oz piece	250	23	5

Note: Fat is lost in broiling/pan frying.
(Cooked wt. = approx. 60-70% raw wt.)

Smoked Sausage

	C	F	Cb
Average All Brands: 2 oz link	170	15	0
3 oz link	255	22	0
Ball Park, Turkey, Bun Size, 2 oz	45	0	5
Butterball			
(w. Turkey), 2 oz	100	6	4
Eckrich, 2 oz	180	16	2
Healthy Choice, Beef/Polska, 2 oz	80	2.5	6

Breakfast Sausages/Patties

	C	F	Cb
Armour Sizzle 'n Serve			
Pork/Turkey, 3 links, 2.1 oz	210	19	2
Lite Original, 3 links	120	8	3
Beef Sausage, 3 links, 2 oz	230	22	1
Butterball: Turkey Burger Pattie (1)	150	8	0
Turkey Breakfast Links (3)	130	7	0
Jennie-O, Maple Breakfast Ssg. (1)	140	11	3
Jimmy Dean: Pork Ssg. Patties (2)	240	23	1
Pork Sausage Links: Original (3)	170	14	1
Maple (3)	130	14	2
Breakfast Sandwiches: *See Page 94*			
Jones/Golden Brown:			
All Natural Beef Ssg Links (3), 2 oz	200	18	2
Pork Ssg, Hearty Links (1), 1.45 oz	150	14	1
Maple Pork Ssg Patties (1), 1.15 oz	130	12	1
Mild Pork Ssg Links (3), 2.08 oz	250	24	1
Mild Pork Ssg Patties (1), 1.15 oz	120	12	0

Vegetarian Patties:

Boca: *See Page 119*
Garden Burger: *See Page 120*

Bagel, Corn & Hot Dogs

Hot Dogs, Ready-To-Go
(Includes Ketchup/Relish; no Mayo)

	C	F	Cb
Regular (1.5 oz frank, 1.5 oz bun)	260	15	22
Bun Length (2 oz frank, 1.5 oz bun)	290	18	21
Jumbo Dog (2 oz frank, 2 oz bun)	360	20	36
¼ lb Beef Dog (¼ lb dog, 2 oz bun)	480	15	36
Mile Long Dog (2.6 oz dog, 1.5 oz bun)	360	24	23

Weinerschnitzel: *See Fast-Foods*

Corn Dogs

Beef/Pork Frank: Avg., 2.6 oz	170	10	16

Foster Farms

Chili Cheese, 1 dog, 2.7 oz	200	9	24
Crunchy 1 dog 2.7	180	10	15
Mini (4), 2.6 oz	210	12	18

State Fair w. Ball Park Franks,

Beef Corn Dogs (1), 2.7 oz	220	10	25
Mini Beef Corn Dogs (6)	260	15	24

Bagel Dogs

Vienna Beef: 1 Bageldog, 1 oz	70	6	1
Mini, 1 piece, 0.8 oz	50	4	0

Hot Dog Toppings/Extras:

American Cheese, 1 slice, 1 oz	110	9	1
Catsup, 1 Tbsp	16	0	4
Chili (w. Beans), ¼ cup	70	3.5	9
Ketchup, 1 Tbsp	15	0	4
Mustard, 1 Tbsp	20	0	1
Onions, Chopped, 1 Tbsp	5	0	1
Pickle Relish, 1 Tbsp	20	0	5
Sauerkraut, ½ cup	20	0	5

Deli & Lunch Meats

Beef Jerky/Meat Snacks:	C	F	Cb
Bridgeford Beef Jerky, 1 oz	100	0.5	5
Beef Stick (5.5 oz stick), 1 oz	150	13	2
Beef Steak, 1 oz	70	0.5	2
Beef & Cheese (Giant Size),			
½ pkg, 1.5 oz	170	14	1
Pepperoni Sticks (2), 1 oz	160	13	2
Pepperoni (1" diam.), 1 oz	130	12	0
Teriyaki, 1 oz pkg	80	0.5	4
Original; Hot 'n Spicy	70	1	5
Berliner (pork/beef), 1 oz	65	5	1

Beerwurst (Beef):

Small (2.75"diam), ¹⁄₁₆" slice	20	2	0
Large (4"diam), ⅛" slice	75	7	0.5

Deli & Lunch Meats

Beerwurst (Pork):	C	F	Cb
Small (2.75"diam), ¹⁄₁₆" slice	15	1	0
Large (4"diam), ⅛" Slice	55	4	0.5
Bologna: 1 Slice, 1 oz	65	6	1
Fat-Free, 1 slice, 1 oz	20	0	2
Beef Bologna: 1 slice, 1 oz	90	8	1
Light, 1 slice, 1 oz	60	4	2
Light (*Oscar Mayer*), 1 sl., 1 oz	60	4	2
Fat Free (*Osc. M.*), 2 sl., 1.6 oz	40	0	1
Ring (*Boar's Head*), 2 oz	150	13	1
Turkey, average, 1 oz	60	5	0.5
Blood Sausage, 1 oz	100	9	0.5
Bratwurst: Average, 1 oz	80	7	1
Boar's Head, cook., 1 wurst, 4 oz	300	25	0
Bob Evan's, Beer, 2.6 oz link	270	21	1

Braunschweiger (Pork/Liver/Sausage),

Oscar Mayer, 1 oz sl.	110	10	1

Chicken, *Average All Brands*

1 thick or 2 thin slices, 1 oz	30	1	1
Chicken Roll, 1 slice, 2 oz	90	4	1.5
Corned Beef: Average, full fat, 1 oz	60	5	0.5
Hillshire Farm, 1oz	30	1	0
Loaf, jellied, 1 oz	45	2	0
Hash, canned, average, 1 oz	50	3	3
Dutch Brand Loaf, average, 1 oz	70	5	1.5

Ham, Sliced:

Baked/Boiled, sliced, 1 oz	30	1	0.5
Chopped: *Eckrich* (97% FF), 1 oz	25	1	1
Armour: Canned, 1 oz	35	1.5	0.5
97% Fat Free, 1 oz	25	1	1.5
Healthy Choice, 2 sl., 2 oz	60	1.5	1
Oscar Mayer, 1 oz slice	60	2	0.5
Honey/Brown Sugar: Avg., 1 oz	30	1	1
Healthy Choice Deli Traditions:			
Hearty Slices, 2 slices, 2 oz	60	1.5	2
Prosciutto, average, 1 oz	70	5	0
Ham & Cheese Loaf, avg., 1 oz	70	5	1
Italian Sausage, 2.6 oz	250	20	3
Kielbasa (Polish Sausage), 1 oz	65	5	1
Beef, 2 oz link	190	17	1
Boar's Head, 1 oz	60	5	0

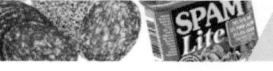

	C	**F**	**Cb**
Kippered Beefsteak:			
Hickory Farms, 3 slices,	50	1	1
Knockwurst, 1 oz	90	8	0.5
Linguica (Gaspar's), 2 oz	180	8	1
Liverwurst, 1 oz	65	5	2
Liver Pate, fresh, average, 1 oz	90	8	1
Luncheon Loaf (Foods Co), 1 oz	65	5	2
Mortadella, 1 oz	105	9	0
Olive Loaf: Average, 1 oz	70	5	3
Oscar Mayer, 1 oz	75	6	2
Pastrami (Beef):			
Healthy Deli, 2 oz	70	2	1
Hillshire (DeliSelect), 6 sl., 2 oz	60	1	0
Boar's Head, 2 oz	70	4	2
Peppered Beef, 1 oz slice	40	2	1
Pepperoni, 5 slices, 1 oz	140	13	0
Pickle Loaf, avg., 1 oz	70	5	5
Pickle & Pimento Loaf			
Oscar Mayer, 1 oz	75	6	3
Proscuitto/Proscuitti: Avg., 1 oz	70	5	1
Hormel, 1 oz	90	7	1
Roast Beef: Lean, 1 oz	40	2	0
Healthy Choice, all types, 2 oz	60	1.5	1
Salami: Beef, average, 1 oz	80	7	1
Beer Salami, average, 1 oz	50	4	0.5
Cotto: Oscar Mayer, 1 sl., 1 oz	70	6	1
Dry: Hard, avg., 4 slices, 1 oz	110	10	3
Oscar Mayer, 2 slices, 1.6 oz	100	8	1
Genoa: Average, 1 oz	120	9	1
Stick (Best's Kosher), 2, 1.75 oz	180	15	2
Italian (Bridgeford), 1 oz	120	11	0
Turkey, average, 1 oz	55	4	1
SPAM (Hormel): Per 2 oz Serving			
Classic: 2 oz serving	180	16	1
7 oz can	630	56	3
12 oz can	1030	96	6
Spam Lite: 2 oz	110	8	1
12 oz can	660	48	6
Other Spam Products:			
Hickory Smoked, 2 oz	170	15	2
Hot & Spicy, 2 oz	180	16	2
Oven Rstd Turkey, 2 oz	80	4	2
Spam w. Bacon, 2 oz	180	16	1
Spam w. Cheese, 2 oz	170	15	1
Spam Spread, 2 oz	140	12	1
25% Less Sodium	180	16	1
Spam Singles:			
Classic, 3 oz pkg	250	22	2
Lite, 3 oz pkg	160	11	2

	C	**F**	**Cb**
Summer Sausage:			
Bridgeford, 1 oz	100	9	1
Oscar Mayer, 1 sl., 1 oz	90	7	1
Treet (Armour), canned, 1 oz	100	9	1.5
Turkey: Average, 1 oz slice	30	1	0.5
¾ oz slice	22	0.5	0.5
Turkey Breast:			
Butterball Fat Free, 3 sl., 2 oz	60	0	4
Hillshire Deli Select, 6 sl., 2 oz	50	0.5	2
Healthy Choice: Deli Thin: Per 4 Slices, 52g (1.8 oz)			
Oven-Roasted	60	1.5	2
Smoked/Rotisserie Seasoned	60	1.5	3
Honey Roasted & Smoked	60	1.5	4
Hearty Deli Sliced:			
Oven Rstd Turkey Brst. 1 sl., 1 oz	30	1	1
Turkey Ham, 1 slice, 1 oz	35	1.5	0.5
Turkey Pastrami, 1 oz	35	1.5	1
Turkey Roll, 1 oz	40	2	0.5
Turkey Loaf, 1 oz	30	1	0.5
Vegetarian Deli (Worthington, Yves): See Page 76			

Meat Spreads

Average All Brands: Per ¼ Cup (2 oz)	**C**	**F**	**Cb**
Chicken	90	10	2
Ham, Deviled	140	11	0
Liverwurst	190	16	2
Roast Beef	130	10	2
Sandwich Spread	140	10	9
Turkey	110	7	2

Paté

	C	**F**	**Cb**
Boar's Head Liverwurst Pate, 2 oz	145	12	0
Les Trois Petit Cochons: Per 2 oz			
Black Peppercorn	240	24	1
Chicken Livers & Black Truffle	140	11	2
Country Pate	240	26	2
Duck Liver with Port Wine	130	11	2
Smoked Salmon	110	9	2
Marcel Henri			
Pate de Champagne	210	18	2
Chicken Liver w. Port Wine, 2 oz	210	18	2
Duck Truffle w. Port Wine, 2 oz	240	24	2
Old Wisconsin Pate			
All types, 2 oz	210	18	3
Underwood: Per 2 oz			
BBQ Chicken	130	8	2
Chicken, White Meat	130	8	2
Deviled Ham	180	15	1
Liverwurst	160	13	4
Roast Beef	130	10	2
Turkey, White Meat	140	9	2

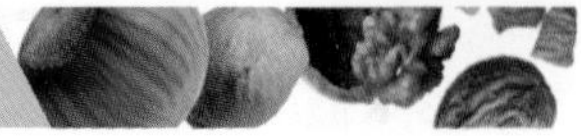

Nuts

	C	F	Cb
Acorns, raw 1 oz	110	7	12
Almonds, Dried/Dry Roasted:			
Whole, 24-28 med., 1 oz	170	15	5.5
½ cup, 2½ oz	420	37	13
Chopped, ½ cup, 2¼ oz	380	34	12
Sliced, ½ cup, 1⅔ oz	280	25	9
Choc. coated (5-6), 1 oz	150	10	15
Oil Rstd *(Blue Diamond)*, 1 oz	170	16	5
Honey Roasted, 1 oz	170	14	8
Almond Meal (partially defatted)			
1 cup (not packed), 2¼ oz	260	11	11
Brazil Nuts, 8 medium, 1 oz	185	19	3.5
Cashews, Dry or Oil Roasted:			
14 large/18 med./26 small, 1 oz	165	14	9
½ cup, 2.4 oz	375	31	20
Honey Roasted, 1 oz	165	13	10
Chestnuts, avg. all: Dried, 1 oz	105	1	22
Raw/Fresh, 5-6 nuts, 1 oz	60	0	13
Canned, water chestnuts,			
sliced/whole/drained, 1 oz	30	0	7
Coconut: Fresh,			
1 piece, 2"x2"x ½", 1 oz	100	10	4.5
Shredded, fresh, ½ cup, 1.4 oz	140	13	6
Dried (Desiccated):			
Unsweetened, 1 oz	185	18	7
Sweetened: Shredded, 1 oz	140	10	13
Grated, ½ cup, 1.3 oz	185	12	18
Cream (canned), ½ cup, 5.2 oz	285	26	12
Milk (canned), ½ cup, 4 oz	225	24	3
Water (center liq.), ½ c., 4¼ oz	25	0	4.5
Filberts or Hazelnuts:			
Shelled, 18-20 nuts	180	17	4.5
Chopped, ¼ cup, 1 oz	180	18	5
Ground, ¼ cup, 0.6 oz	120	12	3
Ginkgo Nuts, can., 14 med., 1 oz	32	0.5	6.5
Hickory, 30 small nuts, 1 oz	200	18	5
Macadamia Nuts, shelled:			
Raw, 7 med./14 small, 1 oz	200	21	4
½ cup, 2.3 oz	480	51	10
Dry Roasted, 1 oz	205	22	4
½ cup, 2.4 oz	480	51	9
Choc. coated, 2-3 pces, 1 oz	170	12	14
Mixed Nuts: 18-22 nuts, 1 oz	170	15	7
Planters: Dry Roasted/Honey	160	12	9
Oil Roasted, all types	170	16	6
Sweet Roasts, 26 pces, 1 oz	160	12	10
Nut Toppings: Chopped, 1 T., ¼ oz	40	4	1.5

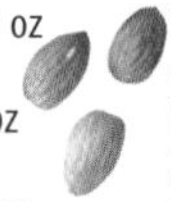

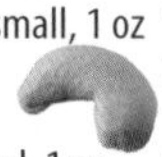

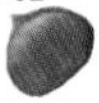

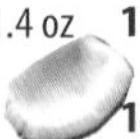

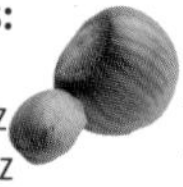

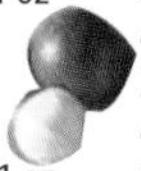

	C	F	Cb
Peanuts:			
Raw/Dried:			
In shell, 1 oz	117	10	3
Shelled, 1 oz	160	14	4.5
Boiled, shelled, ½ cup, 3.1 oz	285	20	19
Roasted: 30 lge./60 sml., 1 oz	165	14	6
1 cup, 5.1 oz	860	76	22
Chopped, 3 Tbsp, 1 oz	165	14	6
Planters: Cocktail, 1 oz	170	14	6
Rich Roasted in Choc., 2½ oz	220	14	19
Roasted in Shell, Salted, 1 oz	160	14	5
Dry Roasted, 1oz	160	13	6
Honey/ & Dry Roasted, 1 oz	160	13	8
Spanish Raw, 1 oz	150	13	6
Spanish Redskin, 1 oz	180	14	5
Sweet N' Crunchy, 1 oz	140	7	16
Pecans: Kernel halves, 1 oz	195	20	4
(20 Jumbo or 31 large halves)			
1 cup halves, 3.8 oz	755	78	15
Chopped, ½ cup, 2 oz	380	39	7.5
Oil Roasted, 15 halves, 1 oz	205	20	4
Honey Roasted, 1 oz	200	21	4
Pilinuts, dried, ¼ cup, 1 oz	215	24	1
Pine Nuts, dried, 1 Tbsp, 10g	70	7	1.5
Pistachios: Unshelled, ½ cup, 2 oz	165	14	7
Shelled, ¼ cup, 45 nuts, 1 oz	170	14	8.5
Lance, 1.1 oz package	95	7	4
Sesame Nut Mix: *Planters,* 1 oz	160	13	9
Soy Nuts: Dry Roasted, 1 oz	130	6	9
½ cup, 3 oz	390	18	28
Dr Soy: Choc coated, 1 oz pkg	140	7	13
Flavors, average, 1 oz	150	8	8
Trail Mix *(Planters):* Fruit & Nut, 1 oz	140	9	14
Golden Nut Crunch, 1 oz	160	11	12
Honey Nut & Caramel, 1 oz	160	10	16
Mixed Nuts & Raisins, 1 oz	150	11	10
Nut & Chocolate, 1 oz	160	10	16
Nuts, Seeds & Raisins, 1 oz	160	12	11
Spicy Nuts & Cajun Sticks, 1 oz	150	10	13
Sweet & Nutty, 1 oz	150	10	14
Walnuts:			
Black: 15-20 halves, 1 oz	175	17	3
Chopped, ¼ cup, 1.1 oz	195	18	3
English/Persian:			
14 halves, 1 oz	185	18	4
Chopped, ¼ cup, 1 oz	190	19	4
Ground, ¼ cup, 0.7 oz	130	13	3

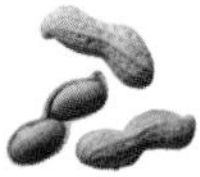

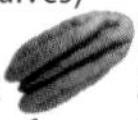

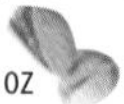

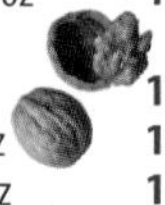

Updated Nutrition Data ~ www.CalorieKing.com
Persons with Diabetes ~ See Disclaimer (Page 24)

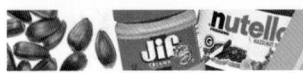

Quick Guide

	C	F	Cb
Peanut Butter: *Average All Brands*			
1 level tsp, 6g	35	3	1.5
1 level Tbsp, 0.6 oz	105	8.5	3.5
2 level Tbsp, 1.2 oz	210	17	7
1 oz Quantity	170	14	6
½ cup, 5 oz	850	70	30
Jif: Reduced Fat, 2 Tbsp	190	12	15
Creamy; Crunchy; Simply, 2 Tbsp	190	16	7
Peanut Butter & Honey, 2 Tbsp	190	15	11
Laura Scudder's: Reg./Org., 2 T, 1.1 oz	210	16	6
Reduced-Fat, 2 T, 1¼ oz	200	12	12
Peanut Wonder, 2 Tbsp	100	2.5	13
Peter Pan: Creamy; Crunch, 2 Tbsp	190	16	6
Whipped, 2 Tbsp	140	12	5
Smucker's Goober,			
Grape/Strawb. 3 Tbsp	240	13	24
Skippy: Reduced Fat, 2 Tbsp	180	12	15
Roasted Honey Nut Creamy, 2 T.	190	16	7

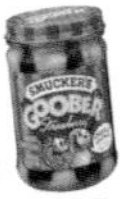

Peanut Butter & Jelly Sandwich

	C	F	Cb
1 sandwich, with 2 oz Bread:			
Light Spread:	310	10	48
(1 Tbsp. P'nut Butter + 1 Tbsp Jelly)			
Thick Spread:	480	19	67
(2 Tbsp. P'nut Butter + 2 Tbsp Jelly)			
With **Goober Grape**, 3 Tbsp, 2 oz	380	15	52

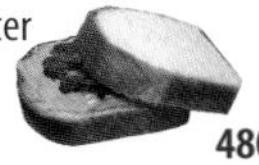

Nutella

	C	F	Cb
Nut & Chocolate Spread			
1 Tbsp, 0.7 oz	100	5.5	11
2 Tbsp, 1.3 oz	190	11	22

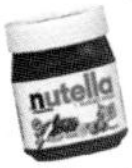

Note: *Nutella* contains approximately 50% sugar and only 13% hazelnuts

Other Nut & Seed Butters

	C	F	Cb
Almond Butter, 1 Tbsp, ½ oz	100	10	3.5
Almond Butter Honey Rstd, 1 T.	90	7	5.5
Beanut Butter, 1 Tbsp, ½ oz	90	5.5	7
Cashew Butter, 1 Tbsp, ½ oz	95	8	4.5
Hazelnut Butter, 1 Tbsp, ½ oz	105	10	2.5
Pecan Butter, 1 Tbsp, ½ oz	110	10	2
Pistachio Butter, 1 Tbsp, ½ oz	90	6.5	4.5
Sesame Butter (Tahini), 1 T., ½ oz	90	8	3
Soy Nut Butter, 1 Tbsp, ½ oz	75	5	4
Tahini ~ *See Sesame Butter*			

Seeds

	C	F	Cb
Alfalfa Seeds,			
sprouted, ½ cup, ½ oz	5	0	1
Caraway, Fennel, 1 tsp	7	0.5	1
Cottonseed Kernels,			
roasted, 1 Tbsp	50	3.5	2
Flax Seeds,			
3 Tbsp, 1 oz	140	9	9
Lotus Seeds,			
dried, ½ cup, ½ oz	55	0.5	10
Poppy Seeds, 1 tsp	15	1	1
Pumpkin & Squash Seeds, whole:			
Roasted/Tamari, 1 oz	150	12	4
½ cup, 4 oz	590	48	15
Dried, (hulled), ¼ cup, 1 oz	155	13	5
Safflower Kernels,			
dried, 1 oz	150	11	10
Sesame Seeds:			
Dried, 1 Tbsp, 9g	50	4.5	2
Roasted/Toasted, 1 oz	160	14	7.5
Sunflower Kernels/Seed:			
Dried, ¼ cup without hulls, ¼ oz	200	18	7
Dry Roasted, 1 Tbsp, 8g	45	4	2
¼ cup, 1 oz	165	14	7
Oil Roasted, ⅕ cup, 1 oz	170	14	6.5
Watermelon Seeds, dried,			
¼ cup, 1 oz	150	13	4

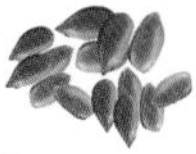

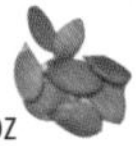

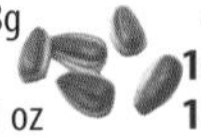

*N*ut eaters are healthier and live longer, say scientists.

Nuts are a nutritious source of protein, vitamins, minerals, fiber, healthy fats, and antioxidants.

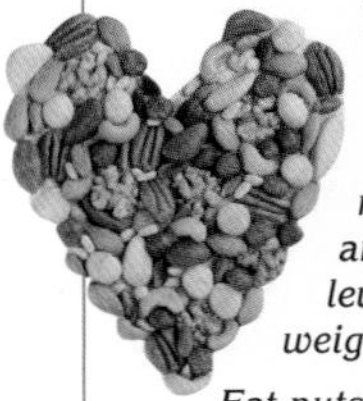

The fat and fiber of nuts can help reduce blood cholesterol. Their protein and fiber also promotes meal satiety (fullness) and reduces hunger levels – of benefit in weight control.

Eat nuts instead of high-sugar snacks, candy and soft drinks. Add chopped nuts to breakfast cereals.

Quick Guide | C | F | Cb

Pancakes

	C	F	Cb
Plain: *Average All Types*			
Small (3" diam.), ¾ oz	50	2	6
Medium (4" diam.), 1¼ oz	85	3.5	11
Large (5" diam.), 2½ oz	175	7.5	22
Add Extra for Syrups/Butter			
Pancake Syrup: Regular, 1 Tbsp	50	0	13
¼ cup, 4 Tbsp	210	0	52
Lite, 1 Tbsp	25	0	6
¼ cup, 4 Tbsp	100	0	26
Butter/Margarine: Regular, 1 T.	100	11	0
Whipped, 1 Tbsp	70	7.5	0

Waffles

	C	F	Cb
Homemade: 7" waffle, 2½ oz	245	13	26
From Mix: 7" waffle, 2½ oz	205	8	28

Frozen Breakfasts

Aunt Jemima

	C	F	Cb
Pancakes: Buttermilk (3)	240	6	41
Homestyle (3)	240	6	41
Low-Fat (3)	200	3	39
Whole Grain (3)	240	6	42
Mini Pancakes (11)	240	4.5	44
Frozen Breakfasts:			
French Toast, Cinnamon, 2 slices	220	4.5	37
French Toast, Homestyle, 2 slices	220	4.5	37
French Toast, Sticks, 5 sticks	360	12	58

Eggo *(Kellogg's)*

	C	F	Cb
Bake Shop Strawb. Swirlz (1), 2.2 oz	150	3	28
French Toast: Toaster Swirlz, set of 4	120	3	20
French Toaster Sticks, avg., (2)	225	6	37
Stuffed French Toaster Sticks (2)	300	7	54
Pancakes: Buttermilk (3)	280	9	44
Minis (11)	260	8	31
Nutri-Grain (3)	240	7	40

Krusteaz

	C	F	Cb
Pancakes: Mini (8)	160	2	30
Buttermilk (2)	140	2	27
French Toast: Homestyle/Thick, 1 sl.	150	3	27
Sticks, Griddled (4)	230	5	41

Pillsbury

	C	F	Cb
Pancakes: Buttermilk Mini (11)	240	4	45
Chocolate Burst (3)	280	7	51
Toaster Strudel, avg. (1)	190	9	26

Pancake Brands | C | F | Cb

	C	F	Cb
Aunt Jemima Mixes: *Prepared*			
Buttermilk, 4 x 4"	180	5	23
Original Complete, 2 x 4"	160	1.5	32
Original, 4 x 4" pancakes	250	6	33
Whole Wheat Blend, 3 x 4" pancakes	200	5	26
Betty Crocker Pancake Mixes			
Complete Original/Buttermilk, 3	200	2.5	40
Bisquick (Shake 'N Pour), 3	220	3	42
Hungry Jack Pancakes			
Mixes: *Per ⅓ Cup, Prepared*			
Complete: Buttermilk, 3 x 4"	150	1.5	31
Extra Light & Fluffy, 3 x 4"	150	2	30
Original, w. 2% Milk, Oil, Egg	250	8	37
w. Skim Milk, Oil, Egg Whites	180	1	37
Easy Packs: *Per ½ Cup Dry Mix, Prepared*			
Blueberry	200	2.5	40
Buttermilk	200	2.5	40
Northern Pines: (3), 3 x 4"	220	4	41

Frozen Waffles

	C	F	Cb
Aunt Jemima: Buttermilk (2)	200	6	33
Homestyle (2); Blueberry (2)	190	6	31
Low-Fat (2)	160	3	30
Eggo *(Kellogg's):* Minis, avg. (3)	250	8	39
Original: Choc. Chip (2)	210	7	32
French Van. (2)	200	8	28
Other, avg. (2)	190	6	30
Flip Flops, avg. (2)	200	7	31
Homestyle	190	7	27
Nutri-Grain: Avg. (2)	170	4.5	27
Low-Fat (2)	140	2.5	27
Special K, 99% Fat-Free (3)	160	2.5	29
Waf-Fulls, Strawberry (1)	170	5	27
GO-LEAN *(Kashi):* Average (1)	85	1.5	16
Nature's Path: Flax Plus, avg. (2)	180	7	24
Homestyle (2)	180	7	26
Mesa Sunrise (2)	200	7	34
Van's: Belgian Homestyle (2)	220	9	31
Hearty Oats: Berry Boost (2)	190	8	26
Maple Fusion (2)	190	9	26
Mini: Chocolate Chip (12)	240	9	35
Homestyle (12)	210	8	32
Original 97% Fat Free (2)	140	2	26
Wheat Free Minis (12)	210	7	35

Updated Nutrition Data ~ www.CalorieKing.com
Persons with Diabetes ~ See Disclaimer (Page 24)

- Pasta includes all shapes and sizes;
  (e.g. spaghetti, fettuccini, elbows, shells,
  twists, sheets, cannelloni, tubes, ziti,).
- All regular pasta products have the same
  cals/fat/carb. on a weight basis.
- 1 oz Dry = approx. 2½ -3 oz cooked.

Dry Spaghetti/Pasta

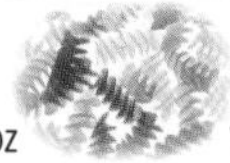

	C	F	Cb
1 oz quantity	105	0.5	21
1lb box/pkg., 16 oz	1685	7	339
Elbows, 1 cup, 3¾ oz	380	2	80
Shells, small, 1 cup, 3¼ oz	330	1.5	69
Spirals, 1 cup, 3 oz	305	1.5	64

Cooked Spaghetti/Pasta

	C	F	Cb
Plain, All Types (no added fat):			
Firm/Al Dente (8-10 mins.), 1 oz	42	0.5	8.5
Medium (11-13 mins.), 1 oz	37	0.5	7.5
Tender (14-20 mins.), 1 oz	32	0.5	7
(Longer cooking increases water absorbed)			
Spaghetti, ½ cup, 2 ½ oz	90	0.5	18
Medium serving, 1 cup, 5 oz	225	1.5	44
Large Serving, 2 cups, 10 oz	450	3	88
Extra Large, 3 cups, 15 oz	675	5	132
Elbows/Spirals, 1 cup, 5 oz	220	1.5	43
Small Shells, 1 cup, 4 oz	180	1	36
Protein-fortified: Dry, 1 c., 3⅓ oz	350	2	63
Cooked, 1 cup, 5 oz	230	0.5	45
Spinach/Vegetable: Dry, 1 c., 3 oz	310	1	61
Cooked, 1 cup, 5 oz	180	0.5	38
Whole-wheat: Dry, 1 c., 3¾ oz	365	1.5	79
Cooked, 1 cup, 5 oz	175	1	37

Fresh Pasta (Refrigerated)

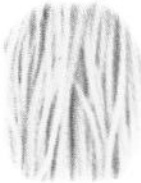

		C	F	Cb
Plain/Spinach/Tomato, average:				
As purchased, 4.5 oz		370	3	70
Cooked, 1 cup, 5 oz		185	1.5	35
Home-made, without egg:				
Cooked, 1 cup, 5 oz		175	1	35
Buitoni				
Cut Pasta: *Per ⅓ of 9 oz Pkg*				
Angel Hair		230	2.5	43
Fettuccine		260	3	46
Linguine		240	2.5	45
Whole Wheat Linguine		240	3	41
Ravioletti, Three Cheese, 1 c., 90g		270	5	43

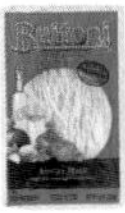

	C	F	Cb
Buitoni (Cont):			
Ravioli: Four Cheese, 1¼ cups	330	10	45
Light Four Cheese, 1¼ cups	260	4.5	41
Whole Wheat Four Chse, 1¼ cups	320	11	40
Tortellini: Herb Chkn, 1 cup, 4 oz	350	10	52
Spinach Cheese, 1 cup, 3.7 oz	320	7	49
Three Cheese, 1 cup, 3.7 oz	320	7	50
Tortelloni: Chse & Rstd Garlic, 1 c.	270	8	37
Other varieties, avg., 1 cup	330	10	47
Pasta Sauces: *See Page 148*			

Macaroni & Cheese

	C	F	Cb
Packaged: *Kraft/Hormel ~ See Page 114-115*			
Restaurant, average: Side, 6 oz	265	13	26
Medium serving, 1 cup, 9 oz	350	17	34
Large serving, 2 cups, 18 oz	700	34	68

Noodles

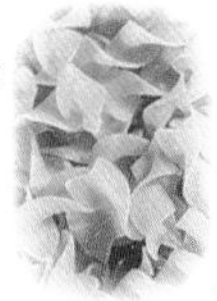

	C	F	Cb
Plain/Egg: Dry, 1 oz	110	1.5	20
1 cup, 1⅓ oz	145	1.5	27
Cooked: 1 oz	40	0.5	7
½ cup, 2¾ oz	110	1.5	20
1 cup, 5½ oz	220	3.5	40
Stir-Fried: 1 cup, 5½ oz	270	9	40
2 cup serving, 11 oz	540	18	80
Yolk Free (Cooked): *Per Cup*			
'No Yolks' (Foulds), 2 oz	210	0.5	41
Passover Gold (Manischewitz)	200	0	41
Chinese: Cellophane/Rice, dry, 1 oz	100	0	25
Chow Mein/hard, dry, 1 oz	150	9	16
Japanese: Soba, dry, 1 oz	95	0.5	21
cooked, 1 cup, 4 oz	115	0.5	24
Somen, dry, 1 oz	100	0.5	21
cooked, 1 cup, 6 oz	230	0.5	49
Japanese Style Pan Fried:			
Maruchan's Yaki-Sobu, 5.6 oz cup	260	3	50
Ramen Noodles (Maruchan/Nissin): *See Page 116*			
Rice Noodles: Dry, 3.5 oz	365	0.5	83
Cooked, 1 cup, 6.2 oz	190	0.5	44
Stir Fry (Yakisoba), 3.5 oz serving	430	6	52
Udon (Chikara), avg., 7.5 oz pkt	250	1	52
Simply Asia/Thai Kitchen ~ Page 117			

Egg Roll/Won Ton Wrappers

	C	F	Cb
Egg/Spring Roll (1), 0.8 oz	65	0	15
Won Ton Wrapper (1), ¼ oz	20	0	4

Quick Guide

Fruit Pies: *Average All Brands (9")*

Apple; Blueberry; Cherry: C F Cb

	C	F	Cb
Small, ⅛ pie, 4¾ oz	320	15	46
Medium, ⅙ pie, 6⅓ oz	425	20	61
Large, ¼ pie, 9½ oz	640	30	92
Whole Pie (9"), 38oz	2560	120	368

Other Pies: *Per Serving (⅙ of 8" Pie)*

Chocolate Cream Pie	345	22	38
Custard; Coconut Custard	270	14	31
Lemon Chiffon Pie	360	14	50
Lemon Meringue	360	13	57
Pecan Pie	440	23	57
Pumpkin Pie	300	12	42
Strawberry Pie	230	9	37

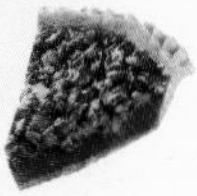

Brands ~ *Per Serving* C F Cb

	C	F	Cb
Denny's: Apple Pie, 7 oz	510	23	72
French Silk, 7 oz	770	57	59
Hostess: Fruit; Cherry, 4.5 oz pie	480	20	68
Lemon, 4.5 oz pie	490	22	69
Long John Silver's: Pecan Pie	370	15	23
Chocolate Cream Pie	310	22	34
Pineapple Cream Pie	290	13	39
Marie Callender's			
Cobbler, avg., ⅛ pie	330	17	44
Mrs Smith's: Peach Cobbler, ⅛ pie	240	8	41
Deep Dish Apple, ¹⁄₁₂ pie	290	14	40
Slices: Apple; Peach, 1 pce	270	13	36
Dutch Apple, 1 piece	250	10	40
Sara Lee			
Pies: Choc Dream Pie, ⅛ pie	420	24	47
Choc Mint Creme Pie, ⅛ pie	420	27	44
Key West Lime Pie, ⅛ pie	380	18	50
Peach Pie, ⅛ pie	310	15	42
Southern Pecan Pie, ⅛ pie	470	23	62
Oven Fresh Pies (9", 37 oz Box): *Per Slice (4.6 oz)*			
Apple Pie, ⅛	340	16	47
Cherry Pie, ⅛	340	16	45
Mince Pie; Blueberry Pie, ⅛, avg.	380	17	53
Pumpkin Pie, ⅛	260	10	39
Southern Sweet Potato Pie, ⅛	280	9	45
Simple Sweets: Apple Pie, ¼ pie	290	15	37
Cherry Pie, ¼ pie	330	16	45
Tastykake: Apple Pie	270	11	31
Coconut Cream Pie	370	20	42
Lemon Pie	300	14	32
Strawberry Pie	340	12	31

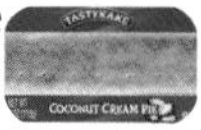

Croissants C F Cb

Average all Brands

	C	F	Cb
Plain/Butter/Cheese: Mini, 1 oz	115	6	13
Small, 1½ oz	170	9	19
Medium, 2 oz	230	12	26
Large, 2½ oz	290	15	32
Extra Large, 3 oz	330	19	37
Sweet Croissants:			
Almond Filled, 3 oz	330	18	39
Chocolate Filled, 3 oz	360	19	43
Dunkin' Donuts: Plain Croissant	310	16	35
Sara Lee: French Style Petite, 2 oz	230	11	26
French Style Original, 1½ oz	170	8	20
Croissant Sandwiches: *See Page 172*			

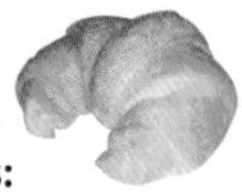

Pastry & Pie Crust C F Cb

	C	F	Cb
Pie Crust: Baked, 9" diameter shell			
1 Pie Shell, 6½ oz	970	64	87
2-crust Pie, 9", 11¼ oz	1660	109	150
Filo Pastry: 4 sheets, 2½ oz	210	2.5	40
Athens: 5 sheets, 2 oz	180	1	37
Pepp. Farm, 2 sheets, 1½ oz	120	1	25
Puff *(Pepp.Farm),* ½ sheet, 4.5 oz	510	33	42
⅙ sheet, 1½ oz	170	11	14
Bake & Fill Shell, 1.7 oz	190	13	16
Arrowhead Mills, Pie Crust, ⅛, avg.	110	6	14
Bisquick: Baking Mix,			
Original, ⅓ cup, 1½ oz	160	5	26
Heart Smart, ⅓ cup, 1½ oz	140	2.5	27
Keebler:			
Ready Crust: Chocolate, ⅛ pie	100	4.5	14
Graham Cracker, ⅛ of 9"	110	5	14
Reduced Fat, ⅛	100	3.5	15
Shortbread Crust, ⅛	110	5	14
Graham Crackers Minis (1)	110	5	15
Marie Callendars Deep Dish Pie Shell, ⅛ pie, 1 oz	140	10	11
Mrs Smith's			
Deep Dish, 9", ⅛	130	7	14
Nabisco Oreo, ⅙ ,1oz	130	7	19
Honey Maid Graham, ⅙, 1 oz	150	8	18
Nilla Pie Crust, ⅙, 1 oz	140	8	18
Pillsbury (All Ready), ⅛ pie, 1 oz	110	7	12
Trader Joe's, Pie Crust, ⅛ pie	190	13	17

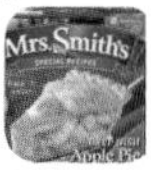

Pie Fillings (Canned)

Fruit: *Average all Fruits*
(Apple/Blueberry/Cherry/Strawberry)

Sweetened: ⅓ cup, 3.2oz	90	0	22
1 cup, 9½ oz	270	0	66
1 can, 21 oz	600	0	150
Light/Lite, ⅓ c., 3.2 oz	60	0	15
Unsweetened, ⅓ cup, 3.2 oz	35	0	8
Lemon Cream/Creme, ⅓ c., 3.2 oz	130	1.5	28

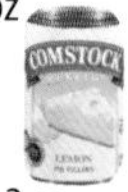

Updated Nutrition Data ~ www.CalorieKing.com
Persons with Diabetes ~ See Disclaimer (Page 24)

Pizzas ~ Ready-To-Eat 🅒 🅕 🅒ᵇ

Average All Retail Outlets/Restaurants

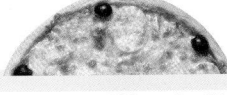

Cheese Pizza
Medium Size (12"):

Thin Crust:

	C	F	Cb
⅛ Pizza (1 slice)	200	8	22
½ Pizza (4 slices)	800	32	88
Whole Pizza (8 slices)	1600	64	172

Deep Dish/Pan:

	C	F	Cb
⅛ Pizza (1 slice)	270	13	27
½ Pizza (4 slices)	1080	52	108
Whole Pizza (8 slices)	2160	104	216

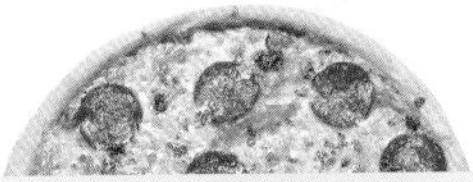

Pepperoni
Medium Size (12"):

Thin Crust:

	C	F	Cb
⅛ Pizza (1 slice)	210	10	23
½ Pizza (4 slices)	840	40	84
Whole Pizza (8 slices)	1680	80	168

Deep Dish/Pan:

	C	F	Cb
⅛ Pizza (1 slice)	280	15	27
½ Pizza (4 slices)	1120	60	108
Whole Pizza (8 slices)	2240	120	216

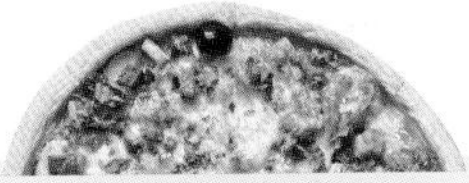

Supreme:
Medium Size (12"):

Thin Crust:

	C	F	Cb
⅛ Pizza (1 slice)	240	11	23
½ Pizza (4 slices)	960	44	92
Whole Pizza (8 slices)	1920	88	184

Deep Dish/Pan:

	C	F	Cb
⅛ Pizza (1 slice)	310	16	28
½ Pizza (4 slices)	1240	64	112
Whole Pizza (8 slices)	2480	128	224

Meat Deluxe
Medium Size (12"):

Thin Crust:

	C	F	Cb
⅛ Pizza (1 slice)	310	18	23
½ Pizza (4 slices)	1240	72	92
Whole Pizza (8 slices)	2480	144	184

Deep Dish/Pan:

	C	F	Cb
⅛ Pizza (1 slice)	380	22	28
½ Pizza (4 slices)	1520	88	112
Whole Pizza (8 slices)	3040	176	224

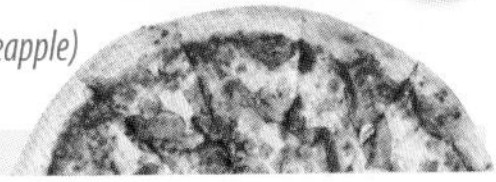

Hawaiian *(Ham & Pineapple)*
Medium Size (12"):

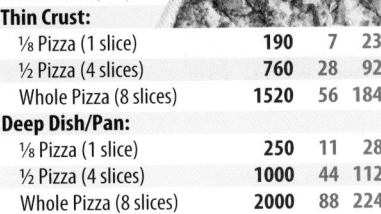

Thin Crust:

	C	F	Cb
⅛ Pizza (1 slice)	190	7	23
½ Pizza (4 slices)	760	28	92
Whole Pizza (8 slices)	1520	56	184

Deep Dish/Pan:

	C	F	Cb
⅛ Pizza (1 slice)	250	11	28
½ Pizza (4 slices)	1000	44	112
Whole Pizza (8 slices)	2000	88	224

Veggie:
Similar to Hawaiian

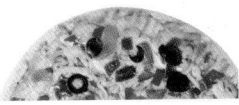

Single Slices
(Extra Large): 🅒 🅕 🅒ᵇ
(Example: Sbarro's)

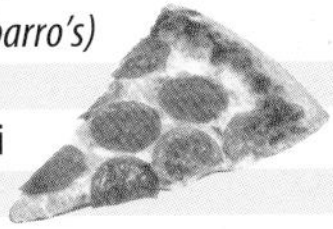

	C	F	Cb
Cheese	460	13	60
Pepperoni	730	37	61
Sausage	670	31	60
Supreme	630	27	63

Individual Pizza (6")
Deep Dish/Pan

(Approx. 9 oz weight):

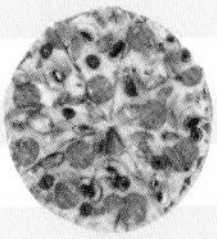

	C	F	Cb
Cheese	600	24	69
Hawaiian	570	21	70
Meat Deluxe	900	50	70
Pepperoni	650	30	67
Veggie	560	22	70

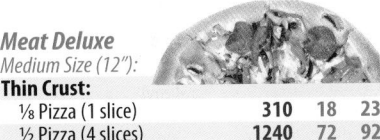

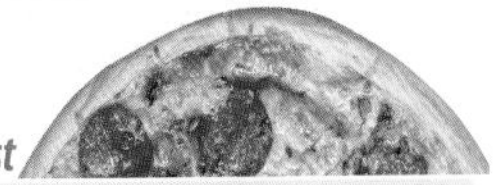

Large (14") Thin Crust

	C	F	Cb
Cheese: ⅛ Pizza	290	12	30
½ Pizza	1160	48	120
Hawaiian: ⅛ pizza	260	9	33
½ Pizza	1040	36	132
Pepperoni: ⅛ Pizza	310	15	30
½ Pizza	1240	60	120
Supreme: ⅛ Pizza	340	17	32
½ Pizza	1360	68	128
Meat Deluxe: ⅛ Pizza	440	26	31
½ Pizza	1760	104	124
Veggie: ⅛ Pizza	260	10	32
½ Pizza	1040	40	128

Frozen Pizzas	C	F	Cb
Amy's: *Per 1/3 Pizza*			
Cheese Pesto	360	18	37
Cheese Pizza	290	12	33
Mushroom & Olive	250	9	33
Pesto	320	16	34
Roasted Vegetable	270	9	42
California Pizza Kitchen			
Crispy Thin Crust: *Per 1/3 Pizza*			
Margherita	290	13	31
Sicilian Recipe	310	14	30
White	290	12	31
For One: Four Cheese, 6.9 oz	510	17	69
Margherita, 6 oz	420	18	45
Sicilian, 5.5 oz	450	22	42
Self Rising Crust: *Per 1/3 Pizza*			
BBQ Chicken, 4.3 oz	270	9	33
Five Cheese & Tomato, 4.3 oz	320	15	29
Thai Chicken 4.3 oz	280	10	34
Celeste			
Pizza For One: Original, 1 pizza	350	17	39
Deluxe; Pepperoni; Chseburger	410	21	42
Meatball	440	24	40
Original/Zesty 4 Cheese, avg.	360	16	48
Sausage & Pepperoni; Suprema	470	26	44
DiGiorno			
Crispy Flatbread Pizza: *Per Slice*			
Italian Sausage & Onion, 5.5 oz	400	26	27
Mushroom Medley, 4.3 oz	320	19	26
Pepperoni & Roasted Peppers, 4.5 oz	340	20	26
Tuscan Style Chicken, 4.7 oz	280	14	25
Deep Dish: *Per 1/6 Pizza*			
Pepperoni	340	18	32
Supreme; Three Meat, avg.	315	15	33
For One: *Per Pizza*			
Garlic Bread Crust: Pepperoni	840	44	81
Thin Crust, Grilled Chicken & Veg.	520	17	64
Traditional Crust: Pepperoni	770	35	83
Supreme	790	36	85
Microwave: *Per 1/2 Pizza*			
Rising Crust: Four Cheese	370	15	44
Supreme	410	18	45
Three Meat	420	19	44
Thin Crispy Crust, Four Cheese	320	12	38

DiGiorno (Cont)	C	F	Cb
Rising Crust: *Per 1/6 Pizza*			
Four Cheese	310	11	40
Pepperoni; Supreme, avg.	360	16	40
Thin Crispy Crust: *Per 1/5 Pizza*			
Four Meat	320	13	37
Grilled Chicken Tomato & Spinach	260	8	33
Ultimate Thin Crust: *Per 1/5 Pizza*			
Four Cheese	330	14	33
Four Meat; Pepperoni, avg.	390	20	33
Freschetta			
Naturally Rising: *Per 1/5 of Large Pizza*			
4 Cheese, 1/5 pizza	360	13	43
4 Meat, 1/5 pizza	380	14	44
Pepperoni, 1/5 pizza	360	14	44
Can. Bacon P'apple, 1/5	310	9	44
Supreme, 1/5 pizza	320	13	37
PizzAmore:			
Original Crust:			
6 Cheese, large, 1 piece	210	8	25
10 Topping Supreme, 1 pce	240	10	25
Pepperoni Duo, 1 pce	240	11	25
Thin Crust: 3 Chse w/ Tom., 2 pce	340	14	36
Chicken, Spinach & Mushr. 2 pce	310	11	37
12" Ultra Thin: Supreme, 3 slices	350	19	27
5 Cheese; Pepperoni, 3 slices	330	17	25
Stuffed Breadsticks: Garlic (1)	110	3	19
Cinn. w. Cream Cheese (1)	140	4	23
Healthy Choice: *Per Pizza (6 oz)*			
French Bread Pizza, Average	350	4	54
Jeno's: *Per Pizza (7 oz)*			
Crispy 'N Tasty: Cheese	450	21	51
Sausage; Pepperoni, average	485	25	50
Home Run Inn (Chicago):			
Classic Large: Cheese, 1/6, 4.5 oz	340	18	30
Sausage, 1/6, 5 oz	360	19	29
Sausage & Pepperoni, 1/6, 5.15 oz	380	20	30
Signature, Ssg Supreme, 5½ oz	360	18	31
Kashi, average, 1/3 pizza	290	9	38
Lean Cuisine			
French Bread Pizza: Cheese, 6 oz	340	7	53
Deluxe; Pepperoni, average	335	9	46
Casual Eating:			
Deluxe, 6 oz	340	10	46
Four Cheese, 6 oz	360	6	51
Mushroom, 6 oz	300	5	47
Roasted Vegetable, 6 oz	320	5	52
Flatbread Melt: Chkn Philly, 6.4 oz	330	8	41
Other varieties, average 6.4 oz	330	9	41
Lean Pockets Pizza, average (1)	280	7	39

Updated Nutrition Data ~ www.CalorieKing.com
Persons with Diabetes ~ See Disclaimer (Page 24)

Frozen Pizzas (Cont) C F Cb

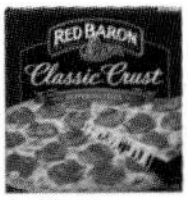

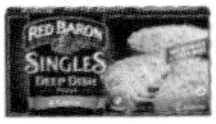

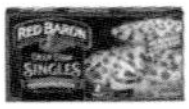

Private Selection
Flat Bread: *Per Pizza*

	C	F	Cb
BBQ Seasoned Chicken	550	16	77
Margherita	600	22	70

Thin Crust: BBQ Chicken, ⅓ pizza

	C	F	Cb
BBQ Chicken, ⅓ pizza	340	14	33
Extra Pepperoni, ⅓ pizza	410	23	29
Margherita, ⅓ pizza	290	12	30

Red Baron
Classic (Large):

	C	F	Cb
4 Cheese, ¼ pizza	380	16	40
Pepperoni, ¼ pizza	370	16	40
Supreme, ⅕ pizza	310	14	33
Sausage & Pepperoni, ¼ pizza	400	19	41
Special Deluxe, ¼ pizza	380	18	41

Garlic Crust: *Per ⅕ pizza*

	C	F	Cb
4 Cheese; Pepperoni	390	15	48

Stone Hearth Fire Baked: *Per ¼ pizza*

	C	F	Cb
Pepperoni	370	17	39

Thin & Crispy Pizzeria Style: *Per ⅓ pizza*

	C	F	Cb
5 Cheese	360	16	39
Pepperoni	410	20	40

Singles

	C	F	Cb
Classic Crust: 4 Cheese (1)	720	38	61
Pepperoni (1)	770	43	61
Deep Dish: 4 Cheese (1)	410	18	45
Meat Trio (1)	410	19	45
Pepperoni (1)	420	19	47
Supreme (1)	420	19	45
Deep Dish Mini Pizza: Cheese (4)	430	21	44
Pepperoni (4)	470	26	43
French Bread:			
Pepperoni (1)	360	15	41
Supreme (1)	360	15	42
Three Meat (1)	370	15	41
5 Cheese & Garlic (1)	410	22	39

Reggio's
Individual Pizza: Cheese (1)

	C	F	Cb
Cheese (1)	250	8	33
Pepperoni, 1 pizza	290	13	33
Sausage & Mushroom (1)	280	10	34

Dinner Size: Cheese, ¼ pizza

	C	F	Cb
Cheese, ¼ pizza	330	12	41
Pepperoni & Sausage, ¼ pizza	400	18	41
Sausage; Supreme, average, ¼	380	16	41

Safeway Select
Thin and Crispy: *Per ⅕ Pizza*

	C	F	Cb
Four Cheese	310	11	37
Supreme	360	16	38

Ultra Thin Crust: *Per ⅓ Pizza Unless Indicated*

	C	F	Cb
BBQ Chicken ¼ Pizza	250	10	23
Margherita	330	17	28
Primo Italiano Meat	330	17	28

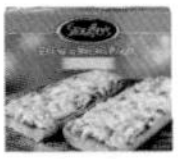

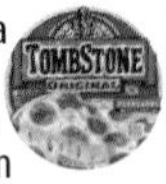

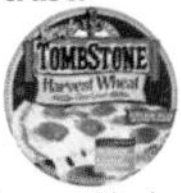

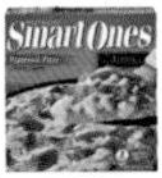

Stouffer's: *Per ½ Pkg*
French Bread Pizzas: Deluxe

	C	F	Cb
Deluxe	430	21	44
Extra Cheese	400	18	44
Pepperoni	410	20	43
Ssg & Pepperoni	460	24	43

Tombstone
Original: *Per ⅕ of Large 12" Pizza Unless Indicated*

	C	F	Cb
4 Meat	310	14	30
Canadian Style Bacon, ¼ Pizza	320	12	37
Deluxe	290	12	31
Extra Cheese, ¼ Pizza	350	15	37
Pepperoni, ¼ Pizza	390	20	37
Pepperoni & Sausage	370	17	37
Sausage/& Mushroom	290	13	30
Supreme	300	14	31

Double Top: Sausage, ⅙ pizza

	C	F	Cb
Sausage, ⅙ pizza	310	16	27
Sausage & Pepperoni, ⅙ pizza	330	18	26

Harvest Wheat Thin Crust:

	C	F	Cb
Cheese, ⅓ pizza	300	10	37
Pepperoni, ¼ pizza	260	10	29
Supreme, ¼ pizza	260	10	29
Light Vegetable	230	6	31

Thin Crust: Three Cheese, ¼ pizza

	C	F	Cb
Three Cheese, ¼ pizza	310	15	28
Pepperoni; Sausage, avg., ¼	325	18	29

Brick Oven Style: Cheese, ⅓ pizza

	C	F	Cb
Cheese, ⅓ pizza	350	15	38
Other varieties, average, ¼ pizza	310	16	29

Tony's
Original Crust: Cheese, ⅓ pizza

	C	F	Cb
Cheese, ⅓ pizza	290	12	37
Pepperoni, ⅓ pizza	310	14	36
Ssg & Pepperoni; Supreme, avg. ⅓	340	17	77

Deep Dish (Individual)**:** Cheese (1)

	C	F	Cb
Cheese (1)	400	16	47
Pepperoni (1)	470	24	49

Totino's
Crisp Crust Party Pizza: *Per ½ Pizza*

	C	F	Cb
Cheese	320	15	34
Pepperoni	370	20	35

Pizza Rolls: Cheese (6), 3 oz

	C	F	Cb
Cheese (6), 3 oz	200	8	26
Pepperoni (6), 3 oz	220	11	24

Trader Joe's:

	C	F	Cb
3 Cheese, ⅓ pizza	270	10	35
Parlanno, ¼ pizza	340	16	34
Spinach, ⅓ pizza	300	12	38

Weight Watchers (Smart Ones): *Per Pizza*

	C	F	Cb
Fajita Chicken	380	7	58
Four Cheese	370	10	56
Pepperoni	390	8	58

Wolfgang Puck
All Natural Pizzas: *Per ⅓ Pizza*

	C	F	Cb
BBQ Chicken	360	15	40
Cheese	340	16	33
Four Cheese Tomato & Pesto	330	17	30
Margherita	330	16	33
Uncured Pepperoni	360	19	32

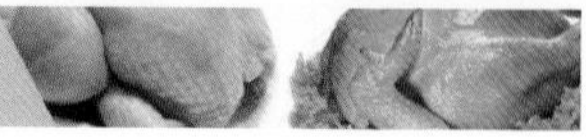

Quick Guide

Chicken	C	F	Cb
From 3lb ready-to-cook chicken			
Breast/Wing Quarter			
Roasted: With skin	300	15	0
Without skin	185	5	0
Fried, batter dipped	530	30	17
Leg Quarter:			
Thigh & Drumstick			
Roasted: With skin, 4 oz	265	15	0
Without skin, 3.35 oz	180	8	0
Fried, batter dipped	430	25	14
(*KFC: See Fast-Foods Section*)			

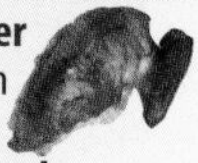

Per 4 oz Edible Portion

	C	F	Cb
Average of Light Meat: *Per 4 oz (no bone)*			
Roasted: with skin	250	12	0
without skin	175	4.5	0
Stewed: with skin	230	12	0
without skin	180	4.5	0
Fried: Batter-dipped, 4 oz	315	17	11
Flour-coated, 4 oz	280	14	2
Average of Dark Meat: *Per 4 oz (no bone)*			
Roasted: with skin	290	18	0
without skin	235	11	0
Stewed: with skin	265	17	0
without skin	220	10	0
Fried: Batter-dipped, 4 oz	340	21	11
Flour-coated, 4 oz	325	19	5

Chicken Parts

Broilers or Fryers: Edible Weights (no bone)	C	F	Cb
Breast: *Per ½ Breast*			
Raw: With skin, 5 oz	250	14	0
Without skin, 4¼ oz	130	1.5	0
Roasted: With skin, 3½ oz	195	8	0
Without skin, 3 oz	140	3	0
Stewed: With skin, 4 oz	200	8	0
Without skin, 3¼ oz	145	3	0
Fried: Batter-dipped, 5 oz	365	19	13
Flour-coated, w. skin, 3½ oz	220	9	2
Drumstick: *Per Drumstick*			
Roasted: With skin, 2 oz	115	6	0
Without skin, 1½ oz	75	2.5	0
Fried: Batter-dipped, 2½ oz	195	11	6
Flour-coated, 1¾ oz	120	7	1
Stewed: With skin, 2 oz	115	6	0
Without skin, 1½ oz	80	3	0

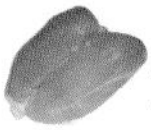

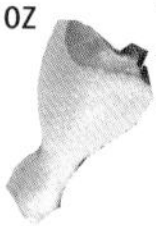

Thigh Portion: Edible Wt. (no bone)	C	F	Cb
Raw: With skin, 3.3 oz			
(4¼ oz with bone)	200	14	0
Without skin, 2.4 oz	80	3	0
Roasted: With skin, 2¼ oz	155	10	0
Without skin, 2 oz	110	6	0
Stewed: With skin, 2½ oz	160	10	0
Without skin, 2 oz	105	5	0
Fried: Batter-dipped, 3 oz	240	14	8
Flour-coated, 2¼ oz	165	9	2
Wing: *Per Wing*			
Raw Weight 3.2 oz (with bone)			
Raw: With skin	110	8	0
Without skin	35	1	0
Roasted: With skin	100	7	0
Without skin	45	2	0
Fried: Batter-dipped	160	11	5
Flour-coated	105	7	1
Stewed: With skin, 4 oz	100	7	0
Buffalo Wings: *See Fast-Foods Section*			
Neck: Simmered, with skin	95	7	0
Without skin	30	2	0
Skin Only: *Skin from ½ Chicken*			
Raw skin, 2¾ oz	275	26	0
Roasted skin, 2 oz	255	23	0
Stewed skin, 2½ oz	260	24	0
Fried, Flour-coated, 2 oz	280	24	5
Fried, Batter-dipped, 6¾ oz	750	55	44
Roasters			
Average of Light & Dark Meat:			
Roasted: With skin, 4 oz	250	15	0
Without skin, 4 oz	190	8	0
Light Meat: Without skin, roasted	175	5	0
Dark Meat: Without skin, roasted	200	10	0
Stewing Chicken			
Average of Light & Dark Meat: *Per 4 oz Stewed*			
With skin	325	22	0
Without skin	270	14	0
Light Meat: Without skin	240	9	0
Dark Meat: Without skin	290	17	0
Capon Chicken			
Roasted: With skin, 4 oz	260	13	0
½ Chicken, with skin	1460	74	0

Chicken Offal & Stuffing	C	F	Cb
Giblets: Simmered, 1 cup	230	7	0.5
Fried, flour-coated, 1 cup	400	20	6
Gizzard, simmered, 1 cup	210	4	0
Heart, simmered, 1 cup	270	12	0.2
Liver: Raw, 4 oz	130	5.5	0
Simmered, 1 cup	215	8.5	1
Liver Pate Fresh, 1 Tbsp, ½ oz	30	2	1
Stuffing: Average, ½ cup	180	9	22

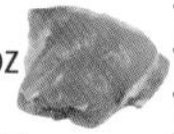

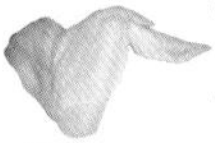

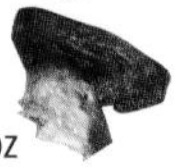

Updated Nutrition Data ~ www.CalorieKing.com
Persons with Diabetes ~ See Disclaimer (Page 24)

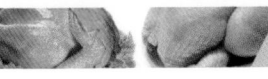

Chicken Products **C F Cb**

Bumble Bee: *Per 4oz Pouch*
Chicken Breast, Skinless fillet:

	C	F	Cb
Garlic & Herb	110	1.5	1
w. Barbeque Sauce	170	1.5	10
w. Southwest Seasoning	120	1	0

Foster Farms

	C	F	Cb
Grilled Chicken Breast Strips, 3 oz	110	2.5	2
Wings: Chipotle, 4 wings, 2.9 oz	190	14	1
Honey BBQ, 4 wings, 2.9 oz	170	10	5
Hot & Spice, 4 wings, 2.9 oz	170	13	1

Tyson:

	C	F	Cb
Breaded Nuggets (5)	270	17	15
Breast Nuggets (5)	220	13	15
Southern Style Nuggets (6)	270	21	11
Breast Patties: Reg., 2.6 oz	200	12	13
Southern Style (1), 2.6 oz	240	18	10
Wings: Flavored, avg. (4)	220	15	1
BBQ Style (4), 3½ oz	200	13	7

Duck, Goose, Quail

	C	F	Cb
Duck: Roasted, with skin, 3 oz	290	24	0
Without skin, 3 oz	170	10	0
½ whole duck, with skin	1290	108	0
Goose: Roast, with skin, 3 oz	260	19	0
Without skin, 3 oz	200	11	0
Pheasant, cooked, 3 oz	210	10	0
Quail, cooked, 1 whole, 6 oz	400	24	0

Turkey

Fryer-Roasters: *Per 3 oz Serving*

	C	F	Cb
Roasted: Light Meat, with skin	140	4	0
without skin	120	1	0
Dark Meat: with skin	155	6	0
without skin	140	4	0

½ of Whole Turkey: (Approx. 3¼ lbs raw wt. w/out neck and giblets; 1.8 lbs cooked wt.)

	C	F	Cb
Roasted: with skin	1650	74	0
without skin	1125	31	0

Ground Turkey, Raw: (4 oz raw wt. = 3 oz ckd wt.)

	C	F	Cb
Regular (85% lean), 4 oz	170	10	0
Lean (93% lean), avg., 4 oz	160	8	0
Foster Farms (94% lean), 4 oz	150	7	0
Jennie-O (93% lean), 4 oz	170	8	0
Trader Joe's (93% lean), 4 oz	150	8	0
Breast, no skin, 4 oz	115	1	0
Patties: Small, 3 oz	130	7	0
Medium, 4 oz	170	10	0
Large, 5.3 oz	225	13	0

Turkey Parts **C F Cb**

Roasted, Edible Weights (no bone)

Breast (½): (from 17¼ oz raw wt. w/bone)

	C	F	Cb
With skin, 12 oz (no bone)	525	11	0
Without skin, 10¾ oz	415	2	0

Back (½):

	C	F	Cb
With skin, 4½ oz	265	13	0
Without skin, 3½ oz	165	6	0

Leg (Thigh & Drumstick):
(from 1 lb raw wt. w/bone)

	C	F	Cb
With skin, 8½ oz (no bone)	410	13	0
Without skin, 7¾ oz	355	8.5	0

Wing: (from 7¼ oz raw wt. w/bone)

	C	F	Cb
With skin, 3 oz (no bone)	185	9	0
Without skin, 2 oz	100	2	0

Neck: Simmered, 1 neck,

	C	F	Cb
(9 oz w. bone)	275	11	0
Giblets, simm., 1 cup, 5 oz	240	7	3

Young Hens (Roasted)

	C	F	Cb
Light Meat: With skin, 3 oz	175	8	0
Without skin, 3 oz	135	3	0
Dark Meat: With skin, 3 oz	200	11	0
Without skin., 3 oz	165	7	0

Young Toms — Similar to Young Hens

Turkey Products

Banquet: *See Frozen Meals, Page 119*

	C	F	Cb
Foster Farms: Meatballs (3)	160	9	3

Hormel: Turkey Chunks (canned), ckd:

	C	F	Cb
White Turkey, 2 oz	60	1.5	0
White & Dark Turkey, 2 oz	70	2.5	0
Jennie-O, Turkey Bacon, 1 slice	35	2.5	0
Turkey Bratwurst, lean, 4 oz	170	10	2
Turkey Meatballs, Italian Style, 3 oz	170	11	1

John Morrell, Off the Bone,

	C	F	Cb
Oven Roasted Turkey Strips, 4 oz	140	5	10
Spam, Oven Roasted Turkey, 2 oz	80	4	2

Swanson: *Frozen Meals, Page 123*

	C	F	Cb
Trader Joe's, Turkey Meatloaf, 3 oz	140	8	5

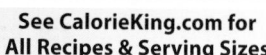

**See CalorieKing.com for
All Recipes & Serving Sizes**

Starters/Appetizers:

Cheesy Grape Balls (1)	20	1.5	1
Shiitake Summer Rolls (1)	120	1	24
Spring Rolls (1)	135	4.5	15

Soups:

Beef Stew	435	8	35
Cheesy Broccoli Potato Soup, 1 cup	150	5	16
Chicken Soup with Rice Dumplings	155	0.5	31
Chili Con Carne	360	15	25
Creamy Butternut Squash Soup	115	3	22
Spicy Pumpkin Soup	205	5	29
Sweet Potato Soup	130	3	22

Salads:

Apple Raspberry Salad	95	2.5	11
Cherry and Smoked Turkey Salad	265	9	31
Citrus Fruit Salad	125	0.5	30
Green Bean Potato Salad	185	5	32
Hot Rosemary Potato Salad	180	2	37
Watermelon Salad	40	0	10

Meat Entrees:

Beef and Mushroom Burgers (2)	450	14	51
Gr. Marinated Lamb Filet, 3½ oz	150	7	1
Lamb and Rosemary Kebobs (1)	220	9	3
Mustard Steak with Tuscan Salad	235	8	8
Veal and Mushrooms	235	7	11

CALORIE KING TIPS
TO REDUCE CALORIES:

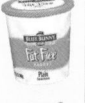

- **Use non-fat milk** in place of whole or 2% milk
- **Use low-fat yogurt** in place of sour cream
- **Skim fat** from surface of soups and casseroles after cooling
- **Add extra vegetables** to soups and hot entrees
- **Cakes/cookies/muffins:** Replace most or all the fat/oil with applesauce and/or prune puree (Example: *Sunsweet Lighter Bake*)

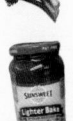

- **Drinks:** Replace sugar with no-calorie sweeteners such as *Equal, Stevia, Splenda and Sweet 'N Low*

Chicken Entrees:

Baked Chicken with Mushrooms	155	2	4
Baked Rosemary Drumsticks (2)	320	11	22
Basil & Lemon Chicken Thighs (1)	150	9.5	3
Chicken Cacciatore	345	7	40
Chicken Kiev	315	8	26
Easy Chicken Pot Pie	275	12	23
Lemon Chicken with Olives	200	9	8
Mushroom & Chicken Coq au Vin	360	9	9

Fish Entrees:

Fish Cutlets in Herb Tomato Coulis	300	4.5	5
Grilled Fish with Corn & Leek, 4 oz	245	10	12
Stir-Fry Mixed Seafood & Noodles	250	4	28
Thai Fish Cakes	260	4	36
Tuna-Mayo Wrap	250	3.5	26

Vegetarian:

Avocado Tacos (1)	100	3	17
Coconut Vegetable Curry	200	11	12
Eggplant Stuffed with Tofu	215	5	40
Fettuccini w/Tomato & Basil Sauce	340	8	56
Gourmet Vegetable Pizza	170	5	24
Nutty Soy 'n Rice Burgers (1)	140	3.5	23
Slow Cooker Veggie Lasagna	185	8.5	14
Vegetable Burgers (1)	185	6.5	18
Zucchini Moussaka	260	5	36

Desserts:

Angel Food Cake	85	0	18
Apple and Rice Pudding	110	0.5	25
Brandy Pumpkin Flan	145	5	17
Fruit Salad Dessert Cake	175	8.5	23
Low-Fat Carrot Cake	185	2	39
Melon Sorbet	100	2	21
Non-Fat Brownies (1)	115	0	26
Non-Fat Chocolate Cupcakes (1)	105	0	22
Non-Fat Vanilla Ice Cream	60	0	11
Watermelon Blueb. Banana Split	175	1	42

Drinks: Per 1 Cup, 8 fl.oz

Apple and Fruit Frappe	135	0	33
Banana Daiquiri	190	2	44
Fruity Iced Tea	50	0	12
Mocha Shake	95	0	14
Pineapple Float	180	0	44
Watermelon Coconut Margarita	235	6	34
Watermelon Kiwi Smoothie	115	0	24

Updated Nutrition Data ~ www.CalorieKing.com
Persons with Diabetes ~ See Disclaimer (Page 24)

White Rice

	C	F	Cb
Raw: Short/Med. Grain, 1 c., 7 oz	715	1	158
Long Grain, 1 cup, 6½ oz	675	1	148
Glutinous, 1 cup, 6½ oz	685	1	151
Cooked Rice (Boiled/Steamed):			
Short/Medium Grain:			
½ cup, 3¼ oz	135	0	30
1 cup (½ Pint), 7.2 oz	270	0.5	59
2 cups (1 Pint), 13 oz	480	1	106
Long Grain: ½ cup, 2¾ oz	105	0	22
1 cup, 5½ oz	205	0.5	44
Glutinous/Sticky, ckd, 1 c., 6 oz	170	0.5	37
Parboiled, cooked, ½ cup, 3 oz	105	0.5	22
Precook./Instant: Dry, ½ c., 3½ oz	370	0	80
Cooked, ½ cup, 3 oz	90	0	20
Wild Rice: Raw, 1 cup, 5½ oz	570	2	120
Cooked, 1 cup, 5¾ oz	165	0.5	35

Brown Rice

	C	F	Cb
Average of Short or Long Grain			
Raw/Dry: ½ cup, 3¼ oz	340	2.5	71
1 cup, 6½ oz	685	5.5	143
Cooked: ½ cup, 3½ oz	110	1	22
1 cup, 7 oz	220	2	46

Rice Dishes

	C	F	Cb
Chinese Fried Rice:			
½ cup, 2½ oz	140	4.5	21
1 cup, (½ Pint), 5 oz	280	9	42
2 cups, (1 Pint), 10 oz	565	18	84
Mexican Rice: 1 cup	500	12	90
Taco John's, 1 serving (6 oz)	250	5	45
Taco Time, 1 serving (4 oz)	160	2	30
Rice-A-Roni: *See Page 116*			
Rice w. Raisins/Pinenuts, 1 cup	400	11	60
Rice Pilaf: Restaurant, 1 cup	275	7.5	46
O'Charley's, 1 order	200	5	31
Rice Pudding (*Kozy Shack*),			
Original, ½ cup	130	3	22
Risotto, 1 cup	420	12	70
Saffron Rice, 4 oz	175	7	25
Spanish Rice: 1 cup	390	9	72
El Pollo Loco, small, 5 oz	160	1	35
Taco Cabana, 4 oz	180	5	30
Sticky Rice, 5 oz	155	0.5	34
Sushi Rice: 1 Tbsp	25	0	5
1 cup, 5.2 oz	390	0	77

Other Packaged Rice Products:
Rice-A-Roni: See Page 116
Uncle Ben's / Zatarain's: See Page 118

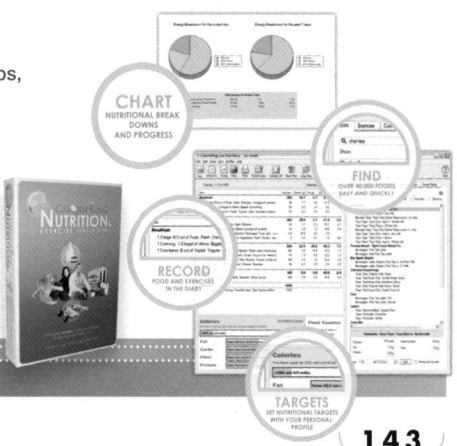

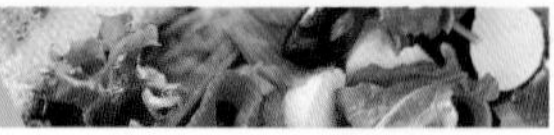

Deli Salads

	C	**F**	**Cb**
General Average, All Outlets			
Antipasto Salad, ½ c,	135	8	13
3-Bean Salad, ½ cup	110	4	17
Bulgur Salad, ½ cup	70	2	12
Caesar Salad, Classic, 1 c.	200	14	15
Side Salad, no Dress,	25	0	6
Carrot Raisin: No Dressing, ½ cup	20	0	5
with Dressing, ½ cup	135	12	6
Chef's Salad: Regular, no Dress.	620	37	8
w. 2 oz 1000 Island	860	61	8
Chicken Salad, ½ cup/scoop, 4 oz	280	21	2
Coleslaw: Traditional, ½ c.	150	8	18
w. Low Cal Dressing, ½ c.	50	2	8
Corn, Mexican, ½ cup	240	12	33
Cucumber: Non-Oil Dressing, ½ c.	60	0	14
w. Oil Dressing, ½ cup	140	12	8
Eggplant Salad, ½ cup	75	5	7
Fettucini w. veges, ½ cup	135	6	16
Garden Salad, no Dress., 1 c.	10	0	2
Greek Salad, 1 cup	105	8	7
Greek Vegetables, 1 c.	110	8	6
Lettuce, hearts, ½ head	15	0	2.5
Lobster Salad, ½ c., 4 oz	250	21	11
Macaroni Salad, ½ cup, 5 oz	360	26	26
Nicoise, 1 cup	450	32	18
Pasta Salad, ½ cup	200	11	19
Potato Salad: Dijon, 3 oz	120	7	13
w. Mayonnaise, ½ cup, 4 oz	215	15	17
Lowfat, ½ cup	110	1.5	21
Rice Salad, ½ cup	150	10	13
Saffron Rice, 4 oz	175	7	25
Spinach Salad, 1 cup	180	13	13
Tabouli, ½ cup	125	7	13
Three Bean Salad, ½ cup	90	4.5	12
Tomato & Mozzarella, ½ cup	180	14	10
Tortellini w. Basil Pesto, ½ cup	150	9	15
Waldorf w. Mayo, ½ cup	110	7	12
Signature Salads: Per 6 oz Serving			
(Supplied to Deli's and Institutions)			
Antipasto Salad, 6 oz	510	50	4
Artichoke Salad, marinated	400	41	8
California Medley	120	7	15
Cheese Agnolotti	250	8	23
Chicken Salad	420	33	11
Crabmeat Flavored	450	38	20

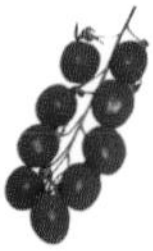

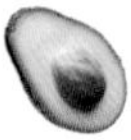

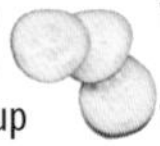

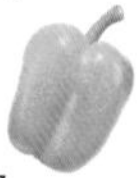

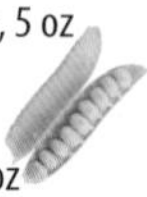

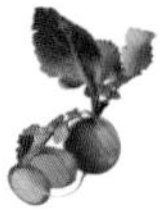

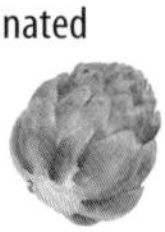

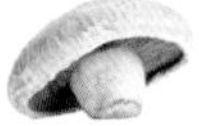

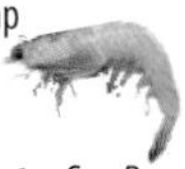

Signature Salads (Cont): *Per 6 oz Serving*	**C**	**F**	**Cb**
Egg Salad	300	23	14
Fresh Button Mushroom	190	16	6
Garden Olive	630	67	3
Ham Salad	400	32	14
Prima Pasta Salad	360	30	18
Seafood Pasta Del Mar	170	10	21
Seafood w. Crab & Shrimp	420	34	20
Shrimp Salad	360	32	8
Tuna Salad	450	36	14
Fast-Food Restaurants: *See Page 182*			

Fast-Food Restaurants: *See Page 182*

Fresh Salad Packs

Pre-Packaged (Supermarkets)	**C**	**F**	**Cb**
Dole: Caesar Kit, 3½ oz	160	13	7
Asian Crunch Kit, 3½ oz	130	7	14
Hearty Italian, 3½ cups	180	13	10
Regular Salad Packs: *Without Added Dressing*			
Classic Cole Slaw, 3 oz	25	0	5
Classic Iceberg, 3 oz	15	0	4
Packaged Salad: *With Dressing*			
Broccoli Ranch, 1½ cups	230	13	25
Cheddar Bacon Ranch, 1½ c.	370	22	35
Garden Vegetable, 1½ cups	240	14	25
Fresh Express			
Complete Salad Kits: *Per Serving, Prepared*			
Asian Supreme, ¼ bag	120	5	17
B.L.T. Caesar, ⅓ bag	170	14	8
Caesar: ⅓ bag	150	13	8
Lite, ⅓ bag	100	7	8
Supreme, ⅓ bag	140	12	7
Mediterranean Supreme, ⅓ bag	150	10	16
Pacifica! Veggie Supreme, ½ bag	220	15	18
Salsa! Ensalada Supreme, ¼ bag	120	8	10

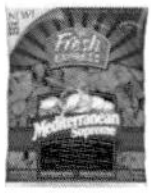

Salad Toppings

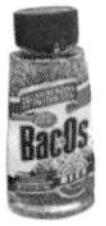

	C	**F**	**Cb**
Bacon Bits: Bacos, 1 Tbsp	30	1.5	2
Hormel, 1 Tbsp	25	1.5	0
Chow Mein Noodles, dry, ½ c.	120	7	13
Croutons, 2 Tbsp, 10g	40	1	7
Olives, 5 medium	25	2	0
Sunflower Seeds, 1 Tbsp, 8 g	45	4	1.5
Toasted sliced Almonds, 2 T., ½ oz	85	7	3
Tortilla Chips, 12 chips, 1 oz	140	7	19

Updated Nutrition Data ~ www.CalorieKing.com
Persons with Diabetes ~ See Disclaimer (Page 24)

Quick Guide

Salad Dressings
Average All Brands
Per 2 Tbsp (Approx 1 fl.oz)

	C	F	Cb
Balsamic Vinaigrette: Regular	90	9	3
Light, 2 Tbsp	45	4	2
Fat Free, 2 Tbsp	25	0	6
Blue Cheese: Regular, 2 Tbsp	150	16	2
Regular, ¼ cup, 2 oz	300	32	4
Light, 2 Tbsp	30	1	4
Caesar: Regular, 2 Tbsp	155	17	1
Regular, ¼ cup, 2 oz	310	34	2
Light, 2 Tbsp	70	8	5
Coleslaw: Regular, 2 Tbsp	125	11	8
Regular, ¼ cup, 2 oz	245	21	15
Light, 2 Tbsp	110	7	14
French/Italian: Regular	150	14	5
Regular, ¼ cup, 2 oz	290	28	10
Light, 2 Tbsp	65	4	9
Fat/Oil-Free, 2 Tbsp	40	0	10
Ranch: Regular, 2 Tbsp	145	16	2
Regular, ¼ cup, 2 oz	290	31	4
Light, 2 Tbsp	80	3	7
Fat-Free, 2 Tbsp	50	0.5	11
Thousand Island: Regular	120	11	5
Regular, ¼ cup, 2 oz	230	22	9
Light, 2 Tbsp	60	4	7
Fat-Free, 2 Tbsp	40	0.5	10

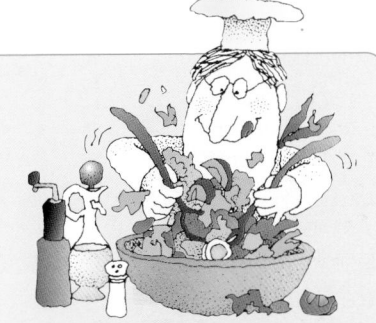

*Enjoy a healthy salad
but don't drown it
in high-fat salad dressings.
Use 'light' dressings to halve
the fat and calories.*

Brands ~ Salad Dressings

	C	F	Cb
Annie's Naturals: *Per 2 Tbsp*			
Artichoke Parmesan	130	13	1
Goddess	120	12	2
Lemon & Chive	150	16	1
Shiitake & Sesame	130	14	1
Tuscany Italian	80	7	5
Vinaigrette: Balsamic	110	11	2
Roasted Red Pepper	70	6	3
Lite, Honey Mustard	40	3	5
Organic: Buttermilk	70	7	1
Creamy Asiago Cheese	80	9	0
Green Goddess	130	13	2
Thousand Island	80	7	4
Vinaigrette, Red Wine & Olive Oil	140	15	0
Bernstein's: *Per 2 Tbsp*			
Creamy Caesar	120	13	1
Herb Garden French	130	12	6
Italian	110	12	1
Restaurant Recipe Italian	120	12	1
Other varieties, average	110	11	2
Fat-Free Cheese & Garlic Italian	10	0	2
Light Fantastic: Cheese Fantastico	25	1.5	3
Roasted Garlic Balsamic	45	3.5	3
Best Foods			
Dijonnaise, 1 tsp	5	0	1
Mayonnaise: *Per 1 Tbsp*			
Canola	45	4.5	0
Low-Fat	15	1	2
Light	35	3.5	1
Real Mayonnaise	90	10	0
Tartar Sauce, 2 Tbsp	80	7	4
Bob's Famous: *Per 2 Tbsp*			
Bleu Cheese	140	15	1
Lite	80	8	1
Ranch Country	150	16	1
Roquefort	140	15	1
Thousand Island	140	14	4
Bolthouse			
Creamy Yogurt Dressings: *Per 2 Tbsp*			
Caesar Parmigiano	80	6.5	3
Chunky Blue Cheese	70	6.5	2
Classic Ranch	80	7.5	3
Brianna's: *Per 2 Tbsp*			
Blue Cheese	120	11	5
Blush Wine Vinaigrette	120	7	14
French Vinaigrette	130	14	0
New American	160	17	6
Rich Santa Fe Blend	25	0	5
Zesty French	150	15	4
Other varieties, average	155	14	8

Brands ~ Salad Dressings (Cont)

Per 2 Tbsp (Approx 1 fl.oz)

	C	F	Cb
Cardini's			
Caesar, 2 Tbsp	160	17	1
Fat-Free Caesar	40	0	9
Light Caesar	80	7	5
Honey Mustard	140	13	5
Italian	120	13	1
Parmesan Ranch	150	15	2
Roasted Asian Sesame	120	10	7
Vinaigrette Dressing:			
Balsamic	100	8	5
Lite: Balsamic	50	3	5
Caesar	60	5	2
Greek	50	4.5	2
El Torito: Cilantro Pepita Caesar	140	14	1
Emeril's: *Per 2 Tbsp*			
House Herb Vinaigrette	100	10	1
Kicked Up French	80	5	8
Girard's: *Per 2 Tbsp*			
Caesar	140	15	1
Light Caesar	90	8	5
Champagne	150	16	1
Light Champagne	60	5	2
Olde Venice Italian	130	13	2
Fat-Free: Balsamic/Red Wine, avg.	25	0	6
Caesar	40	0	9
Raspberry	60	0	14
Vinaigrette: Blue Cheese	100	10	3
Hidden Valley: *Per 2 Tbsp*			
Regular Ranch: Italian Ranch	140	14	2
Old-Fashioned Buttermilk Ranch	140	14	2
Bacon Ranch	140	14	1
Cracked Peppercorn Ranch	120	12	2
Cole Slaw	150	15	5
Light, Original Ranch	80	7	3
Fat-Free, Original Ranch	30	0	6
Ken's Steak House Dressings: *Per 2 Tbsp*			
Balsamic & Basil Vinaigrette	110	12	1
Chunky Blue Cheese	150	16	1
Country French	150	12	10
Creamy Caesar	160	18	0
Peppercorn Ranch	180	19	1
Ranch	140	15	2
Italian w. Aged Romano	120	12	2
Thousand Island	140	13	4
Lite: Caesar/Olive Oil Vinaigrette, avg.	65	6	3
Ranch	90	7	5

Kraft

	C	F	Cb
Regular Dressings: *Per 2 Tbsp*			
Honey Dijon	100	9	6
Coleslaw Maker	110	9	7
Creamy Italian	100	11	2
Light Raspb. Vinaigrette	60	4	5
Ranch	120	12	3
Roka Brand Blue Cheese	120	13	1
Thousand Island w. Bacon	100	8	7
Tuscan House Italian	120	12	2
Kraft Free (Fat-Free): Italian	20	0	4
Classic Caesar Italian	50	0	11
Honey Dijon	50	0	12
Light Done Right!:			
Red Wine Vinaigrette	45	4	3
Special Collection:			
Caesar Vinaigrette with Parm.	70	5	3
Greek Vinaigrette	110	12	2
Sundried Tomato	60	5	4
Sweet Honey Catalina	130	10	8
Tangy Tomato 7 Bacon	100	6	10
Seven Seas: Viva Robust It.	90	9	2
Red Wine Vin. & Oil	45	4	3
Kroger: *Per 2 Tbsp*			
3 Cheese Ranch/Creamy Ranch	130	14	2
Balsamic Vinaigrette	90	9	2
California Honey French	140	12	9
Chunky Bleu Chse; Crmy Cucumber	150	16	3
Creamy Italian	120	13	3
Peppercorn Ranch	110	12	2
Poppy Seed	160	14	8
Thousand Island	90	8	5
Zesty Italian	90	9	3
Fat-Free: Creamy Ranch	30	0	7
French	35	0	9
Honey Dijon	30	0	7
Thousand Island	45	0	10
Zesty Italian	20	0	4
Lite: Creamy Caesar	80	8	3
Creamy Ranch	70	6	3
Zesty Italian	35	2	4
Litehouse: Caesar	130	13	2
Chunky Bleu Cheese	150	16	1
Coleslaw	100	8	8
Jalapeno Ranch	120	12	2
Lite Bleu Cheese	70	6	2
Roquefort	80	8	2
Tangy Orange Citrus	50	0	13
Thai Peanut	60	3	6

Updated Nutrition Data ~ www.CalorieKing.com
Persons with Diabetes ~ See Disclaimer (Page 24)

Brands ~ Salad Dressings (Cont)

Maple Grove: Per 2 Tbsp, 1 fl.oz	C	F	Cb
Regular: Honey Mustard	100	8	8
Sweet-N-Sour	90	6	10
Fat Free: Balsamic Vinaigrette	5	0	1
Caesar	10	0	3
Greek	15	0	3
Honey Dijon; Poppyseed Vin., avg.	40	0	10
Other varieties, avg.	25	0	6
Lite: Caesar	60	4.5	4
Honey Mustard	70	4	8

Marie's: Per 2 Tbsp			
1000 Island	150	15	4
Caesar	170	19	1
Chunky Blue Cheese	160	17	0
Creamy Ranch	170	19	1
Honey Dijon	130	12	5
Poppy Seed	150	13	8
Sesame Ginger	100	8	7
Premium, Spinach Salad	70	1.5	13

Marzetti's			
Asiago Peppercorn	160	16	1
Asian Ginger	120	12	4
Bistro Blue Cheese	180	19	1
Chunky Blue Cheese	150	15	1
Honey Balsamic	120	11	4
Original Slaw	160	15	6
Ranch	160	17	1

Nasoya: Per 2 Tbsp			
Vegi-Dressing (Tofu Base/Dairy Free):			
Thousand Island	60	5	2
Other flavors	60	7	1
Nayonaise: Original	70	7	2
Fat-Free, 2 Tbsp, 1 oz	20	0	4

Newman's Own: Per 2 Tbsp			
Balsamic Vinaigrette	90	9	3
Creamy Caesar	150	16	1
Family Recipe Italian	120	13	1
Olive Oil & Vinegar	150	16	1
Parmesan Roasted Garlic	110	11	2
Ranch	140	15	2
Two Thousand Island	140	14	4
Lighten Up: Light Italian	60	6	0
Light Raspberry & Walnut	70	5	7
Light Balsamic Vinaigrette	45	4	2

San-J: Per 2 Tbsp	C	F	Cb
Tamari Peanut	70	2	9
Tamari Sesame	40	2	5
Fat-Free, Tamari Ginger	25	0	5

Seven Seas:			
Creamy Italian	110	12	2
Viva Robust Italian	90	9	2

Spectrum: Per 2 Tbsp			
Organic Omega-3:			
Asian Ginger	130	13	2
Creamy Garlic Ranch	120	13	1
Golden Balsamic Vin.	110	11	3
Pomegranate Chipotle	130	13	2
Vegan Caesar	100	10	2

Wishbone			
Creamy: Chunky Blue Cheese	150	15	2
Creamy Caesar	170	18	1
Creamy Italian	110	10	4
Deluxe French	120	11	5
Garlic Ranch	140	15	2
Ranch	120	13	2
Russian	120	6	14
Sweet 'n Spicy	130	12	6
Thousand Island	130	12	6
Light: Blue Cheese	50	2	6
Creamy Caesar	50	2	7
Country Italian	30	1.5	3
Honey Dijon	50	2	8
Italian	35	2	4
Parmesan Peppercorn Ranch	50	2	7
Ranch	40	2	5
Thousand Island	50	2	9
Fat-Free:			
Chunky Blue Cheese	35	0	7
Italian	20	0	4
Ranch	30	0	7
Oil & Vinegar: Balsamic Vinaigrette	50	5	3
House Italian	100	10	3
Red Wine Vinaigrette	80	5	9
Robusto Italian	80	7	4
Light Vinaigrette: Balsamic & Basil	60	5	3
Asian w. Sesame & Ginger	70	5	6
Raspberry Walnut	80	5	7
Salad Spritzers: All flavors,			
10 sprays (¼ fl.oz) for 1 cup salad	10	1	1

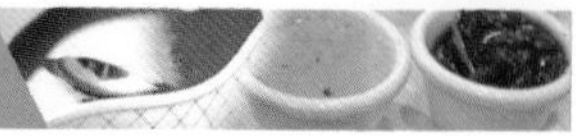

Gravy

	C	F	Cb
Homemade Gravy, avg:			
Thin, little fat, 2 Tbsp, 1 oz	20	1	3
Thick, 2 Tbsp, 1¼ oz	50	2	9
¼ cup, 2½ oz	100	4	18
Pillsbury (Gravy Mixes): *Prepared*			
Brown; Homestyle, ¼ cup, 2 oz	15	0	3
Chicken, as prep., ¼ cup, 2 oz	20	0	4

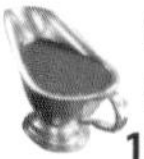

Gravy-In-Jars-Homestyle

Boston Market, ¼ c., 2 oz	40	2	3
Franco-American (In Jars):			
99% Fat Free, ¼ cup, 2 oz	25	0.5	3
Heinz, reg., all flav., ¼ c., 2 oz	25	0	4
Fat Free Roast Turkey, ¼ c., 2 oz	20	0	4
Vons, all types, ¼ c., 2 oz	20	0.5	4

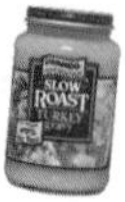

Tomato Products

	C	F	Cb
Whole/Chopped/Crushed/Diced			
1 cup, 8½ oz	50	0	10
In Aspic, ½ cup	50	0	12
w. Green Chili, 1 c., 8½ oz	60	0	16
Stewed, ½ cup, 1.7 oz	40	1.5	6.5
Wedges in Tom Juice, 1 cup	70	0.5	18
Salsa, average, 1 Tbsp	15	0	3.5
Tomato Ketchup:			
Regular: 1 Tbsp, ½ oz	15	0	4
Single Serve, 1 pkt	10	0	3
One-Carb *(Heinz)*, 1 Tbsp, ½ oz	5	0	1
Tomato Paste, 2 Tbsp, 1 oz	25	0	6
Regular, ¾ cup, 6 oz	140	1	32
Tomato Puree, ½ cup, 4½ oz	50	0	10
Tomato Sauce:			
Regular, ½ cup, 4.4 oz	50	0	11
Spanish Style, ½ c., 4.3 oz	40	0	9
w. Mushr., ½ c., 4.3 oz	45	0	10
w. Onions, ½ c., 4.3 oz	50	0	12
Tomato Seasoning, 3 tsp	20	0	4
Sundried Tomatoes:			
Natural, 5-6 pces, 0.4 oz	22	0	5
In Oil, drained, 6 pces, ½ oz	40	2.5	4

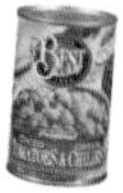

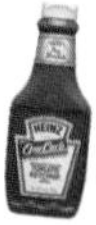

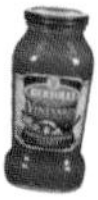

Sauces ~ Brands

	C	F	Cb
A-1			
Steak & Marinades Sauce: *Per Tablespoon (½ oz)*			
Bold & Spicy; Teriyaki; New York	20	0	5
Carb Well Steak Sauce	5	0	1
Chicago	20	1	3
Jamaican Jerk	25	0.5	5
New Orleans Cajun	25	0	5
Steak Sauce	15	0	3
Barilla: *Per ½ Cup*			
Green & Black Olives	80	3	10
Roasted Garlic	60	1	12
Other varieties, average	70	2.5	12
Bertolli: *Per ½ Cup*			
Italian Sausage	100	3	15
Olive Oil & Garlic	90	3	14
Marinara; Rst Pepper, avg.	80	2	13
Portobello w/ Merlot	80	2.5	12
Tomato & Basil	80	2	13
Vineyard Selection, Marinara	80	2	14
Best Foods/Hellmann's: *Per 2 Tbsp*			
Tartar Sauce	80	7	4
Buitoni			
Pasta Sauces: *Per ½ Cup Serving, 4½ oz*			
Arrabbiata	90	6	8
Alfredo	130	11	4
Light Alfredo	90	6	5
Marinara	70	3	10
Pesto: with Basil	300	28	6
with Sun Dried Tomatoes	210	18	9
Roasted Garlic Marinara	60	1.5	10
Tomato Herb Parmesan	130	8	10
Vodka	100	7	7
Bull's Eye: *Per 2 Tbsp*			
Original BBQ Sauce	50	0	13
Sweet & Tangy	60	0	13
Catelli			
Garden Select Pizza Sce, avg.,1 fl.oz	65	0.5	1
Meat Sauce, ½ cup, 4 oz	85	2.5	11
Garden Select 6 Vege Recipe Sauce: *Per ½ Cup*			
Parmesan & Romano	80	2.5	12
Thick & Chunky, Diced Tomato & Basil	70	1.5	12
Other varieties, avg.	80	1.5	13
Cento: *Per ½ Cup*			
Sauces: Passata Tomatoes	30	0	5
All Natural: Pasta	50	3	3
Pizza	40	1.5	6
Tomato: Arrabbiata	140	9	12
Marinara	120	9	9
Puttanesca	140	9	12
White Clam	170	15	4

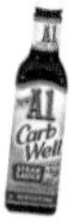

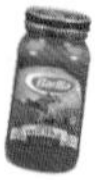

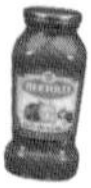

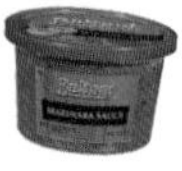

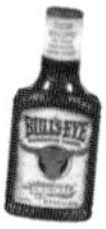

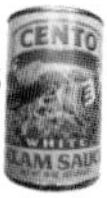

Updated Nutrition Data ~ www.CalorieKing.com
Persons with Diabetes ~ See Disclaimer (Page 24)

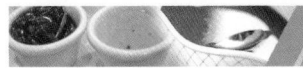

Sauces (Cont)

	C	F	Cb
Classico: *Per ½ Cup Unless Indicated*			
Organic Spinach & Garlic	60	1	10
Rstd Red Pepper Alfredo, ¼ c.	60	5	3
Spicy Tomato & Basil	90	3.5	12
Signature Recipes Sauce:			
Cabernet Marinara with Herbs	70	1.5	12
Caramelized On. & Rstd Garlic	85	2.5	13
Creamy Alfredo, avg., ¼ cup	80	7	3
Fire Rstd Tom. & Garlic	50	1	8
Florentine Spinach & Cheese	80	3.5	9
Mushrooms & Ripe Olives	60	1.5	10
Pesto, Sun-Dried Tomato, ¼ cup	90	5	8
Pesto, Traditional Basil, ¼ cup	230	21	6
Spicy Red Pepper	60	2.5	8
Spicy Tomato & Pesto	90	5	10
Sun-Dried Tomato	80	4	11
Traditional Favorites Sauce: *Per ½ Cup*			
Four Cheese	80	3	12
Italian Sausage w. Peppers & Onions	80	2.5	10
Roasted Garlic	50	1	9
Colgin, Liquid Smoke	0	0	0
Contadina: *Per ¼ Cup*			
Pizza Sauce: Flavored w. Pepperoni	35	1	5
Original; Four Cheese, avg.	30	0.5	6
Cooking Sauce: Sweet & Sour, 1 T.	40	1	8
Tomato Sauce, avg., ¼ cup	20	0	4
Crosse & Blackwell: *Per 1 Tbsp*			
Ham Glaze	30	0	7
Mint Sauce	5	0	2
Del Monte			
Spaghetti Sauces: *Per ½ Cup*			
w. Four Cheeses	70	1.5	15
w. Meat/Mushrooms, avg.	60	1	14
Other varieties, avg.	75	1	16
Chunky Sce: Garlic & Herb	60	1.5	11
Italian Herb	60	1	12
Sloppy Joe Sauce, Original, ¼ cup	50	0	11
Enrico's			
Sicilian	80	2.5	13
Traditional Italian Style	60	1.5	12
Mushroom Onion, ½ cup	70	1.5	13
Pizza, ¼ cup	40	1.5	6
Other varieties, ½ cup	60	1	12

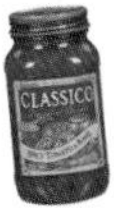

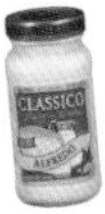

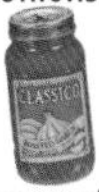

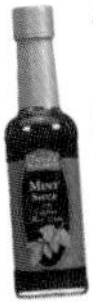

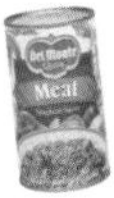

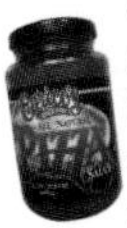

Emiril's	C	F	Cb
Pasta Sauces: *Per ½ Cup*			
Homestyle Marinara	90	3	14
Kicked Up Tomato	70	3	9
Puttanesca	80	5	9
Roasted Gaaahlic	80	3.5	12
Roasted Red Pepper	60	3	7
Vodka Sauce	130	8	13
Francesco Rinaldi: *Per ½ Cup*			
Traditional: 3-Cheese	80	2	15
Original	80	3	12
Meat/Mushroom	80	3	12
Other varieties, average	70	2.5	12
French's			
Worcestershire Sauce, 1 tsp	60	0	1
Heinz: *Per 1 Tbsp, Approx. ½ oz*			
57	20	0	4
Barbecue Sauces, all flavors	35	0	9
Chili Sauce	20	0	5
Horseradish Sauce	75	6	2
Tomato Ketchup: Regular	15	0	4
Reduced Sugar	5	0	1
Worcestershire Sauce, 1 Tbsp	10	0	1
Original Cocktail Sauce			
¼ cup, 2.2 oz	60	0	15
House of Tsang: *Per 1 Tbsp (Approx. ½ oz)*			
Bangkok Peanut	45	2.5	4
Classic Stir Fry	25	1	4
Ginger Soy	20	0	4
Hot General Tsao	45	0.5	10
Hibachi Grill: Kobe Steak Grill	50	4	3
Spicy Hunan Smokehut	40	1	8
Sweet Ginger Sesame	40	1	8
Thai Peanut	50	3	5
Tokyo Teriyaki	40	0	10
Hoisin, 1 tsp	15	0	4
Imperial Citrus Stir-Fry	25	0	5
Korean Teriyaki Stir-Fry	35	1.5	5
Mandarin Marinade	25	0	6
Oyster	30	0	7
Saigon Sizzle Stir-Fry	45	2	7
Spicy Brown Bean	15	0	3
Sweet & Sour Stir-Fry	35	0	9
Szechuan Spicy Stir-Fry	25	1	4

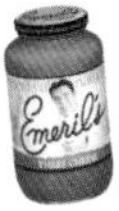

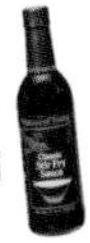

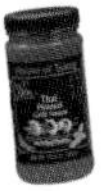

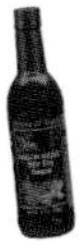

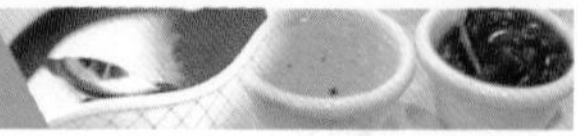

Brands (Cont)

	C	F	Cb
Hunt's			
BBQ Sauce: Original, 2 Tbsp	60	0	15
Hickory & Brown Sugar, 2 T.	70	0	18
Manwich Sloppy Joe Sce, ¼ cup	30	0	7
Spaghetti Sauce: *Per ½ Cup*			
Classic Italian: Four Cheese	50	1	10
Garlic & Herb	40	1	8
Zesty & Spicy	60	2	10
Original Style: Traditional	50	1	10
Meat Flavor	60	1	11
Jack Daniel's			
Original No. 7 BBQ Sce, 2 Tbsp	50	0	12
Hickory Brown Sugar, 2 Tbsp	50	0	13
Honey Smokehouse, 2 T.	50	0	12
Jim Beam			
Hot Wing Sauce, 2 Tbsp	20	2	0
KC Masterpiece: *Per Tbsp.*			
Marinades: Garlic & Herb	30	1	5
Honey & Teriyaki w/ Sesame	40	0.5	9
Steakhouse	40	1.5	7
Kikkoman Marinades			
Black Bean Sce, 2 Tbsp	50	1	6
Hoisin Sce, 2 Tbsp	80	1.5	17
Honey Mustard, 1Tbsp	30	0	6
Roasted Garlic & Herbs, 1 Tbsp	20	0	4
Teriyaki, 1 Tbsp	15	0	2
Teriyaki Roasted Garlic, 1 Tbsp	25	0	4
Knorr			
Classic Sauce: *Per 2 Tbsp*			
Bernaise:			
Prep'd with Whole Milk	65	5.5	3
Prep'd with Non-Fat Milk	60	4.5	3
Hollandaise:			
Prep'd with Whole Milk	65	5.5	3
Prep'd with Non-Fat Milk	60	4.5	3
Classic Gravy, avg., ¼ cup	25	0	4
Kraft			
Sauce: Cocktail, 2 Tbsp	60	0.5	11
Horseradish, 1 tsp	15	1.5	1
Sandwich & Burger Spread, 1 T.	45	3.5	3
Sweet 'n Sour, 2 Tbsp	60	0	13
Tartar: 1 Tbsp	60	4.5	4
Hot & Spicy, 1 Tbsp	70	6	4
Fat-Free Tartar, 1 Tbsp	25	0	5
Barbecue Sauces, average, 2 Tbsp.	50	0.5	12
Las Palmas			
Red Chile Sauce, ¼ cup, 2 oz	15	0.5	2
Enchilada Sauce: Green Chile	25	1.5	3
Hot Red Original, ¼ cup, 2 oz	15	0.5	2

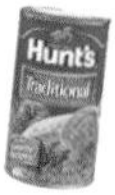

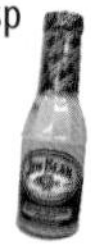

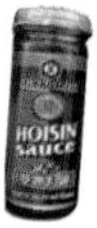

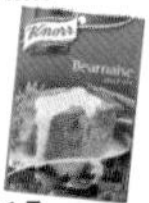

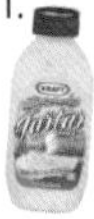

	C	F	Cb
Lawry's 30 Minute Marinade: *Per Tbsp*			
Caribbean Jerk; Teriyaki	20	0	5
Herb & Garlic	10	0	2
Lemon Pepper	10	0	2
Mesquite	5	0	1
Sesame Ginger	30	0	7
Steak & Chop	5	0	1
Packet Seasonings: *Per 2 teaspoons (Dry)*			
Fajitas; Taco, average	10	0	3
Average other flavors	20	0	4
Lea & Perrins			
Worcestershire Sauce, 1 tsp	5	0	1
Monterey			
Pesto Sauce, ¼ cup, 2 oz	280	28	4
Mr Yoshida's			
Original Gourmet Swt Teriyaki, 2 T.	90	0	20
Hawaiian Sweet & Sour, 2 T.	70	0	18
Mrs. Dash Marinades (Salt-Free)			
Garlic Lime, 1 Tbsp	30	1.5	4
Lemon Herb Peppercorn, 1 T.	25	2	2
Southwestern Chipotle, 1 T.	20	1.5	2
Spicy Teriyaki, 1 Tbsp	25	1	5
Muir Glen: *Per ½ Cup*			
Organic Pasta Sauce:			
Mushroom; Portobello Mushroom	50	0	10
Other varieties, average	50	1	11
Newman's Own: *Per ½ Cup*			
Bombolina (Tomato & Basil)	90	4.5	13
Five Cheese	80	3	10
Fra Diavolo	70	3	10
Marinara; Sockarooni	70	2	12
Roasted Garlic & Peppers	70	2.5	11
Vodka	110	5	11
O Organics			
Tomato Salsa, 2 Tbsp	15	0	3
Old El Paso			
Enchilada Sauce:			
Green Chile, ¼ cup	20	1	3
Other varieties, ¼ cup	25	1	3
Sauce Mixes, 2 tsp	10	0	2
Picante Sauce, 2 Tbsp	10	0	2
Taco Sauce, 1 Tbsp	5	0	1
Salsas, Thick & Chunky:			
Make Mine Medium, 2 Tbsp	10	0	2
Wild for Mild, 2 Tbsp	10	0	2
Pace: *Per 2 Tbsp*			
Picante Sauce	10	0	2
Chunky Salsa	10	0	2
Mexican Four Cheese Salsa Con Queso	90	7	5

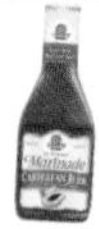

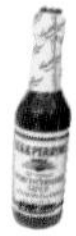

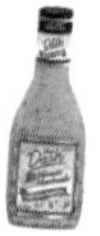

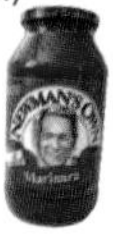

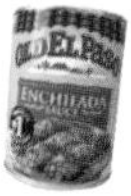

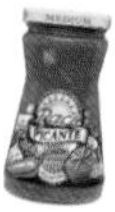

Updated Nutrition Data ~ www.CalorieKing.com
Persons with Diabetes ~ See Disclaimer (Page 24)

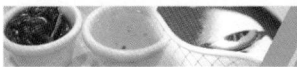
Brands (Cont)	C	F	Cb
Prego: *Per ½ Cup*			
Classic Italian Sauce: Marinara	100	5	11
Flavored w. Meat	130	5	19
Fresh Mushroom	90	3	14
Italian Sausage & Garlic	100	3.5	13
Mini Meatball	110	5	13
Mushroom & Garlic	80	2.5	13
Roasted Garlic Parmesan	70	1	13
Three Chse; Tom. Basil & Garlic, avg.	80	2	13
Traditional	80	3	13
Chunky Garden:			
Combo	70	1.5	13
Mushroom Supreme	90	3	13
Other varieties, avg.	90	3	13
Heart Smart: Traditional Italian	90	3	13
Mushroom Italian	100	3	15
Premier Japan			
Ginger/Wasabi Tamari, 1 T.	5	0	1
Garlic	10	0	2
Ragu: *Per ½ Cup (Unless Indicated)*			
Pizza Quick Sauce: *Per ¼ Cup*			
Traditional	40	2	6
Homemade Style	30	1	5
Thick & Zesty	40	1.5	5
Cheese Creations: *Per ¼ Cup*			
Classic Alfredo	110	10	2
Light Parmesan Alfredo	70	5	3
Roasted Garlic	110	10	3
Chunky: *Per ½ Cup*			
Mushroom & Green Pepper	80	2.5	12
Other varieties, average	80	2.5	12
Light varieties, average	50	0	10
Old World Style: Margherita	70	2	10
Meat Flavor	70	3	9
Mushroom; Traditional	70	2.5	10
Organic: Garden Combination	80	2.5	12
Cheese; Traditional	80	3	11
Robusto!: 7-Herb Tomato	80	3	12
Chopped Tom. Olive Oil & Garlic	95	5	10
Roasted Garlic	80	2.5	13
Sauteed Onion & Garlic	90	3.5	12
Six Cheese	90	3	12

Safeway Select	C	F	Cb
Salsa: *Per 2 Tbsp*			
Chipotle	15	0	3
Garlic Lover's	10	0	3
Peach Pineapple	20	0	4
Salsa Verde	20	0	4
Southwest	10	0	2
Sauces:			
Fiesta Fajita, 2 Tbsp	15	0	2
Enchilada, ¼ cup, 2.2oz	20	0	4
Green Taco; Red Taco 2 Tbsp	10	0	2
Roasted Tomato, 2 Tbsp	15	0	2
Select Sauces: *Per ½ Cup*			
Arrabbiata	110	8	10
Artichoke Pesto	60	2	9
Four Cheese	70	3	10
Garlic Basil	70	4	6
Marinara	60	2	10
Spicy Red Bell Pepper	50	1	9
Sundried Tomato & Olive	70	0	12
Tomato Alfredo	130	10	9
Vodka	130	10	9
Seeds of Change: *Per ½ Cup*			
Tomato Basil Genovese	60	3.5	9
Marinara di Venezia	60	3.5	6
Vodka Americana	120	10	8
The Wizard's			
Hot Stuff, 1 Teaspoon	0	0	0
Vegetarian Worcestershire, 1 tsp	0	0	1
Timpone's: *Per ½ Cup*			
Mom's	70	3	7
Tony Roma's			
Wing Sauce, 1 Tbsp	15	1	1
Trader Joe's BBQ Sauce,			
Kansas City Style, 2 Tbsp	60	0	15
Walnut Acres: *Per ½ Cup (125g)*			
Marinara & Zinfandel	50	1	9
Tomato & Basil	50	0	9
Low Sodium	40	0	9
Tomato & Mushroom	50	1	9

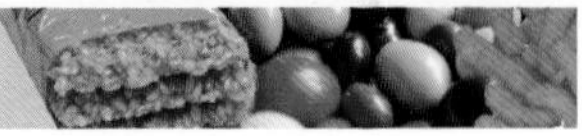

Home-Popped Popcorn

	C	F	Cb
Popping Corn Kernels:			
2 Tbsp, 1 oz	110	1	26
(makes approx. 5 cups)			
Air-popped (no oil), plain, 1 oz	110	1	22
1 cup (6g)	20	0	5
Oil-popped, plain, 1 oz	145	8	16
1 cup (11g)	55	3	6
Popcorn Oil, 1 Tbsp	120	14	0

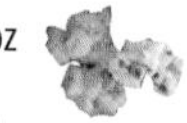

Microwave Popcorn

	C	F	Cb
Average All Brands (Popped)			
Butter: Regular, 1 cup	35	2	4
Light, 1 cup	25	1	4
Act II Popcorn:			
Butter, 1 cup, 0.3 oz	30	2	4
5 cups, popped, 1 oz	160	10	18
Light Butter, 1 cup, 0.2 oz	25	1	4
5 cups, popped, 1 oz	110	4.5	19
Butter Lovers,1 cup, 0.3 oz	35	2.5	4
4½ cups, 1 oz	170	12	16
94% Fat-Free Butter, 1 cup	30	1.5	4.5
4½ cups, 1 oz	130	2.5	28
American Fare (K-Mart):			
Butter, 1 cup, 0.3 oz	40	2	5
3 cups, 1 oz	120	2	23
Theater Butter, 1 cup	40	2	5
3.5 cups	140	8	15
Jolly Time: America's Best, 1 cup	20	0	4
Blast O Butter: Regular, 1 cup	45	3	5
Light, 1 cup	30	1.5	4
Healthy Pop: Butter Flavor, 1 cup	20	0	4
Caramel Apple, 1 cup	20	0	5
Mallow Magic, 1 cup	60	5	6
Newman's Own: Butter, 3½ cups	130	5	18
Light Butter Flavor, 3½ cups	120	4	19
Orville Redenbacher's:			
Movie Theater Butter, 1 cup	35	2	3
4½ cups, popped, 1 oz	160	9	14
Smart Pop!: Butter, 7 cups	105	0	21
100 Calorie Mini Bags (1)	100	2	24
Tender White, 1 cup	40	3	3
Pop Secret Popcorn:			
1-Step, Cheddar, 1 cup	40	2.5	3
100 Calorie Pop, Butter, 1 c.	15	0.5	3
Butter, 1 cup	40	2.5	3
Extra Butter, 1 cup	40	2.5	3
Homestyle, 1 cup	20	1	3
Light Butter, 1 cup	20	1	3
Movie Theater Butter, 1 cup	40	2.5	4
94% Fat-Free: Butter, 1 c.	20	0	4
Kettle Corn, 1 cup	15	0	4
Smart Balance, 1 cup	25	1	3

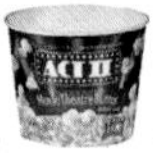

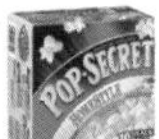

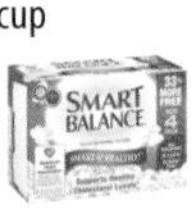

Bagged Popcorn

	C	F	Cb
Average All Brands (Ready-to-Eat)			
Regular/Plain: ½ oz pkg	80	5	8
1 oz pkg	160	10	16
4 oz pkg	640	40	64
2 oz Box (store/airport)	320	16	32
3 oz Bag (9" high x 5" wide)	480	24	48
Caramel Popcorn,			
without nuts, 1 cup, 2 oz	240	4	46

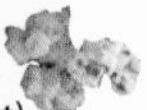

Brands ~ Bagged Popcorn

	C	F	Cb
7-Select (7-11): Popcorn, 1.5 oz pkg	230	16	21
Boston's: Lite, 3½ cups, 1 oz	130	4.5	20
Gourmet Super Prem., 2 c., 1 oz	160	11	13
Homestyle, 2½ cups, 1 oz	160	9	18
40% Less Fat, 2¾ cups, 1 oz	140	6	17
Cracker Jack: Original,			
½ cup, 1 oz	120	2	23
1 cup, 2 oz	240	4	46
99-Cents Pkg, 3⅜ oz	410	7	78
Crunch 'N Munch			
Caramel			
⅔ cup, 1 oz	150	6	23
1 cup, 2 oz	300	12	46
4 oz box	600	24	92
7.5 oz box	1125	45	172
Fiddle Faddle:			
Butter Toffee/Caramel			
1 oz qty	120	3.5	22
1 cup, 2 oz	240	7	44
8 oz box	960	28	176
Jay's: Fat Free Caramel Corn, ¾ cup	110	0	26
Korn Krunch: *(Kornfections Treasures):*			
Almond Pecan (Sugar Free), 1 oz	150	8	19
Orville Redenbacher's:			
Popcorn Cakes, Minis, avg. (8)	60	1	12
Poppycock: Pecan Delight, ½ cup	150	8	20
Original Clusters, ½ cup, 1 oz	160	8	20

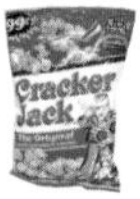

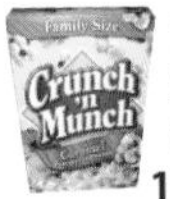

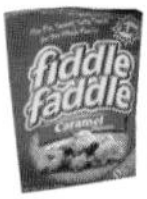

Movie Theater Popcorn

	C	F	Cb
Small (7 cups): Plain	385	21	44
with Butter (3 pumps, ¾ oz)	570	42	44
Medium (15 cups): Plain	825	45	94
with Butter (4 pumps, 1 oz)	1075	73	94
Large (20 cups): Plain	1100	60	124
with Butter (6 pumps, 1½ oz)	1485	102	124
Butter: 1 Pump, ¼ oz	65	7	0
4 Pumps (2 Tbsp), 1 oz	250	28	0

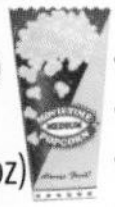

Updated Nutrition Data ~ www.CalorieKing.com
Persons with Diabetes ~ See Disclaimer (Page 24)

Corn & Tortilla Chips

Average All Brands
Corn Chips:

	C	F	Cb
Avg. all types, 1 oz	150	8	18
8 oz bag	1200	64	144
Doritos: 13 chips, avg., 1 oz	140	7	18
White Nacho Cheese, 1 oz	150	8	17
Fritos, 32 chips, 1 oz	160	10	15

Tortilla Chips: Average, 1 oz — **140** / 7 / 18
(1 oz = approx. 12 chips or 13 strips)

	C	F	Cb
Doritos: 13 chips, 1 oz	140	7	18
Reduced Fat, 13 chips, 1 oz	130	5	19
Baked! Nacho Cheese, 15 chips,1 oz	120	3.5	21
Snyder's, Multigrain, 1 oz	130	5	20
Stacy's, Baked, Pita Chips (14), 1 oz	130	5	19
Utz Red.-Fat Baked, 10 chips, 1 oz	140	7	18

Tostitos: Regular, 1 oz — **140** / 7 / 19

	C	F	Cb
Light, 1 oz	90	1	20
6.75 oz bag	610	6	135

Potato Chips/Crisps

Average All Brands — C | F | Cb
Regular:

	C	F	Cb
Plain or flavored, 2 chips	15	1	1.5
1 oz pkg (20 chips)	150	10	15
4 oz quantity	600	40	60
14 oz pkg	2100	140	210

Brands:

	C	F	Cb
Lay's Classic, 1 oz	150	10	15
Lay's Stax, avg. all, 1 oz	150	10	15
Pringles: Original 14 Chips, 1 oz	150	9	15
Large, 6.41 oz can	960	58	96
Minis, 1 bag, 0.8 oz	140	9	16
Selects, avg., 28 chips, 1 oz	145	9	16
Snack Stack, 23g tub	120	8	12
Extreme, avg., 15 chips, 1 oz	150	9	15
Ruffles, 12 chips, 1 oz	160	10	14

Reduced Fat:

	C	F	Cb
Pringles, 16 Chips, 1 oz	140	7	17
Sun Chips; Terra, avg.,			
16 chips, 1 oz	140	6	18

Low-Fat/Baked:

	C	F	Cb
Lay's Baked!, 15 chips, 1 oz	120	2	23
Ruffles Baked!: Orig. 9 chips, 1 oz	120	3	21
Cheddar Sour Crm, 10 chips, 1 oz	120	3	22
Baked! Tostitos Scoops (15) 1 oz	120	3	22

Fat Free: *Lay's Light,* 1 oz — **75** / 0 / 17

	C	F	Cb
Pringles (Fat-Free), 15 chips, 1 oz	70	0	15

Pretzels

Average All Brands — C | F | Cb
Hard-Baked Pretzels:

	C	F	Cb
1 oz quantity	100	0	22
Sticks, thin, 2¼" (9/oz), 1	12	0	3
Twists, thin, ¼" thick, (5/oz),1	25	0	5
Dutch (2¾"x 2⅝") ½ oz, 1	55	1	11
Sourdough *(Snyder's),* ¾ oz, each	100	0	22

Soft Pretzels (Twists) average:

	C	F	Cb
Plain: Regular, 2.2 oz	210	2	43
King Size, 5.1 oz	485	4.5	99
New York Street Vendors, 7 oz	660	6	135
Big Cheese, 1.76 oz	130	3	22

Peanut Butter filled *(Tr. Joe's)* 1 oz — **150** / 8 / 14
Choc-coated *(Snyders),* 1 oz — **140** / 6 / 18

	C	F	Cb
White Choc covered, 7 pces, 1 oz	140	6	19

Brands ~ Pretzels — C | F | Cb

7-Select:
Choc Covered Pretzels

	C	F	Cb
10 pces, 2 oz	265	13	35
1 pkg (4 oz), actual weight, 4.75 oz	630	30	84

Rold Gold *(Frito-Lay)*

	C	F	Cb
Braided Twists (8), 1 oz	110	1	23
Classic: Pretzel Sticks, 1 oz	100	0	23
Rods, 1 oz	110	1	22
Tiny Twists, 1 oz	110	1	23
Fat-Free, Tiny Twists, 1 oz	100	0	23
Tiny Twists: Cheddar Cheese, 1 oz	110	1	22
Honey Mustard, 1 oz	110	1	23

Snyder's of Hanover Pretzels

	C	F	Cb
100 Calorie Pack, Snaps, 0.9 oz	100	0.5	22
Multigrain:			
Pretzel Sticks/Twists, 1 oz	120	2	23
Pretzel Nibblers,			
Honey Mustard, 1 oz	140	5	20
Homestyle (15), 1 oz	120	1	25
Mini (20), 1 oz	110	0	25
Nibblers, (16), 1 oz	120	0	25
Rods (3), 1 oz	120	1	24
Southern Style BBQ, 1 oz	140	7	17
Thins, 1 oz	110	0	23

SuperPretzel: Soft Pretzels (1) — **160** / 1 / 34

	C	F	Cb
Softstix (2)	130	3	22
Soft Pretzel Bites (5)	150	0.5	32

Pretzelfils: Pizza (2) — **120** / 2 / 20

	C	F	Cb
Pepperjack; Mozzarella, (2), avg.	130	4.5	19

Utz: Pretzels, avg., 1 oz — **110** / 1 / 21

	C	F	Cb
Real Choc-covered Pretzels (2)	120	8	17

Snacks   C F Cb

Note: Actual weight of packaged snacks is usually 5-10% more than label Net Wt. For accuracy, weigh snack and allow extra calories, fat and carbs for any extra weight.

	C	F	Cb
Apple Chips (Seneca), 1 oz	150	9	18
Bagel Crisps (N.Y. Style) 6 crisps, 1 oz	130	5	17
Banana Chips, ¼ cup, 13 chips, 1 oz	150	7	21
Beef Jerky (Lance), average, 1 oz	70	1	4
Beef Sticks (Lance) 1 oz	130	10	4
Bugles, Original, 1⅓ cup, 1 oz	160	9	18
Cheese Balls (Utz), 1 oz pkg	150	9	16
Cheese Crackers (Lance) (6), 1.4 oz	190	11	22
Cheese Curls: 1 cup, 1 oz	150	8	16
Cheese Nips, 1.25oz pkg	170	7	22
Cheese Puffs: Avg., 1 oz	160	10	15
American Fare, 1½ cup, 1 oz	160	11	13
Snyder's Multigrain, 1 oz	130	6	19
Cheese Twists, (27), 1 oz	160	12	13
Cheerios, Snack Mix, avg., ⅔ cup, 1.1 oz	125	3.5	22
Cheetos: Regular, all flavors, 1 oz	160	10	15
4 oz pkg	640	40	60
Baked!, cheese flavored, 1 oz	130	5	19
Cheez Balls, 27 balls, 1 oz	150	9	11
Cheez-It Crackers:			
Avg. all flavors, 1 oz	150	8	18
1.25 oz pkg	165	7	23
3 oz pkg	450	24	54
Reduced Fat, 1 oz	130	4	20
Party Mix, 1 pouch, 0.74 oz	100	3.5	15
Chex Mix (General Mills):			
100 Calorie Pouch, avg.	100	3	18
Bold Party Blend, ½ cup, 1 oz	120	4.5	18
Traditional, ½ cup, 1 oz	110	3	19
Chips Ahoy! 1.4 oz pkg	190	9	27
Mini: 1.25 oz pkg	170	8	24
Go-Pak!, 4 oz cup	550	27	77
Snak-Saks, 8 oz pkg	1100	51	154
Churros (Mex. Pastry) 10", 1	100	5	12
Combos (Oven Baked):			
Crackers, ⅓ cup, 1 oz	140	6	18
1 cup, 3 oz	420	18	54
Pretzels, ⅓ cup, 1 oz	130	4.5	19
1 cup, 3 oz	390	14	57
Cookies: See Pages 83-89			
Cool Cuts, Carrot & Ranch, 2.3 oz	70	5	5
Corn Chips: See Page 153			
Corn Crunchies/Spirals, 1 oz	95	0	22
Corn Nuts: ⅓ cup, 1 oz	130	4.5	20
1.7 oz pkg	220	7.5	34
Corn Puffs: (Pirate's Booty), 1 oz	130	5	18
Wotsits (Walker), ¾ oz pkg	105	6.5	11
Dunkin Stixs (Hostess), 3, 4oz	490	25	63

Snacks (Cont)   C F Cb

	C	F	Cb
Fig Newtons: Regular, 2 oz pkg	200	4	40
Fat-Free, 2.1 oz pkg	180	0	44
Minis, Fig/Strawb., avg, 1.34oz pkg	130	3	27
Flavor Twists (Fritos), 1 oz	160	10	16
French's Potato Sticks ¾ c., 1 oz	180	12	16
Funyuns, Onion flavor (13), 1 oz	140	7	18
Genisoy Soy Crisps, avg., 1 oz	120	3	17
Garden Harvest Tst'd Chips, avg., 1 oz	120	3.5	20
Goldfish (Pepperidge Farm) 1 oz	140	5	20
Gold-N-Chees (Lance), 1 oz	150	8	17
Honey Mustard Onion Pieces			
(Snyder's) 1 pkg, 2 oz	280	14	36
Hot Peanuts (Lays), 3½ oz	310	25	10
Jerky (Beef), 1 oz stick	70	1	4
Lance Sandwich, avg., 1.4 oz pkg	200	10	22
Munchies (Frito-Lay):			
Cheese Fix, 1 pkg	250	12	31
Flaming/Totally Ranch, ¾ c.	140	6	19
Munchos, 16 pieces, 1 oz	160	10	16
Nibblers: Garlic Bread (13), 1 oz	130	3	24
Fat Free (16), 1 oz	120	0	25
Nutter Butter: Single Sve, 1.9 oz pkg	250	10	37
Bites: 1.25 oz pkg	170	7	24
Choc-Covered, 2.54 oz pkg	350	17	48
Onion Rings (T.G.I. Friday), 1 oz	130	6	19
Oreo: 100 Calorie Pack, 0.84 oz	100	4	15
2 Go! 2 oz, (4 cookies)	270	11	41
Double Stuf, 1.5 oz pkg	210	10	30
Mini Bite Size: 1.25 oz	170	7	25
Go-Pak, 4 oz cup	530	22	81
Snak-Saks, 8 oz pkg	1040	48	168
Oreo Cakesters, 2 oz pkg	250	12	36
Oriental Mix (Rice Snacks), 1 oz	125	3.5	21
Rice Snacks (Trader Joe's), 1 oz	110	0	22
Oyster Crackers (Sunshine), 1 oz	60	1.5	11
Party Mix (Cheez-It), ½ cup, 1 oz	130	4.5	21
Peanut Butter Nuggets (10), 1 oz	140	6	15
Pirate's Booty:			
1 oz bag	130	5	19
4 oz bag	520	20	76
w. Caramel, 2.75 oz bag	330	5.5	63
Pirate's Cannon Balls: 1 oz	130	5	18
5 oz bag	715	27	99
Pita Chips, avg., (9) 1 oz	130	4	18
Popcorn: See Page 152			
Pork Cracklins, 1 oz	180	14	0
Pork Skins/Rinds, 1 oz	160	10	0
Baken-ets, 99c pkg, 1.87 oz	300	19	0
Potato Chips: See Page 153			
Potato Skins (TGI Friday) (16), 1 oz	130	9	24

Updated Nutrition Data ~ www.CalorieKing.com
Persons with Diabetes ~ See Disclaimer (Page 24)

Snacks (Cont)

	C	F	Cb
Quakes Rice Snacks, 1 oz	130	4	26
Quaker Mini Delights, 1 bag, avg.	90	3.5	16
Rice Chips, Bar-B-Q/Onion, 1 oz	140	7	18
Ritz Bits S'wiches: Cheese, 1.5 oz pkg	220	13	24
P'nut Butter, 1.25 oz pkg	170	10	20
Big Bag (99c), Cheese, 3 oz	450	25	50
Carry Me Pack, Cheese, 2 oz	290	17	33
Ritz Crackers, 2 Go!, 1.38 oz	190	9	24
Sandwich Crackers (Austin): Per Pkg			
Chse Cracker w. Pnut Butter, 1.37 oz	190	10	23
Chse Cracker w. Cheddar, 1.37 oz	210	10	26
PB & J Cracker Sandwich, 1.38 oz	190	8	26
Sesame Sticks (Cityfarm), 1 oz	160	9	13
Smart Puffs (Robert's), 1.37 oz bag	180	8	23
Snack Mix (Quaker):			
Baked Cheddar, 1 oz	130	4.5	19
Kids Mix, 1 oz	130	4.5	20
Snackwells Cookies, Pack 2 Go! 1.7oz	210	5	38
Soy Crisps, avg. 1 oz	120	3	17
Soy Nuts: Dry Roasted, ¼ cup, 1 oz	130	6	9
Choc-coated, 1 oz	140	7	13
Dr Soy Soy Nuts BBQ, 1 oz	150	8	8
Sunflower Chips: (Snyders), 1 oz	140	6	20
100 Calorie Snack Pack (1)	100	4	14
Takis Fajitas (12), 1 oz	140	7	17
4 oz pkg	560	28	68
TastyKake:			
Koffee Kake Jr, 71g	280	10	45
Chocolate Jr, 94g	340	12	65
Creme Filled Koffee Kakes (2)	230	10	25
Tings (Robert's), 2 oz bag	300	14	36
Toasted Cheese Crackers, 1 pkg	220	11	23
Tortilla Chips: Page 153			
Tostitos:			
Blue; Yellow; Scoops, avg., 1 oz	140	7	19
Multigrain, 1 oz	150	8	18
Trader Joe's, Cheese Crunchies, 1 oz	130	6	19
7 oz pkg	910	42	133
Trail Mix (Nuts/Seeds/Dried Fruit):			
Regular, 3 Tbsp, 1 oz	140	9	13
Tropical, 3 Tbsp, 1 oz	130	7	16
w. Chocolate Chips, 1 oz	180	12	16
Dr Soy Trail Mix, 1 oz	110	4	12
Turkey Jerky Teriyaki (Oberto), 1 oz	80	1	8
Vegetable Snacks (Snyder's), 1 oz	140	7	19
Veggie Chips, (365/Wholefoods),1 oz	130	7	13
Wasabi Peas, ¼ cup, 1 oz	120	3	19
Wheatables (Keebler):			
Original, (17), 1 oz	140	6	20
Orig.-Red.-Fat (19), 1 oz	140	4	22
Honey Wheat (17), 1 oz	140	6	20
Multigrain (17), 1 oz	140	6	20
Yogurt Pretzels (7), 1.5 oz	190	7	30
Yogurt Raisins (Sun-Maid), 1 oz	120	4.5	20

Fruit Snacks

	C	F	Cb
Betty Crocker: Fruit Gushers, 25g	90	1	20
Fruit by the Foot, 1 roll, 21g	80	1	17
Fruit Roll Ups, 1 roll, 14g	50	1	12
Scooby Doo; G-Force, 25g pkg	80	0	20
General Mills:			
Blues Clues; Dora the Explora (1)	60	0	14
Other varieties	80	0	21
Kellogg's: Disney Fruit Snacks, 25g	80	0	19
Fruit Streamers, 1 Roll	80	1	17
Rolls,1 pouch, 0.63 oz	70	1.5	14
Yogos, 20g	80	1.5	16
Sunkist: Fruit Snacks, 1 pouch	90	1	20
Fruit Smoothie Blitz, 1.3 oz	140	1	32

Vending Machines

	C	F	Cb
Brownie, frosted (Lance), 3 oz	400	18	56
Cheese Balls (Utz), 1 oz	150	9	11
Choc Chip Cookies (Nabisco), 1.4 oz	190	9	27
Choc Milk, 8 fl.oz	260	9	36
Coca-Cola Classic, 12 fl.oz	145	0	40
Diet Coke, 12 fl.oz	0	0	0
Corn Chips, 1 oz	160	10	16
Hostess Sweet Roll, 4¼ oz	400	12	69
Donut, plain, 1.4 oz	160	9	18
Fruit Pie (Hostess), 4½ oz	480	20	68
Granola/Cereal Bars	140	3	26
Hershey's, 1.55 oz bar	210	13	26
Hot Fries (Con Agra), 1 oz	150	7	17
Kellogg's Rice Krispies Treat	90	2.5	17
Lance Captain's Wafers, 1 pkg	70	3	9
M & M's: Plain, 1.7 oz	240	10	34
Peanuts, 1.7 oz	250	13	30
Milk: Whole, 8 fl.oz	160	9	13
Reduced Fat, 2%, 8 fl.oz	140	5	14
Milky Way, 2 oz	260	10	41
Orange Juice, 8 fl.oz	190	14	6
Popcorn, plain, 1 oz	160	10	16
Pork Skins, 1 oz	160	10	0
Potato Chips: 1 oz	150	10	15
Reduced Fat, 1 oz	120	3	21
Pretzels, 1 oz	110	1	23
Raisins, ½ oz pkg	45	0	11
Reese's P'nut Butter Cups, 1½ oz	230	13	23
Snickers, 2.1 oz bar	280	14	35
Tortilla Chips, 1 oz	140	7	18

S Soups

Homemade & Restaurant

Restaurant & Take-Out
Average All Preparations, Per 8 fl.oz

	C	F	Cb
Bean Medley	200	3	34
Beef Consomme	30	0	2
Borscht (w. Sour Cream)	130	8	14
Bouillabaisse	400	15	10
Chicken & Corn	290	14	20
Chicken & Wild Rice	80	4	9
Chicken Consomme	50	0	2
Chicken Curry	180	8	18
Chicken Jambalaya	160	7	8
Chicken Noodle	80	2	12
w. Chicken	160	4	12
Chicken Soup	80	2	6
Chili with Beans	250	12	25
Clam Chowder	240	15	17
Corn & Crab	120	3	18
Corn Chowder	150	8	16
Cream of Broccoli	200	12	20
Cream of Potato	150	6.5	17
Cream of Mushroom	200	13	15
Fish Chowder	220	15	6
French Onion	420	15	25
Gazpacho	50	0	5
Lentil Soup	250	9	28
Lobster Bisque	320	15	10
Matzo Ball (w. 1 large ball)	180	7	24
Minestrone	125	2.5	20
Mulligatawny	300	15	8
Pea & Ham	240	10	25
Potato & Bacon	170	7	19
Pumpkin, Creamy	210	10	26
Shark Fin Soup	100	4	8
Spicy Shrimp Soup, 1 bowl	160	7	10
Split Pea Soup	180	2.5	30
Vegetable (Fat Free)	75	0	18
Vegetable Beef	80	2	10
Vichyssoise	200	9	15
Watercress	90	4	13

Other Soups: *See International & Fast-Foods Sections (Arby's, Au Bon Pain, Boston Market, Dunkin' Donuts, Denny's, Schlotzsky's, Sizzler, Souplantation, Sweet Tomatoes, Zoup!)*

Homemade Soups: Calculate calories, fat and carbohydrates from recipe ingredients.

Bouillon Cubes & Powders

	C	F	Cb
Bouillon Cubes: *Average all Types*			
Regular, 1 cube	5	0	1
Low Sodium (LiteLine)	12	0	1
Powders: Average, 1 tsp	10	0	1
Herb-Ox: Instant Broth & Seasoning,			
Beef, 1 envelope	5	0	1
Chicken; Vegetarian	5	0	1
Herbs, Spices: 1 tsp	5	0	1
Soup Oyster Crackers			
40 small/3 large, ½ oz	60	2	8

Amy's (Organic)

Per ½ Can, 1 Cup, Unless Indicated

	C	F	Cb
Alphabet, Fat-Free	80	0	16
Black Bean Vegetable	130	1.5	25
Chunky Vegetable	60	0	13
Cream of Mushroom, ¾ cup	140	9	13
Cream of Tomato	100	2	17
Curried Lentil	230	8	30
Fire Roasted Vegetable	140	4.5	23
Lentil	180	5	25
Lentil Vegetable	150	4	23
Minestrone	90	1.5	17
No Chicken Noodle	90	3	13
Pasta & 3 Bean	130	5	19
Split Pea	100	0	19
Summer Corn & Vegetable	150	6	23
Thai Coconut	140	10	9
Tuscan Bean & Rice	160	4.5	25
Vegetable Barley	70	1	13
Low Sodium: Butternut Squash	100	2.5	20
Chunky Tomato Bisque	120	3.5	21

'Light in Sodium' Range *(50% less sodium),*
(Calories/Fat/Carb ~ Same as Regular Range)

Andersen's   ~ *Per Cup*

	C	F	Cb
Lentil	110	2	19
Split Pea	130	0	24
Split Pea w. Bacon	140	1	23
Tomato	130	3.5	22

Baxters

Per ½ Can

	C	F	Cb
Luxury: Cream of Asparagus	135	9	12
Cullen Skink	175	7.5	16
Lobster Bisque	90	4	8
Roasted Red Pepper & Tomato	120	6.5	14
Seafood Chowder	155	9	12

Updated Nutrition Data ~ www.CalorieKing.com
Persons with Diabetes ~ See Disclaimer (Page 24)

Bean Cuisine | C | F | Cb
Per Cup (Prepared as Directed)

	C	F	Cb
13 Bean Bouillabaisse; Lentil, avg.	220	0	26
Island Black Bean	180	4	19
Santa Fe Corn Chowder	160	0	24
White Bean Provencal	200	0	20

Bear Creek ~ *Per Cup*

	C	F	Cb
Cheddar Potato	180	7	28
Chicken Noodle	120	1.5	22
Creamy Potato	150	3.5	27
Hot & Sour	80	1	16
Minestrone	110	0	23
Navy Bean	130	0.5	26
Split Pea	110	2	19
Tortilla	90	0.5	22
Vegetable Beef	110	0.5	22

Campbell's

Condensed Soup: *Per ½ Cup*

	C	F	Cb
Bean w. Bacon	170	4	25
Beef w. Vegs/Barley; Minestrone, avg.	90	1.5	16
Cheddar Cheese	100	5	11
Chicken & Dumplings	70	2.5	10
Chicken Won Ton	60	1	8
Cream of Asparagus	110	7	9
Cream of Broccoli	90	3.5	12
Cream of Chicken & Mushroom	80	6	7
Cream of Mushroom	70	2	10
Cream of Onion	100	6	10
Cream of Potato	90	2	15
Cream of Shrimp	90	5	8
Creamy Chicken Noodle	120	7	11
French Onion	45	1.5	6
Green Pea	180	3	28
Manhattan Clam Chowder	70	0.5	12
New England Clam Chowder	90	2.5	13
Old Fashioned Vegetable	80	1.5	14
Split Pea w. Ham & Bacon	180	3.5	27
Tomato	90	0	20
Tomato Bisque	130	3.5	23
Vegetable	100	0.5	20

Healthy Request Condensed: *Per ½ Cup*

	C	F	Cb
Chicken Rice	70	1.5	13
Vegetable Beef	90	1	15

Campbell's (Cont) | C | F | Cb

Kids Condensed Soup: *Per ½ Cup*

	C	F	Cb
Dora; Jimmy Neutron	80	2	13
Chicken Alphabet; Chicken & Stars	70	2	11
Chicken Noodle O's	90	2.5	15
Curly Noodle	80	2	11
Goldfish Pasta	80	2	12
Goldfish Pasta & Meatballs	90	3	11

Chunky: *Per 8 fl.oz Cup*

	C	F	Cb
Baked Pot. w. Cheddar & Bacon Bits	160	6	23
Classic Chicken Noodle	120	3	16
Gr. Chkn & Sausage Gumbo	140	2.5	21
Hearty Beef Barley	170	2.5	26
Manhattan Clam Chowder	120	3.5	19

Select Harvest: *Per 8 fl.oz Cup*

	C	F	Cb
Beef w. Roasted Barley	130	1	21
Carmelized French Onion	80	2	12
Chicken Vege. Medley	120	1	20
Chicken w. Egg Noodles	120	4	12
Creamy Chicken Alfredo	220	13	15
Creamy Potato w. Rstd Garlic	180	10	20
Harvest Tomato w. Basil	100	0	22
Italian Saus. w. Pasta & Pepperoni	160	7	18
Italian-Style Wedding	140	5	16
New England Clam Chowder	170	10	15
Potato Broccoli Cheese	150	9	15
Savory Chicken & Rice	110	0.5	20
Savory Bean w. Rstd Ham	170	1.5	30
Slow Roasted Beef & Veg.	100	0.5	16
Split Pea w. Roasted Ham	150	1	29
Tomato Garden; Vegetable Medley	100	0.5	20

Select Harvest Bowls: *Per Cup*

	C	F	Cb
Chicken w. Egg Noodles	120	4	12
Italian-Style Wedding	130	4	16
Mexican-Style Chkn Tortilla	130	2.5	19
Minestrone	100	1	19
Savory Chicken & Rice	110	1	18
98% Fat-Free, New Eng. Clam Chowder	110	2.5	17

Microwavable Bowls: *Per Cup*

	C	F	Cb
Chicken Noodle Soup	70	2	10
Creamy Tomato Soup	160	5	25
Tomato Soup	110	0	24

Soup at Hand Sippable: *Per Container*

	C	F	Cb
Chicken w. Mini Noodles	80	2	11
Cream of Broccoli	150	7	17
Creamy Tomato	180	4	32
New Eng. Clam Chowder	160	10	13
Vegetable Beef	60	1	10

Dr McDougall's

	C	F	Cb
Big Cup Soups/Meals: *Per Cup*			
Hot & Sour Noodle	320	1	34
Miso Soup w. Noodles	180	1	34
Pad Thai Noodle, average	200	1	42
Black Bean & Lime	340	2	60
Minestrone & Pasta	200	1	40
Ramen Chicken Flavor	200	1	40
Split Pea w. Barley	240	1	42
Tamale Soup w. Baked Chips	200	2	36
Tortilla Soup w. Baked Chips	200	2	34
Light Sodium: *Per Container*			
Chicken Noodle, Vegan	140	0.5	28
Chinese Chicken Noodle	140	1	28
Lentil Couscous	190	1	37
Split Pea	200	1	35
Tomato, Basil Pasta	100	0.5	21
White Bean & Pasta	170	1	34

Dixie Diners' Club

Per Cup (Prepared as Directed)

Carb Counters, Dine 'n Dash:			
Broccoli & Cheese	70	5	3
Chicken Cheese Enchilada	95	6	4
Chicken Noodle	40	1	3
Cream of Mushroom	50	4	2

Fantastic Cup Soups

Simmer Soups: *Per Cup, Prepared*			
Blarney Stone Creamy Potato	220	4.5	15
Dutch Split Pea	120	1	21
New Eng. Vege. Chicken Noodle	90	1	14
Vegetarian Soup Cups: *Per Container*			
Baja Black Bean Chipotle	130	0.5	31
Buckaroo Bean Chili	160	2	33
Classic French Onion	90	2.5	15
Creamy Potato Leek	120	2.5	22
Great Lakes Cheddar Broccoli	100	3	15
Green Onion Miso w. Tofu	140	1.5	26
Hot & Sour	170	2	33
Mama's Minestrone	160	2.5	30
Sesame Miso	140	2	27
Spicy Thai	150	0.5	32
Split Pea	140	0.5	28
Three Onion Noodle	180	2	36
Vegetarian Chicken Noodle	90	1	17

Health Valley

	C	F	Cb
Per Cup, Prepared			
Broths: Chicken: Fat-Free	20	0	0
Low-Fat	35	1.5	0
Vegetable, Fat-Free	20	0	5
Fat-Free Soup:			
Chicken Flav. Noodles w. Veggie	110	0	24
Creamy Potato with Broccoli	80	0	17
Lentil with Couscous	130	0	28
Zesty Black Bean with Rice	100	0	22
Organic Soup: 14 Garden Vegetable	80	0	18
Lentil & Carrot	110	0	24
Low-Sodium: Corn & Vegetable	80	0	20
Vegetable Barley	80	0	20
No Salt Added: Minestrone	70	0	17
Split Pea	110	0	23
Tomato	80	0	18
Vegetable	90	2	16

Healthy Choice

Per Cup			
Bean & Ham	180	2	29
Chicken & Dumplings	140	2.5	21
Chicken w. Rice Soup	110	1.5	17
Chicken Tortilla Style	160	2	25
Country Vegetable	110	1	19
Fiesta Chicken	120	2	20
Garden Vegetable	120	0.5	24
Hearty Chicken	130	2	20
New England Clam Chowder	110	1	19
Old Fashioned Chicken Noodle	100	1.5	13
Split Pea and Ham	170	2	22
Vegetable Beef	130	1	22
Zesty Gumbo	100	2	16

Imagine

Per Cup			
Bistro: Corn Chipotle	100	1	22
Cuban Black Bean	170	3.5	30
Fire Roasted Tomato	120	2.5	24
Canned Organic:			
Chicken Pot Pie	160	4.5	22
Classic Minestrone	120	3.5	20
Country Split Pea	180	2.5	30
Italian White Bean	160	2.5	28
Roasted Garlic Potato	120	3	22
Tortilla	160	4	25

Updated Nutrition Data ~ www.CalorieKing.com
Persons with Diabetes ~ See Disclaimer (Page 24)

Imagine

	C	F	Cb
Per Cup			
Garden Natural Soup, Creamy:			
Acorn Squash & Mango	70	1.5	14
Chicken	70	1.5	12
Portobello Mushroom	80	3	10
Potato Leek	110	3	18
Sweet Corn	120	3	20
Sweet Pea	80	1.5	14
Tomato	80	1	15
Tomato Basil	90	1.5	17

Kikkoman

	C	F	Cb
Dry Mixes, Prepared as Directed			
Chinese Style Egg Flower: 1⅓ tsp	40	1	7
Hot & Sour, 1⅓ tsp	30	0	6
Instant Miso:			
Shiro (White): 1 pkt	35	1	4
w. Tofu, 1 pkt	35	1	3

Knorr

	C	F	Cb
Recipe Mix: *Dry Mix*			
Cream of Spinach, 2 T.	60	1.5	11
French Onion, 2 Tbsp	45	1	8
Spring Vegetable, 2 Tbsp, 0.3 oz	25	0	6
Tomato w. Basil, 3 Tbsp, 0.7 oz	70	1	15
Bouillon Cubes: *Per ½ Cube, 1 Cup, Prepared*			
Beef; Chicken, average	20	1.5	0.5

Lipton

	C	F	Cb
Cup-a-Soup: *Per Envelope*			
Cream of Chicken	70	1.5	14
Chicken Noodle	80	0.5	17
Recipe Secrets: *Per Dry Mix*			
Beefy Onion, 1 Tbsp	25	0.5	5
Onion, 1 Tbsp	20	0	4
Onion Mushroom, 1⅔ Tbsp	25	0	7

Manischewitz

	C	F	Cb
Condensed: *Per ½ Cup*			
Chicken Broth, Clear	15	0	2
Chicken w. Kreplach	40	1	6
Chicken w. Matzo Balls	80	3.5	9
Quart Jars: *Per 8 fl.oz, Prepared*			
Borscht w. Beets	90	0	21
Borscht Low Calorie	25	0	6
Ready To Serve: Matzo Balls in Broth	220	9	27
Dry Mixes: *Per Cup*			
Matzo Ball & Soup Mix	40	0.5	9
Split Pea Cello	140	0	25
Vegetable Soup	120	0	22

Maruchan

	C	F	Cb
Instant Lunch,			
Avg. all flavors, 1 pkg	290	12	38
Ramen, all flavors, ½ pkt, 1½ oz	190	7	26

Miso Cup

	C	F	Cb
Per Cup, Prepared as Directed			
Golden Vegetable; Savory Seaweed	30	1	3
Savory Seaweed	30	1	3
Traditional with Tofu	35	1	4
Reduced Sodium	25	1	3

Nile Spice ~ *Per Cup*

	C	F	Cb
Black Bean; Lentil	170	1.5	35
Couscous Lentil Curry	200	1.5	36
Couscous Minestrone	180	1.5	34
Potato Leek	110	3	19
Sweet Corn chowder	110	2	22
Low-Fat: Split Pea	200	1	35
Chicken Flavored Vegetable	110	1.5	21

Nissin ~ *Per Whole Package*

	C	F	Cb
Low-Fat: Choice Ramen,			
Slow Stewed Beef	280	2	56
Top Ramen: Beef Flavor	380	14	54
Chicken Flavor	380	14	52

Pacific Foods ~ *Per Cup*

	C	F	Cb
Chicken Broth	15	0	1
Natural, Beef Broth	20	0	1
Vegetable Broth	15	0	3
Creamy Organic: French Onion	30	1	5
Butternut Squash	90	2	17
Cashew Carrot Ginger	120	5	19
Curried Red Lentil	140	4.5	19
Tomato	100	2	16
Light Sodium: Rstd Pepper & Tom.	110	2	16
Tomato	100	2	17
Hearty Artisan Soups:			
Beef Steak & Fusilli Pasta	100	3.5	13
Chicken Fajita	160	2.5	26

Pritikin ~ *Per Cup*

	C	F	Cb
Fat-Free Chicken Broth	5	0	0
Hearty Vegetable	80	0	15
Split Pea	180	0.5	32
Vegetarian Vegetable	80	0	17

Progresso

	C	F	Cb
Microwaveable Bowls: *Per Cup*			
Chicken & Wild Rice/Noodle, avg.	100	1.5	16
Minestrone Soup	90	1.5	17
Vegetable Soup	80	0.5	16
Rich & Hearty: *Per Cup*			
Chicken & Homestyle Noodles	110	2.5	14
Chicken Corn Chowder	200	9	23
Chicken Pot Pie Style	150	5	19
New England Clam Chowder	180	8	22
Savory Beef Barley Veg.	130	1.5	21
Slow Cooked Veg. Beef	120	1	20
Steak & Homestyle Noodles	110	2	16
Steak & Sauteed Mushrooms	110	2	18
Other varieties, average	125	2	21
Traditional: *Per Cup*			
Beef Barley	120	2.5	17
Chickenn Herb Dumpling	100	2.5	14
Hearty Chicken & Rotini	100	2	13
Homestyle Chicken	100	2	14
Italian-Style Wedding	120	4	11
Roasted Garlic Chicken	100	2	13
Southwestern Style Chicken	120	2.5	19
Split Pea w/ Ham	140	1	24
Vegetable Classic: *Per Cup*			
French Onion	50	1.5	8
Green Split Pea with Bacon	160	2	28
Garden Vegetable	90	0	20
Hearty Tomato	110	1	23
Lentil; Tomato Basil, avg.	155	2.5	29
Minestrone	100	2	20
Tomato Rotini	130	0.5	28
Vegetable	80	0	15
Light, Low-Fat/Low-Carb:			
Beef Pot Roast	80	1	12
Southwestern-Style Veg., 8.5 oz	60	0	12
Vegetable & Noodle, 8.75 oz	60	0.5	13

Shelton's

	C	F	Cb
All Natural: *Per Cup*			
Black Bean & Chicken	190	4	28
Chicken Corn Chowder	110	1	22
Chicken Chili Mac	200	3	27
Chicken Noodle	80	2	9
Chicken Rice	90	1	14
Chicken Tortilla	120	1.5	18
Turkey Chili Mac	190	2.5	27
Broth, Chicken, Regular	35	2.5	0

Signature (Safeway)

	C	F	Cb
Signature Soups: *Per Cup*			
Baked Potato	410	27	28
Broccoli & Cheesy Cheddar	270	18	18
Chunky Chicken Noodle	160	5	14
Coconut & Red Curry	240	9	26
Fiesta Chicken Tortilla	100	2	12
Italian-Style Wedding	160	7	15
Pacific Coast Clam Chowder	340	24	21
Stompin' Steakhouse Chili	260	9	24
Tuscan Tomato & Basil Bisque	330	22	27

Simply Asia

	C	F	Cb
Noodle Soup Bowls: *Per Bowl*			
Miso Tofu	420	3.5	82
Sesame Chicken	430	4.5	82
Soy Ginger, ½ bowl	330	5	61
Spring Vegetable	420	2.5	84
Szechwan Hot & Sour	480	7	88

Spice Hunter

	C	F	Cb
Mixes ~ Per Bowl			
Beef Barley	180	2	32
Chicken Noodle	140	1.5	25
Chicken Vegetable	160	1	31
Creamy Thai Noodle	200	5	34
Miso Udon	160	1.5	31
Split Pea	250	1.5	43

Swanson

	C	F	Cb
Per Cup			
Vegetable Broth	15	0	3
99% Fat Free, Chicken Broth	10	0.5	1
Organic: Beef Broth	15	0.5	1
Chicken Broth	15	0.5	1

Tabatchnick

	C	F	Cb
Per Pouch			
101 Calories: *Per Pouch*			
Cabbage	90	1	21
Barley Mushroom; Wild Rice, avg.	80	1	17
Onion	60	1.5	11
Broths: *Per ½ Pouch*			
Chicken with Noodles & Dumplings	150	6	19
New York Style Chicken	70	1	13
Dairy: *Per Pouch*			
Corn Chowder	130	4.5	21
Cream of Broccoli	90	4	12
New England Potato	140	4	24

Updated Nutrition Data ~ www.CalorieKing.com
Persons with Diabetes ~ See Disclaimer (Page 24)

Tabatchnick (Cont)	C	F	Cb
Gluten Free: *Per Pouch*			
Old Fashioned Potato	100	1.5	21
Split Pea	140	0	34
Southwest Bean	220	5	35
Vegetarian Chili	180	3.5	28
Low Sodium: *Per Pouch*			
Barley Mushroom	80	1	17
Pea	140	0	34
Vegetable	90	1.5	17
Meat: *Per Pouch*			
Frenchman's Onion	60	1.5	11
Wilderness Wild Rice	80	0.5	16
Parve: *Per Pouch*			
Balsamic Tomato & Rice	110	3.5	18
Black Bean	230	2.5	39
Minestrone	100	1.5	18
Vegetable	90	1.5	17

Thai Kitchen			
Rice Noodle Soup Bowls: *Per Bowl*			
Hot & Sour	250	4.5	51
Lemongrass & Chili	250	4	50
Thai Ginger	260	4.5	51

Trader Joe's			
Canned: *Per 8 fl.oz Cup Unless Indicated*			
Barley w. Vegetables	110	3	19
Chunky Minestrone, low fat	110	2.5	19
Lentil & Vegetable	140	3	21
Condensed, Clam Chowder, ½ cup	80	2	11
Organic: Per Cup unless indicated			
Black Bean, 1 cup	130	1.5	25
Lentil Vegetable, ½ can	130	3.5	19
Split Pea	100	0	19
Light Sodium, Tomato Bisque	130	4	21
Low Sodium: Minestrone, 10¾ can	200	4	37
Chkn & Mafalde Pasta, 10¾ can	110	3	19
Low Fat, Chicken Noodle, 8 fl.oz	90	1	14
Cartons, 32 fl.oz: *Per 8 fl.oz Cup*			
Butternut Squash	90	2	16
Carrot Ginger	80	1	17
Creamy Corn & Roasted Pepper	110	2	23
Garden Patch Veggie	60	0	14
Latin Style Black Bean	70	1	12
Sweet Potato Bisque	130	1	28
Organic: Butternut Squash	70	0	17
Creamy Tomato	90	3.5	15
Tomato & Roasted Red Pepper	100	3.5	15

Westbrae Natural	C	F	Cb
Instant Miso, all flavors	35	1.5	3
Ready-to-Eat: *Per Cup, 8 fl.oz*			
Fat-Free: Old World Split Pea	150	0	28
Alabama Black Bean Gumbo	140	0	26
Hearty Milano Minestrone	120	0	24
Louisiana Bean Stew	130	0	25
Mediterranean Lentil	140	0	24
Santa Fe Vegetable	160	0	31
Spicy Southwest Vegetable	130	0	25
Low-Fat, New York UnChicken Ndle	60	1	10
Semi-Condensed: *Per ¾ Cup, 6 fl.oz*			
Monte Carlo Creamy Mushroom	70	3	10
Low-Fat, California UnChicken Broth	15	0.5	2
Fat-Free, Tuscany Tomato	70	0	16

Whole Foods			
Per Cup			
Canned: Chicken Noodle	110	3	16
Chicken with Wild & Red Rice	110	2.5	17
Italian Style Wedding	150	6	19
Vegetable	90	1	21
Vegetable Beef	130	3.5	21
365 Organic: Black Bean	150	1	25
Chicken Noodle	90	2	11
Cream of Mushroom	100	6	11
Lentil	120	1	16
Minestrone	120	2	21
Vegetable	70	1	11

Wolfgang Puck			
Per Cup			
Original: Chicken and Egg Noodles	130	6	11
Chicken and Dumpling	220	13	17
Creamy Roast Chicken with Rice	200	10	16
New England Clam Chowder	170	7	18
Old Fashioned Beef Barley	120	3.5	17
Organic: Butternut Squash	200	11	22
Chicken with Egg Noodle	110	5	11
Corn Chowder	210	13	20
Classic Tomato w. Basil	130	6	18
Old Fashioned Potato	200	14	17

Wylers			
Dry Mix: Mrs Grass Onion, 7g	20	0	4
Homestyle Vegetable, 12g	35	0	7
Mrs Grass Soup Mix:			
Chicken Noodle, 1 cup	70	1.5	10
Beef Vegetable, 1 cup	90	0.5	18

Soybean Products — C · F · Cb

Cheeses (Soy): *See Page 80*

Miso Soy Bean Paste

	C	F	Cb
Cold Mountain: Light Yellow, 1 tsp	10	0	1
Mellow Red, 1 tsp	15	0	3
Red, 1 tsp	10	0	1
Miso Soup (dry mix), avg.			
1 Tbsp., dry mix	35	1	5
1 cup, prepared	35	1	5
Natto, ½ cup, 3 oz	160	7	14
Okara (Tofu fiber residue), ½ c., 2 oz	47	1	8
Tempeh: 1 piece, 3 oz	180	8	12
Fried, 3 oz	250	14	14
Seitan *(White Wave),* Trad., 3 oz	90	1	3
Soybean Protein *(TVP),* 1 oz	95	0	8
Soy Bean Paste, 1 tsp	10	0	2

Soy Beans: *See Page 167*

Soy Drinks: *See Page 48*

Tofu ~ Packaged — C · F · Cb

	C	F	Cb
Tofu Stir-Fried, average all, 4 oz	120	8	3
Azumaya Tofu: Soft (Silken), 3.2 oz	40	2	1
Soft, Light (Silken), 3.2 oz	40	1	3
Firm; Extra Firm, 2.8 oz	70	4	2
Light Extra Firm, 2.8 oz	60	2	3
Seasoned Tofu, avg., 3 oz	90	5	3
House Foods			
Premium Tofu: Soft (Silken), 3 oz	50	2.5	2
Medium Firm (Regular), 3 oz	60	3	1
Firm, 3 oz	70	3.5	2
Extra Firm, 3 oz	80	4	1

Tofu ~ Packaged (Cont) — C · F · Cb

	C	F	Cb
House Foods (Cont)			
Organic Tofu: Firm, 3 oz	60	3	0
Extra Firm, 3 oz	90	4.5	0
House Tofu: Tokusen Kinugoshi, 3 oz	90	4	3
Sukui/Soon (Extra Soft), 3 oz	45	2	2
Yaki Tofu: Yaki (Broiled), 3 oz	90	5	2
Tofu Steak: Grilled, 3 oz	90	5	2
Garlic & Pepper, 4.8 oz	90	4	1
Mori-Nu Tofu (Silken)			
Soft, 3 oz, 1" slice	45	2.5	2
Firm, 3 oz, 1" slice	50	2.5	2
Extra Firm, 3 oz, 1" slice	45	1.5	2
Organic Firm 3 oz, 1" slice	60	2.5	2
Lite, Firm, 3 oz, 1" slice	30	0.5	1
Seasoned Tofu: *Per 3 oz*			
Japanese Miso	60	2.5	3
Chinese Spice	50	2	3
Nasoya Tofu: Soft, ⅓ pkg, 2.8 oz	60	3	1
Silken, 3.2 oz	45	2	1
Firm, ⅓ pkg, 3.2 oz	70	3	2
Extra Firm, ⅓ pkg, 2.8 oz	80	4	2
Chinese Spice, ¼ pkg, 3 oz	90	5	3
Garlic & Onion, ¼ pkg	90	5	1
White Wave: Baked Tofu, 1 sq. avg.	95	5	2
Soft/Firm Tofu, ⅓ block, 3.2 oz	90	6	1
Reduced Fat, ⅓ block, 3.2 oz	90	4	4
Tofu Tenders, Light Tamari, ½ pkg	120	7	15

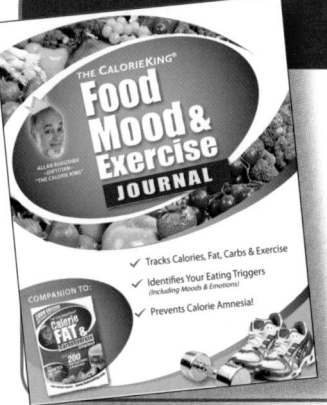

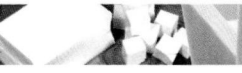

Spices & Herbs

	C	F	Cb
Per Teaspoon: Average all types	5	0	1
All Purpose, 1 tsp	0	0	0
Allspice, ground	5	0	1
Chili Powder	8	0	1
Cinnamon, ground	6	0	2
Curry Powder	6	0	2
Garlic Powder	9	0	2
Nutmeg, ground	12	0	1
Onion Powder	7	0	2
Parsley, dried	4	0	1
Pepper, avg.	6	0	1
Saffron	2	0	0
Salt-Free Blends, 1 tsp	0	0	0
Tumeric, ground	8	0	1
Seeds: Fenugreek	12	1	2
Mustard, Poppyseed	15	1	1
Other types, average	7	0	1

Seasonings & Flavorings

	C	F	Cb
Accent Flavor Enhancer, 1 tsp	0	0	0
Angostura Bitters, 1 tsp	15	0	4
Bacon Bits, average, 1 Tbsp	35	2	2
Bacon Chips (Durkee), 1 T., 7 g	30	1	2
Bac-Os (Betty Crocker), 1½ Tbsp, 7g	20	1	1.5
Bragg Liquid Aminos, 1 tsp	0	0	0
Butter Buds, 1 tsp	5	0	2
Garlic Bread Sprinkle, 1 tsp	8	0.5	1
Garlic Salt, 1 tsp	2	0	0
Italian Seasoning, 1 tsp	4	0	1
Lemon Pepper Seasoning, 1 tsp	7	0	1
Meat Tenderizer, avg., 1 tsp	7	0	1
Molly McButter, 1 tsp	5	1	1
Mrs Dash Blends, 1 tsp	0	0	0
Salad Crunchies (*McCormick*), 1 tsp	10	0.5	2
Salt: Regular, Sea Salt, Lite Salt	0	0	0
Seasoning Mixes, avg., ¼ pkg	70	1	9
Taco Seasoning, avg., ¼ pkg	30	0.5	4
Old El Paso: Chili Season. Mix, 1 T.	8	0.5	1.5
Cheesy Taco Season. Mix, 1 Tbsp	10	0.5	2
Taco/Burrito Seasoning Mix, 2 tsp	15	0	4
Fajita Seasoning Mix, 1 tsp	5	0	1.5
Vegit Seasoning Mix, ¼ tsp	0	0	0

Supplements

	C	F	Cb
Aloe Vera Juice, undiluted, 2 fl.oz	5	0	1
Brewer's Yeast: Tablets, 2 tabs	4	0	0.5
Flakes, 1 heaping Tbsp, ⅓ oz	30	0.5	4
Powder, 1 heaping Tbsp, ½ oz	50	0.5	6
Calcium Chews: *CVS,* 1 chew	20	0	3
Trader Joe's, Choc., 1 chew	20	1	3
Cod Liver Oil, 1 Tbsp	125	13	0
Fiber Choice, 2 tabs	15	0	4
Fibersure, 1 heaping tsp	25	0	6
Fish Oil Capsules, average, 1	10	1	0
Flax Oil: Capsules, 2	10	1	0
Barlean's, 3 softgels	110	11	0
Garlic Tablets/Capsules, each	3	0	0
Glowelle:			
Beauty Drink, 8 fl.oz	100	0	24
Powder Stick (1)	50	0	12
Lecithin Granules, 1 T., 10g	55	4	0.5
***Metamucil* Powder:**			
Orange (Smooth Texture) 1 rounded Tbsp, 11g	45	0	12
Sugar-Free, 1 rounded tsp, 6g	20	0	5
Pink Lemonade, Sugar-Free, 1 rounded teasp, 6 g	20	0	5
Fiber Wafers (2)	120	5	17
Capsules:			
Heart & Digestive (6)	10	0	3
Strong Bones (5)	10	0	3
Protein, Powders, avg., 1 oz	100	0.5	0
Seaweed: Dried, 1 oz	85	0.5	22
Soaked, drained, 1 oz	15	0.5	3
Spirulina, 1 tablet	2	0	0.5
Vitamins/Minerals: Tabs/Caps, 1	2	0	0
Vitamin E Capsules, each	5	0.5	0
***Viactiv* Chews** (1)	20	0.5	4

Cough & Pharmaceutical

	C	F	Cb
Antacids: Avg., 1 tablet	4	0	1
Liquid, 1 Tbsp	6	0	1
(Antacid Sodium Counts ~ See Page 293)			
Cough/Cold Syrups:			
Regular: w. sugar, 1 Tbsp	35	0	9
w. alcohol, 1 Tbsp	46	0	9
Sugar-Free *(Diabetic Tussin),* 1 T.	0	0	0
Cough Drops/Lozenges: See Page 77			
***Sudafed* Syrup,** 1 tsp	14	0	3
***Tylenol* Liquid:** Child, 1 tsp	17	0	4
Extra Strength, 1 tsp	11	0	3

Sugar

	C	F	Cb
White Sugar, granulated:			
1 level teaspoon, 4g	15	0	4
1 heaping teaspoon, 6g	25	0	6
Single portion, 1 pkg	10	0	3
1 Tablespoon, 12g	50	0	12
1 ounce, 1 oz	110	0	28
1 cup, 7 oz	770	0	200
1 pound	1760	0	464
Single Portion Packages:			
1 Stick, 4g	15	0	4
Square Pkg, 6g	25	0	6
Starbucks, 8g	30	0	8
1 cube, ½", 6g	25	0	6
Brown Sugar: 1 Tbsp, 13g	50	0	13
1 ounce, 1 oz	110	0	28
1 cup, not packed, 5 oz	540	0	140
1 cup, packed, 7¾ oz	845	0	218
Powdered/Confectioners:			
Sifted, 1 cup, 3½ oz	385	0	98
Unsifted, 1 cup, 4¼ oz	460	0	117
Cinnamon Sugar, 1 tsp, 4g	15	0	4
Dextrose, 1¼ tsp	15	0	4
Fructose: Dry, 1 tsp, 4g	15	0	4
Liquid, 1 oz	80	0	21
Glucose, 1 oz	110	0	27
Glucose Tablets (1), 5g	20	0	5
Palm Sugar, 3 Tbsp, 12g	45	0	11
Piloncillo (Brown Sugar), 3oz cone	325	0	81
Turbinado Sugar, 2 Tbsp, 1 oz	110	0	27
Unrefined Cane Sugar, 1 oz	110	0	27

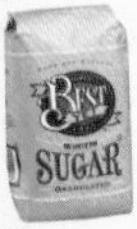

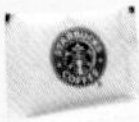

Sugar Substitutes

	C	F	Cb
DiabetiSweet, 1 teaspoon	9	0	4
(Carbohydrate as Sugar Alcohol)			
Equal: Tablet (2)	4	0	0.5
Granular, 1 tsp	4	0	0.5
Packet (1)	4	0	0.5
Flavored, 1 stick	4	0	0.5
Natra Taste; Sweet One, 1 pkt	4	0	1
NutraSweet, 1 tsp	4	0	0
Splenda:			
Granular: 1 tsp	5	0	0.5
1 cup	95	0	24
Packet, all flavors	5	0	0.5
Sugar Blend,Orig/Brown, ½ cup	385	0	96
Stevia, Single Serving	0	0	0
Sugar Twin: 1 pkt	3	0	0.5
Sweet 'N Low, 1 pkt	2	0	0.5
Walgreens Wal-Sweet, 1 pkt	0	0	0
Weight Watchers, 1 pkt	4	0	1
Whey Low, 1 tsp	3	0	3

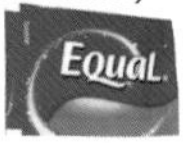

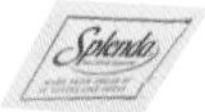

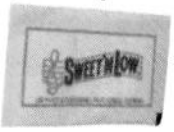

Syrups, Molasses, Agave

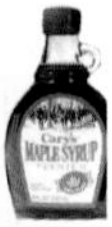

Syrups: *Average All Brands*
(Corn/Rice/Maple/Pancake/Sundae/Waffle)
Includes Aunt Jemima, Cary's, Karo, Hershey's,
Hungry Jack, Log Cabin, Mrs Butterworth's

	C	F	Cb
Regular/Dark/Light Color:			
1 Tbsp, ½ fl.oz	55	0	14
¼ cup (4 Tbsp)	220	0	55
Single Portion: 1½ oz pkg	170	0	42
Lite: 1Tbsp	25	0	6
¼ cup (4 Tbsp)	100	0	25
Sugar-Free: *Cary's,* 2 Tbsp, 1 oz	18	0	5
Cozy Cottage, 2 Tbsp, 1 oz	10	0	3
Da Vinci, 2 Tbsp, 1 oz	5	0	1
Honey Cream Syrup, ¼ c., 2 oz	220	0	55
Molasses: Dark/Light: 1 T., ¾ oz	55	0	14
1 cup, 11½ oz	880	0	224
Blackstrap, 1 Tbsp, ¾ oz	47	0	13
Agave Nectar, avg., 1 Tbsp, ¾ oz	60	0	15

Ice Cream Toppings

	C	F	Cb
Average All Types & Brands			
(Hershey's, Smuckers)			
Butterscotch, Caramel, 2 T.	140	1	30
Chocolate: Hot Fudge, 2 T.	140	4	22
Fat Free Chocolate, 2 T.	100	0	23
Pineapple, Strawberry, 2 T.	110	0	28
Smuckers: Lite, 2 T.	90	0	23
Magic Shell, 2 Tbsp	210	15	18
Milky Way, 2 Tbsp	130	4	23

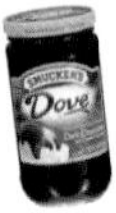

Honey, Jam, Preserves

	C	F	Cb
Average All Brands			
Honey: 1 tsp, ¼ oz	22	0	5.5
1 Tbsp, ¾ oz	65	0	17
1 ounce, 1 oz	85	0	23
1 cup, 12 oz	1030	0	269
Single Portion, ½ oz pkg	45	0	11
Jams/Jellies/Marmalade/Preserves:			
Regular, 1 tsp, ¼ oz	20	0	5
1 Tbsp, ¾ oz	55	0	14
1 ounce, 1 oz	80	0	20
Single Portion, ½ oz pkg	40	0	11
Apple/Fruit Butters, 1 T., 0.6 oz	20	0	6
Fruit Spreads: Regular, 1 tsp	15	0	4
Low Sugar, 1 tsp	8	0	2
Low Cal. *(Featherweight),* 1 tsp	8	0	2
Jelly: Regular, average, 1 tsp	18	0	4.5
Imitation, Low Calorie, 1 tsp	4	0	1

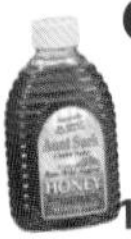

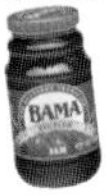

Updated Nutrition Data ~ www.CalorieKing.com
Persons with Diabetes ~ See Disclaimer (Page 24)

Vegetables

	C	F	Cb
Alfalfa Sprouts, ½ cup, ½ oz	5	0	0.5
Artichokes, Globe/French:			
1 medium, 4½ oz	60	0	13
1 large, 5.7 oz	75	0	17
Artichoke Heart, plain, 2 pieces	15	0	3
Asparagus, raw/frozen:			
3 medium spears	10	0	2
Cuts & Tips *(Del Monte)*, ½ cup, 4.3 oz	20	0	3
Bamboo Shoots, ckd, ½ cup, 2 oz	7	0	1
Beans: Green/Snap/String, ½ c., 2 oz	20	0	4
10 beans (4" long), 2 oz	20	0	4
Dried Beans, *average all types:*			
(Kidney, Brown, Lima, Navy, Pinto, White)			
Raw: 2 Tbsp, 1 oz	95	0.5	18
1 cup, 7 oz	665	3	126
Cooked: 1 oz	35	0	7
½ cup, 3 oz	105	0	21
Bean Sprouts, avg., ½ cup, 2 oz	15	0	3.5
Beets (Beetroot):			
Raw, 1 beet (2" diam), 4 oz	35	0	8
Cooked, 1 cup, slices, 3 oz	35	0	8
Canned ~ See Page 168			
Beet Greens, ckd, ½ c., 2½ oz	20	0	4
Bell Pepper: *See Peppers*			
Bitter Melon/Gourd, 1 c. pces, 1½ oz	15	0	1.5
Blackeye Peas, ckd, ½ cup, 3 oz	100	0.5	18
Bok Choy (Chinese Chard), ckd., 3 oz	10	0	1.5
Breadfruit, ¼ small fruit, 3 oz	100	0	26
Broadbeans (Fava Beans):			
Green (in pod): raw: 4 pods			
(3½ oz w. shells; 1.2 oz beans)	30	0	6
1 cup beans (no shell), 4½ oz	110	1	22
Mature Seeds: Raw, 1 cup. 5.3 oz	510	2.5	87
Cooked, ½ cup, 3 oz	95	0	17
Broccoflower, ⅕ head, 3½ oz	35	0	7
Broccoli: Raw, chopped,1 cup, 3 oz	30	0	6
3 Florets, 2½ oz	25	0	5
1 Spear (5" long) 1.1 oz	10	0	2
1 Whole: Medium size, 14 oz	135	1.5	26
Large, 21 oz	205	2	40
1 Head (no stalk), 11 oz	105	1	21
1 Stalk, small (5" long), 5.3 oz	50	0.5	10
Brocco Sprouts, ½ cup, 1 oz	15	0	2
Brussels Sprouts: ckd, ½ cup, 2.8 oz	30	0.5	6
2 Sprouts, 1½ oz	15	0	3
Butterbeans, cooked, ½ cup, 3 oz	90	0	16
Cabbage, All types/colors, avg.:			
Raw: 1 Leaf, large, 1 oz	5	0	2
Shredded, 1 cup, 2½ oz	15	0	4
½ Lge Head (7" diam), 22 oz	150	1	35
Cooked, shredded, ½ cup, 2½ oz	15	0.5	3.5

Vegetables (Cont)

	C	F	Cb
Cactus Leaf (Nopales)			
1 leaf, 4½ oz	20	0	4
1 cup, slices, 3 oz	15	0	3
Carrots: Regular thick variety,			
1 small, 4 oz	45	0	11
1 medium, 6 oz	70	0	16
1 large, 8 oz	95	0	22
Chopped, 1 cup, 4½ c	50	0	12
Grated, 1 cup, 4 oz	45	0	11
Slices, 1 cup, 4½ oz	50	0	12
Sticks (4"), 4-5, 1½ oz	20	0	4
Long thin variety, 1 medium, 2.2 oz	25	0	6
Baby: Snack size, 3 medium, 1 oz	10	0	2.5
Snack Pack, 3 oz	30	0	7
Cauliflower, Raw: 1 cup (pces), 3½ oz	25	0	5
½ medium head, 10 oz	70	0	15
Cooked, 3 florets, 2 oz	10	0	2
Celeriac, ½ cup, raw, 2¾ oz	35	0	7
Celery: 1 large stalk, 11", 2.2 oz	10	0	2
1 small stalk, 5", ½ oz	2	0	0.5
4 Strips/thin sticks, ½	5	0	1
Chopped, 1 cup, 3½ oz	15	0	3
Chard (Swiss), ½ cup, ckd, 3 oz	20	0	3.5
Chayote Squash: 1 med., 7 oz	40	0	9
1 cup pieces, 4½ oz	25	0	6
Chick Peas			
Dry, 1 cup, 7 oz	730	12	121
Cooked, 1 cup, 6 oz	270	4	45
Chicory Greens, 1 cup, 1 oz	7	0	1.5
Chili Peppers: *See Peppers*			
Chinese Long Bean, sliced, 1 c., 3.2 oz	45	0	8
Chives, chopped, 1 Tbsp	1	0	0
Choy Sum, 3 oz	15	0	3
Cilantro (Coriander), 1 cup	5	0	0.5
Collards, cooked, ½ cup, 3 oz	25	0	5
Corn, yellow/white:			
Raw: Kernels, ½ cup, 3 oz	80	0.5	19
Ear (5"x 1¾"), raw, 5½ oz	153	1	37
Cooked: Kernels, ½ cup, 3 oz	77	0.5	18
Cob, cooked: Small, 2¼ oz	60	0.5	14
Large ear, 5½ oz	120	1	28
Courgette: *See Zucchini*			
Cowpeas: *See Blackeye Peas*			
Cress, Garden, raw, 1 cup, 1¾ oz	15	0	3
Cucumber: 1 whole, 11 oz	45	0.5	11
½ cup slices, 2 oz	10	0	2
Mini/Lebanese (1), 3 oz	15	0	3
Daikon Radish, ½ cup, slices, 2 oz	9	0	2
Dandelion Greens, raw, ½ cup, 1 oz	10	0	2.5
Edamame *(Immature green soybeans):*			
Shelled, ½ cup, 2.6 oz	110	5	8
With shells, 10 pods, 1¼ oz	30	1	3

Vegetables (Cont)

	C	F	Cb
Eggplant: Raw, ¼ med, 4 oz	30	0	7
Raw, ½ cup, 1" pieces, 1½ oz	10	0	2
1 slice, fried, 1 oz	75	4	10
Endive, Belgian/French: Raw,			
1 med. head (6"), 2½ oz	12	0	3
Fennel, 1 cup, sliced, 3 oz	25	0	7
Gai Choy Cabbage, ckd, 1 cup, 6 oz	20	0	3
Gai Lan (Chinese Kale), ckd, 1 cup	35	0.5	7
Garlic, 1 clove	4	0	1
Ginger: ¼ cup slices, 1 oz	20	0	5
Crystallized (sugared), 7 pce, 1½ oz	130	0	35
Horseradish, raw, 1 pod, ½ oz	5	0	1
Jerusalem Artichoke, raw, ½ cup	55	0	13
Jicama, raw, sliced, ½ cup, 2¼ oz	25	0	6
Kale, 1 cup, chopped, 2½ oz	35	0.5	7
Kohlrabi, ½ cup, cooked, 1¾ oz	17	0	5
Leek, cooked, 1 whole, 4½ oz	40	0	9
Lentils, green/brown: Dry, 1 oz	100	0.5	17
Dry, 1 cup, 6¾ oz	680	2	115
Cooked, ½ cup, 3½ oz	115	0.5	20
Lettuce: 1 cup, chop./shred., 2 oz	7	0	1
Butterhead, 2 leaves, ½ oz	2	0	0.5
Cos/Romaine, shred'd, 1 c., 1.7 oz	10	0	2
Iceberg: 1 outer leaf, ½ oz	2	0	0.5
1 medium head, 16 oz	75	1	16
Lima Beans, baby, ckd,½ c., 3 oz	105	0	20
Lotus Root, 10 slices, ckd, 3 oz	60	0	14
Mung Bean Sprouts, ½ cup, 2 oz	15	0	3
Mushrooms: Raw, 1 medium, 0.6 oz	4	0	0.5
Raw, 1 large, sliced, ¾ oz	5	0	1
Raw, ½ cup pieces, 1¼ oz	8	0	1
Cooked, ½ cup pieces, 2½ oz	20	0.5	4
Fried/Sauteed, 6 oz	220	16	11
Mustard Greens, Raw, ½ cup, 1 oz	7	0	2
Nopales: *See Cactus Leaf*			
Okra: Raw, 8 pods, 4 oz	30	0	7
Cooked, ½ cup, slices, 2¾ oz	20	0	4
Onions, Raw: 1 small, 2½ oz	30	0	7
1 medium, 4 oz	50	0	11
1 large, 5½ oz	65	0	15
1 jumbo, 16 oz	190	0.5	46
Chopped: Raw, ½ cup, 3 oz	35	0	8
1 Tbsp, 0.4 oz	5	0	1
Slices: 1 cup, 4 oz	50	0	12
1 medium slice (⅛"), ½ oz	5	0	1
1 large slice (¼"), 1⅓ oz	15	0	4
Dehydrated flakes, ¼ c, ½ oz	50	0	12
Rings, breaded/fried, 2 rings	80	5	9
Scallions, ½ cup, 2 oz	15	0	3
Spring, ½ cup, chopped, 2 oz	15	0	3

(*French's* Fried Onions: *See Page 114)*
Blossom/Blooming: See Fast-Foods (Chili's/Outback)

Vegetables (Cont)

	C	F	Cb
Parsley, chopped, ½ cup, 1 oz	10	0	2
Parsnip: 1 medium, 4 oz	85	0	20
Cooked, ½ cup slices, 2¾ oz	55	0	13
Peas: Raw, Green, ¼ cup, 1½ oz	30	0	5
Raw, with pods, ½ lb	70	0	13
Snow Peas, 10 pods, 1.2 oz	15	0	3
Split: Dry, hulled, 1 oz	100	0.5	17
Cooked, 1 cup, 7 oz	230	1	42
Peppers: Sweet, 1 medium, 4.2 oz	30	0	7
Bell: 1 medium, 4.2 oz	30	0	7
½ cup, chopped, raw, 2½ oz	20	0	5
2 rings (5" diam. x ¼" thick)	3	0	1
Chili: Green/Red, 1½ oz	20	0	5
Habanero, 1 only, 8g	10	0	2
Pigeon Peas, cooked, ½ cup, 3 oz	95	1	17
Pimientos, 3 medium, 3½ oz	25	0	5
Poi, ½ cup, 4.2 oz	135	0	33
Potatoes: Raw (with skin)			
1 Baby, 2 oz	45	0	10
1 Small, 6 oz	135	0	30
1 Medium, 8 oz	180	0	40
1 Large, 12 oz	270	0	60
1 Extra large, 16 oz	360	0	80
Baked (no added fat): large, 10 oz (raw wt):			
Plain, with skin, 7 oz (ckd wt)	185	0	42
without skin, 5½ oz (ckd wt)	145	0	34
w. Skin/Toppings:			
+ 2 tsp fat	270	8	58
+ Sour Cr./Chives, 2 Tbsp	320	6	60
+ Plain Yogurt, 2 Tbsp	260	1	60
+ Grated Cheese, 1 oz	370	9	58
Mashed:			
w/ milk plus fat, ½ cup, 4 oz	120	4.5	18
KFC Style w/o gravy, 4 oz	100	3	16
Loaded (fat/cream/cheese/bacon):			
Side serving, 6 oz	180	9	22
Large serving, 12 oz	360	18	44
Potato Skins: (Baked w/ Cheese topping),			
½ whole, 4 oz	240	13	22
French Fries: Small svg, 2.6 oz	250	13	30
Medium svg., 4 oz	380	20	47
Froz., uncooked, 18 fries, 4 oz	165	5.5	28
Oven-heated, 18 fries, 4 oz	165	5.5	28
Take-Out, 1 cup, 5 oz	440	25	60
McDonald's ~ See Page 222			
Fried, 18 pcs, 4 oz	165	5.5	28
Au Gratin, ½ c., 4.3 oz	160	9	14
Pancakes, 2 small, 2 oz	120	6.5	12
Puffs, fried, 4 puffs, 1 oz	55	2.5	8
Scalloped: 1 cup, 8½ oz	220	9	26

Ore-Ida Frozen Potatoes: See Page 168

Updated Nutrition Data ~ www.CalorieKing.com
Persons with Diabetes ~ See Disclaimer (Page 24)

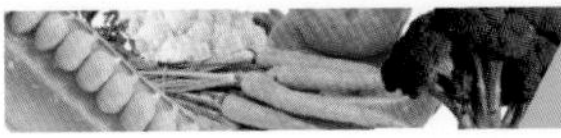

Vegetables (Cont)

	C	F	Cb
Potato Salad, ½ cup, 4½ oz	180	10	14
Pumpkin:			
Raw, 1″ cubes, 1 cup, 4 oz	30	0	7
Cooked:			
Mashed: 1 scoop, 2 oz	10	0	2
½ cup, 4⅓ oz	25	0	6
Baked, without fat, 4 oz	90	7	9
Pumpkin Flowers, 1 cup, 1.2 oz	5	0	1
Purslane: Cooked, ½ c., 2 oz	10	0	2
Raw, 1″ cubes, 1 cup, 1.5 oz	5	0	1.5
Radicchio: 2 leaves, ½ oz	5	0	1
Shredded, 1 cup, 1½ oz	20	0	4
Radishes: 1 small	0	0	0
10 med./5 large, 1.6 oz	5	0	1
½ cup slices, 2 oz	10	0	2
Rhubarb, raw, ½ cup, 2 oz	15	0	3
Rutabaga, ckd., ½ c. cubes, 3 oz	30	0	7
Salsify, ckd, ½ c. slices, 2½ oz	50	0	11
Sauerkraut, ½ cup, 2½ oz	15	0	3
Seaweed: Dried, 1 oz	5	0	2
Soaked, drained, 1 oz	15	0	4
Nori/Laver, dried, 6 sheets, ½ oz	35	0	5
Shallots, chopped, 1 T,, ½ oz	5	0	1
Sorrel, raw, ½ cup, 4 oz	20	0	4
Soybeans: Mature, dry, 1 oz	120	5.5	9
Dry, ½ cup, 3.3 oz	390	18	28
Cooked, ½ cup, 3 oz	150	7.5	8
(Soy Products/Tofu/Tempeh: See Page 162)			
Spinach: Cooked, ½ cup, 3 oz	20	0	4
Raw: 3 leaves/1 cup, 1 oz	7	0	1
1 Bunch, 12 oz	80	1.5	12
Creamed, avg., ½ cup, 4½ oz	190	15	8
Squash: Summer, raw, ½ c., 2½ oz	10	0	2
Cooked, ½ cup slices, 3 oz	15	0	3
Winter, cooked,			
Acorn, ½ cup cubes, 3½ oz	35	0	9
½ medium (10 oz raw wt.)	115	0	30
Butternut, ½ c. cubes, 3½ oz	40	0	10
¼ medium (9 oz raw wt.)	115	0	30
Spaghetti, ½ cup, 1¾ oz	15	0	3
Succotash, ckd, ½ cup, 3⅓ oz	110	1	23
Sweetcorn: *See Corn*			
Sweet Potatoes:			
Cooked with skin (no fat)			
1 medium, 4 oz	105	0	24
No skin, mashed, ½ c., 5½ oz	125	0	29
Swiss Chard, ckd, chopped, 1 c., 6 oz	35	0	7
Taro, cooked, ½ cup, 2⅓ oz	95	0	23

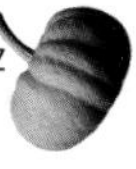
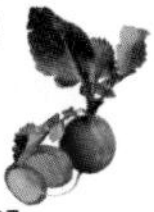
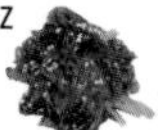
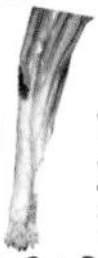
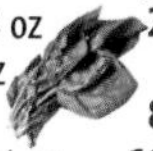
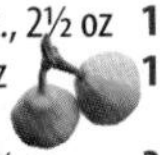
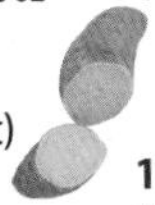

Vegetables (Cont)

	C	F	Cb
Tomatoes: 1 small (2¼″ diam.), 3 oz	15	0	3
1 medium (2¾″ diam.), 5 oz	25	0	5
1 large (3½″ diam.), 8 oz	40	0.5	9
1 extra lge (3″ diam.), 12 oz	60	0.5	14
Chopped, 1 cup, 6½ oz	35	0.5	7
Extra Listings: *Page 103*			
Tomatillo, 1 medium, 1.2 oz	10	0	2
Turnip: ckd, ½ cup, 2¾ oz	15	0	4
Greens, cooked, ½ cup, 2½ oz	15	0	3
Water Chestnuts: 5-6 nuts, 1 oz	56	0.5	13
½ cup slices, 2¼ oz, raw	60	0	15
Canned, 1 oz	15	0	3
Watercress, 10 sprigs, 1 oz	3	0	0.5
Yams: Cooked, ½ cup, 2½ oz	80	0	19
Baked, 1 medium (6″) 8 oz	265	0.5	63
1 large (9″) 12 oz	400	0.5	94
Yardlong Bean, 1 pod, ½ oz	5	0	1
Yucca Root, ½ cup, 3½ oz	165	0.5	39
Zucchini: 1 medium, 7 oz, raw	30	0.5	7
½ cup slices, cooked, 3 oz	15	0	4

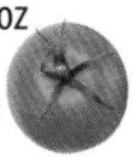
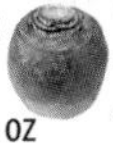
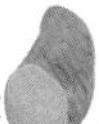
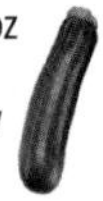

Frozen Vegetables

	C	F	Cb
Birds Eye			
Petite Varieties:			
Brussels Sprouts, (10), 3 oz	45	0	8
Peas: ⅔ cup, 3 oz	70	0	12
with Pearl Onions, ⅔ c., 3.2 oz	60	0	11
Sweet/White Corn, ⅔ c., 3.2 oz	100	1	21
Ultimate Mixed Vege, ¾ cup, 3 oz	50	0	10
Whole Beans, 1 cup, 3 oz	35	0	5
Whole Onions, ⅔ cu, 3 oz	30	0	6
Steamfresh:			
Asian Medley, 1 cup, 3.3 oz	50	2	6
Asp., Corn & Baby Carrots, ⅔ c., 3.1 oz	70	0.5	13
Broccoli & Cauliflower, 1 c. 3.4 oz	30	0	4
w. Carrots, ¾ cup, 3 oz	30	0	5
Broc., Crts., Peas, Wtr. Ches., ¾ c.	35	0	6
Garlic Baby Peas & Mushr., ¾ c.	80	2	12
Sugar Snap Peas, ⅔ cup, 3 oz	40	0	7
Whole Green Beans, 1 cup, 3 oz	35	0	5
Singles: *Per 3.25 oz Bag*			
Baby Brussels Sprouts	50	0	9
Super Sweet Corn	80	1	14
Sweet Peas	70	0	13
Steamfresh Vegetables & Sauce:			
Asian, 1 cup	60	1	12
Green Bean & Almonds, ¾ cup	80	4	8

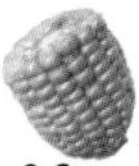

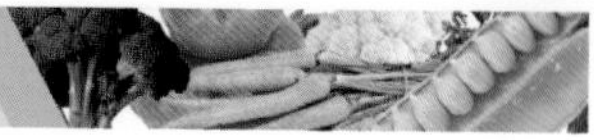

Frozen Vegetables (Cont) · C · F · Cb

Green Giant
Just for One,

	C	F	Cb
Broccoli & Cheese Sauce, 4.25 oz	45	1.5	7
Vegetables: Asparagus Cuts, ⅔ c.	20	0	3
Corn: Nibblers, ½ ear, 2.2 oz	70	0.5	14
Extra Sweet Niblets, ⅔ cup	70	1	13
Shoepeg, no sauce, ½ cup	70	1	15
Honey-Glazed Carrots, 1 cup	90	3	15
Spinach, no sauce, ½ cup, 3½ oz	25	0	3
Rice & Vegetables: *Per ½ Pkg, Prepared*			
Cheesy Rice & Broccoli	135	2.5	21
Rice Medley	140	2	26
Rice Pilaf	115	1.5	22
White & Wild Rice	140	3	25
Valley Fresh: *Per ½ Cup, Prepared*			
Rstd Red Pot., Green Beans w.Sce	80	1	16

Ore-Ida (As Purchased):

	C	F	Cb
French Fries: Country, 13 fries, 3 oz	130	4.5	20
Crispers 20 pces, 3 oz	210	12	23
Crispy Crowns (11), 3 oz	170	10	21
Extra Crispy Crinkles (13), 3 oz	150	6	32
Fast-Food Fries, 27 fries, 3 oz	160	6	23
Waffle Fries, 8 fries, 3 oz	160	6	22
Golden Fries, 14 pces, 3 oz	130	3.5	21
Oven Chips, 7 pces, 3 oz	160	7	22
Roasted, Original ¾ cup, 2.65 oz	130	4.5	18
Shoestrings, 32 pces, 3 oz	140	5	22
Steak Fries, 7 fries, 3 oz	110	3	19
Zesties, 12 pces, 3 oz	150	5	22
Hash Browns: Toaster, 2 patties	220	12	25
Golden Patties (1), 2.63 oz	140	8	15
Potatoes & Onion, 1 cup, 3.2 oz	90	3.5	13
Potatoes O'Brien, ¾ cup, 3 oz	60	0	14
Southern Style, ⅔ cup, 3 oz	70	0	16
Onion Rings: Gourmet, 3 pces, 3 oz	170	9	23
Onion Ringers, 6 pces, 3.2 oz	220	12	25
Sweet Potatoes: 4 oz	80	0	18

Steam n' Mash

	C	F	Cb
Cut Russet, ¾ Cup, 3.3 oz	80	0	17
Garlic Seasoned Potatoes, ¾ cup	110	4	17
Three Chse Potatoes, ¾ c.	80	0.5	16
Tater Tots: 9 pces, 3 oz	170	8	20
ABC (9), 3 oz	160	8	22
Extra Crispy, 12 pces, 3 oz	170	9	20
Ultimate Bake: with Butter, 5 oz	170	5	27
with Cheese, 5 oz	190	6	28

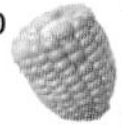

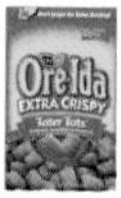

Canned/Bottled · C · F · Cb

Solids & Liquid

	C	F	Cb
Artichoke Hearts *(Fanci Foods)*:			
Plain, 1 oz (1)	8	0	1
Marinated, ¼ bottle, 1 oz	25	1.5	2
Asparagus: Drained, 3 spears	10	0	1.5
Pieces, ½ cup, 4.3 oz	25	0.5	3
Bamboo Shoots, 1 cup, 4½ oz	25	0	4
Bean Salad, ½ cup, 4⅓ oz	90	0	20
Beans: Green, ½ c., 2½ oz	15	0	3
Baked Beans, ½ c., 4½ oz	120	0.5	27
Butter Beans, ½ c., 4½ oz	90	0	16
Italian, ½ c., 4½ oz	30	0	6
Kidney Beans, ½ c., 3½ oz	105	0.5	19
Lima Beans, ½ cup, 4½ oz	80	0	15
Pinto Beans, ½ cup, 4½ oz	105	1	18
Beets: Sliced, ½ cup, 3 oz	25	0	6
Crinkle/Pickled *(Del Monte)* ½ cup	80	0	20
Carrots: Sliced, ½ cup, 2½ oz	20	0	4
Honey Glazed *(Del Monte)* ½ cup	75	0	18
Corn: Kernels, ½ cup, 4½ oz	80	0.5	18
Creamed style, ½ cup, 4½ oz	90	0.5	23
Garbanzo/Chick Peas, ½ c., 4.2 oz	145	1.5	27
Green Chilies, diced, 2 Tbsp, 1 oz	6	0	1.5
Hearts of Palm (1), 1.2 oz	7	0	1
Mushrooms: ½ c., 2½ oz	20	0	4
in Butter Sauce, 2 oz	20	1	2
Onions: Pickled, 1 med., ½ oz	10	0	2
Cocktail, 1 onion	0	0	0
French's Fried Onions: *See Page 114*			
Peas, ½ cup, 3 oz	60	0.5	10
Peppers: Hot Chili, Jalapeno, (1), 1 oz	5	0	1
Sweet, undrained, 2½ oz	13	0	3
Jalapeno, w. liquid, ½ cup chopped	20	0.5	3
Fried, drained, 2 Tbsp, 1 oz	60	5	3
Salsa, average all types, 2 Tbsp	10	0	2
Sauerkraut, drained, 1 cup, 5 oz	25	0	6
Spinach, ½ cup, 3½ oz	25	0.5	3.5
Succotash: w. Cr. Style Corn, ½ c.	100	0.5	23
w. whole kernels, undrained, ½ c.	80	0.5	18
Sweetcorn: *See Corn*			
Sweet Potato: ½ cup, 3½ oz	90	0	24
Tomatoes, Sundr.: Natural, 5-6 pce	20	0	5
In Oil, drained, 6 pces, ½ oz	40	2.5	4
Tomato Products: *See Page 148*			
Vegetables, mixed, ½ cup, 4 oz	45	0	8
Yams: in Light Syrup, ½ cup, 4 oz	105	0	25
Candied, ½ cup, 5 oz	170	0	46
Zucchini in Tom. Sce., ½ c., 4 oz	30	0	8

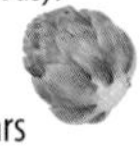

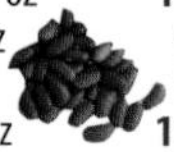

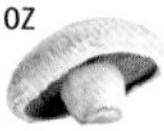

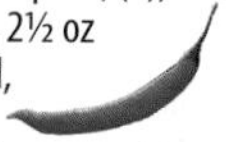

Quick Guide

	C	F	Cb
Yogurt			
Average All Brands: Per 8 oz Cup			
Plain Yogurt: Whole	140	8	10
Low-Fat	145	3.5	16
Fat-Free	125	0.5	17
Fruit Flavored: Whole, 8 oz	225	8	32
Low-Fat	230	3	43
Fat-Free, regular	215	0.5	43
Fat-Free, no sugar added	80	0	15

Yogurt Parfait/Deli Cups	C	F	Cb
With Fruit Pieces:			
(⅔ Yogurt + ⅓ Fruit)			
Small, 8 oz cup	140	3	20
Large, 12 oz cup	210	4.5	30
With Fruit + Granola:			
Small, 8 oz cup (+ ¾ oz Granola)	235	7	30
Large, 12 oz cup (+ 1½ oz Granola)	400	13	58

Yogurt ~ Brands	C	F	Cb
Alta Dena: Low-Fat: Plain, 8 oz	170	4.5	20
All Natural, avg., other flavors	215	2	41
Non-Fat: Fruit Flavors	190	0	38
Plain, 8 oz	110	0	16
Vanilla, 8 oz	160	0	30
Blue Bunny			
Light, avg. fruit flav., 6 oz	100	0	14
No Sugar Added, 6 oz	80	0	14
Superfruit, avg., 6 oz	100	0	14
Omega 3, avg., 4 oz cup	80	1	15
Breyers			
Creme Savers, avg., 6 oz	170	1.5	22
Fruit On The Bottom, avg, 6 oz	160	1.5	32
Inspirations: Choc Chip/Mint, 4 oz	140	3.5	23
Strawberry/Vanilla Bean, 4 oz	110	1	22
Light, avg all flavors, 6 oz	80	0	12
Smooth & Creamy, avg., 6 oz	170	1.5	34
YoCrunch: Light, avg., 6 oz	120	1	22
Low-Fat w/ Granola, fruit, avg.	190	2	38
M&M's/Reese's/Crunch, avg.	200	4.5	35
100 Calorie Pack: Strawberry	100	0.5	23
Vanilla, Cheesecake	100	2	21
Brown Cow			
Cream Top: Plain, 6 oz	130	7	9
Fruit Flavors, average, 6 oz	175	6	27
Low-Fat: Plain, 8 oz cup	130	3	15
Flavors, average, 6 oz	150	2	27
Non-Fat: Plain, 8 oz cup	110	0	16
Fruit Flavors, avg., 6 oz	135	0	26
Greek: Plain, 5.3 oz cup	80	0	6
Strawberry, 5.3 oz cup	130	0	18

Cabot	C	F	Cb
Non-Fat: Plain, 8 oz	100	0	19
Fruit flavors, 8 oz	130	0	24
Greek Style: Reg., 6 oz	210	17	9
Low-Fat (2%), 6 oz	160	3	25
Cascade Fresh:			
Low-Fat, all flavors, 6 oz	140	2	23
Fat-Free, all flavors, 6 oz	110	0	20
Whole Milk: Plain, 8 oz	170	8	12
Flavors, average, 8 oz	200	7	24
Colombo			
Light, all flavors, 6 oz	90	0	16
Classic: Banana Strawb.	180	0	39
Vanilla, 6 oz	130	0	25
Fat-Free, Plain, 8 oz	100	0	15
Dannon:			
Activia Yogurt:			
Plain, 8 oz	170	4.5	20
Light, avg. all flav., 4 oz	70	0	13
Fiber, all flav., 4 oz cup	110	2	19
Drinks, all flavors 5.75 fl.oz	160	3	27
All Natural:			
Low-Fat, avg., 4 oz cup	120	1	22
6 oz Cups: Flavors	150	2.5	25
Plain, Non-Fat	80	0	12
Danimals: Crush Cups, 4 oz	100	1.5	17
Drinkables, 3.1 fl.oz	70	0.5	15
Fruit Blends, avg., 6 oz cup	170	1.5	33
Fruit On The Bottom, avg., 6 oz	150	1.5	28
Light & Fit: 6 oz Cups, (80 calories)	80	0	16
60 Calorie Packs, 4 oz	60	0	11
Quarts, Strawb./Vanilla,			
8 oz serving	110	0	21
Smoothies, 7 fl.oz	70	0	14
Carb & Sugar Control: 4 oz cup	50	1.5	3
Smoothies, 7 fl.oz bottle	60	2.5	4
Emmi Swiss (Low-Fat):			
Fruit flavors, 6 oz	160	2.5	26
Bircher Muesli, 6 oz	180	3	30
Fage			
Classic: Peach/Cherry/Strawb., 5.3 oz	210	12	18
Honey, 5.3 oz	250	12	28
0%, 8 oz	120	0	9
2%: Plain 8 oz	150	4.5	9
Fruit, 5.3 oz	130	2.5	18
Honey, 5.3 oz	180	2.5	29
Horizon Organic			
Fruit on Bottom, all varieties, 6 oz	140	0	27
Low-Fat: Blended, avg. all flav., 6 oz	150	1.5	27
Yogurt Tuberz (1)	60	0.5	11
32 oz Carton: Fat-Free, Plain, 8 oz	80	0	12
Cream on Top: Plain, 8 oz	160	7	14
Vanilla, 8 oz	220	6	32

Brands (Cont)

	C	F	Cb
Jewel: *8 oz Ctn (Low-Fat)*			
Fruit On The Bottom, avg.	240	2.5	46
Swiss, average	200	2	38
Vanilla	210	2	40
32 oz Tubs: Plain, 1 cup, 8 oz	170	3	20
Plain, Non-Fat, 1 cup, 8 oz	130	0	19
Kemps: '100 Calories' (Non-Fat), 5 oz	100	0	22
Light '80 Calories', 6 oz ctn	80	0	16
Yo Stix, average, 2.25 oz tube	80	2	13
Yo-J Drink, average, 8.3 fl.oz	150	0	35
Kirkland, Low-Fat:			
Blueb./Peach/Strawb. 8 oz	240	2	48
Knudsen: 70 Calories, 6 oz	70	0	11
Free, average, 6 oz	170	0	33
Kroger:			
Blended, Flavors: 6 oz	190	2	35
8 oz	250	2.5	47
Carb Master, avg. all flavors, 6 oz	80	1.5	4
Fruit On The Bottom, avg all flav.	170	2	30
Lite, avg. all flavors, 8 oz	100	0	17
Fat-Free, Plain, 8 oz	120	0	17
Low-Fat, Plain, 8 oz	140	4	16
La Yogurt:			
Original, average, 6 oz	150	2	30
Light, average, 6 oz	90	0	15
Rich & Creamy, 6 oz	160	2	30
Enriched, average, 6 oz	160	2	30
Fruit on the Bottom, avg., 8 oz	220	2.5	43
Sabor Latino: Dulche De Leche, 6 oz	190	1.5	36
Fruit Flavors, average, 6 oz	170	2	34
LALA, Classic Blended:			
Fruit Flavors, avg., 8 oz	200	4	36
Smoothies, avg., 9 fl.oz	200	4	34
Lucerne			
Low-Fat: Plain, 6 oz	150	3.5	18
Fruit flavors, avg., 6 oz	170	2	32
Vanilla, 6 oz	170	2	33
Fat-Free: Plain, 6 oz	80	0	13
Light Fat-Free, fruit, 6 oz	130	0	19
Meadow Gold, avg., 6 oz ctn	85	0	16
Mountain High			
Original Style, Plain, 8 oz	180	8	17
Strawb./Vanilla, 8 oz	210	7	27
Low-Fat: Classic, all flav., 6 oz pkg	140	1.5	25
Large Containers: Plain, 8 oz	140	2.5	18
Lemon; Raspberry, 8 oz	190	2	33
Fat-Free: Plain, 8 oz	120	0	18
Strawberry/Vanilla, avg., 8 oz	160	0	29

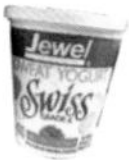

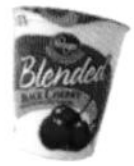

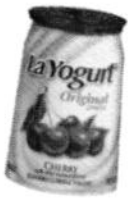

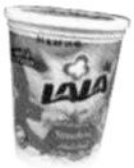

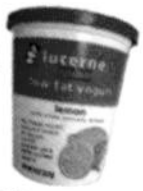

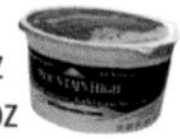

	C	F	Cb
Nancy's			
Whole Milk: Honey, plain, 8 oz	170	8	17
w. Fruit on Top, avg, 8 oz	230	5	41
Low Fat: Plain/Lemon, 8 oz, avg	150	3	16
Other flavors, average, 8 oz	175	3	27
Non-Fat: Plain, 8 oz	120	0	17
Vanilla (32 oz ctn), swtn'd, 8 oz	220	0	40
Soy Cultured: (6 oz ctn): Plain	150	3	25
Berry flavors, average	140	3.5	24
O Organics (Safeway),			
Low-Fat, avg., 6 oz	140	2.5	23
Oikos, Greek Yogurt:			
Plain, 5.3 oz cup	80	0	6
1 cup, 8 oz	130	0	9
Blueberry, 5.3 oz cup	120	0	16
Honey, 5.3 oz cup	120	0	18
Vanilla, 5.3 oz cup	110	0	12
Publix: Fat-Free, Plain, 8 oz	140	0	23
Swiss Style, Low-Fat, 8 oz	240	2.5	41
Ralphs: *Same as Kroger*			
Roberts:			
Plain, 8 oz	130	2.5	15
Lemon, 8 oz	200	2	34
Fat-Free, all flav., 8 oz	90	0	14
with splenda, 6 oz	70	0	11
Silk (Soy): Plain, 1 c., 8 oz	150	4	22
Vanilla, 6 oz	150	3	25
Other flavors, avg, 6 oz	150	2	30
Stater Bros: Plain, 8 oz	140	2	19
Fruit on the Bottom, avg., 8 oz	220	2	44
Blended Low-Fat, avg., 8 oz	240	2	48
Stonyfield Farm (Organic)			
Fat-Free: Plain, 6 oz	80	0	12
Choc. Underground, 6 oz	170	0	37
Fruit Flavors, avg., 6 oz	120	0	24
Lowfat: Apple Pie, 6 oz	130	1.5	21
Plain, 6 oz	90	1.5	11
Other fruit flavors, 6 oz, avg.	130	1.5	22
Whole Milk Yogurt: French Van. 6 oz	170	6	23
Other fruit flavors, 6 oz, avg.	160	6	21
O'Soy: Choc.; Vanilla, 6 oz	155	3	25
Strawberry & Peach, 4 oz	100	2	14
YoKids, all flavors, 4 oz cups	80	1	13
Trader Joe's			
European Style (32 oz Container):			
Whole Milk, Plain, 8 oz	170	7	14
Non-Fat : Plain, 8 oz	120	0	17
Chocolate; Mocha, 5.3 oz	130	2	20

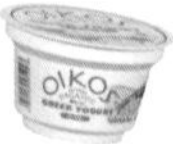

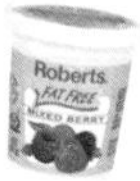

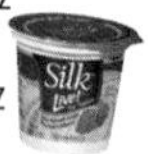

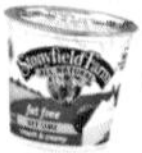

Updated Nutrition Data ~ www.CalorieKing.com
Persons with Diabetes ~ See Disclaimer (Page 24)

Brands (Cont) — C F Cb

Trader Joe's (Cont):

	C	F	Cb
French Vanilla, Non-Fat, all flav., 6 oz	130	0	26
Low-Fat Pre-Stirred, Fruit Flav. 8 oz	220	3	40
Greek Style: *Per 8 oz Container*			
Apricot Mango; Honey	300	15	28
Fig; Strawberry	310	18	27
Non-Fat: Pomegranate, 5.3 oz	110	0	12
Blueberry, 5.3 oz cup	120	0	16
Weight Watchers, all flav., 6 oz ctn	100	0.5	17
Wildwood: Soyogurt Plain, 6 oz	110	3.5	14
Other flavors, avg., 6 oz	130	3	23

Whole Foods (365)

	C	F	Cb
365: Non-Fat, Plain, 6 oz	90	0	13
Fruit flavors, avg., 6 oz	145	0	30
Vanilla, 6 oz	130	0	23
365 Organic:			
Fruit flavors, avg., 6 oz	150	0	29
Whole Soy: Plain, 6 oz	150	3.5	27
Berry; Strawb. Ban., 6 oz	180	3.5	35
Other flavors, avg., 6 oz	160	3.5	30

YoCrunch: *Low-Fat, 6oz Cup*

	C	F	Cb
With Oreo Cookies	180	3.5	33
With Granola	190	2	38
Vanilla w. Candy pces	200	4.5	35

Yoplait

	C	F	Cb
Original, average all flavors, 6 oz	170	1.5	33
Fiber One, average all flavors, 4 oz	50	0	13
Go-Gurt!, 2.25 oz tube	70	0.5	13
Light, Fruit Flavors, 6 oz	100	0	19
Thick & Creamy, all flavors, 6 oz	190	3.5	32
Light Thick & Creamy, 6 oz	100	0	20
Large 2lb Container, 99% Fat-Free, 1 cup, 8 oz	200	1.5	39
Yo-Plus, avg., all flav., 4 oz	110	1.5	21
Trix, Fruit Flavors, 4 oz	90	0.5	18
Whips!: Choc. Flavors, 4 oz	160	4	26
Fruit Flavors, 4 oz	140	2.5	25
Yoplait Kids: 4 oz cup	80	1	13
Squeezers, 2 oz	60	1	11

Yogurt Drinks & Probiotics

Dairy Delite:

	C	F	Cb
Blueberry, 16 fl.oz	420	7	82
Peach, 16 fl.oz	420	7	82
Strawb./Banana, 16 fl.oz	380	7	74

Dannon:

	C	F	Cb
Activa, 5.75 fl.oz	160	3	27
Danimals, 3.1 fl.oz	70	0.5	15
DanActive, 3.1 fl.oz	80	1.5	13
Light 'n Fit Smoothies:			
Regular, 7 fl.oz	70	0	14
Carb/Sugar Control, 7 fl.oz	60	2.5	4

	C	F	Cb
Glen Oaks, all flavors, avg., 8 fl.oz	190	3.5	35
Good Belly Probiotic, 2.7 fl.oz bottle	50	0	12

Kemps, Yo-J Drink,

	C	F	Cb
Orange Cream, 8.3 fl.oz	150	0	35
Raspberry Orange, 8.3 fl.oz	150	0	34
Strawberry Banana, 8.3 fl.oz	150	0	34
Wild Berry, 8.3 fl.oz	150	0	34

Promise Activ: *Per 3.3 fl.oz*

	C	F	Cb
Supershots: Blueberry	70	3.5	8
Strawberry Banana	50	0	10
Vanilla	70	3.5	8

Ralphs:

	C	F	Cb
Active Lifestyle, Average all flavors, 7 fl.oz	120	0	24
Smoothies:			
Peach, 7 fl.oz	200	2.5	37
Raspberry, 7 fl.oz	210	2.5	40
Strawberry, 7 fl.oz	190	2.5	35

Stonyfield Farm

	C	F	Cb
Smoothies, avg., 10 oz	230	3	40
Wildwood, Probiotic Drink, 8 fl.oz	185	2.5	32

Yonique: *Per 6 fl.oz Container*

	C	F	Cb
Low-Fat: Guava	130	1.5	27
Mango	140	1.5	28
Pina Colada	160	3.5	26
Strawberry Banana	140	1.5	28
Strawberry	150	1.5	32

Yoplait Smoothies,

	C	F	Cb
All Flavors, 8 fl.oz	220	3	43

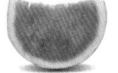 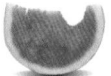 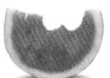 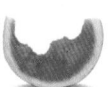 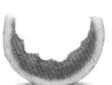 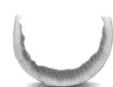

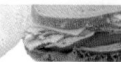

Cafeteria-Style Foods | C | F | Cb

Average All Preperations

	C	F	Cb
Beef Stroganoff, 5 oz	195	13	7
Beef Stroganoff w. 4 oz noodles	350	14	36
Chicken Lasagna, 1 piece	300	11	32
Chicken Chop Suey w. 4 oz rice	245	4	37
Deep Dish Burrito, 7 oz	265	13	20
Grnd Beef Casserole, 2 scoops, 6 oz	245	13	17
Italian Meat Sce for Spagh., 5 oz	150	9	9
w. 5 oz Spaghetti	350	10	49
Lasagna, 1 piece	275	11	25
Meatloaf, 3 oz	205	13	4
Ranch Beans, 2 scoops, 6 oz	350	11	45
Red Beans & Rice, 7 oz	280	9	37
Scalloped Potato/Ham, 2 scp, 6 oz	160	6	20
Stuffed Shells in Sauce (1)	105	3	17
Swedish Meatballs (3)	205	12	9
Sweet & Sour Pork/Rice, 9 oz	240	3	40
Swiss Steak w/Mushr. Gravy, 6 oz	280	11	4
Tator Tot Casserole, 2 scoops, 6 oz	260	15	20
Tenderloin Tips/Mushr. Gravy, 5 oz	210	13	3
w. 5 oz noodles	395	15	38
Tuna Noodle Casserole, 2 scp, 6 oz	180	6	17
Turkey Tetrazzini, 2 scoops, 6 oz	195	7	17
Vegetable Lasagna, 1 piece	250	13	21

Croissants

	C	F	Cb
Unfilled: Medium 1½ oz	180	10	21
Filled: w. Ham (2 oz), garnish	280	14	24
w. Ham (2 oz), Cheese (2 oz)	470	30	20
w. Chick (2 oz) Cheese (2 oz)	470	30	20
w. Turkey/Ham/Chse (2 oz ea.)	580	36	20
Au Bon Pain: Ham & Cheese	340	10	46
Spinach & Cheese	250	9	32

7-Eleven: *Page 244*

Bagels

	C	F	Cb
Plain: Large, 4 oz (no filling)	320	2	65
with 2 oz Cream Cheese	500	27	54
with 2 oz Lox (Smoked Salmon)	400	4	65

Also see Bagels Section: *Page 58*
Fast-Foods Restaurants: *Page 183*
Au Bon Pain: *Page 185*
Bruegger's: *Page 192*
Einstein Bros Bagels: *Page 206*

Sandwiches | C | F | Cb

No Spreads Unless Indicated
(Includes 2 Slices Bread ~ 3 oz)

	C	F	Cb
BLT (5 strips Bacon, 2 Tbsp Mayo)	600	40	46
Breaded Chicken & garnish	540	28	46
Chicken Salad w. Mayo., 5 oz	580	30	49
Chopped Liver, Egg, Mayo.	630	25	44
Corned Beef w. Mustard., 5 oz	560	28	44
Egg Salad w. Mayonnaise	570	29	49
Egg Salad Club w. Bacon, Mayo.	780	53	49
Grilled Cheese (3 oz)	540	30	44
Ham (4 oz); Cheese (4 oz), Mayo.	910	56	44
Lobster Salad (4 oz) w. Mayo.	530	25	45
Overstuffed Tuna Salad (7 oz)	870	39	75
Philadelphia Cheese Steak S'wich	550	23	42
Reuben (6 oz Beef/Pastrami, 2 oz Cheese, 2 Tbsp Dressing)	920	60	28
Roast Beef (4 oz) w. Mustard	460	12	45
Roast Pork (4 oz) w. Apple Sauce	500	16	55
Shrimp Salad Club w. Bacon, Mayo.	800	57	48
Sloppy Joe w. Sauce (7 oz)	600	30	45
Steak Sandwich (5 oz cooked)	680	32	41
Triple Cheese (4 oz) Melt	720	45	46
Tuna Salad w. Mayo., 5 oz	610	30	49
Turkey Breast (5 oz) w. Mayo.	460	18	44
Turkey Breast (5 oz) w. Mustard	360	7	44
Turkey Club w. Bacon, Mayo.	830	38	31
Vegetarian w. Avocado, Cheese	820	49	72

7-Eleven: *Page 244*
Schlotzsky's: *Page 246*
Subway: *Page 257*

Wraps & Roll-Ups | C | F | Cb

Average All Types
(Meat/Chicken/Fish/Veggie)

	C	F	Cb
Small size, approx. 9 oz	500	25	48
Regular, approx. 15 oz	830	40	80
Large, approx. 22 oz	1400	70	134

Fast-Foods Restaurants: *Page 182*
Au Bon Pain: *Page 185*
Sonic Drive-In: *Page 251*
Subway: *Page 257*
WAWA: *Page 266*

Updated Nutrition Data ~ www.CalorieKing.com
Persons with Diabetes ~ See Disclaimer (Page 24)

Fair & Carnival Foods

	C	F	Cb
Mexican			
Burritos w. Bean/Beef, 17 oz	1100	41	104
Carne Asada, 14.5 oz	820	44	58
Fish Tacos, 1 taco, 5 oz	270	13	31
Nachos w. Cheese, 9" plate	860	59	70
Taco Chicken, 3.3 oz	210	12	16
Tamale (1), 3.5 oz	180	8	21
Taquitos, 5 oz	370	17	43
Greek			
Baklava, 2" square	245	13	32
Falafel, 11.6 oz	660	27	85
Greek Salad, 14 oz	520	48	17
Gyros, 7.5", 12 oz	680	40	55
Spanakopita, 8 oz	200	7.5	23
Italian			
Garlic Bread, ½ loaf, 10 oz	1135	40	147
Pizza Bread, Pepperoni, ½ loaf, 12 oz	1115	32	151
Pizza on a Stick, 1 piece	535	28	55
Personal Pizza, 7": Cheese (1)	670	24	80
Pepperoni (1)	795	35	80
Ham & Pineapple (1)	800	31	87
Low Carb			
Beef Patty, wrapped in lettuce, 4 oz	480	33	0
Sandwiches: *Per 7½" Roll*			
Ham, 11 oz	645	39	47
Hot Pastrami, 9 oz	760	17	62
Roast Beef, 11 oz	620	36	46
Philadelphia Cheese Steak, 13 oz	680	36	49
Tuna, 12 oz	830	60	46
Turkey, 11 oz	665	24	65
Veggie, 11 oz	490	23	49
Oriental: Fried Egg Roll, 6 oz	400	19	44
Rice Bowl: Beef, 6" Bowl	880	13	136
Chicken, 6" Bowl	870	15	135
Hamburgers			
⅓ Pound Burger, 7.5 oz	670	41	26
Cheeseburger, 6 oz	550	36	25
Hot Dogs/Franks: *With Bun*			
Hot Dog: Regular, (1)	215	14	28
with Chili, 6 oz	450	32	32
with Chili & Cheese, 7.3 oz	500	36	31
⅓ Pound Hot Dog	550	41	31
Foot Long Hot Dog	470	26	41
Corn Dog: Regular, 4 oz	250	14	23
Jumbo, 6 oz	375	21	36
Jumbo Franks w. Bun:			
Bratwurst; Sausage; Kielbasa, avg.	800	60	28

Fair & Carnival Foods (Cont)

	C	F	Cb
Barbeque Items *(Weights with Bone)***:**			
Chicken, 15 oz	740	24	34
Corn on the Cob, 8" (1), 16 oz	200	1	42
Pork Ribs, 18 oz	1360	68	21
Smoked Turkey Legs (w/ skin), 19 oz	1135	54	0
Beef Stew over Rice, 2 cups	440	14	61
Cheese Curds, Breaded/Fried, Estimate *(Culver's)*, 6.7 oz	670	38	54
Potatoes & Fries			
Australian Battered Potato, 12 oz	1290	66	155
Baked Potato, 14 oz	435	0.5	100
Fries: French, 7 oz	560	24	70
Cheese Fries, 10 oz	645	38	62
Chili Fries, 10 oz	700	36	83
Chili/Cheese Fries, 13 oz	745	45	57
Curly Fries, 7 oz	620	30	78
Tasti Chips, 40 chips, 6.5 oz	780	33	117
Sweet Potato, 14 oz	405	0.5	97
Ranch Dip, 3 oz	165	14	9
Finger Foods			
Artichoke: Steamed, 6 pieces	65	0	16
Fried, 9 pieces	250	14	24
Chicken Nuggets (6)	340	17	26
Chicken Strips (4), 4.5 oz	445	21	33
Finger Steaks (2), 4 oz	400	20	26
Mushrooms, Fried, 10-12 pieces	395	26	34
Onion Rings, 3 rings	310	13	40
Onion Flower	1320	72	140
Shrimp, Fried, 10-12 pieces, 5 oz	555	30	36
Sweet Potato Strips, Fried, 4 pces	750	30	106
Zucchini, Fried, 4 slices	620	40	42
Salads/Sides			
Baked Beans, 4 oz	140	2	38
Chili, 1 cup	280	11	24
Cole Slaw, 5 oz	350	21	37
Pickle, whole (6")	30	0	8
Potato Salad, 5 oz	290	15	35
Popcorn:			
Plain: Small, 3 oz	450	24	48
Large, 6 oz	900	48	96
Kettle Corn: Small, 5 oz	600	15	110
Large, 10 oz	1200	30	220
Cakes, Donuts, Cookies			
Funnel Cake: Plain	760	44	80
Toppings: Cinn. & Sugar, 2 tsp	30	0	8.5
Apple Cinnamon, 2 oz	85	3	36
Strawberries & Cream, 2 oz	70	0	16
Cinnamon Roll, large	730	24	114
Churro, 1½ oz	165	8	21
Donuts, Jumbo Twist, 7.5 oz	905	49	109

173

Eating Out – Fair ◊ Carnival ◊ Stadium

Fair & Carnival Foods (Cont)

Cakes, Donuts, Cookies (Cont)	C	F	Cb
Fried Snicker Bar, 5 oz	445	29	42
Fried Oreos, 3 cookies	300	10	33
Fried Twinkie, 1	420	34	45
Cotton Candy, 5½ oz bag	625	0	156
Red Rope Licorice, (24"), 2 oz	200	0	46
Cream Puff, 4.3 oz	500	43	22
Puff-on-a-Stick (4), 8.6 oz	995	86	44
Strawberry Crepe, 4.3 oz	280	14	36
Choc. Dipped Strawberry, 1 pce	125	7	15
Fudge, 1.5 oz	200	11	25
Twinkie Dog (Sundae)	500	14	89
Key Lime Pie Bar, 6 oz	635	40	59
Cheesecake on a Stick, 6 oz	655	47	56
Cobbler, 5 oz	350	10	62
Soft Pretzel, 4.5 oz	340	2	70
Candied Apple, 7 oz	330	0.5	80

Ice Cream & Frozen Treats

	C	F	Cb
Dippin' Dots Ice Cream: Small, 4 oz	150	7	17
Medium, 8 oz	305	14	35
Large, 16 oz	600	28	70
Snow Cone (includes 3 oz syrup)	270	0	68
Frozen Yogurt in sugar cone, 14 oz	475	2	94
Ice Cream: Small, sugar cone, 10 oz	775	42	83
Large, sugar cone, 14 oz	935	54	96
Sherbet, 8 oz	270	4	59
Frozen Banana, choc cover, 5 oz	240	4	53

Drinks

	C	F	Cb
Lemonade, 18 fl.oz	210	0	52
Orange Julius, 20 fl.oz	490	10	96
Strawberry Julius, 20 fl.oz	430	0	98
Icee, 16 fl.oz	235	0	59
Malt, 16 fl.oz	690	33	85
Slushies, 16 fl.oz	260	0	65
Soft Frozen Lemonade, 12 fl.oz	300	0	78
Smoothies: Berry Flavors, 16 fl.oz	350	1	80

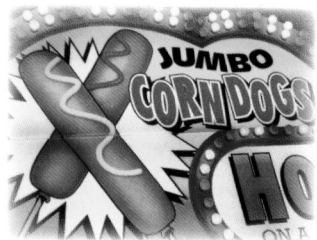

Stadium Foods

Sandwiches	C	F	Cb
Bacon Burger, 8.3 oz	470	25	34
Cheeseburger, 8.3 oz	450	23	33
Chicken Sandwich: w. Cheese, 8.3 oz	510	29	40
no Cheese, 7.7 oz	460	25	40
w. Bacon, 8.3 oz	530	31	41
Hamburger, 7.8 oz	400	19	33
Polish Sausage Sandwich, 7 oz	565	33	46
French Fries, 6.4 oz	470	34	39
Fruit Cup, 6 oz	80	0	20

Hot Dogs	C	F	Cb
Chili Dog, 7.7 oz	520	29	45
Hot Dog, 6.4 oz	465	21	50
Jumbo Dog, 6 oz	440	25	38
Kraut Dog w. Sauerkraut , 7.8 oz	490	27	41
Nachos, 40 chips w. 4 oz cheese	1100	59	132

Individual Pan Pizza (6"): *Per 10 oz Pizza*	C	F	Cb
BBQ Chicken	630	24	71
Cheese	630	27	71
Pepperoni	660	30	70

Snacks	C	F	Cb
Brownie, 2.5" x 4.5"	360	18	44
Cheese Sauce, 1.25 oz	100	8	4
Cheetos, 2.75 oz pkg	440	28	42
Chocolate Chip Cookie, 2.3 oz	280	12	40
Churros, 8", 3 oz	325	15	42
Doritos, Nacho, 2.75 oz pkg	390	20	48
King Size Candy:			
Butterfinger, 3.75 oz	485	18	75
Nestle Crunch, 2.75 oz	390	21	85
Lays Chips, 2.75 oz pkg	440	28	42
Peanuts in shell, 8 oz	930	80	24
Popcorn: Small (9 cup size)	575	35	56
Large (15 cup size)	950	58	93
Red Vines, 5.5 oz box	560	0	136
Soft Pretzel: Regular, 5.5 oz	490	3.5	101
Giant, 8 oz	710	5	147

Beverages: Orange Juice, 12 fl.oz	C	F	Cb
Beverages: Orange Juice, 12 fl.oz	180	0	2
Beer: Heineken, 16 fl.oz	200	0	16
Light Miller, 16 fl.oz	165	0	10
Miller Draft, 16 fl.oz	205	0	18
Jack Daniels Punch, 12 fl.oz	235	0	34
Wine, White, 9 fl.oz	190	0	6
Soda (with ½ ice), average: 20 fl.oz	160	0	40
32 fl.oz	260	0	65
Snow Cone, 18 oz (incl. 3 oz syrup)	270	0	68
Starbuck's Frappuccino, 12 fl.oz	195	2.5	39

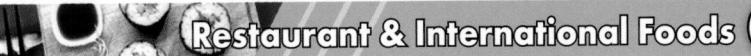
Chinese & Asian Dishes

Appetizers	C	F	Cb
Crab Cake, 2¼ oz	125	10	1
Dumplings: Pork, steamed, 1	80	4.5	5
Pork, fried, 1 dumpling	90	6	5
Vegetable, steamed, 1	35	1	5
Egg Rolls, mini, 3 rolls	100	3	11
Spring Roll: Small, 1½ oz	85	4	9
Medium, 3 oz	170	8	17
Large, 5 oz	290	15	29
Wonton, 1 only	75	4	5
Soup: Egg Flower, bowl 12 oz	90	2	16
Hot & Sour Soup, bowl 12 oz	110	3.5	14
Rice: Plain, 1 cup (½ Pint), 6½ oz	320	2	66
2 cups (1 Pint), 13 oz	640	4	132
Fried: 1 cup, 5 oz	365	11	55
Large dish, 16 oz	950	28	67
Noodles: Chinese Egg, ckd, 1 cup	200	4	37
Entrees & Mains: Per Serving			
Almond Chicken, 6 oz	270	10	21
BBQ Pork 5.5oz	440	23	15
Beef in Black Bean Sce, 8.5 oz	390	17	17
Broccoli Beef, 6 oz	370	21	13
Chicken (sliced) & Broccoli 5.5 oz	160	8	10
Chicken Skewers, 3 oz	210	9	18
Chop Suey: Chicken, 5 oz	140	9	2
Pork, 5 oz	170	12	3
Chow Mein, Beef/Chicken, 8 oz	390	12	59
Crab Puff/Rangoon, 1 dumpling	190	11	13
Crispy Fried Chicken, 8 oz	485	33	12
Egg Drop Soup: w. Noodles, 1 cup	110	3	16
w/out Noodles, 1 cup	60	3	4
Egg Foo Yung w. Sauce, 1 cup	270	15	16
Kung Pao Chicken, 5.5 oz	240	15	12
Lemon Chicken, 5 oz	525	21	57
Lo Mein (stir-fried) 8 oz	705	42	49
Moo Shu Chicken (2)	360	19	25
Omelet, Chicken/Shrimp, 16 oz	990	82	10
Orange Chicken, 5.5 oz	500	27	42
Steamed Whole Fish, ½ sockeye salmon	646	36	23
Sweet & Sour: Fish, 20 oz	1160	58	106
Pork, 5.5 oz	400	23	35
Vegetable Combination, w. oil, 6 oz	367	5	66
Vegetables, Steamed, no oil, 6 oz	137	1	29
Sauces: Mandarin Sauce 1.5 oz	70	0	17
Potsticker Sauce 1.5 oz	35	0	8
Bubble Tea, average, 12 fl oz	280	0.5	68
Fortune Cookie: each	32	0.5	7

Cajun & Creole

	C	F	Cb
Alligator, 4 oz cooked	160	2	0
Baked Herb Chicken, 1 serving	850	53	2
Bouillabaisse	400	15	10
Cajun Fried Turkey, 1 serving	630	25	0
Cocktail Sauce, 2 Tbsp	30	0	6
Couche-couche, ½ cup	80	0	17
Crawfish Bisque, 1 serving	500	10	10
Crawfish, cooked, 2 oz	45	0.5	0
Creole Jambalaya, 1 serving	550	30	15
Frog Legs, steamed (2)	45	0	0
Guinea Fowl, flesh, 4 oz, ckd	160	4	0
Hogshead Cheese, ¼ cup	80	5.5	0
Jambalaya, Shrimp & Crabmeat	520	14	12
Red Beans & Rice, 1 serving	400	17	52
Roasted Quail, w. Bacon on Toast	550	25	15
Remoulade Sauce, 2 Tbsp, 1 oz	110	11	2
Shrimp Creole, 1 serving	450	20	10
Stuffed Smothered Steak, w. 1 cup Rice	890	50	50
Turtle, cooked, 3 oz	120	3	0

Cuban

	C	F	Cb
Bl. Beans w. Rice (Moros con Cristianos)	510	22	76
Black-Eyed Pea Fritters (Bollitos de Carita)	80	5	6
Casserole Corn Tamale	445	20	55
Chkn w. Yellow Rice (Arroz con Pollo)	925	49	87
Cuban Bread (Pan Cubano)	80	1.5	15
Donuts in Syrup (Bunuelos)	170	5	10
with Melado	100	5	10
Grilled Plantains	145	0	40
Gypsy's Arm Cake (Brazo Gitano)	260	18	42
Roast Pork S'wich (Pan con Lechon)	640	30	62
Seasoned Beef w. Olives & Raisins (Picadillo)	435	36	10
Shredded Beef (Ropa Vieja)	550	35	10
Taro Root Mash (Pure de Malanga)	315	3	69
Yuca with Citrus Garlic Dressing (Yuca con Mojo)	190	9	25

French Foods

	C	F	Cb
Blanquette d'Agneau (Lamb Stew)	800	30	17
Brioche, 1 cake	280	14	34
Bouillabaisse (Fish Stew)	400	15	10
Coq au Vin (Chicken in Wine)	800	30	16
Coquilles St. Jacques	320	13	36
Crème Brulée, 1 serving	460	40	21

Restaurant & International Foods

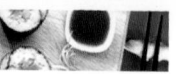

French Foods (Cont)

	C	F	Cb
Baguette, 3 slices, 2.2 oz	150	1	35
Creme Caramel (Caramel Custard)	260	10	38
Crepe Suzette, 1x6" crepe w. sauce	220	10	13
Duck a l'Orange	780	35	47
Escargot (Snails), garlic butter (6)	200	10	4
Frog Legs, fried, 4 med. pairs	400	20	10
Lamb Noisettes, fried, 2 chops	500	40	1
Potage Creme Crecy (Carrot Soup)	360	18	14
Salade Nicoise (Tuna/Oliv./Veg.)	450	13	14
Veal Cordon Bleu (Veal/Ham/Ch)	650	25	18
Vichyssoise (Pot./Leek Soup), 1 c.	200	9	15
Baguette & French Stick: *Page 56*			
Croissants: *Pages 136, 172, 205*			

German

	C	F	Cb
Bavarian Bread Dumpling, 3 small	330	10	28
Beef Goulash with Veggies	520	20	46
Black Forest Cake, 1 slice	380	16	30
Bratwurst, grilled, 1 medium, 6 oz	450	37	2
Chicken: Fried, Viennese-style	530	20	28
Livers w. Apple/On., 6 oz	460	28	10
Herring, Pickled: Rollmops, 4 oz	260	16	3
with Sour Cream, 4 oz	310	20	3
Hot Sausage Curry	300	7	6
Kugelhupf Cake, 1 lge slice, 4 oz	400	23	40
Sauerbraten Pork (Pot Roast)	650	35	15
Torte: Linzer (Alm./Raspb. Jam)	430	18	58
Sacher (Choc./Apricot Jam)	260	12	23
Weiner Schnitzel, 1 medium	750	35	38

Greek

	C	F	Cb
Baklava Pastry: Small	240	13	32
Large, 3¾ oz	400	21	45
Calamari, deep fried, 1 cup	300	13	17
Chicken Kebob Plate	345	13	8
Dolmades (Stuffed Grape Leaves)			
2 rolls, 6 oz	200	5	13
Galactobureko, 1 only			
(Filo, Custard, Pastry in Syrup)	360	15	48
Greek Chicken Salad	400	18	9
Gyros: 6" Pita, 8 oz	475	32	35
7½" Pita, 12 oz	680	40	55
Hummus & Pita, 4 oz	260	12	30
Kataifi, (Filo, Nut, Pastry in Syrup)	350	11	56
Moussaka: Small serving, 8 oz	350	22	22
Large serving, 16 oz	700	44	44
Soup: Avgolemono (Egg Lemon Soup			
with Chicken & Rice), 1 cup	85	6	5
Souvlaki (Lamb), each, 2 oz	120	6	1

Greek (Cont)

	C	F	Cb
Stuffed Tomatoes, 2 only	250	12	17
Taramosalata, 1 Tbsp, ½ oz	40	3	2
Tyropita (Filo/Egg/Cheese Pastry)	350	26	31
Tzatziki (Cucumber/Yog. Dip), 1 oz	40	2	2
Daphne's Greek Cafe: *See Fast-Foods Section*			

Hawaiian

	C	F	Cb
Ahi Tuna, grilled (6 oz fillet), no fat	220	2	0
Chicken Long Rice, 1 cup, 7 oz	240	14	12
Gyoza, 1 only	55	2	6
Haupia (Coconut Pudd.), 1 pce (4"x 2½")	120	6	17
Hawaiian Sweet Bread, ½" sl., 2 oz	180	4.5	29
Kalua Chicken, 4 oz	280	16	0
Pork, 4 oz	350	24	0
Kim Chee (pickled cabbage), ½ c., 4 oz	20	0	5
Kulolo (Taro Pudding), 1 slice	125	5	19
Lau Lau: Chicken (1) 7 oz	280	21	3
Pork (1) 7 oz	320	26	5
Loco Moco (rice/burger/egg/gravy)	650	27	63
Lomi Salmon, ¼ cup, 4 oz	20	1	2
Malasadas (Donut), 2 oz	240	13	26
Manapua (Char Siu Pork Bun), 2.3 oz	180	8	25
Poi (mashed ckd taro), 1 c., 8½ oz	270	0.5	65
Poke, avg all types, 3 oz	90	1	0
Portuguese Sausage, 2 oz	180	15	2
Potato Salad, ½ cup, 5 oz	170	10	17
Shave Ice *(Matsumoto),* all flavors:			
w. Icecream, 1 large	300	4	64
w. Beans, 1 large	290	0	72
Spam Musubi: w. Regular Spam	265	11	34
(4 oz rice+1.3 oz Spam/7-Eleven Hawaii)			
Homemade: w. Lite Spam (50% less fat)	220	5	34
Taro Pancake Mix, ⅓ cup (makes 2)	140	2	26
Plate Lunches:			
Chicken Katsu (9 oz) w. 2 scp Rice	1110	48	108
+ Macaroni Salad, ¾ cup	1360	68	123
or Tossed Salad + Fr. Dress. (2 T.)	1240	61	111
Hamburger (5 oz) w. 2 scoops Rice	710	24	81
Gravy + Macaroni Salad	1135	49	112
MahiMahi (7 oz) w. 2 scoops Rice	650	12	90
+ Macaroni Salad + Tartar Sce	1150	58	109
or Macaroni Salad, no Tartar Sce	935	34	108
or Tossed Salad + Fr. Dress. (3 T.)	815	27	96
or Tossed Salad, no dressing	670	12	93
Teri Beef (5 oz) w. 2 scoops Rice	790	23	94
+ Macaroni Salad, ¾ cup	1095	47	113
or Tossed Salad, no dressing	800	23	95

Updated Nutrition Data ~ www.CalorieKing.com
Persons with Diabetes ~ See Disclaimer (Page 24)

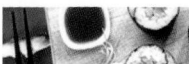

Indian & Pakistani

	C	F	Cb
Per Serving			
(Meat dishes allow 4 oz meat/serving)			
Aloo Samosa, each	155	12	12
Alu Gosht Kari (Meat/Pot. Curry)	600	40	23
Chicken Korma	500	35	6
Chicken Pilaf (Murgh Biriyani)	700	53	50
Chicken Tikka	260	16	2
Chicken Vindaloo	400	20	8
Chapati/Roti, 7" diam. piece	60	0.5	11
Dahl (Lentil Puree): 1 cup, no oil	230	1	37
1 Tbsp Tadka (oil topping)	120	13	0
Dhakla (Lentil Dish), 1" sq., 1 oz	105	5	13
Dhansak, ½ cup	105	3.5	11
Gosht Kari (Meat Curry/Tom./Pot.)	460	25	17
Lamb Pilaf	520	35	40
Lassi (Sweet or Mango), 1 cup, 8 oz	160	4	24
Masala Gosht (Beef/Tom./Gravy)	400	25	18
Mulligatawney Soup, average	300	15	8
Murgh Tikka, 1 cup	300	4	7
Naan Bread, ¼ (8" x 2"), 1 oz	75	2	11
Pappadum, 1 large/2 small	50	3	5
Pesrattu (Lentil Crepe), 9", 2.6 oz	130	5	15
Pork Vindaloo Curry w/o Rice	620	47	3
Rajmah (Kidney Bean Curry), 1 cup	225	5	35
Rogan Josh (Lamb/Yogurt Sce),			
without Rice/Potatoes	500	30	3
Shahi Korma (Braised Lamb)	430	28	3
Tandoori Chicken: Breast	260	13	5
Leg/Thigh portion	300	17	6

Italian Dishes

	C	F	Cb
Baked Ziti: Small	370	27	32
Regular	575	42	49
Breadstick (1), 2 oz	120	2.5	25
Broccoli Fettucine Alfredo, reg.	815	23	125
Bruschetta, 2 slices	380	17	53
Calzones, average, all types	840	34	101
Cannelloni, 1 tube, 6 oz	280	15	18
Cheese Breadstick (1), 2.4 oz	180	8	20
Cheese Ravioli w. Sauce	495	17	65
Chicken Alfredo	775	29	82
Chicken Parmigiana, 11 oz	520	22	16
Chicken Scallopine, dinner	1110	71	68
Eggplant Parmigiana	900	39	78
Fettucine Alfredo: Small	525	15	80
Lunch	775	22	119
Dinner	1130	81	68
Linquine & Seafood, dinner	1130	71	79
Manicotti Formaggio	800	38	57
Meat Lasagne: Small, 10 oz	440	23	39
Large, 16 oz	700	36	60
Meat Ravioli	725	22	102
Minestrone Soup, 1 bowl	110	2	18
Penne Rustica: Lunch	1300	71	76
Dinner	1540	80	101
Ravioli, over-stuffed, average	990	67	57
Spaghetti & Meatballs:			
With Tomato Sauce: Kids	500	20	58
Medium/Lunch	1080	63	89
Large/Dinner	1430	81	119
With Meat Sauce: Kids	550	25	56
Medium/Lunch	1300	79	84
Large/Dinner	1700	103	110
Veal Marsala, dinner	1320	66	132
Veal Parmigiana, dinner	1270	65	116
Vegetable Primavera	610	8	116
Macaroni & Cheese ~ *Page 135*			
Panini S'wich (Restaurant):			
Chicken, 16 oz	900	38	81
Meats, avg., 18 oz	940	39	81
Vegetarian, 15 oz	750	31	83
Pizza: Ready-To-Eat ~ *Page 137*			
Gourmet Deep Dish (*Gino's East*) ~ *Page 209*			
Desserts: Lemon Ice	180	0	45
Gelato: Vanilla (Milk Base), ½ cup	200	15	18
Choc. Hazelnut (Milk), ½ cup	370	29	26
Water Base, ½ cup	100	0	25
Tiramisu, 1 piece, 5 oz	400	29	30
For more listings see Fast-Foods Section			

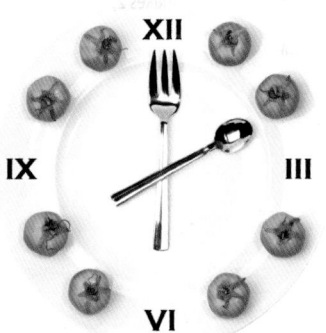

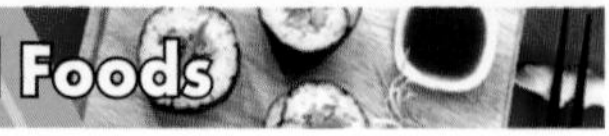

Japanese

	C	F	Cb
Sushi Rice: cooked, 1 Tbsp	**25**	0	5
1 cup, 5¼ oz	**380**	3	82
Sushi (Maki) Rolls: *Per Piece*			
Average all types (California Rolls; Crm Cheese w. Crab; Eel; Salmon; Shrimp; Tuna; Yellowtail; Vegetable)			
Small (1⅛" diam. x 1⅛" high), 0.8 oz	**25**	0.5	3.5
Med. (1¾" diam. x 1¾" high), 1.6 oz	**50**	1	7
Large (2¼" diam. x ⅞" high), 2 oz	**60**	1.5	9
Sushi Packs: *Per Pack*			
Average all types: 6 large pces	**370**	5	55
9 medium pieces	**360**	6	60
12 small pieces	**265**	3	45
Futomaki (thick roll), 6 pieces	**380**	5	72
Hand Roll (Cone) 4 oz	**120**	2	18
Inari (rice filled soybean pocket), 4 pce	**420**	9	73
Sushi-Nigiri (fish on rice):			
average all types, 1 piece	**70**	0.5	12
Sushi Plate: Assorted, 6 pieces	**420**	3	36
Combination (Sushi & Sushi Rolls)			
2 Sushi + 6 sm. & 3 med. rolls	**400**	7	72
Sashimi (Sliced Raw Seafood/Beef)			
Ika (Squid), 4 oz	**105**	2	0
Hamachi (Yellowtail), 4 oz	**165**	6	0
Maguro (Yellowfin Tuna), 4 oz	**120**	1	0
Niku (Beef), 5 oz	**200**	10	0
Saba (Mackerel), 4 oz	**160**	7	0
Suzuki (Sea Bass), 4 oz	**110**	0.5	0
Tako (Octopus), 4 oz	**95**	1	0
Dipping Sauces: Average, 2 Tbsp	**30**	0	7
Ginger Vinegar Dressing, 2 Tbsp	**20**	0	5
Edamame (young green soybeans):			
Steamed (in pods), 4 oz	**60**	3	5
Boiled beans (no pods), 4 oz	**160**	7	12
Katsu-don Pork w. Rice	**1100**	39	141
Miso Soup w. Tofu pces, 1 cup	**85**	3	11
Seaweed Salad, 1.5 oz	**20**	2	0
Sukiyaki (Beef/Tofu/Veg.), 8 oz	**400**	24	32
Tempura (Batter-fried Shrimp & Veggies)			
3 large shrimp & veggies	**320**	18	25
1 shrimp only	**60**	4	3
Teppan Yaki (Steak, Seafood & Veggies)			
10 oz serving	**470**	30	15
Teriyaki: Beef, 4 oz serving	**350**	25	4
Chicken, 4 oz serving	**260**	9	7
Salmon, medium, 6 oz serving	**270**	8	3
Sake Wine (16% alc.), 3 fl.oz	**115**	0	7
Yakatori, 1 skewer, 2½ oz	**140**	5	1

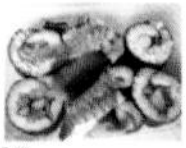

Kosher/Deli Foods

	C	F	Cb
Bagel/Bialy, 1 small, 2 oz	**160**	2	32
Beiglach (Cheese Knish)	**350**	17	35
Blintzes: Average, 1 only	**120**	1	25
w. Sour Cream. & Preserves	**370**	10	30
Borscht: (no sour cream), 1 cup	**85**	3	14
Diet/Reduced Cal., 1 cup	**30**	1	7
Cabbage Roll (meat/rice), 5 oz	**170**	6	21
Chicken Broth: 1 cup	**80**	8	0
with vegetables	**100**	8	5
with noodles	**150**	9	16
Lowfat, plain, 1 cup	**25**	1	0
Cholent, 1 med. serving, 1 cup	**350**	16	48
Chopped Liver: 1 serving, 3 oz	**110**	6	5
with Egg Salad, ¼ cup	**100**	7	3
Farfel, dry, ½ cup	**90**	0.5	21
Hallah (Yeast Bread), 1 sl., 1 oz	**85**	2	14
Gefilte Fish Balls: Reg., medium, 2 oz	**55**	2	4
with jelled broth	**80**	2	6
Cocktail size, 1 oz	**30**	1	2
Sweet, medium, 2 oz	**65**	2	4
with jelled broth	**95**	2	9
Herring: Smoked, 2 oz	**120**	8	0
in Sour Cream, 2 oz	**150**	10	0
Kasha, cooked, ½ cup	**100**	0.5	20
Kipfel (Vanilla/Almd. Cookie), 1 pce	**60**	2	7
Knaidlach ~ See Matzo Balls			
Knish: Kasha/Potato, 1 only	**130**	4	22
Cheese, 1 only	**350**	17	35
Kreplach, beef, 1 piece	**40**	1	6
Kugel, potato/noodle, 1 serving	**300**	20	25
Latkes (Potato Pancake), 2 oz	**200**	11	22
3 Latkes w. Sour Cr./Apple Sce	**750**	25	95
Lochshen: Plain, 1 cup	**130**	2	26
Pudding, 1 cup	**380**	13	48
Lox (Smoked Salmon), 2 oz	**65**	2	0
Mandelbrot (Almond Bread),			
1 slice, ¼" thick	**45**	2	5
Matzo *(See Page 90)*, 1 oz board	**110**	0.5	21
Matzo Balls: 2 small, or 1 large, 2"	**90**	3	12
Extra large ball, 3"	**180**	6	24
Matzo Ball Soup:			
Cup w. 2 small or 1 large ball	**150**	5	27
Bowl with Chicken & Noodles	**325**	13	34
Jerry's Deli, large bowl	**560**	17	56
New York Cheesecake, 4 oz	**350**	24	26
Pierogi, potato/cheese, 1 pce	**90**	4	11
Reuben S'wich w. ½ lb corned beef	**920**	60	28
Schmaltz (Rend'd chick. fat), 1 T.	**90**	10	0

Updated Nutrition Data ~ www.CalorieKing.com
Persons with Diabetes ~ See Disclaimer (Page 24)

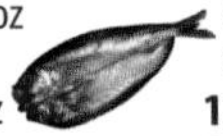

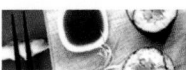

Korean Food

	C	F	Cb
Bibimbab (Veggies & Beef on Rice), 1 cup	565	15	89
Bulgogi (Barbeque Beef), 3.5 oz	325	12	15
Galbi (Short Ribs), 16 oz	975	61	16
Gujeolpan (Pancake w. Meat & Vegetables), cup w. 1 pancake	340	11	39
Japchae (Noodle w. Veggies & Meat), 1¼ cup	365	19	34
Sides:			
Kimchee (Cabbage Relish), ½ cup	30	0	6
Namool (Assorted Veggies) 1 cup	125	6.5	9
Soups: *Per Serving*			
Muguk (Radish & Chive Soup), 6 oz	105	7	6
Samgyetang (Ginseng Chicken Soup)			
no Chicken Skin, 1 cup	520	11	60
w. Chicken Skin, 1 cup	725	35	60
Yuk Gae Jang (Spicy Beef Soup), 1¼ cup	180	13	5

Lebanese/Middle East

	C	F	Cb
Baba Ghannouj, 2 Tbsp, 1 oz (Eggplant/Sesame Dip)	70	6	2
Baklava, 1 pastry, 1¾ oz (Pastry, Nuts, Syrup)	245	18	18
Cabbage Rolls, 1 roll, 3 oz (Cabbage Leaf, Meat, Rice)	100	3	12
Cous Cous, 1 serving (Semolina, Milk, Fruit, Nuts)	400	21	43
Felafel (Chick Pea Fritter):			
Fried, 1 medium, 1 oz	60	4	4
Hummus, ¼ cup, 2.2 oz	105	3	5
Fried Kibbi, 1 piece, 3 oz (Wheat, Meat, Pinenuts)	180	8	15
Kafta, 1 skewer, 1½ oz (Ground Lamb Ssg. on Skewer)	85	5	2
Kibbeh Naye, 1 cup, 9 oz (Raw Lamb, Bulgur & Spices)	450	18	28
Lebanese Omelet, 1 serving, 4 oz (Egg, Spinach, Pinenuts, Onion)	200	12	13
Pilaf, 1 cup (Rice, Onion, Rais., Apr. Spice)	400	11	60
Shawourma, 1 serving, 4 oz (Spit-Roast Beef)	280	15	2
Shish Kabob, 1 stick, 2½ oz	130	7	2
Spinach Pie, 1 piece, 3½ oz	290	21	20
Sweet Almond Sanbusak, 1 pce (Pastry, Almonds, Spices)	200	15	11
Tabouli, 1 serving, 4 oz	125	7	13
Tahini Sauce, avg., 1 Tbsp	90	8	2

Mexican

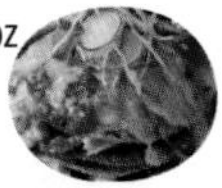

	C	F	Cb
Black Bean Soup, 1 bowl	200	3	34
Burritos *(Taco Bell):* Bean	370	10	55
Supreme® Beef	440	18	50
Chili, plain, ¼ cup	90	6	8
Chili con Carne: w. Beans, 1 cup	310	17	15
w/o Beans, 1 cup	370	28	10
Chimichangas, Beef, 5 oz	400	19	43
Chorizo Sausage, 2 oz	265	23	0
Churros, 1½ oz	150	8	18
Corn Chips, ½ c., 1 oz	160	10	17
Costillas Ribs, 6 oz	675	52	0
Enchilada, average	330	10	49
Fajitas, Chicken	200	7	20
Guacamole, avg., 2 Tbsp, 1 oz	45	4	2
Horchata: *Don Jose,* 1 cup, 8 fl. oz	140	4	25
Cacique, 1 pint bottle, 16 fl. oz	320	7	62
Margarita (w. 1½ oz Tequila)	160	0	6
Masa (Pre-mixed for Tamales), 1 oz	80	5	9
Menudo, ½ cup	55	1.5	10
Nachos: *Del Taco,* Regular	395	24	40
Macho Nachos	1145	63	113
Taco Bell: BellGrande®	760	43	80
Supreme®	470	26	42
Nachos: with cheese, peppers, 1 portion (6-8 nachos), 7 oz	600	33	60
with cheese, beans, ground beef, peppers, 1 portion (6-8 nachos), 9 oz	570	31	56
Nopal Cactus Salad, 1 serving	130	9	11
Papas Fritas (Fried Potatoes) (1), 6 oz	325	18	40
Piloncillo (Brown Sugar): 1 Tbsp, 13g	50	0	13
Cone, small, 3″, 3 oz	325	0	81
Quesadilla, Cheese *(Taco Bell)*	490	28	39
Queso Fresco, ¼ cup	80	4.5	8
Refried Beans, ¾ cup, 6 oz	160	3	26
Rice Pudding (Arroz Con Leche), 4 oz	140	3	24
Sopes (Gorditas), 2 oz	120	0	27
Taco *(Taco Bell):* Regular, Crispy	170	10	13
Ranchero Chicken	270	15	21
Taco Supreme®	220	14	14
Double Decker® Taco	340	14	39
Taco Salad w. Salsa	840	52	85
Taco Sauce, average, ¼ cup	15	0	3
Taco Shell, regular	50	2	8
Tamales, Beef/Chicken, avg, 4.5 oz	250	11	27
Taquitos, Beef & Cheese, 4.5 oz	330	15	36
Tostada *(Taco Bell)*	250	10	29
Tortilla, Corn, 6″ diam.	70	1	14
Tortilla Chips, 1 oz	150	8	18

Extra Listings of Mexican Dishes:
• **Fast-Foods Section** *(Taco Bell, Del Taco)*
• **Canned Bean/Chili Products:** *See Pages 113-118*

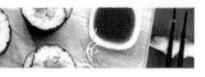
Mexican (Cont) | C | F | Cb

	C	F	Cb
Breads: Bolillos, 1 roll, 3½ oz	240	4	42
Telera, 2 oz	150	1.5	19
Mexican Cornbread, 4" square	210	11	19
Cakes, Cookies, Pastries			
Banderilla (Pastry Puff), 1 shell	140	10	8
Bigotes, 7"	570	22	44
Calvos, 2½ oz	320	18	38
Capirotada (Bread Pudding), 10 oz	810	38	107
Cinnamon Cookies, 2	125	8	13
Cocadas, 1 oz	120	6	15
Cortadillo, 1 cookie, 1.9 oz	300	11	48
Concha (All Colors):			
Small (3" diam), 2½ oz	250	8	38
Medium (4" diam), 3½ oz	350	11	53
Large (5" diam), 5½ oz	550	18	84
Cream Puff with Custard, 4¼ oz	255	14	25
Cuerno, 2 oz	200	4.5	34
Cuerno Fine, 2¾ oz	330	17	40
Donut, large, 4", 3½ oz	440	21	58
Elotes, 3½ oz	450	24	51
Empanadas (Average all types):			
Small, 2 oz	230	10	28
Regular, 3 oz	300	14	42
Fiesta Cookie, 2¼ oz	280	8	47
Galletas Mixtas (1), 1 oz	100	2.5	16
Guayaba, 3¼ oz	360	14	53
Jelly Rolls, 3¼ oz	240	4	46
Mantecadites (Almond Shortbread), 4½ oz	670	42	64
Mini Pound Cake, 3 oz	260	12	33
Mini Cupcakes, 1¾ oz	180	8	25
Muffins/Nino Enbuelto, large, 6 oz	465	11	48
Nuez, 3¼ oz	380	17	52
Ojo De Buey, 4 oz	360	15	55
Oreja (Elephant Ear), 3 oz	310	15	38
Pan Dulce (Mexican Sweet Bread), 1 bun	330	10	45
Panquecitos, 2½ oz	260	11	36
Piedras, 4 oz	470	15	76
Polvorones, 3 oz	370	18	48
Puerquitos, 5 oz	600	24	88
Rebanadas, 3½ oz	390	18	51
Roles De Canela (Cin. Roll), 4½ oz	490	15	81
Roscas, 2¾ oz	360	18	44
Semitas, 3 oz	300	10	46
Sopapillas (flaky pastry puffs), 1 pce	100	7	10
w. Honey & Cream	200	14	18
Strawberry Crema Roll (⅙), 2½ oz	240	5	45

Extra Food Listings ~ See CalorieKing.com

Polish | C | F | Cb

	C	F	Cb
Cabbage Rolls w. Sour Cr., 2 sm.	220	10	30
Chicken Casserole w. Mush., 1 cup	520	27	5
Kielbasa (Sausages, Onions, fried), 2 large	350	28	2
Meatballs in Sour Cream, 3 x 1½" balls	300	16	11
Pierogi, Fruit/Veg, 3" ball	80	2	15
Pork Goulash (Pork/Veg. Stew)	550	21	38
Pot Roast with Vegetables	630	21	28

Soul Foods | C | F | Cb

	C	F	Cb
Breakfast Sausage, fried, 2 patties	250	17	0
Brunswick Stew, 1 cup, 8.5 oz	320	14	19
Cornbread, homemade, 3 oz	200	7.5	28
Fatback, raw, ¼ oz	60	6.5	0
Ham Hock	90	6.5	2
Hog Maw	45	2.5	0
Hominy, cooked, ¾ cup	110	0.5	25
Hush Puppies, 5 pieces	260	12	35
Kale, cooked, ½ cup	20	0.5	4
Oxtail	70	3.5	0
Pig's Ear, ¼ ear	50	3	0
Pig's Foot, ½ foot	70	4.5	0
Pig's Tail, ⅓ tail	115	10	0
Poke Salad, cooked, ½ cup	16	0.5	3
Pork Brains	40	2.5	0
Pork Chitterlings, simmered, 3 oz	260	25	0
Pork Cracklings, ½ oz	80	6	0
Pork Neck Bones	65	4	0
Pork Skin, 1 cup	70	4.5	0
Pork Tongue, ⅓ tongue	75	5.5	0
Possum	65	3	0
Sousemeat	60	4.5	0
Succotash, ½ cup	80	1	17
Sweet Potato Pie, ⅛ of 9" pie	250	12	34
Tripe, 2 oz	55	2	0
Vienna Sausage, 2 small	90	8	1
small	45	4	0.5

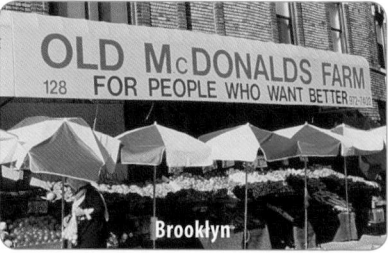

Brooklyn

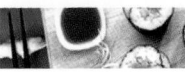

Spanish

	C	F	Cb
Arroz Abanda (Fish with Rice)	340	8	31
Arroz Con Pollo (Rice/Chick. Sal)	500	23	50
Clams Marinara, 8 clams	330	16	22
Cochifrito (Lamb w. Lemon/Garlic)	650	25	5
Cochinillo Asado, 2 sl. (Rst Suckling Pig)	300	15	3
Cocido Madrileno (Madrid-Style Boiled Dinner)	450	27	18
Flan de Leche (Caramel Custard)	325	9	52
Fritadera de Ternera (Sauteed Veal)	450	27	2
Gazpacho, 1 bowl	60	0	15
Paella a la Valenciana (Chicken & Shellfish Rice)	900	42	70
Pollo a la Espanola (Chicken)	475	30	4
Ternera al Jerez (Veal w. Sherry)	660	29	6
Zarzuela (Fish & Shellfish Medley)	530	27	40

Thai Foods

	C	F	Cb
Appetizers: Satay Pork, 1 oz	100	4	2
Spring Roll, 1¼ oz	110	6	13
Soups: Tom Yam (Hot & Sour):			
Spicy Shrimp/Seafood, 1 cup	100	4	6
1 bowl	160	7	10
Vegetarian, 1 cup	50	0	11
Curries: Chicken w. Ginger, 1 cup	390	34	4
Thick Red Curry w. Beef, 1 cup	600	50	7
Thai Chicken Curry, 1 cup	340	23	4
Massaman Curry, 1 cup	680	57	8
Green Curry w. Pork, 1 cup	480	44	5
Pad Thai, Large serving, 18 oz	990	38	125
Fish: Steamed w. Spicy Thai Sce	450	8	46
Crispy Fried, 5 oz	290	15	9
Spicy Chicken (w. veggies), stir-fry	450	22	14
Spicy Garlic Tofu w. veggies, stir-fry	340	18	18
Sticky Thai Rice: Plain 1 cup, 6 oz	170	0.5	36
w. Coconut & Sesame Seeds, 1 cup	880	28	120
Stir-fried Rice Noodles, 1 c., 5½ oz	270	9	40
Stir-fried Vegetables, 1 cup	100	3	18
Salads: Green Papaya Salad	160	0	40
Spicy Prawn, 9 shrimp	170	3	15
Thai Chicken, 1 serving	330	9	17
Thai Beef Salad, 1 serving	260	9	15
Thai Noodle, 1 serving	410	13	45
Satay Chicken & Peanut Sauce:			
1 satay stick	390	24	20
Sauces: Peanut Satay, ½ cup, 4 oz	160	10	13

Vietnamese

	C	F	Cb
Banh Cuon (Steam Rice w. Pork), 1 roll	105	7	8
Bo Nuong (Beef Satay), 2 sticks	265	9	4
Bo Xao Dau Phong (Ginger Beef w.Onion, Fish Sce.)	750	30	10
Ca Chien Gung (Whole Snapper/Ging.)	600	16	6
Canh Chay (Veg./Tofu Soup)	80	3	13
Cari (Curry) Chicken, 1 cup	475	29	16
Cari (Curry) Chicken, w. Rice Noodle, cup curry & cup cooked noodles	660	29	60
Cari (Curry) Chicken, w. Steam Rice, cup curry & cup rice	650	29	55
Cuu Xao Lan (Curried Lamb, Veggies in Coconut)	900	40	80
Ga Chien (Crisp Chick + Plum Sce)	900	40	105
Ga Nuong (Chicken Satay + Sce)	240	10	4
Ga Xao Rau (Marinated Chicken Braised w. Veg.)	800	26	100
Gio Lua (Lean Pork Pie), ⅙ of pie	245	12	0
Goi Cuon (Cold Spring Rolls), each	60	1	7
Rau Cai Xao Chay (Stir Fried Vege.)	400	15	65
Thit Bo Vien (Beef Balls), 6 balls	225	14	2
Thit Heo Goi Baup Cai, each (Spicy Cabbage Rolls w. Pork)	200	7	11
Soup: *Per Bowl (1½ Cup)*			
Bun Bo Hue (Hot & Spicy Soup no Pork Feet	340	9	35
w. Pork Feet	830	45	35
Chicken & Rice Noodle Soup	400	3	55
Pho Bo (Beef Noodle Soup)	410	7	59
Pho Ga (Chicken Noodle Soup)	460	7	58
Pho Tai (Rare Beef & Noodle Soup)	440	7	73
Salad: *Per ½ Cup*			
Goi Du Du (Green Papaya Salad)	155	3	29
Sauce: Nuoc Cham (Hot Sauce)	5	0	1

Gourmet & Miscellaneous

	C	F	Cb
Ants Eggs/Larvae, 1 Tbsp	20	0	0
Ants, Choc. coated, 3 Tbsp	140	7	2
Bee Maggots, canned, 3 Tbsp	65	2	0
Caviar, black/red, 1 Tbsp	40	3	0
Caterpillars, canned, 2 oz	60	2	0
Frog Legs, fried, 1 pair (large)	125	7	0
Haggis, boiled, 4 oz	350	24	22
Locusts, roasted, 1 oz	35	1	0
Silkworms, raw, 1 oz	60	2	0
Snails in garlic butter, 6 large	200	10	4
Snake, roasted, 4 oz	160	6	0

Fast - Foods & *Restaurants*

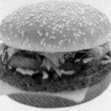

©2009
Allan Borushek
FOR MORE RESTAURANTS
See www.CalorieKing.com

For Complete Menu Listings
& Extended Nutritional Data
~ See CalorieKing.com

A&W; Applebee's	**Page 183**	Hungry Howies Pizza	**Page 213**	Round Table Pizza	**Page 241**
Arby's	184	In-N-Out Burger	213	Roy Rogers	242
Arthur Treachers	185	IHOP; Jack's	213	Rubio's Fresh Mexican Grill	242
Atlanta Bread Co.	185	Jack in the Box	214	Ruby Tuesday	242
Au Bon Pain	185	Jamba Juice; Jersey Mike's	215	Runza	243
Auntie Anne's	186	Jimmy John's; Johnny Rockets	216	Ryan's Family Steakhouse	244
Back Yard Burgers; Baja Fresh	187	KFC; Koo Koo Roo; Kolache	217	7-Eleven	244
Baskin-Robbins	188	Krispy Kreme; Krystal	218	Sammy's; Samurai Sam's	245
Big Apple Bagels	188	La Rosa's Pizzeria; La Salsa	219	Sandella's Flatbread Cafe	245
Big Boy; Blimpie	189	Little Caesar	220	Sbarro's; Schlotzsky's	246
Bob Evans	190	Lone Star	220	Shakey's; Sheetz	247
Bojangles; Boston Market	191	Long John Silver's	221	Shoney's	248
Boston Pizza	192	Macaroni Grill	221	Sizzler	249
Braum's; Bruegger's Bagels	192	McDonald's	222	Skyline Chili	250
Buck's Pizza; Burgerville	192	Manhattan Bagel	224	Smoothie King	250
Burger King	193	Max & Erma's; Mazzio's Pizza	224	Snappy Tomato	251
Captain D's Seafood	194	Mimi's Cafe; Miami Subs	225	Sonic Drive-In	251
Caribou Coffee; Carl's Jr	194	Mr. Goodcents; Mr. Hero	225	Souper Salad	252
Carvel Ice Cream; Charley's	195	Mrs Fields Cookies	226	Souplantation	252
Checkers	195	Nathan's; Noodles & Co	226	Southern Tsunami	253
Cheesecake Factory; Chevy's	195	Ninety Nine; O'Charley's	226	Spaghetti Warehouse	254
Chick-Fil-A; Chili's	196	Old Country Buffet	227	Starbucks	254
Chipotle; Church's Chicken	197	Olive Garden	228	Steak Escape; Steak 'n Shake	256
Cinnabon; Cinnamonster	198	Old Spaghetti Factory	228	Sub Station; Submariner	257
Chuck E. Cheese; Cici's Pizza	198	On The Border	229	Subway	257
Cosi; Costco; Cousins Subs	198	Orange Julius	229	Sweet Tomatoes	258
Cold Stone Creamery	198	Outback Steakhouse	229	Swiss Chalet	258
Culvers; D'Angelo's	198	Panda Express; Panera Bread	230	Taco Bell	259
Dairy Queen	200	Papa Gino's	230	Taco Cabana; Taco John's	260
Daphne's; Davanni's	200	Papa John's; Papa Murphy's	231	Taco Mayo; Target Food Court	261
Del Taco; Denny's	201	Pei Wei Asian Diner	231	Taco Time; Tacone	261
Dippin' Dots; Donato's	202	Pepe's Mexican	232	TCBY; Teriyaki Stix	262
Domino's Pizza	203	Perkin's; Peter Piper	232	Taco Maker; ThunderCloud Subs	262
Don Pablos; Dunkin' Donuts	204	P.F. Chang's; Piccadilly	233	Tim Horton's; T.J. Cinnamons	263
Eat 'N Park	205	Pita Pit	234	Togo's Eatery; Topz	264
Edo Japan; Einstein Bros	206	Pizza Hut	234	Tropical Smoothie Cafe	264
El Pollo Loco; Fatburger	207	Pizza Ranch	235	Tubby's; Una Mas	265
Fazoli's Italian Food	207	Planet Smoothie; Pollo Tropical	236	Uno Chicago Grill	265
Firehouse Subs	208	Popeye's; Port of Subs	236	Villa Pizza	265
Freshens	208	Pret A Manger	237	Vocelli Pizza	265
Frisch's; Gino's; Godfather's	209	Pretzelmaker; Pretzel Time	237	Wahoo's Fish Taco	266
Gold Star Chili; Golden Corral	209	Qdoba; Quizno's Subs	238	WAWA	266
Great American Bagel	210	Rally's Hamburgers; Ranch 1	239	Wendy's; Western Sizzlin	267
Green Burrito	210	Red Lobster; Rita's; Robeks	240	Wienerschnitzel	267
Great Steak & Potato Co	210	Rocky Rococo	241	Whataburger; White Castle	268
Haagen-Dazs; Hardee's	211	Roly Poly	241	Winchell's	269
Harvey's; Heavenly Ham	212			Yoshinoya	269
Hot Dog On A Stick	213			Zaxby's; Zero's; Zoup!	270

A&W® (Sept '09)

Burgers	C	F	Cb
Hamburger	380	19	33
Cheeseburger	420	21	37
Double Cheeseburger	680	38	44
Bacon Cheeseburger	530	30	39
Bacon Double Cheeseburger	760	45	45
Papa Burger	690	39	44
Papa Single Burger	470	25	38
Sandwiches: Crispy Chicken	550	25	52
Grilled Chicken	400	15	31
Chicken Strips: 3 pieces	500	29	32
Hot Dogs: Plain	310	19	23
Coney Chili Dog	340	20	26
Coney Chili Cheese Dog	380	23	28
Corn Dog Nuggets: 5 pieces	180	8	20
8 pieces	280	13	32
Fries/Sides:			
French Fries: Small/Kids, 2.5 oz	200	8	28
Regular, 4 oz	310	12	45
Large, 5.5 oz	430	17	61
Cheese Fries: 6 oz	390	18	50
Chili Cheese Fries, 7 oz	410	17	52
Cheese Curds, Breaded/Fried: 5 oz	570	40	27
Onion Rings: Reg., Breaded, 4 oz	350	16	45
Large, 5.5 oz	480	27	62
Dipping Sauces: BBQ, 1 oz	40	0	10
Honey Mustard, 1 oz	100	6	12
Ranch, 1 oz	160	17	2
Desserts: Per Small Serving			
Polar Swirl: M&M/Oreo, avg.	700	25	107
Reese's	740	31	97
Sundaes: Choc./Caramel/Fudge, avg	340	9	55
Strawberry	300	8	47
Soft Serve, Vanilla cone, 5.5 oz	260	7	41
Milkshakes: Strawb., small, 16 fl.oz	670	29	90
Chocolate/Vanilla, avg., 16 fl.oz	710	30	100
Medium, 20 fl.oz	890	38	123
Floats: **A&W Root Beer:** 20 oz	350	5	77
Large, 32 fl.oz	640	10	136
Diet, 20 oz	170	5	30
Freeze, A&W Root Beer, 16 oz	430	9	79
Sodas			
Sodas/Pepsi Avg.: Small, 11 fl.oz	140	0	39
Medium, 14 fl.oz	180	0	49
Large, 22 fl.oz	280	0	77
A&W Root Beer: Medium, 14 fl.oz	290	0	76
Diet, 20 fl.oz	0	0	0
Tea: Lipton Raspberry, Med., 14 fl.oz	140	0	37

Applebee's® (Sept '09)

(Author Estimates)	C	F	Cb
Appetizers/Starters			
Buffalo Chicken Wings:			
With Dressing	1025	87	15
Without Dressing	670	50	10
Boneless Buffalo Wings: w/ Dressing	1105	81	48
w/o Dressing	735	42	44
Mozzarella Sticks (9) plus dip	1005	57	72
Sandwiches & Burgers			
A1 Steakhouse Burger: w/ Fries	1545	85	134
w/o Fries	1085	60	80
Bruschetta Burger, w/o Fries	1280	90	53
California Turkey Club: w/ Fries	1255	72	100
w/o Fries	820	49	49
Cheeseburger: w/ Fries	1000	51	89
w/o Fries	720	37	50
Cowboy Burger: w/ Fries	1450	80	111
w/o Fries	1100	64	64
Fire Pit Bacon Burger: w/ Fries	1235	79	78
w/o Fries	855	59	33
Surf 'N Turf Burger w. Russian Dress:			
w/ Fries	1290	73	102
w/o fries	820	48	46
Entree Meals: Includes Sides/Sauce			
Cajun Lime Tilapia			
w. Rice Pilaf & Vegetables	380	7.5	40
Cheddar-Jack Mac & Cheese			
w. Chicken & Toasted Bread	1000	39	83
Chicken Broccoli Alfredo Bowl			
w. Toasted Side Bread	1515	98	115
Chop Steak			
w. Vegetables & Mashed Potatoes	985	59	50
Fiesta Lime Chicken w. Sides	1110	58	91
Applebee's Riblets:			
w/ Fries & Cole Slaw	2225	151	93
w/o Fries & Cole Slaw	1610	116	25
Fajitas: *Includes 4 Tortillas*			
Chicken	1150	58	97
Steak	1165	60	99
Flour Tortilla 8", each, 1.6 oz	145	3	25
Salads: Full Serving with Dressing			
Apple Walnut Chicken Salad	1165	92	26
Grilled Shrimp 'N Spinach	940	74	30
w/o Bacon Vinaigrette	465	31	13
Oriental Chicken Salad	985	67	37
Sizzling Fajitas: Includes 4 Tortillas			
Average all types	1900	76	174
Flour Tortilla (8"), each, 1.6 oz	145	3	25
Soup, French Onion Soup	150	8	10
Cakes/Desserts: Per Serving			
Sizzling Apple Pie w. Ice Cream	1085	56	146
Triple Chocolate Meltdown Cake	725	31	107

Arby's® (Sept '09)

Roast Beef Sandwiches: *W/o Mayo*	C	F	Cb
Roast Beef Sandwich:			
Regular, 3 oz beef	320	14	34
Medium, 5 oz beef	415	21	34
Large, 7 oz beef	550	28	41
Super, 3 oz beef	400	19	41
Beef 'n Cheddar Sandwich: Reg.	440	20	43
Medium	540	27	44
Large	660	36	46
Roastburger: All American	420	18	46
Bacon Cheddar	440	18	44
Bacon Bleu	470	23	44
Chicken Sandwiches:			
Chicken Bacon & Swiss: Crispy	540	23	50
Roast	440	16	40
Chicken Fillet: Crispy	480	23	47
Roast	380	16	37
Melts:			
Arby's Melt, w/o Arby's Sauce	300	12	36
Ham & Swiss Melt, w/o Horsey Sce	280	6	35
Market Fresh Sandwiches:			
Corned Beef Reuben	610	33	55
Pecan Chicken Salad	870	47	92
Roast Ham & Swiss	690	31	75
Roast Turkey & Swiss	710	30	74
Roast Turkey Ranch & Bacon	820	38	74
Ultimate BLT	780	45	75
Toasted Subs:			
Classic Italian	600	27	61
French Dip & Swiss	510	16	63
Philly Beef	590	26	59
Turkey Bacon Club	580	21	60
Regular Combos: Includes Med. Fries & 22 fl.oz Pepsi			
Beef 'n Cheddar Sandwich	1150	49	159
Chicken Bacon & Swiss Crispy	1250	52	166
Chicken Fillet Sandwich, Roast	1090	45	153
Corned Beef Reuben Sandwich	1320	62	171
Pecan Chicken Salad Sandwich	1580	76	208
Popcorn Chicken, large	1120	47	150
Roast Turkey & Swiss Sandwich	1420	59	190
Market Fresh Chopped Salads: w/o Dressing			
Farmhouse Crispy Chicken	390	19	26
Italian	430	31	11
Turkey Club	250	12	10
Sides & Sidekickers:			
Cheddar Fries, Medium	550	33	62
Curly Fries, Small, 3.7 oz	360	21	24
Medium, 5.5 oz	500	29	58
Large, 6.7 oz	600	36	70
Jalapeno Bites, 5 bites	310	21	29
Loaded Potato Bites, 5 bites	350	22	27
Mozzarella Sticks, 4 sticks	430	28	38
Potato Cakes, 2 cakes	250	18	26

Popcorn Chicken:	C	F	Cb
Regular, 4.5 oz	330	15	27
Large, 6.5 oz	410	18	34
Kids Menu: Curly Fries, 2.3 oz	230	14	27
Popcorn Chicken	240	11	20
Jr Roast Beef Sandwich, w/o Mayo	270	9	34
Breakfast: Per Serving			
Blueberry Muffin, 3 oz	320	12	49
Biscuits: Plain	275	15	28
Bacon, Egg & Cheese	460	30	30
Ham, Egg & Cheese	445	26	31
Sausage, Egg & Cheese	555	40	30
Croissants: Plain	190	10	21
Bacon & Egg	335	22	23
Ham & Cheese	280	15	22
Sausage & Egg	435	32	23
French Toastix, 4.4 oz	310	13	44
Sourdoughs: Bacon, Egg & Cheese	435	21	40
Egg & Cheese	390	17	40
Ham, Egg & Cheese	440	19	41
Sausage Egg & Cheese	555	33	40
Wraps: Bacon, Egg & Cheese	515	29	50
Sausage, Egg & Cheese	690	45	50
Sauces: Arby's, 1 packet, 0.5 oz	15	0	4
Cheddar Cheese, 0.7 oz	25	2	2
Horsey, 0.5 oz	60	5	3
Marinara, 1.5 oz	30	2	4
Spicy Three Pepper, 0.5 oz	20	1	3
Tangy Southwest, 1½ oz	250	26	3
Mayo Packet, ½ oz	105	11	0
Dipping Sauces: BBQ, 1 oz	45	0	11
Bronco Berry, 1½ oz	90	0	23
Buffalo, 1 oz	10	1	2
Honey Mustard, 1 oz	130	12	6
Desserts:			
Turnovers: Apple with Icing	380	17	64
Cherry Turnover with Icing	380	16	64
Shakes: 17 fl.oz			
Chocolate; Jamocha; avg.	645	17	109
Vanilla	550	17	83
Drinks:			
Iced Fruit Tea: Mandarin Peach, 20 fl.oz	90	0	23
Passion Fruit, 20 fl.oz	100	0	25
Mountain Dew; Pepsi, 16 fl.oz, av.	160	0	43
Sweet Tea, 16 fl.oz	120	0	32

184

Arthur Treachers® (Aug '09)

Meals: With Triple Chips

	C	F	Cb
Boats: Chicken, 9.8 oz	520	33	53
Fish, 10.2 oz	560	29	57
Shrimp, 9.8 oz	610	29	72

Sides: Per Ala Carte Serving

	C	F	Cb
Baked Potato, 8 oz	210	0	48
Batter Dip't Chkn, 2.6 oz	190	6	26
Batter Dip't Fish, 3.7 oz	260	7	35
Chips: 1 Regular, 6.5 oz	370	20	46
1 Triple, 15 oz	850	45	105
Cole Slaw, 3.5 oz	140	9	15
Hushpuppies, 6 pieces, 7 oz	830	30	127
Onion Rings, 1 regular, 4.6 oz	260	1.5	56

Atlanta Bread Co® (Sept '09)

Sandwiches

	C	F	Cb
Chicken Salad on Sourdough	440	19	42
Honey Maple Ham on Honey Wheat	410	5	64
Kid's Peanut Butter & Jelly on French	550	15	89
Kid's Grilled Cheese on French	390	15	46
Turkey Bacon Rustica on Ciabatta	960	56	62
Tuna Salad on French	630	33	57
Turkey on Nine Grain	370	6	50
Veggie on Nine Grain	500	25	52
Signature Sandwiches On Focaccia			
Bella Chicken	610	38	34
California Avocado	930	50	98
Chicken Waldorf	450	29	26
ABC Special	750	38	57
NY Hot Pastrami	660	29	59
Paninis: Chicken Pesto	710	26	80
Chicken Cordon Bleu	670	19	80
Cubano	650	19	80
Italian Vegetarian	570	16	84
Turkey Club	710	24	81

Salads: Without Dressing

	C	F	Cb
Caesar	150	9	7
Balsamic Bleu Salad	330	18	35
Chopstix Chicken	240	10	22
Greek Salad	240	16	15
House Salad	90	2	13
Salsa Fresca Salmon Salad	560	29	40

Soups: Per 1¼ Cup

	C	F	Cb
Broccoli Cheese	250	17	14
Chicken & Sausage Gumbo	190	6	24
Chili, Beef/Frontier, avg	290	10	30
Tomato Fennel & Dill	290	23	18
Wisconsin Cheese	290	15	24

For Extra Menu Items ~ see CalorieKing.com

Au Bon Pain® (Sept '09)

Bagels: Per Bagel

	C	F	Cb
Asiago Cheese	340	6	56
Cinnamon Crisp	410	7	27
Everything	340	5	61
Jalapeno Double Cheddar	340	10	52
Honey 9 Grain	350	4	69

Cream Cheese Spreads: Per 2 oz

	C	F	Cb
Lite Cream Cheese	120	9	5
Honey Pecan, 2.5 oz	200	16	10
Vegetable	170	16	3

Breakfast Sandwiches

	C	F	Cb
Egg on a Bagel	360	4	60
with Bacon	420	8	60
with Bacon & Cheese	510	16	61
with Cheese	450	10	61
Prosciutto & Egg	520	16	60
Salmon & Wasabi	430	11	64

Croissants, Filled: Almond

	C	F	Cb
Almond	600	38	55
Apple	270	11	44
Chocolate	430	22	58
Raspberry Cheese	360	17	46
Spinach & Cheese	290	16	28

Café Sandwiches

	C	F	Cb
Arizona Chicken	690	28	60
Baja Turkey	650	24	68
BBQ Brisket	660	21	81
Caprese	680	32	65
Chicken Pesto	650	23	65
Mozzarella Chicken	680	24	66
Spicy Tuna	470	16	60

Hot Sandwiches and Melts

	C	F	Cb
Steakhouse on Ciabatta	710	30	73
Tuna Melt	670	29	68
Turkey Melt	780	32	77
Wraps: Chicken Caesar Asiago	610	28	61
Mediterranean Wrap	610	29	73
Southwest Tuna	750	44	66
Thai Peanut Chcken	530	17	79

Harvest Rice Bowls:

	C	F	Cb
BBQ Brisket	790	19	118
w/ Brown Rice	740	21	103
BBQ Chicken	690	11	120
w/ Brown Rice	650	12	105
Mayan Chicken	560	12	87
w/ Brown Rice	510	13	73

Breads

	C	F	Cb
Artisan Honey Multigrain Baguette	340	5	66
Bread Bowl (1)	620	3	123
Farm House Rolls (1)	350	7	60
Focaccia (1)	360	7	62
Rosemary Garlic Breadstick	190	5	31

Au Bon Pain® cont... (Sept '09)

	C	**F**	**Cb**
Soups: Per Medium 12 oz Bowl			
Baked Stuffed Potato	350	20	29
Carrot Ginger	140	5	22
Chicken Gumbo	180	8	21
Corn & Green Chili Bisque	260	15	27
Cream of Chicken & Wild Rice	240	14	22
Italian Wedding	170	7	19
Southern Black-Eyed Pea	170	2	29
Southwest Vegetable	170	5	28
Tomato Florentine	170	4	25
Vegetarian Black Bean	260	1	46
Wild Mushroom Bisque	190	9	22
Macaroni & Cheese: Kids, 6 oz	250	14	18
Medium, 12 oz	500	29	36
Salads: Per Container			
Chef's Salad, 8.9 oz	240	15	8
Chickpea, Tom. & Cucumber, 10.6 oz	230	12	23
Garden Salad, 7 oz	70	2	12
Grilled Chicken Asiago, 8.5 oz	300	13	18
Mandarin Sesame Chicken, 9.7 oz	310	17	29
Mediterranean Chicken, 10.3 oz	290	16	12
Smoked Turkey Cobb, 11 oz	330	19	15
Thai Peanut Chicken, 11 oz	240	8	19
Tuna Garden, 10.5 oz	240	12	15
Turkey & Strawberry, 8.9 oz	110	4	11
Dressing: Hazelnut Vinaig., 2 oz pkg	270	25	11
Sesame Ginger	230	20	12
Cookies: Blondie (1), 4 oz	460	33	59
English Toffee (1), 1.6 oz	230	13	26
Palmier (1), 3.5 oz	440	23	53
Shortbread (1), 2.3 oz	310	18	34
Desserts: Apple Strudel, 4.2 oz	430	24	48
Cherry Strudel	460	26	49
Creme de Fleur	490	25	57
Muffins: Blueberry	490	17	74
Carrot Walnut	520	25	66
Cranberry Walnut	500	23	61
Low-Fat Triple Berry	290	2	67
Raisin Bran	480	11	85
Scone, Chocolate Orange Pecan	580	28	74
Cakes: Lemon Pound Cake, 5 oz	520	27	64
Banana Nut Pound Cake, 4.7 oz	520	28	60
Mint Chocolate Pound Cake, 5 oz	530	28	65
Beverages: Caffe Latte, 16 fl.oz	260	14	21
Coffee Blast, 16 fl.oz	440	21	71
Froz. Watermelon Lemonade, 16 fl.oz	260	0	64
Hot Chocolate, 16 fl.oz	460	15	74
Peach Iced Tea, 22 fl.oz	240	0	61
Strawberry Smoothie, 16 fl.oz	310	1	66

For Complete Nutritional Data ~ see CalorieKing.com

Auntie Anne's® (Aug '09)

	C	**F**	**Cb**
Pretzels: With Butter			
Almond	390	6	74
Cinnamon Sugar	470	12	84
Garlic	350	5	65
Jalapeno	330	5	63
Original	340	5	63
Original Stix, 6 sticks	340	5	65
Sesame	400	10	67
Sour Cream & Onion	360	5	68
Pretzels: Without Butter			
Almond Pretzel; Whole Wheat	350	2	74
Cinnamon Sugar	380	1	84
Garlic Pretzel; Sour Crm & Onion	310	1	65
Jalapeno	300	1	63
Original	310	1	65
Original Stix, 6 sticks	310	1	65
Sesame	360	6	67
Dipping Sauces			
Caramel Dip, 1.5 oz	130	3	23
Chse Sce; Hot Salsa Chse, avg., 1.1 oz	90	7	2
Cream Cheese, 1¼ oz	80	6	1
Heated Marinara Sauce, 2 oz	20	0.5	5
Sweet Dip, 1.4 oz	130	0	32
Sweet Mustard, 1¼ oz	60	2	10
Beverages: Per Serving			
Auntie Anne's Lemonade, 21 fl.oz	260	0	66
Dutch Ice (20 fl.oz): Kiwi-Banana	220	0	53
Blue Raspberry	240	0	62
Lemonade	300	0	76
Mocha	390	12	73
Orange Creme	270	0	69
Pina Colada	300	0	73
Strawberry	230	0	58
Wild Cherry	280	0	69
Dutch Smoothie: *Per 20 fl.oz*			
Blue Raspberry	440	15	72
Kiwi-Banana	420	15	66
Lemonade	470	15	81
Mocha	540	22	79
Orange Creme	460	15	76
Pina Colada	470	15	79
Strawberry	430	15	69
Wild Cherry	460	15	76

Back Yard Burgers® (Sept '09)

Burgers	C	F	Cb
American Cheeseburger ⅓ lb	780	48	47
Back Yard Burger ⅓ lb	680	39	47
Bacon Cheddar	850	54	48
Black Jack	780	49	48
Bleu Cheeseburger: ⅓ lb	780	47	47
⅔ lb	1270	86	47
Cheddar Cheeseburger: ⅓ lb	790	48	47
⅔ lb	1290	88	47
Jr Burger	530	27	47
Mushroom Swiss	790	49	45
Pepper Jack, ⅓ lb	740	45	47
Swiss Cheeseburge: ⅓ lb	790	48	47
⅔ lb	1290	88	47
Chicken Sandwiches			
Blackened Chicken	540	24	53
Crispy Chicken	590	26	65
Grilled Chicken	350	4.5	47
Hawaiian Chicken	450	11	59
Specialities: Big Dog	500	33	32
Bak-Pak: Chicken Tender Meal	1110	71	91
Dog	320	18	29
Chicken Tender Meal	1260	79	102
Chili Cheese Big Dog	630	44	34
Garden Veggie Burger	400	8	57
Sides: Per Serving			
Chili	150	9	8
Seasoned Fries: Regular, 6 oz	640	45	58
Large, 9 oz	960	68	87
Salads: Without Dressing			
Blackened Chicken	330	15	25
Fried Chicken	410	19	41
Garden Fresh	100	2	20
Grilled Chicken	220	4	23
Side Salad	30	0	6
Dressings: Per Serving			
Bleu Cheese	220	24	1
Honey Mustard	240	23	7
Ranch	150	15	2
Desserts: Per Serving			
Cobblers: Apple	360	14	59
Blackberry	290	8	51
Cherry	350	12	59
Peach	330	11	56
Shakes: Per 12 fl.oz			
Chocolate; Strawberry	560	26	79
Vanilla	540	26	71

For Complete Nutritional Data ~ see CalorieKing.com

Baja Fresh® (Sept '09)

Burritos: No Tortilla Chips	C	F	Cb
Baja Burrito: with Chicken	790	38	65
with Steak	850	46	67
Bare Burrito: with Charbroiled Chkn	640	7	97
Veggie and Cheese	580	10	101
Bean & Cheese Burrito: with Chkn	970	35	96
with Steak	1030	43	97
Vegetarian	840	33	96
Burrito Mexicano: with Chicken	790	13	117
with Steak	860	21	118
Burrito Ultimo: with Chicken	880	36	84
with Steak	950	44	85
Grilled Vegetarian	800	33	94
Fajitas			
Chicken with Corn Tortillas	860	24	105
Chicken with Flour Tortillas	1140	33	147
Nachos: with Charbroiled Chicken	2020	110	164
with Charbroiled Steak	2120	118	163
with Cheese	1890	108	163
Quesadilla: with Charboiled Chkn	1330	80	84
with Charbroiled Steak	1430	87	84
with Cheese	1200	78	84
Vegetarian	1260	78	96
Tacos: No Tortilla Chips			
Baja Fish Taco, Fried	250	13	27
Grilled Mahi Mahi Taco	230	9	26
Original Baja Style Taco: w/ Chicken	210	5	28
with Charbroiled Shrimp	200	5	28
with Charbroiled Steak	230	8	28
Salads: No Dressing or Tortilla Chips			
Baja Ensalada:			
with Charbroiled Chicken	310	7	18
with Charbroiled Shrimp	230	6	18
with Charbroiled Steak	450	18	18
Tostadas: Charbroiled Chicken	1140	55	98
Charbroiled Fish	1130	55	99
Charbroiled Shrimp	1120	55	99
Charbroiled Steak	1230	63	98
Savory Pork Carnitas	1180	62	100

For Complete Nutritional Data ~ see CalorieKing.com

Baskin Robbins® (Sept '09)

Ice Creams: Per 4 oz Scoop

	C	F	Cb
Classic Flavors: Cherries Jubilee	240	12	30
Chocolate	260	14	33
French Vanilla	280	18	26
Jamoca Almond Fudge	270	15	31
Mint Chocolate Chip	270	16	28
Old Fashioned Butter Pecan	280	18	24
Orange Sherbet	160	2	34
Oreo Cookies 'n Cream	280	15	32
Pralines 'n Cream	280	14	35
Rainbow Sherbet	160	2	34
Reese's P'nut Butter Cup	300	18	31
Very Berry Strawberry	220	11	28
World Class Chocolate	280	16	31
Premium Churned: Per 2.5 oz Scoop			
Light: Milk Chocolate	130	4.5	20
Raspberry Chip	140	4	24
Vanilla	130	4.5	19
Frozen Yogurt, Fat-Free Van., 4 oz	150	0	32
Fruit Blast Bars, all flavors, av.	50	0	14
Ice, all flavors, 4 oz scoop	135	0	34
Sorbets: Per 4 oz Scoop			
Lemon, Strawberry	130	0	34
Mango	120	0	32
Sundaes:			
Classic Sundaes: Banana Royale	620	28	87
Brownie Sundae	920	47	119
Classic Banana Split	1010	34	173
Premium Sundaes:			
Chocolate Chip Cookie Dough	990	43	138
Oreo Outrageous	1130	55	158
Reese's Peanut Butter Cup	1120	80	109
Snickers 1000		46	138
Soft Serve Sundaes: Per 10 oz Regular			
Caramel	580	21	89
Strawberry	450	18	59
Sundae Cups: Oreo	330	15	45
Peanut Butter Cup	390	24	36
Pralines 'n Cream	330	16	43
Soft Serve, '31 Below' Blends: Per 16 oz Cup			
Chocolate Oreo	1290	55	187
Fudge Brownie	1390	58	199
Heath	1160	54	151
Oreo	1000	41	143
Reese's P'nut Butter Cup	1220	67	134
Strawberry Banana	710	23	112
White Chocolate Strawberry	820	34	114
Soft Serve, Cups:			
Vanilla: Regular, 6 oz	280	11	37
Large, 9 oz	430	17	58
Kid's, 3 oz	140	6	19
Fruit Cream:			
Strawberry: Medium, 16 fl.oz	630	19	102
Large, 24 fl.oz	860	25	144
Mango/Peach: Medium, 16 fl.oz	635	18	110
Large, 24 fl.oz	880	24	154

Baskin Robbins cont... (Sept '09)

Beverages

	C	F	Cb
Freezes w. Orange Sherbet:			
Small	370	4	82
Medium	510	5	112
Large	740	8	164
Cappuccino Blast: Per Medium, 24 fl.oz			
Original	480	19	72
Original with Whipped Cream	500	21	74
Original, Non-Fat	340	0	78
Caramel	670	23	111
Mocha	610	19	104
Oreo 'n Cookies	740	29	113
Fruit Blast: Per Medium, 24 fl.oz			
Peach Passion	370	0.5	94
Strawberry Citrus	330	0	83
Wild Mango	470	1.5	116
Fruit Blast Smoothie: Per Medium, 24 fl.oz			
Mango	620	2	148
Peach Banana	540	1	131
Strawberry Banana	560	1	135
Ice Cream Soda: Per Medium			
with Vanilla Ice Cream	720	30	103
Ice Cream Float: Per Medium			
w. Vanilla Ice Cream & Root Beer	680	30	99
Milk Shakes: Per Medium, 24 fl.oz			
Choc Chip Cookie Dough	1030	42	137
Vanilla	980	45	125
Choc with Vanilla Ice Cream	990	44	131
Strawberry w. Strawb. Ice Cream	770	31	105
Cones: Cake	25	0	5
Sugar	45	0.5	9
Waffle	160	4	28

For Complete Nutritional Data ~ see CalorieKing.com

Ben & Jerry's®

Ice Cream & Frozen Yogurt ~ See Page 106
Novelty Bars ~ See Page 110

Big Apple Bagels® (Aug '09)

	C	F	Cb
Bagels: All types, avg., 5 oz	340	2	68
½ bagel, 2.5 oz	170	1	34
Choice Bagels: Per Bagel			
Blueberry Cobbler	390	8	70
Cheddar Nacho	350	6	60
Cinnamon Apple Pie	385	8	68
Cinnamon Bun	400	8	70
Cinnamon Danish	395	8	72
French Toast	370	4	74
Quiche Lorraine	355	8	54
Strawberry White Chocolate	365	4	72
Swiss Melt	370	8	68
White Chocolate Swirl	395	8	70

Big Apple cont... (Aug '09)

Cream Cheese: *Per 2 Tbsp , 1 oz*

	C	F	Cb
Plain	90	9	2
Plain, Lite	60	4.5	3
Other varieties, avg	90	8	2
Whipped: Classic Plain	70	7	1
Brown Sugar Cinnamon	70	5	5
Reduced-Fat Spring Veggie	60	5	2

My Favorite Muffin: *Per Jumbo, 5.8 oz*

Regular: Blueberry	505	24	63
Chocolate Chip	635	33	81
Cinnamon Swirl Cheesecake	640	33	84
Pumpkin Spice	545	24	78
Fat Free: Blueberry	325	0	78
Chocolate Marble	375	0	87
Cinnamon Bun	505	0	126

Sandwiches:

Big Apple Club	795	37	75
Classic Reuben, Overstuffed	960	43	57
Grilled Chicken Bruschetta Pizzaah	345	21	24
Morning Classic	485	11	73
Roast Beef Parmesan Grinder	585	15	76

For Complete Nutritional Data ~ see CalorieKing.com

Big Boy

~ Same Menu and Data as Frisch's Big Boy ~ Page 209

Biggby Coffee (Sept '09)

Hot Drinks: *Per 16 fl.oz Unless Indicated*

	C	F	Cb
Caffe Latte: with 2% Milk	175	7	16
with Non-fat Milk	115	0	16
with Soy	145	5	15
Cappuccino: with 2% Milk	105	4.5	9.5
with Non-Fat Milk	70	0	9.5
with Soy	90	3	9
Chai Latte: with 2% Milk	350	7	58
with Non-fat Milk	295	0	58
Cocoa Caramella: with 2% Milk	300	9	48
with Whipped Cream	380	15	52
Mocha Mocha: with 2% Milk	275	7.5	46
with Whipped Cream	355	14	50
Nutty Buddy, with 2% Milk, no sugar	165	7	18

Cold Drinks: *Per Tall, 16 fl.oz*

Banana/Berry Creme Freeze, av.	345	10	67
Berry Fruizen-T	335	0	84
Chai Big Chill	415	11	74
Chocolate Magic Milk	385	18	44
Mocha Big Chill	405	20	56
Original Big Chill	190	9	27

Extra Menu Listings ~ See CalorieKing.com

Blimpie® (Aug '09)

	C	F	Cb

Cold Deli Subs: *Per 6" Sub on White*

Blimpie Best, with Provolone	420	14	49
BLT, without Cheese or mayo	345	11	46
Club, with Swiss	385	10	49
Cuban, with Swiss	415	11	43
Ham & Swiss Cheese	390	10	50
Roast Beef & Provolone	410	11	47
Seafood, without Cheese	335	7	56
Tuna without Cheese	485	21	46
Turkey & Provolone	395	10	49
Wraps: Chicken Caesar	605	29	56
Steak & Onion	775	47	62
Zesty	570	26	59

Hot Deli Subs: *Per 6" Sub on White*

Meatball, with Provolone	605	32	51
Pastrami, with Swiss	435	16	42
VegiMax, with Provolone	520	20	56

Salads: *Regular*

Chef Salad	175	7	10
Macaroni Salad Side	330	22	28
Seafood Salad	120	4	17
Tuna Salad	270	18	7

Dressings & Sauces: *Per 1.5 oz*

Creamy Caesar	210	21	2
Creamy Italian	180	18	4

Soups: *Per 8.6 oz Serving*

Chicken Noodle	130	4	18
Cream of Broccoli & Cheese	190	8	15
Garden Vegetable	80	0.5	14
Harvest Vegetable	100	1	19
Minestrone	90	3	14
New England Clam Chowder	170	3	28
Cookies: Oatmeal Raisin	170	7	26
Sugar	325	17	41
Other varieties, average	195	11	22

For Complete Nutritional Data ~ see CalorieKing.com

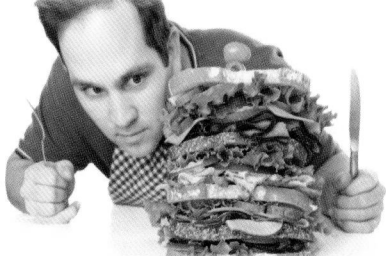

Bob Evans® (Aug '09)

Breakfast

	C	F	Cb
Country Biscuit	665	46	39
Ham & Cheese Benedict	835	53	44
Pot Roast Hash Breakfast	700	45	34
Farm Fresh Eggs: Hard Cooked (1)	55	4	1
Over Easy (1)	100	8	1
Scrambled (3)	240	16	3
Hotcake: Blueberry (1), w/o topping	345	10	58
Buttermilk (1), w/o topping	335	10	56
Omelets: Three Cheese	490	37	4
Border Scramble	620	44	16
Lite (with No Cholesterol Eggs)	440	25	15
Farmer's Market	620	43	14
Ham & Cheddar	475	33	4
Western	485	32	7
Crepes: Plain (1)	345	25	25

Sandwiches & Burgers

	C	F	Cb
Burgers: Bacon Cheeseburger	720	38	35
Cheeseburger	650	31	35
Hamburger	540	22	34
Sandwiches: Fried Chicken Club	635	31	47
Bob-B-Q Pulled Pork	600	25	67
Grilled Chicken Club	585	31	34
Grilled Chicken, plain	440	19	34
Pot Roast	555	26	51
Turkey Bacon Melt	590	28	47

Dinners: As Served

Beef:

	C	F	Cb
Pot Roast Beef Stew, 20 oz	725	34	67
Steak Tips & Noodles, 27.8 oz	945	54	50
Steak Tips Stir-Fry, 31.6 oz	1010	43	87

Chicken:

	C	F	Cb
Chicken-N-Noodles: Deep-Dish	785	38	66
Slow-Roasted, 11 oz	290	16	23
Chicken Parmesan, 25 oz	690	28	65
Chicken Stir-Fry, 27 oz	635	20	78
Fried Chicken Strips (1), 1.5 oz	135	8	10
Grilled Chicken Breast, 4½ oz	250	14	0
Garlic Butter Grilled Chkn Breast	240	14	1
Turkey, Slow-Roasted Turkey, 4 oz	135	5	1
Fish: Pot.-Crusted Flounder, 5 oz	220	12	9
Salmon Stir-Fry, 29½ oz	760	28	78
Wildfire Salmon, 9 oz	355	14	15

Seniors:

	C	F	Cb
Country Fried Steak: with Gravy	550	37	37
w/o Gravy, 5.3 oz	495	33	31
Chicken Parmesan, 17 oz	550	25	41
Meatloaf, 9 oz	435	22	22
Open Faced Roast Beef, 9½ oz	475	24	22

Bob Evans® (Aug '09)

Dinners (Cont)

	C	F	Cb
Pasta: Garden Vegetable Alfredo	810	48	72
Garden Veg. & Chicken Alfredo	850	46	60
Garden Veg. & Salmon Alfredo	975	54	60
Italian Sausage & Pepper	695	40	54
Vegetarian: Vegetable Stir-Fry	505	14	87
Side Dishes: Baked Potato, 10½ oz	220	3	51
Bread & Celery Dressing, 3 oz	150	8	16
Coleslaw, 3½ oz	210	14	19
Corn, 3½ oz	165	11	17
Garden Vegetables, 6½ oz	160	11	15
Glazed Carrots, 3½oz	75	3	13
Green Beans, 4 oz	45	2	6
Grilled Mushrooms, 7 oz	85	5	10
Loaded Baked Potato, 11.8 oz	390	16	53
Mashed Potatoes, 5½ oz	190	7	16
Rice Pilaf, 6 oz	135	5	21
Fries: French Fries, 4½ oz	320	13	46
Home Fries, 5 oz	185	6	28
Sauces/Condiments: Apple Sce, 4 oz	85	0	9
Beef Gravy, 2 oz	25	1	3
Chicken Gravy, 2 oz	55	4	3
Cranberries, 0.7 oz	70	0	17
Hollandaise Sauce, 1 oz	25	1	3
Marinara Sauce, 3 oz	35	1	5
Mayonnaise, ½ oz	90	10	0
Pancake Syrup, 3 oz	215	0	55
Pork-Roasted Gravy, 2 oz	65	5	3
Sour Cream, ½ oz	35	3	1
Tarter Sauce, 0.7 oz	115	12	1
Wildfire BBQ Sauce, 1 oz	60	0	15
Kid's Menu: Mac & Cheese, 6½ oz	320	11	44
Mini Cheeseburger (1)	285	15	22
Plenty-O-Pancakes, 5½ oz	335	12	52
Smiley Face Potatoes, 3 oz	270	16	29
Salads: Cobb, 14½ oz	570	37	10
Country Spinach, 11 oz	480	31	12
Cranb. Pecan Chicken, 10½ oz	675	45	38
Garden Salad, 3 oz	60	1	9
Heritage Chef Salad, 12½ oz	400	25	10
Specialty Garden Salad, 3.7 oz	125	7	10
Wildfire Grilled Chicken, 13.7 oz	440	19	37

Desserts, Pies, Sundaes

	C	F	Cb
Pie: Apple Pie, N.S.A., 1 slice	500	30	56
Coconut Cream Pie, 1 slice	530	28	64
Kids Sundae: Fudge Blast, 4 oz	215	9	31

Bojangles® (Sept '09)

Cajun & Southern Style Chicken	C	F	Cb
Breast, average	280	17	12
Leg, average	120	16	11
Thigh, average	310	23	11
Wing, average	160	25	11
Sandwiches			
Cajun Filet: no Mayo	335	11	41
w. Mayonnaise	435	22	41
Grilled Filet: no Mayo	235	5	25
w. Mayonnaise	335	16	25
Snacks: Buffalo Bites	180	5	5
Chicken Supremes, 4 pieces	335	16	26
Biscuit Sandwiches: Biscuit, plain	245	12	29
Bacon Biscuit	290	17	26
Bacon, Egg & Cheese Biscuit	550	42	27
Cajun Filet Biscuit	455	21	46
Country Ham Biscuit	270	15	26
Egg Biscuit	400	30	26
Sausage Biscuit	350	23	26
Smoked Sausage Biscuit	380	26	27
Steak Biscuit	650	49	37
Fixins': Botato Rounds	235	11	31
Cajun Pintos	110	0	18
Dirty Rice	165	6	24
Green Beans	25	0	5
Macaroni & Cheese	200	14	12
Marinated Cole Slaw	135	3	26
Potatoes, no Gravy	80	1	16
Seasoned Fries	345	19	39
Sweet Biscuits: Bo Berry	220	10	29
Cinnamon	320	18	37

For Complete Nutritional Data ~ see CalorieKing.com

Boston Market® (Sept '09)

Sandwiches & Burgers	C	F	Cb
Boston Chicken Carver	750	29	64
Boston Turkey Carver	700	26	65
Crispy Country Chicken S'wich, 14 oz	1020	42	114
Half Boston: Chicken Carver	375	15	32
Sirloin Dip Carver	450	23	31
Turkey Carver	350	13	32
Meatloaf Open-Faced	670	38	48
Roasted Sirloin Open-Faced	410	15	32

Boston Market® cont... (Sept '09)

Individual Meals	C	F	Cb
BBQ Brisket, 6.5 oz	400	20	28
Crispy Country Chicken w. Gravy, 8 oz	480	23	36
Half BBQ Chicken, 14.5 oz	730	30	28
Pastry Top Chicken Pot Pie, 15 oz	800	48	59
Meatloaf, 7.6 oz	520	36	21
Roasted Turkey, 4 oz	150	2.5	0
Salads, Entree			
Caesar Salad: w/o dressing, 6 oz	140	8	7
with 2 oz Dressing	420	38	9
with 1.5 oz Lite Ranch Dressing	210	12	15
Market Chopped Salad:			
w/o Dressing	200	10	22
with 2 oz Dressing	480	40	24
Add Extra for:			
5 oz Rotisserie Chicken	180	3	0
3 oz Roasted Turkey	110	2	0
3 oz Roasted Sirloin	160	6	0
3 oz Crispy Country Chicken	220	11	16
Sides			
Baked Beans, 7.7 oz	270	1.5	53
Caesar Salad, 2.2 oz: w/o Dressing	40	2	3
with 1 oz Dressing	180	17	4
Cinnamon-Apples, 5 oz	210	3	47
Coleslaw, 6.7 oz	300	20	27
Cornbread	180	5	31
Creamed Spinach, 6.7 oz	280	23	12
Fresh Steamed Vegetables, 4.8 oz	60	2	8
Fresh Vegetable Stuffing, 4.8 oz	190	8	25
Garlic Dill New Potatoes, 5.5 oz	140	3	24
Gravy: Beef, 3 oz	35	1.5	4
Poultry, 4 oz	50	2	7
Green Beans, 3.2 oz	60	3.5	7
Macaroni & Cheese, 7.8 oz	300	11	35
Mashed Potatoes, 7.8 oz	270	11	36
Potato Salad, 7 oz	390	29	26
Seasonal Fresh Fruit Salad, 5 oz	60	0	15
Sweet Corn, 6.2 oz	170	4	37
Sweet Potato Casserole, 7 oz	460	16	77
Soups			
Chicken Noodle, 14 oz	250	8	23
Chicken Tortilla: with toppings	410	26	30
without toppings	160	8	13
Desserts			
Apple Pie, 5.7 oz	580	30	74
Chocolate Cake, 5.1 oz	580	34	67
Choc. Chip Fudge Brownie, 2 oz	320	13	49

For Complete Nutritional Data ~ see CalorieKing.com

Fast - Foods & *Restaurants*

Boston Pizza® (Sept '09)

	C	F	Cb
Starters: Cactus Cut Potatoes/Dip	830	70	38
Boston's Pizza Bread, no sauce	500	12	84
Oven Rstd Boston's Wings	480	30	18
Soup: Baked French Onion	310	14	35
Salads: *Includes Dressing*			
Caesar Salad, starter size	210	19	7
Citrus Chicken, grilled	780	16	119
Crispy Chicken Pecan	1150	93	32
Sandwiches:			
Boston Cheesesteak	1140	49	113
Chicken Parmesan	850	45	66
New York Steak	560	34	20
Pizzas (Medium): *Per Slice*			
BBQ Chicken	190	6	25
Boston Royal	210	6	26
Bruschetta	250	11	27
Great White North	240	9	24
Hawaiian	210	5	28
Meateor	260	11	25
Rustic Italian	240	10	28
The Pepper	220	9	25
Pastas: *Full Order, Without Garlic Bread*			
Baked Seven Cheese Ravioli w. sce	490	26	34
Chicken & Mushroom Fettuccini	1460	79	139
Spicy Italian Penne	1530	88	137
Desserts: *Includes Ice Cream*			
Apple Crisp	740	19	138
Chocolate Explosion	870	49	98

For Complete Nutritional Data ~ see CalorieKing.com

Braum's® (Sept '09)

	C	F	Cb
Frozen Yogurt: Per ½ Cup			
Choc. Peanut Butter Cup	180	10	19
Other flavors, average	130	5	19
Ice Cream: Per ½ Cup			
Carb Watch: Chocolate Chip	180	10	17
Other flavors, average	155	11	17
Light: Average all varieties	130	4	19
Premium: Peanut Butter Cup	200	14	17
Other flavors, average	160	9	18

For Complete Nutritional Data ~ see CalorieKing.com

Buck's Pizza® (Sept '09)

	C	F	Cb
Pizzas (14"): Per Slice, ⅛ Pizza			
Canadian Bacon	315	9	47
Cheese	295	8	47
Pepperoni	360	14	47
Sausage	360	14	47

Bruegger's Bagels® (Sept '09)

	C	F	Cb
Bagels			
Average all flavors, 4.3 oz	330	3	65
Breakfast S'wiches: With Plain Bagel			
Egg & Cheese	420	18	71
with Bacon	460	23	65
with Ham	460	18	73
with Sausage	640	30	63
Smoked Salmon	460	10	22
Spinach & Cheddar Omelet	540	17	65
Western	760	56	66
Deli Sandwiches: Plain Bagel			
BLT	570	23	72
Chicken Salad	630	26	73
Garden Veggie	400	2.5	82
Ham	460	7	76
Roast Beef	730	39	71
Tuna Salad	620	27	73
Turkey	510	14	70
Signature & Classic Sandwiches:			
Herby Turkey, Sesame	600	14	80
Leonardo da Veggie, Asiago	590	17	83
Roma Roast Beef	770	44	62
Tarragon Chicken Salad	770	41	73
Thai Peanut Chicken	580	11	91
Turkey Chipotle Club	800	51	57
Salads: With Dressing			
Caesar	270	17	22
Chicken Caesar	370	20	23
Mandarin Chicken Medley	450	21	37
Sesame Chicken	480	28	30
Cookies: Chocolate Chip	390	17	52
Double Chocolate	390	19	51
Everything	380	18	49
Dessert Bars: Seven Layer	650	43	58
Chocolate Chunk Brownie	330	18	40
Toffee Almond	400	19	53

For Complete Menu & Data ~ see CalorieKing.com

Burgerville® (Sept '09)

	C	F	Cb
Hamburger	320	17	30
Cheeseburger	380	20	30
Double Beef Cheeseburger	450	27	30
Half Pound Colossal	750	45	43
Colossal Cheeseburger	540	30	43
Tillamook Cheeseburger	640	39	42
Sandwiches: Crispy Chicken	460	19	54
Chicken Strips, 5 pieces	340	17	27
Grilled Chicken, Low-Fat	330	5	45
Nine Grain Turkey Club	540	32	36
French Fries: Regular, 5 oz	360	15	52

For Complete Menu & Data ~ see CalorieKing.com

Updated Nutrition Data ~ www.CalorieKing.com
Persons with Diabetes ~ See Disclaimer (Page 24)

Burger King® (Sept '09)

Breakfast:	C	F	Cb
Cheesy Bacon BK Wrapper	390	24	29
Ham Omelet Sandwich	290	12	33
French Toast Sticks: 3 Piece	230	11	29
5 Piece	380	18	49
Cini-minis (4)	400	18	52
Vanilla Icing for Cini-minis	90	0	22
Biscuits			
Bacon, Egg & Cheese	430	25	34
Ham, Egg & Cheese	410	23	34
Sausage	420	27	32
Sausage, Egg & Cheese	560	37	35
Croissan'wich: Bacon Egg & Chse	350	19	27
Ham Egg & Cheese	340	17	28
Sausage & Cheese	380	24	26
Double Croissan'wich			
with Bacon, Egg & Cheese	430	26	28
with Ham, Bacon, Egg & Cheese	430	24	29
with Ham, Sausage, Egg & Chse	550	36	30
with Sausage, Egg & Cheese	690	50	30
Hash Browns: Small, 5 oz	420	27	40
Medium, 7 oz	610	39	58

Sandwiches & Burgers:			
Burgers:			
BK Stackers: Double	620	39	32
Triple	820	55	33
Quad	1010	70	34
BK Veggie: Burger	420	16	46
with Cheese	470	20	47
Cheeseburger	340	16	31
Double Cheeseburger	510	29	31
Hamburger	290	12	30
Steakhouse Burger	950	59	55
XT: 3 Cheese Steakhouse	1050	71	52
Mushroom & Swiss	870	49	54
Steakhouse	970	61	55
Chicken & Fish Sandwiches			
Original Chicken, with Mayo	630	39	46
BK Big Fish with Tartar Sauce	640	32	66
Spicy Chick'N Crisp	450	30	34
TenderCrisp Chicken	800	46	68
TenderGrill Chicken	490	21	51
Whopper Sandwiches			
Original	670	40	51
Double Whopper	920	58	51
Triple Whopper	1160	76	51
Whopper JR.:	370	21	31
with Cheese	420	25	31

Salads: Without Dressing or Croutons	C	F	Cb
Garden: with TenderCrisp Chicken	410	23	27
with TenderGrill Chicken	210	7	8
Kids Menu:			
BK Burger Shots, 2-pack	220	11	18
BK Fresh Apple Fries w. Dipping Sce	70	0.5	16
Sides:			
BK Chicken Fries, w/o Buffalo Sce:			
6 pieces, 4 oz	250	15	16
9 pieces, 5.5 oz	380	22	24
Cheesy Tots: Small, 6 pces, 2.7 oz	220	12	21
Medium, 9 pieces, 4 oz	330	18	31
Chicken Tenders:			
4 pces, 2.2 oz	180	11	13
8 pieces, 4.3 oz	360	21	25
French Fries: Small, 4.1 oz	340	17	44
Medium, 5.6 oz	480	23	61
Large, 6.8 oz	580	28	74
Onion Rings: Value, 1.5 oz	150	8	17
Small, 3.2 oz	310	17	36
Medium, 4.6 oz	450	24	52
Large, 5.3 oz	510	27	60
Sauces & Condiments: Per 1 oz Container			
Dipping Sauces: Barbecue	40	0	11
Buffalo	80	8	2
Honey Mustard	90	6	8
Ranch	140	15	1
Sweet & Sour	45	0	11
Zesty Onion Ring	150	15	3
Desserts/Pies:			
Dutch Apple Pie	320	13	47
Hershey's Sundae Pie	310	19	32
Beverages:			
Apple Juice, 6.67 fl.oz	100	0	23
Mocha Iced Coffee, 16 fl.oz	360	10	66
Icee, Coca-Cola: Small, 16 fl.oz	110	0	31
Medium, 22 fl.oz	140	0	40
Shakes:			
Chocolate: Small, 16 fl.oz	450	15	79
Medium, 22 fl.oz	670	21	119
Large, 32 fl.oz	990	31	178
Strawberry: Small, 16 fl.oz	440	15	77
Medium, 22 fl.oz	650	20	116
Large, 32 fl.oz	960	29	173
Vanilla: Small, 16 fl.oz	360	15	57
Medium, 22 fl.oz	480	20	76
Large, 32 fl.oz	720	29	113
Oreo Sundae Shakes: *Per Medium, 22 fl.oz*			
Chocolate	1010	35	171
Strawberry	980	34	168

For Complete Nutritional Data ~ see CalorieKing.com

Fast - Foods & *Restaurants*

California Pizza Kitchen
~ See CalorieKing.com

Captain D's Seafood® (Sept '09)

Dinners/Platters: Includes Standard Sides, Cracklins
& Hush Puppies

	C	F	Cb
Catfish Feast	1050	63	87
Clam Platter, ½ lb	1450	87	133
Coastal Fried Flounder	1530	93	115
Deluxe Seafood Platter	1485	85	112
Seafood Scampi	670	13	84
Seasoned Tilapia Dinner	610	13	84
Shrimp Lover's Trio	935	30	89
Ultimate Shrimp Platter	1270	65	69
Salads:			
Fried Chicken Salad	215	10	20
Side Salad	60	0	14
Wild Alaskan Salmon Salad	185	1	10
Sides			
Baked Potato, plain	240	0	54
Broccoli, 3.5 oz	40	1	5
Mac. & Cheese, 4 oz	160	7	17

Caribou Coffee® (Sept '09)

Without Whipped Cream Unless Indicated

Classic: *Per Medium, 16 fl.oz*			
Coffee, with Steamed 2% Milk	90	3.5	9
Coffee Of The Day with 2% Milk	20	0.5	1
Cold: *Per Medium, 21 fl.oz*			
Iced Americano	5	0	0
Iced Coffee, Cold Pressed	5	0	0
Iced Latte with 2% Milk	150	6	14
Iced Mocha with 2% Milk	210	2.5	44
Coolers: *Per Medium, 20 fl.oz*			
Caramel with Whipped Cream	500	16	88
Chocolate with Whipped Cream	510	19	88
Coffee with Whipped Cream	420	17	67
Espresso with Whipped Cream	370	16	57
Espresso: *Per 16 fl.oz Unless Indicated*			
1 medium, 3 shots, 6 fl.oz	0	0	0
Breve	510	45	17
Cappuccino w. 2% Milk	70	3	6
Macchiato with 2% Milk, 6 fl.oz	20	1	1
Smoothies: *Per Medium, 20 fl.oz*			
Passion Fruit Green Tea	290	0	70
Pom-a-Mango	350	0.5	85
Strawberry Banana	350	0	84
Snowdrift: *Per Medium, 20 fl.oz*			
Cookies 'n' Cream with 2% Milk	550	15	95
Mint with 2% Milk	410	9	71
Wild: *Per Medium with Whipped Cream, 20 fl.oz*			
Hot Apple Blast	400	11	76s
Mint Condition with 2% Milk	460	17	68

For Complete Menu & Data ~ see CalorieKing.com

Carl's Jr.® (Sept '09)

Charbroiled Burgers:	C	F	Cb
Big Hamburger	460	17	54
Chili Cheeseburger	780	41	58
Famous Star	600	34	53
with Cheese	660	39	53
Kids Hamburger	230	10	24
Super Star with Cheese	920	58	54
Western Bacon Cheeseburger	720	33	69
Double	960	52	70
The Six Dollar Burger: Original	890	54	58
Bacon Cheese	950	62	49
Chili Cheese	1000	56	59
Guacamole Bacon	1040	70	53
Low-Carb	570	43	7
Western Bacon	1020	53	81
Chicken Sandwiches:			
Charbroiled: BBQ Chicken	380	7	49
Bacon Swiss Crispy Chicken	750	40	62
Chicken Club	560	27	44
Santa Fe Chicken	630	35	44
Spicy Chicken Sandwich	420	27	33
Chicken Strips, 5-piece	610	43	32
Chicken Stars, 6-piece	320	24	14
Fish: Fish & Chips	730	39	72
Carl's Catch Fish Sandwich	710	37	74
Breakfast:: Bacon & Egg Burrito	550	32	37
Breakfast Burger	780	41	64
French Toast Dips, 5 pcs, no syrup	460	21	60
Hash Brown Nuggets, 4 oz.	350	23	32
Loaded Breakfast Burrito	780	49	51
Sourdough Breakfast Sandwich	450	21	38
Steak & Egg Burrito	650	36	43
Sunrise Croissant Sandwich	590	44	27
Fries: Chili Cheese, 12.3 oz	990	56	89
CrissCut Fries, 4.9 oz	450	29	42
Natural Cut: Small, 4.2 oz	320	15	42
Medium, 6 oz	460	22	60
Large, 6.5 oz	500	24	65
Onion Rings, 4½ oz	530	28	61
Salads: Without Dressing			
Charbroiled Chicken Salad	250	9	14
Side Salad	50	2.5	4
Dressings: Per 2 oz Pkg			
Blue Cheese	320	34	1
Thousand Island	240	23	7
Low-Fat Balsamic	35	1.5	5
Shakes: Van./Choc./Strawb. avg.	710	33	86
Oreo	730	38	81
Malts, average all flavors	780	35	99

Carvel® (Aug '09)

Ice Creams: Per Regular 7.5 oz

	C	F	Cb
Cups: Chocolate	410	21	48
Vanilla	450	26	47
No Sugar Added, Vanilla	300	7	57
No-Fat, Chocolate/Vanilla	270	0	62
Dashers: Banana Barge	970	46	128
Mint Choc. Chip	800	42	96
Peanut Butter Cup	1060	60	95
Novelties: Brown Bonnet	390	23	43
Deluxe Flying Saucer w. Sprinkles	350	17	49
Flying Saucer, Chocolate	230	10	33

Desserts: Per Regular Sundae

	C	F	Cb
Classic Sundae: Caramel	670	34	81
Bittersweet Fudge	690	38	77
Strawberry	580	33	63
Thinny-Thin Classic Sundae			
No-Fat: Fudge	380	0	81
Strawberry	320	0	69

Fountain: Per Small, 16 fl.oz

	C	F	Cb
Carvelanche: Butterfinger	730	38	92
M&M; Reece's	755	39	87
Fried Ice Cream: Arctic Blender	850	29	132
Light Arctic Blender	630	5	132
Thick Shake: Strawberry	600	31	70
Float-Chocolate	790	34	109
Float-Strawberry	750	39	85
Float-Vanilla	810	39	102

Checkers®

Same Menu & Data as Rally's ~ See Page 239

Cheesecake Factory® (Aug '09)

(Author Estimates)
10" Cheesecake: Per Slice

	C	F	Cb
Adam's P'nut B'cup Fudge Ripple	930	59	93
Banana Cream	860	63	70
Brownie Sundae	970	63	96
Choc Chip Cookie Dough	1910	72	102
Dulce de Leche Caramel	1010	74	83
Kahlua Cocoa Coffee	840	55	80
Key Lime Cheesecake	710	49	64
Original Cheesecake	630	45	53
Vanilla Bean Cheesecake	870	64	69
White Choc. Raspberry Truffle	900	62	80
Appetizer: Avocado Eggrolls, 1 roll	435	27	48

Dinners: Complete Meal

	C	F	Cb
Cajun Jambalaya Pasta	1960	43	290
Chicken Madeira	1430	76	82
Famous Factory Meatloaf	1955	96	162
Fresh Fish Tacos	1130	23	160
Herb Crusted Filet of Salmon	1040	60	68
Lemon-Herb Roasted Chicken	1790	108	94
Salad: BBQ Ranch Chkn, no bread	1415	113	65

Charley's Grilled Subs® (Aug '09)

	C	F	Cb

Subs: Regular 7½" without Dressings/Mayo/Sauce/
Toppings, Unless Indicated

	C	F	Cb
BBQ Cheddar, with Sauce	585	11	70
Bacon 3 Cheese Steak	645	30	55
Buffalo Chicken, with Sauce	530	16	61
Chicken Bacon Club	580	23	54
Cordon Bleu	530	17	55
Chicken Teriyaki	525	16	60
Italian Deli	555	26	55
Mushroom Swiss Steak	520	19	57
Philly Cheesesteak	525	19	58
Philly Chicken	525	16	60
Philly Ham & Swiss	445	13	60
Philly Steak Deluxe	535	19	60
Philly Veggie	460	15	66
Sicilian Steak	620	28	55
Turkey Cheddar	460	12	55
Ultimate Club	515	20	55

Salads: Cheese/Dressings not included

	C	F	Cb
Chicken, Grilled/Teriyaki/Buffalo, avg.	290	5	5
Fresh Garden Salad	140	3	5
Grilled Steak Salad	290	6	5
Dressings, Italian/Ranch, avg., 1 oz	165	18	1
Mayo, 1 Tbsp., ½ oz	100	11	0
Fries: Regular	610	45	41
Ultimate	1250	103	57
Original Lemonade, 16 fl.oz	165	0	40

Extra Menu Items & Data ~ www.CalorieKing.com

Chevys Fresh Mex® (Aug '09)

Sizzling Fajitas: Without Tortillas

	C	F	Cb
Original Famous Chicken	910	31	92
Sizzling Steak	1000	45	90
Grilled Tacos: Chicken	1020	34	121
Fish (Sea Bass)	970	33	121
Steak	1090	43	120
Grande Salads: Santa Fe	670	39	30
Santa Fe w/o Cheese or Bacon	320	11	28
Tostada Salad with Chicken	1550	94	102
w/o Tortilla Strips/Chse/Sour Cream	920	45	80
Tortilla Soup	395	17	36
Sides: Black Beans	190	2	33
Refried Beans	290	15	28
Guacamole, 2 oz	105	10	3
Mexican Rice	210	3	39
Salsa for Chips, 5 oz	40	0	8
Sour Cream, 2 oz	120	12	2
Tamalito (Sweetcorn), 2	180	7	29
Tortilla (El Machino), 2	140	4	22

Chick-fil-A® (Sept '09)

Chick-fil-A Sandwiches	C	F	Cb
Chargrilled Chicken w/o Sauce	260	3	33
Chargrilled Chicken Club w/o Sce	380	12	34
Chicken Salad	500	20	53
Cool Wraps: *Without Dressing*			
Chargrilled Chicken	410	12	49
Chicken Caesar	480	16	45
Spicy Chicken	400	12	47
Breakfast: Chicken Biscuit	450	20	48
Bacon, Egg & Cheese Biscuit	520	29	44
Sausage Biscuit	590	41	42
Burritos: Chicken	410	18	41
Sausage	480	27	38
Chick-n-Minis, 1 box, 3 pces	260	10	29
Chicken, Egg & Cheese Bagel	500	20	49
Cinnamon Cluster	400	15	61
Hash Browns, 3 oz	280	19	25
Salads: *Without Dressing & Condiments*			
Chargrilled Chicken & Fruit	220	6	21
Chargrilled Chicken Garden	170	6	10
Chick-n-Strips	450	22	26
Southwest Chargrilled Chicken	240	9	17
Salad Dressings, Sauces & Condiments:			
Garlic & Butter Croutons, 0.5 oz	60	2	9
Tortilla Strips, 0.5 oz	80	4	8
Dressings: Blue Cheese, 1 oz	150	16	1
Buttermilk Ranch; Caesar, 1 oz	160	17	1
Light Italian, 1.1 oz	15	0.5	2
Thousand Island, 1.1 oz	150	14	5
Sauces: BBQ; Honey Mustard, 1 oz	45	0	11
Buffalo, 0.7 oz	10	0	1
Buttermilk Ranch, 0.7 oz	110	12	1
Chick-fil-A, 1 oz	140	13	6
Honey Roasted BBQ, 0.4 oz	60	5	2
Sides: Carrot & Raisin Salad, 6 oz	260	12	39
Chicken Salad Cup, 6 oz	350	24	6
Cole Slaw, 10.5 oz	600	51	32
Side Salad w/o Dressing, 4 oz	70	4.5	5
Waffle Potato Fries: Small, 3 oz	280	16	31
Medium, 4 oz	370	21	41
Large, 4.5 oz	420	24	46
Soup: Breast of Chicken, 16 oz	240	7	30
Desserts: Cheesecake	310	23	22
Fudge Nut Brownie	370	19	45
Lemon Pie	360	13	58
Icedream Cone w/o Toppings	170	4	31
Milkshake, Chocolate, 18.25 oz	760	28	113

Chili's® (Sept '09)

Start It Off Right: Per Serving	C	F	Cb
Bottomless Tostada Chips w. Sauce	470	39	26
Kickin' Jack Nachos: 12 Nachos	1200	90	62
w. Fajita Beef, w/o guacamole	1380	94	63
with Fajita Chicken, w/o guac.	1340	92	64
On. String & Jalapeno Stack + Ranch	2130	213	34
Skillet Queso w. Tostada Chips	940	77	42
Southwestern Eggrolls w. Dressing	910	57	72
Triple Dipper: Big Mouth Bites (2)	780	51	46
Boneless Wings, Buffalo w. Dress.	740	60	26
Chicken Crisper Bites (2)	690	40	58
Hot Spin. & Artichoke Dip w/ Chips	930	77	42
Meals: Per Serving			
Big Mouth Burgers: *Without Sides*			
Bacon Burger	1090	69	57
Big Mouth Bites	1580	97	104
Chicken: Chicken Club Tacos (3)	1500	76	137
Chicken Tacos (3)	1200	45	144
Country Fr. Chkn Crispers, w/o sce	1490	90	110
Crispy Honey Chipotle Chkn Crispers	1930	108	181
Fajitas: Per Skillet, without Tortillas or Condiments			
Buffalo Chicken	1090	77	50
Classic Chicken	370	11	25
Classic Steak	470	25	25
Fire Grilled Quesadillas:			
Bacon Chicken Ranch	1750	122	95
Chicken Fajita	1480	96	99
Jalapeno Beef	1780	126	98
Guiltless Grill: Per Serving			
Buffalo Chicken Sandwich	390	7	46
Carne Asada Steak	370	10	11
Cedar Plank Tilapia	200	4	8
Chicken Platter	370	2	49
Honey-Mustard Glazed Gr. Salmon	420	20	13
Hot Off The Grill: Incl. Toast, w/o Sides Unless Indicated			
Cajun Ribeye	1000	79	19
Classic Sirloin	540	38	20
Flame-Grilled Ribeye	990	79	19
Country Fried Steak with Sides	1430	82	122
Salads: Includes Dressing Unless Indicated			
Boneless Buffalo Chicken	1070	77	46
Chicken Caesar	900	71	28
Side House Salad, w/o dressing	210	12	17
Quesadilla Explosion	1260	76	84
Southwestern Cobb	1080	71	57
Desserts: Cheesecake, 1 slice	700	42	67
Chocolate Chip Paradise Pie, 1 sl.	1140	66	129
Molten Chocolate Cake, 1 slice	1010	51	131
For Complete Menu & Data ~ see CalorieKing.com			

Chipotle® (Sept '09)

	C	F	Cb
Breads			
Flour Tortillas (13"), 1 tortilla	290	9	44
Flour Tortillas (6"), 3 tortillas	270	8	39
Taco Shells, Crispy, 3 shells	180	6	27
Meal Components			
Barbacoa, 4 oz	170	7	2
Black Beans, 4 oz	120	1	23
Carnitas, 4 oz	190	8	1
Cheese, 1 oz	100	9	0
Chicken, 4 oz	190	7	1
Lettuce, 1 oz	5	0	0
Pinto Beans, 4 oz	120	1	22
Rice, 3½ oz	130	3	23
Steak, 4 oz	190	7	2
Condiments			
Salsa: Corn, 4 oz	80	1.5	15
Green Tomatillo, 2 oz	15	0	3
Red Tomatillo, 2 oz	40	1	8
Tomato, 4 oz	20	0	4
Sour Cream, 2 oz	120	10	2
Vinaigrette, 2 fl.oz	260	25	12
Extras: Chips, serving, 4 oz	570	27	73
Guacamole, 3½ oz	150	13	8

Chuck E. Cheese® (Sept '09)

	C	F	Cb
Appetizers: Includes Condiments			
Buffalo Wings (12)	900	60	48
Italian Bread Stick w/ Dressing (1)	175	9	18
Mozzarella Stick w/ Marinara (1)	95	6	6
Pizzas: Per Medium Slice			
BBQ Chicken	185	6	24
Cheese	155	5	21
Pepperoni	175	7	21
Vegetarian	160	6	22
Individual Pizza: Whole, 6 Slices			
Cheese	540	19	69
Pepperoni	585	24	68
Oven Baked Sandwiches:			
Ham & Cheese	685	27	79
Italian Sub	790	39	78
Roasted Chicken Ciabatta	715	28	80
Hot Dog with Mustard & Relish	310	19	35
French Fries:			
With Ketchup & Ranch: 4 oz	420	20	55
8 oz	840	40	110
Desserts: Apple Dessert Pizza, 1 sl.	190	5	33
Choc. Birthday Cake (8"), 1 slice, ⅒	290	13	41
Cinnamon Sticks, 1 stick	70	2	11

Church's Chicken® (Sept '09)

	C	F	Cb
Chicken: Per Serving			
Original: Breast, 1 piece	200	11	3
Leg, 1 piece	110	6	3
Thigh, 1 piece	330	23	8
Wing, 1 piece	300	19	7
Spicy: Breast, 1 piece	320	20	12
Leg, 1 piece	180	11	8
Thigh, 1 piece	480	35	20
Wing, 1 piece	430	27	17
Tender Strips: 1 piece	120	6	6
Spicy, 1 piece	135	7	7
Sides: Per Regular Serving			
Cajun Rice, 6 oz	130	7	16
Cole Slaw, 6 oz	150	10	15
Corn on the Cob (1)	140	3	24
French Fries, 3½ oz	290	14	38
Honey Butter Biscuits (1), 1.7 oz	240	12	28
Jalapeno Bombers, 4 pieces, 4 oz	240	10	29
Macaroni & Cheese, 6 oz	220	10	24
Mashed Potatoes & Gravy, 6 oz	70	2	12
Okra, 3.4 oz	350	22	36
Whole Jalapeno Peppers (2), 1.3 oz	10	0	2
Sauces: Per Packet			
BBQ; Sweet & Sour	25	0	8
Creamy Jalapeno	80	9	1
Honey Mustard	90	9	3
Purple Pepper	45	0	12
Ranch	105	10	1

Cici's Pizza® (Sept '09)

	C	F	Cb
Buffet: Per ⅒ of 12" Pizza			
Alfredo	120	3.5	18
Bacon Cheddar	110	4.5	19
Bar-B-Que	150	2.5	25
Beef	140	4.5	20
Cheese	150	4	19
Ham & Pineapple	150	3.5	21
Pepperoni & Jalapeno	150	4.5	20
Sausage	140	5	20
Spinach Alfredo	120	3.5	19
Zesty Ham & Cheddar	120	4	19
To-Go: Per ⅒ of 15" Pizza			
Alfredo	150	6	20
Bar-B-Que	240	6	36
Beef	190	8	24
Pepperoni & Jalapeno	210	7	24
Sausage	170	7	24
Spinach Alfredo	170	6	23
Zesty Ham & Cheddar	160	7	23
Zesty Pepperoni	170	9	23
Zesty Veggie	140	6	24

Cinnabon® (Sept '09)

Sweet Rolls:	C	F	Cb
Cinnabon Bites (6)	510	19	77
Classic Cinnamon Roll (1)	815	32	117
Cinnabon Stix, 5 pieces, 85g	380	21	41
Minibon (1) 92g	340	13	49
Caramel Pecanbon (1)	1100	56	141
CinnaPretzel (1)	750	6	156
Sweet Roll Icing: Frosting Cup, 1.4 oz	180	11	109
Drinks: Mochalatta Chill, 16 oz	425	17	63

CinnaMonster® (Sept '09)

Cinnamon Roll: Per Roll	C	F	Cb
Caramel Pecan	840	32	120
Original	880	24	100

Cold Stone Creamery® (Sept '09)

Ice Creams	C	F	Cb
Amaretto: Like it	330	20	33
Love it	530	31	53
Gotta have it	790	47	80
Sorbet: Average all flavors			
Like it	155	0	38
Love it	250	0	62
Gotta have it	380	0	93

Cosi® (Sept '09)

	C	F	Cb
Sandwiches: Buffalo Blue	565	25	47
Italiano	745	42	49
Roasted Turkey & Brie	690	32	62
Sesame Ginger Chicken	480	7	69
Turkey Rustica	620	27	60
TBM	565	34	50
Tuna	540	6	52
Melts: Bacon, Turkey Cheddar	570	24	48
Grilled Chicken Parmesan	620	25	54
Pesto Chicken	670	31	52
Tuna Melt	875	40	51
TBM Melt	705	39	58
Pizza, Individual: Margherita	700	31	96
Pepperoni	805	40	94
Traditional Cheese	665	28	95
Soup: Pollo & Pasta Soup, cup	160	4	14
Tomato Basil Aurora, cup	225	15	20
Three Bean Chili, cup	150	1	36
Salads: No Dresssing			
Greek Salad	270	20	17
Grilled Chicken Caesar	355	16	16
Signature Salad	325	18	34
Dressings: Cosi Vinaigrette, 2 oz	355	39	2
Caesar, 2 oz	265	28	4
Italian, 2 oz	245	26	2
Sherry Shallot Vinaigrette, 2 oz	285	26	9

Costco Food Court (Aug '09)

Pizza: Per Slice	C	F	Cb
Combo, 11oz	680	29	72
Cheese, 10 oz	700	28	70
Pepperoni , 9 oz	620	24	68
Dogs, average, 8 oz	550	32	46
Salad, Chicken Caesar, 20 oz	800	57	32
Meals: Chicken Bake 11.5 oz	810	30	77
Ital. Sausage Sandwich, 12.6 oz	700	42	46
Beverages: Hot Latte, 9.6 fl oz	190	5	24
Hot Mocha, 11.3 fl oz	310	9	45
Mocha Freeze, 16.3 fl .oz	320	7	49
Latte Freeze, 15.3 oz	240	7	32
Churro, 5.2 oz	430	18	62
Smoothies: Fruit Smoothie, 16 fl.oz	290	0	72
Tropical Smoothie	270	0	65
Desserts: Ice cream Bar, 8 oz	870	65	60
Berry Sundae, 12.3 oz	410	0	87
Frozen Yogurt, 12 oz	390	0	82

Cousins Subs® (Sept '09)

7½" Subs	C	F	Cb
BLT	590	38	47
Cheese Steak	505	19	49
Chicken Breast	570	27	50
Chicken Cheddar Deluxe	670	39	51
Club	645	35	51
Double Cheese Steak	745	36	49
Garden Veggie	390	12	51
Gyro	710	41	61
Ham & Provolone	605	34	50
Hot Veggie	470	17	55
Italian Special	815	51	50
Meatball & Provolone	725	38	54
Pepperoni Melt	720	45	50
Philly Cheese Steak	530	19	55
Pizza	710	39	55
Roast Beef	605	30	50
Seafood w. Crab	640	38	60
Three Cheese	685	44	50
Tuna	645	38	39
Turkey Breast	530	28	50
Better Bunch, 5" Mini Subs: Without Mayo, Cheese			
Club	190	2	26
Garden Veggie	135	1	26
Ham	175	2	26
Hot Veggie	145	1	27
Turkey Breast	175	2	26
French Fries: Small, 2.8 oz	250	13	30
Medium, 4 oz	365	19	43
Large, 5.3 oz	485	25	57

Cousins Subs® cont... (Aug '09)

Salads: Without Dressings

	C	F	Cb
Chef Salad	325	14	25
Garden Salad	235	11	24
with Chicken Breast	350	12	25
Italian	405	24	24
Seafood Salad	315	11	34
Side Salad	135	6	14
Tuna Salad	625	46	23

For Complete Menu & Data ~ see CalorieKing.com

Culver's® (Sept '09)

Butter Burgers:

	C	F	Cb
Original: Single, Kids	345	15	35
Double	480	23	36
Triple	615	31	37
Cheddar w. Bacon	870	48	56
Cheese: Single, Kids	400	20	36
Double	580	32	37
Culver's Bacon Deluxe: Single	575	38	34
Double	750	50	34
Culver's Deluxe: Single	495	31	34
Double	670	43	34
Low Carb Butter Burger	445	32	1
Mushroom & Swiss: Single	415	21	33
Double	635	35	35
Sourdough Melt, Single	415	20	33
Wisconsin Swiss Melt, Single	405	20	33
Corn Dog	260	14	26
Chicken Tenders, 4 pieces	440	20	32
Hot Dog	365	22	30
Sides			
French Fries: Small, Kids	275	12	38
Regular	385	17	53
Large	495	22	68
Chili Cheddar Fries, 9.3 oz	660	34	73
Dairyland Cheese Curds, 6.7 oz	670	38	54
Mashed Potatoes w. Gravy	140	2	26
Sandwiches: Angus Philly Steak	520	20	46
Beef Pot Roast	365	16	33
Chicken Salad Wrap	520	26	39
Crispy Chicken Filet	625	29	68
Grilled Chicken Breast	375	8	47
Grilled Ham 'N' Swiss On Rye	495	25	33
Grilled Reuben Melt	590	31	41
North Atlantic Cod Filet	740	42	58
Pork Tenderloin (Breaded)	595	29	62
Turkey Sourdough BLT	560	31	36

Culver's® (Sept '09)

Dinner Plates: Per Serving

	C	F	Cb
Beef Pot Roast	635	24	74
Breaded Shrimp, 8 pcs	1250	61	148
Chopped Steak	685	29	67
Fried Chicken, 2 pieces	1755	94	140
Fish & Chips, 6 pieces	1380	83	104
North Atlantic Cod, Fried, 2 pieces	1830	116	135
Salads			
Chicken Cashew w/ Grilled Chicken	440	25	17
Classic Caesar w/ Grilled Chicken	360	14	15
Cobb Salad	530	31	19
Garden Fresco	225	11	25
Side Salad	85	5	6
Desserts			
Frozen Custard: Chocolate, 1 sc.	295	14	35
Vanilla, 1 scoop	310	18	30
Concrete Mixer, Choc, Medium	990	49	122
Lemon Ice, 7 oz	140	0	35
Turtle Concrete Mixer, medium	1155	71	114
Sundaes: Banana Foster, 2 scoops	785	41	93
Turtle, 2 scoops	975	60	97
Root Beer Float, medium	465	18	70
Malt, Chocolate, medium	970	45	122
Shake, Chocolate, medium	910	44	114

For Complete Nutritional Data ~ see CalorieKing.com

D'Angelo's® (Aug '09)

Sandwiches:

	C	F	Cb
Cheeseburger: Pokket	460	23	35
Sub	530	25	49
Wrap	600	31	52
Chicken Stir Fry: Pokket	400	10	39
Sub	470	12	53
Wrap	550	19	57
Classic Veggie: Pokket	360	13	43
Wrap	520	22	61
Roast Beef: Sub	320	5	46
Wrap	400	12	61
Turkey: Pokket	260	1	31
Sub	330	3	45
Grilled Quesadillas: Number 9	380	19	31
Chicken Stir Fry	360	15	31
Classic Vegetable	290	13	33
Salads: No Dressing Unless Indicated			
Caesar Salad with Dressing	620	54	28
Chicken Caesar Salad	670	53	21
Chicken Cobb Salad	330	18	14
Greek Salad with Dressing	780	70	23
Tossed Salad	60	0	13
Turkey Salad	170	1	10

Extra Menu Items ~ www.CalorieKing.com

Fast - Foods & *Restaurants*

Dairy Queen® (Sept '09)

Burgers/Sandwiches	C	F	Cb
DQ All Beef Hot Dogs: Hot Dog	250	14	21
Chili & Cheese	430	22	39
GrillBurgers: *Per Burger*			
Bacon Cheddar	650	35	41
Classic w/o Cheese	470	21	42
½ lb Burger	720	40	42
½ lb Flame Thrower	1060	75	41
Burgers: Bacon Dbl Cheeseburger	730	41	35
DQ Original Cheeseburger	400	18	34
Hamburger	350	14	33
Double Hamburger	540	26	33
Sandwiches: Crispy Chicken	560	28	48
Grilled Chicken	370	16	32
Chicken			
Chkn Strips Basket (4), with Gravy	1360	63	103
Grilled Chicken Wrap	200	12	9
Iron Gr. Chicken Quesadilla Basket	1070	50	117
Salads: Without Dressing			
Crispy Chicken	460	19	31
Grilled Chicken	280	11	14
Sides			
DQ French Fries, 4 oz	310	13	43
DQ Onion Rings, 4 oz	360	16	47
Desserts: Per Medium			
Blizzard Treats: Banana Cream Pie	780	30	115
Butterfinger	740	26	114
Cappuccino Heath	870	38	112
Choco Cherry Love	730	33	94
Chocolate Chip	880	50	96
Cookie Dough	1010	40	148
Oreo Cookies	680	25	100
Reese's P'nut Butter Cups	760	31	101
Strawberry CheeseQuake	690	28	92
DQ Blizzard Cakes (8"): *Per ⅛ Cake*			
Oreo	760	33	104
Reese's P'nut Butter Cup	720	33	94
Strawberry CheeseQuake	610	27	79
DQ Dipped Cones: *Per 7¾ oz Cone*			
Butterscotch	490	23	59
Chocolate	470	22	60
DQ Sundaes: *Per Medium, 8.2 oz*			
Caramel	430	11	75
Hot Fudge	440	14	66
Strawberry	350	10	56
Malts: Per Medium			
Caramel	960	24	163
Chocolate	900	22	154
Strawberry	770	20	128
Moo Latte: Per 16 fl.oz			
Cappuccino	500	18	71
French Vanilla	560	18	88
Mocha	590	23	82

For Complete Nutritional Data ~ see CalorieKing.com

Daphne's® Greek Cafe (Aug '09)

Lunch: *Without Dressing*	C	F	Cb
Chicken Kabob	425	21	84
Chicken Salad & Soup	570	27	49
Falafel Zesta Lunch	570	36	100
Salad & Soup	470	25	47
Zesta Lunch	545	35	91
Plate: Calamari	565	32	97
Chicken Kabob (2)	525	23	88
Shrimp	440	26	85
Greek Salad: Without Dressing			
Side Portion	330	16	36
Regular Portion	385	19	41
w. Shrimp	585	30	54
Pita Sandwiches: Without Tzatziki Sauce			
Calamari	500	28	44
Chicken	515	22	36
Greek Veggie	485	33	36
Gyros Jr.	475	32	35
Shrimp	405	24	35
Steak	595	41	34
Tzatziki Sauce, 1 oz	75	8	3
Soup, Avgolemono, 1 cup, 8 fl.oz	320	17	33

Davanni's® (Sept '09)

Half Hoagies: Includes 6" White Bun, Cheese, Salad, Butter, Dressing, Mayo & Sauce

	C	F	Cb
3 Cheese	385	28	21
Assorted	390	29	21
BLT	595	48	22
Chicken & Bacon w. Honey Mustard	440	22	30
Chicken Breast	460	29	22
Chicken Parmigiana	365	17	22
Club	385	25	22
Italian Sausage	525	37	28
Pastrami	445	25	22
Pizza	315	18	22
Salami	470	36	21
Southwest Chicken	480	27	25
Tuna Melt	550	42	24
Turkey	355	22	22
Turkey Bacon Chipotle	465	30	22
Veggie	350	23	25
Calzones: Sausage Gr.Peppers	790	42	70
Pepperoni	825	49	66
Pizzas			
5 Meat: Thin, 1 slice	240	12	18
Traditional: 1 slice	300	13	29
Solo Thin	1010	63	45
The Works: Thin, 1 slice	250	14	18
Traditional: 1 slice	310	14	29
Solo Thin	595	32	42
Veggie: Thin, 1 slice	210	9	18
Traditional: 1 slice	265	10	30
Solo Thin	495	22	42

Del Taco® (Sept '09)

Breakfast	C	F	Cb
Breakfast Burrito	280	13	26
Bacon & Egg Quesadilla	430	20	37
Egg & Cheese Burrito	400	18	35
Steak & Egg Burrito	520	25	35
Hash Brown Sticks (5)	210	15	18
Tacos: Big Fat Chicken Taco	330	14	34
Big Fat Steak Taco	390	18	33
Chicken Del Carbon	210	8	18
Chicken Soft Taco	220	12	16
Classic Taco	200	12	10
Crispy Fish Taco	300	17	29
Macho Taco	300	17	16
Steak Taco Del Carbon	210	8	18
Burritos: Del Combo Burrito	510	16	61
Chicken Fajita, Chicken /Veg. only	320	10	37
Del Beef Burrito	470	20	37
Del Classic Chicken Burrito	510	33	37
Deluxe Combo Burrito	570	25	64
Deluxe Del Beef Burrito	510	23	39
Half Pound Red/Green Burrito, avg.	440	10	67
Macho Beef Burrito	1010	44	82
Macho Chicken Burrito	920	30	111
Macho Combo Burrito	990	34	112
Spicy Chicken/Veggie Works, avg.	615	16	96
Quesadillas: Cheddar; Spicy Jack	480	25	37
Chicken Cheddar; Spicy Jack Chkn	570	30	40
Salad:			
Deluxe Taco Salad	850	46	70
Burgers: Cheeseburger	430	22	40
Double Del Cheeseburger	560	35	35
Triple Del Cheeseburger	950	66	40
Nachos: 4 oz	370	21	3
Macho Nachos, 17 oz	1090	53	116
Sides:			
Chips & Salsa, 3 oz	160	8	20
Fries: Small, 5 oz	270	16	31
Macho, 10 oz	550	31	63
Chili Cheese, 10.5 oz	570	33	46
Deluxe Chili Cheese, 12 oz	610	36	48
Shakes: Chocolate, 13.4 fl.oz	630	13	117
Strawberry, 13.4 fl.oz	600	13	108
Vanilla, 13.4 fl.oz	560	13	100

Denny's® (Sept '09)

Breakfast: *Without Sides*	C	F	Cb
Favorites: T-bone Stk & Eggs, 16 oz	780	36	4
Top Sirloin Steak & Eggs, 10 oz	420	21	1
Country Fried Steak & Eggs, 11 oz	660	42	29
Moons Over My Hammy, 13 oz	780	42	50
Two Egg Breakfast, 4 oz	200	15	1
Omelettes: Ham & Cheddar, 10 oz	590	44	4
Ultimate, 12 oz	670	54	8
Veggie-Cheese, 13 oz	500	37	10
Pancakes: *Without Margarine, Syrup or Topping*			
Buttermilk (3), 9 oz	510	6	102
Platter: Belgian Waffle, 8 oz	650	50	31
Fabulous Fr. Toast (3), 15 oz	1010	52	93
Scrambles: Heartland, 20 oz	1150	66	97
Meat Lovers, 19 oz	1130	66	80
Slams: All American, 10 oz	820	69	5
French Toast, 15 oz	940	53	68
Grand Slamwich	1030	66	68
Lumberjack, 15 oz	850	46	60
Burgers & Sandwiches: Without Sides			
Burgers: Bacon Cheddar, 15 oz	1100	72	55
Classic Cheeseburger: w. Chse, 13 oz	930	58	56
w/o cheese,12 oz	770	45	56
Double Cheeseburger, 20 oz	1625	116	56
Mushroom Swiss, 15 oz	900	54	59
Western, with sauce, 17 oz	1300	82	83
Sandwiches: BLT. w. mayo, 6 oz	570	37	36
Club, w. mayo, 11 oz	660	34	55
Grilled Chicken, with dressing	970	58	69
The Super Bird, w/o dress., 10 oz	560	27	43
Melts: Chicken Ranch, 12 oz	920	42	79
Spicy Buffalo Chicken, 14 oz	940	46	81
Meals: Without sides, sauce or bread unless indicated			
Chicken: Strips, (4), 8 oz	560	24	41
Grilled Chicken Dinner, 10 oz	280	4	4
Seafood:			
Fit Fare Grilled Tilapia, 17 oz	600	11	106
Grilled Shrimp Skewer (2), 10 oz	370	10	39
Lemon Pepper Tilapic w/ Rice Pilaf	640	27	41

Continued next page....

Fast - Foods & *Restaurants*

Denny's® cont... (Sept '09)

Meals (Cont):
Without sides, sauce or bread unless indicated

Steak/Beef:

	C	F	Cb
Country Fried Steak w/ gravy	1000	65	54
Meat Loaf w/ gravy, 7 oz	600	46	14
Mshrm. Swiss Chopped Stk w. Gravy	930	75	18
T-bone: 12 oz	740	56	0
w. Shrimp Skewer, Dinner, 12 oz	830	60	0
w. Breaded Shrimp, 13 oz	920	64	20
Top Sirloin Steak, 6 oz	220	6	1
w. Breaded Shrimp, Dinner, 9 oz	440	15	23
w. Shrimp Skewers, 8 oz	310	9	1

Salads: Without Dressing or Bread

Grilled Chicken Deluxe, 17 oz	290	10	15
Chicken Strip Deluxe, 18 oz	590	29	44

Dressings: Per 1 oz

Bleu Cheese	130	13	1
Caesar	100	10	0
French	75	5	8
Honey Mustard	160	15	5
Ranch	130	14	1

Sides

Biscuits & Sausage, 8 oz	580	34	57
Butter Rolls, 2 pcs	260	9	38
Garlic Bread, 2 pcs	170	9	21
Grits & Margarine, 12 oz	260	5	47
Hashed Browns, 5 oz	200	12	20
Pancake Puppies (6)	390	12	67

Condiments

Maple-flav. Syrup, 3 tbsp	145	0	36
Sugar-free, 3 tbsp	25	0	9
Cherry Topping, 3 oz	85	0	21
Whipped Marg., 1 Tbsp	50	6	0

Soups: Without Bread

Chicken Noodle, 12 oz	165	4	19
Clam Chowder, 12 oz	265	17	24
Vegetable Beef, 12 oz	125	1	18

Desserts

Cheesecake, 7 oz	640	41	58
French Silk Pie, 7 oz	770	57	59
Hot Fudge Brownie a la Mode, 9 oz	830	37	122
Oreo Sundae, 9 oz	760	37	103
Oreo Blender Blaster, 14 oz	890	44	113

Beverages:

Milkshakes, Van/Choc, 12 oz	560	26	76
Floats, Root Beer/Cola, 16 oz	430	17	69
Oreo Sundae, 9 oz	760	37	103
Oreo Blender Blaster, 14 oz	890	44	113

For Complete Nutritional Data ~ see CalorieKing.com

Dippin' Dots® (Sept '09)

Flavored Ices	C	F	Cb
All flavors, ½ cup, 3 oz	90	0	23

Frozen Yogurt:

Strawberry Cheesecake, ½ cup	100	0	21

Ice Cream: Per ½ Cup

Average all flavors	180	11	20
Fat-Free, Fudge, No Sugar Added	90	0	18
Red.-Fat, Vanilla, No Sugar Added	125	6	13

Donato's® Pizza (Sept '09)

Thin Crust Pizza: ¼ Large Pizza

Chicken Vegy Medley	495	20	51
Classic Trio	675	37	52
Founder's Favorite	700	38	52
Hawaiian	590	27	56

Thicker Crust Pizza: ¼ Large Pizza

Founder's Favorite	860	42	78
Mariachi Beef	795	36	81
Mariachi Chicken	805	35	81
Pepperoni	800	39	76
Serious Cheese	800	38	77
Vegy	715	29	83
Works	845	41	81

No Dough Pizza - Individual

Chicken Vegy Medley	495	29	20
Classic Trio	530	37	18
Founder's Favorite	560	38	18
Hawaiian	435	26	22
Mariachi Beef	530	34	23
Mariachi Chicken	495	30	21
Pepperoni	500	35	17
Pepperoni Zinger	585	42	17
Serious Cheese	455	31	17
Serious Meat	655	46	19
Works	545	37	21

Stromboli: 3 Meat

	690	31	67
Cheese	695	31	66
Deluxe	615	25	68
Pepperoni	715	34	67
Vegy	605	24	69

Desserts:

Apple Timpano, 2 slices	405	9	72
Cinnamon Timpano, 2 slices	525	22	73

For Complete Nutritional Data ~ see CalorieKing.com

Domino's® Pizza (Sept '09)

C F Cb

12" Classic Hand-Tossed: Per Slice, 1/8 Pizza
	C	F	Cb
Beef	210	8	25
Cheese Only	175	5	25
Green Peppers, Onion & Mushroom	175	5	25
Ham	175	5	25
Ham & Pineapple	180	5	26
Pepperoni	210	8	25
Pepperoni & Sausage	240	11	26
Sausage	215	9	26

12" Crunchy Thin Crust: Per Slice, 1/8 Pizza
	C	F	Cb
Beef	175	10	14
Cheese Only	140	7	14
Green Pepper Onion & Mushroom	140	7	14
Ham	145	7	14
Ham & Pineapple	145	7	15
Pepperoni	175	10	14
Pepperoni & Sausage	205	13	15
Sausage	185	11	15

12" Ultimate Deep Dish: Per Slice, 1/8 Pizza
	C	F	Cb
Beef	265	13	27
Cheese Only	210	10	27
Green Pepper Onion & Mushroom	230	10	27
Ham	235	10	27
Ham & Pineapple	240	10	28
Pepperoni	265	13	27
Pepperoni & Sausage	295	16	28
Sausage	275	14	28

12" Feast Classic Hand-Tossed: Per Slice, 1/8 Pizza
	C	F	Cb
America's Favorite Feast	250	12	26
Bacon Cheeseburger Feast	260	13	25
Barbecue Feast	245	10	30
Deluxe Feast	225	10	26
ExtravaganZZa Feast	280	14	27
Hawaiian Feast	215	7.5	27
MeatZZa Feast	270	13	26
Pepperoni Feast	260	13	26
Philly Cheese Steak Feast	215	8.5	23
Vegi Feast	210	7.5	26

12" Feast Crunchy Thin Crust: Per Slice, 1/8 Pizza
	C	F	Cb
America's Favorite Feast	220	14	16
Bacon Cheeseburger Feast	230	15	15
Barbecue Feast	215	12	20
Deluxe Feast	195	12	16
ExtravaganZZa Feast	250	16	17
Hawaiian Feast	185	10	17
MeatZZa Feast	240	15	16
Pepperoni Feast	230	15	16
Philly Cheese Steak Feast	185	11	13
Vegi Feast	180	10	16

Domino's® Pizza cont... (Sept '09)

C F Cb

12" Feast Ultimate Deep Dish: Per Slice, 1/8 Pizza
	C	F	Cb
America's Favorite Feast	285	15	28
Bacon Cheeseburger Feast	300	16	27
Barbecue Feast	285	13	32
Hawaiian Feast	255	11	29
Pepperoni Feast	300	16	28
Philly Cheese Steak Feast	250	12	25

Oven Baked Sandwiches
	C	F	Cb
Chicken Bacon Ranch	890	45	72
Chicken Parm	770	30	73
Italian	880	45	71
Philly Cheese Steak	690	27	72

BreadBowl Pasta: Per 1/2 Bowl
	C	F	Cb
3-Cheese Mac-N-Cheese, 11 oz	730	28	95
Chicken Alfredo, 10.85 oz	700	25	93
Chicken Carbonara, 11.65 oz	740	28	94
Italian Sausage Marinara, 11.9 oz	730	26	97
Pasta Primavera, 11 oz	670	24	94

Salads: Per Container
	C	F	Cb
Garden Fresh, 8.45 oz	140	8	10
Grilled Chicken Caesar, 11.2 oz	200	9	12

Salad Dressings & Condiments: Per 1.5 oz Package
	C	F	Cb
Blue Cheese	230	24	2
Buttermilk Ranch	220	24	2
Creamy Caesar	210	22	2
Golden Italian	220	23	2
Light Italian	20	1	2

Bread Side Items
	C	F	Cb
Breadsticks: 1 stick, w/o sauce	105	6	11
8 sticks, w/o sauce	850	48	88
Cheesy Bread:			
1 stick, w/o sauce	115	6	11
8 sticks, w/o sauce	910	48	88

Bread Dipping Sauces: Per Container
	C	F	Cb
Garlic	250	28	0
Marinara	25	0	5
Cinna Stix:			
1 stick, w/o icing	120	6	14
8 sticks, w/o icing	945	48	112
Sweet Icing, Dipper Cup	250	2.5	57

Chicken Side Items
	C	F	Cb
Buffalo Chicken Kickers			
w/o Dipping Sauce (2)	105	4.5	7
Buffalo Wings:			
Barbecue, 2 wings, w/o sauce	220	14	6
Hot, 2 wings, w/o sauce	200	14	2

Chicken Dipping Sauces: Per Container
	C	F	Cb
Blue Cheese	210	22	2
Hot	55	4.5	3
Ranch	195	21	2

Fast - Foods & *Restaurants*

Don Pablos® (Sept '09)

Appetizers: Per Serving	C	F	Cb
Beef Taquito (6)	560	34	36
Chicken Flauta (6)	505	31	39
Dips: *Without Chips*			
Queso Blanco, 6 oz cup	340	27	13
Prairie Fire Bean w. Cheese, 6 oz	380	25	23
Nachos (1 order): Taco Beef	1625	113	85
Cheese	1315	98	48
Classic Quesadillas: *Per Serving*			
Cheese Quesadilla, small, 4 slices	810	50	52
Mesquite Grilled Chicken, 4 slices	665	32	55
Mesquite Grilled Steak, 8 slices	1560	91	122
Burritos *(No Sides)*: Chicken	880	48	70
Beef & Bean	1390	73	123
Carnitas: Trad'l Pork with Cold Set	1235	52	137
Chimichangas: *Without Rice & Refritos*			
Spicy Beef Chimi De Oro	1350	68	131
Chicken Chimi	1100	42	114
Rellenos: *With Sauce/Cheese Topping*			
Beef (1)	300	17	20
Cheese (1)	395	26	19
Chicken (1)	235	11	21
Tamales, Chicken w/ Ranchero Sce (1)	220	10	25
Tacos: Crispy Beef	290	18	21
Crispy Chicken	255	14	22
Soft Beef	325	18	29
Soft Chicken	295	14	30
Lunch, *1 Order:* Don Pablo's	755	39	54
Dos Beef Tacos (Soft)	850	37	92
Dos Chicken Enchiladas	730	35	63
Classic Fajitas: *w/o Rice, Beans or Cold Set*			
Chicken	600	20	74
Steak	770	39	83
Quesadillas: Cheese	905	55	61
Mesquite-Grilled Chicken	775	39	63
Salads:			
Chicken Caesar, with Dressing	1565	118	85
Steak Caesar, with Dressing	1790	144	97
Tortilla Salad in Taco Shell, w/o Dress.	550	29	59
Flour Tortilla Taco Shell	485	27	50
Salad Dressing, 3 oz: Ranch	320	34	3
Bleu Cheese	450	48	3
Honey Mustard	315	27	17
Low Fat French	150	4	30
Sides: Chips & Salsa, 1 order	340	17	43
Guacamole, 1¼ oz	50	5	2
Mexican Rice, 3 oz	105	1	21
Refritos, 5 oz	260	10	31
Sour Cream, 1¼ oz	75	7	2
Soup: Tortilla, 12 oz Bowl	260	12	26
White Chicken Chili, 6 oz cup	235	13	23

Extra Menu Items ~ see CalorieKing.com

Dunkin Donuts® (Sept '09)

	C	F	Cb
Donuts: Apple N' Spice	240	11	32
Bavarian Kreme	250	12	31
Boston Kreme	280	12	38
Chocolate Frosted	230	10	32
Chocolate Kreme Filled	310	16	37
French Cruller	250	20	18
Jelly Filled	260	11	36
Old Fashioned Cake	280	18	27
Powdered Cake	300	18	30
Strawberry Frosted	230	10	33
Sugar Raised	190	9	22
Vanilla Kreme Filled	320	17	37
Fancies: Bow Tie Donut	310	15	39
Coffee Roll, avg, all varieties	375	18	50
Eclair,	350	14	53
Fritter: Apple	400	15	63
Glazed	400	15	63
Munchkins: Plain Cake, 4	200	12	20
Glazed, avg all varieties, 4	220	12	32
Jelly Filled, 5	300	13	40
Powdered Cake, 4	240	14	24
Sugar Raised, 5	200	13	25
Bagels: Plain	330	3	71
Cinnamon Raisin	370	4	72
Everything; Poppy Seed	365	6	74
Multigrain	400	9	65
Onion; Wheat	345	3.5	65
Salt	330	3	71
Sesame	370	7	72
Danish: Apple Cheese	330	16	41
Cheese	330	17	39
Strawberry Cheese	320	16	40
Muffins: Chocolate Chip	630	23	98
Blueberry	510	16	87
Reduced Fat	450	10	86
Coffee Cake	620	25	93
Corn	510	17	84
Honey Bran Raisin	500	14	86

Continued Next Page ...

Dunkin Donuts® cont... (Sept '09)

Breakfast **C** **F** **Cb**

Oven Toasted Breakfast Sandwiches:

	C	F	Cb
Bagels: Bacon Egg & Cheese	530	18	76
Ham Egg & Cheese	520	17	75
Sausage Egg & Cheese	660	29	76
Supreme Omelet & Cheese	520	17	77
Biscuits: Sausage Egg & Cheese	600	40	37
Supreme Omelet & Cheese	470	28	37
Croissant: Bacon Egg & Cheese	510	31	39
Ham Egg & Cheese	510	30	39
Sausage Egg & Cheese	640	42	40
Saus. Supreme Omelet & Cheese	680	44	41
Supreme Omelet & Cheese	500	30	41
English Muffin:			
Bacon Egg & Cheese	360	16	35
Ham Egg & Cheese	350	15	35
Sausage Egg & Cheese	490	28	35
Hash Browns, 9 pieces	200	11	22

Sandwiches & Burgers

Dunkin' Deli Sandwiches

Cravings: Chicken Bruschetta	580	26	49
Chipotle Chicken	600	25	50
Pastrami Supreme	750	39	51
Pressed Cuban Sandwich	680	33	50
Deli Classics: Tuna (Albacore)	660	19	56
Turkey & Cheese	450	13	52
Favorites: Steak & Cheese	470	16	50
Toasted Italian	560	25	52
Turkey & Bacon Club	440	13	51

Salads: With Dressing

Dunkin' Deli: Caesar	320	29	11
Chicken Caesar	440	33	11
Garden	180	6	21
Soups: Broccoli Cheddar, 1 cup	190	11	14
Chicken Noodle	130	3	19

Beverages

Cappuccino, 10 fl.oz	80	4	7
Coolatta: Watermellon, 16 fl.oz	250	0	60
Coffee: w. Skim Milk, 16 fl.oz	140	0	30
w. Cream, 16 fl.oz	330	23	28
w. Milk, 16 fl.oz	170	4	29
Strawberry Fruit, 16 fl.oz	300	0	72
Tropical Orange, 16 fl.oz	220	0	52
Hot Chocolate: Small, 10 fl.oz	230	11	35
White, 1 medium, 14 fl.oz	340	13	56
Iced Coffee: 16 fl.oz	10	0	2
Flavored Coffee: Caramel, 10 fl.oz	10	0	2
Toasted Almond, 10 fl.oz	15	0	2

Eat 'N Park® (Sept '09)

Breakfast **C** **F** **Cb**

	C	F	Cb
Egg Beaters (2)	135	7	2
Fruit Cup	60	0.5	15
Hash Browns	200	8	28
Home Fries	210	12	24
Oatmeal with Milk	200	4	33
Omelette: Cheese	390	30	2.5
Chicken Fiesta	565	37	10
Ham & Cheese	535	35	4
Veggie	415	30	8
Western	345	21	7
Pancakes, Buttermilk: Plain (1)	75	1	15
Blueberry (1)	85	1	16
Waffles: Belgian (1)	280	12	35
Strawberry (1)	375	18	48

Burgers:

Black Angus: American Grill	610	37	31
BBQ Bacon Cheddar	865	53	53
Mushroom & Onion	710	41	45
Superburger	1085	73	28
Classic: Black Angus	420	21	22
Bacon Cheeseburger	530	31	22
Cheeseburger	465	25	22
Garden Burger	220	4	33
Original, Superburger	565	38	27

Sandwiches:

BLT	490	15	66
Buffalo Chicken	740	41	59
Chicken Caesar Wrap	500	26	26
Chicken Chargrill	320	6	32
Chicken Portabella Hoagie	845	56	47
Grilled Cheese	725	39	65
Hot Turkey	500	9	71
Reuben on Rye	730	50	31
Santa Fe Turkey & Bacon	880	60	45
Shredded Pot Roast	530	31	28
Turkey Club	835	50	52
Whale of a Cod	880	41	76

Appetizers:

Buffalo Chicken Tenders	635	42	27
Fried Cheese Sticks	535	36	26
Grilled Chicken Quesadillas	905	55	51
Onion Rings	245	16	23

Eat 'N Park® cont... (Sept '09)

	C	F	Cb
Dinners: Baked Lemon Sole, 1 filet	195	10	6
Chargrilled Chicken, 2 pieces	350	9	0
Chicken Fillets (5)	530	26	28
Chicken Parmigiana: Marinara Sce	960	37	100
Meat Sauce	985	40	95
Chicken Stir-Fry	390	9	47
Cod Floridian, 2 filets	240	3	8
Ground Sirloin	425	26	5
Spaghetti Marinara	695	9	129
Spaghetti with Meat Sauce	830	16	145
T Bone Steak	575	39	1
Salads			
Buffalo Chicken Salad	610	35	42
Chicken Fajita	730	43	41
Garden Salad	95	3	15
Grilled Chicken	445	20	30
Grilled Chicken & Strawberry	215	6	13
Grilled Chicken Portobella	320	11	23
Dressings: Per 2 fl.oz			
Bleu Cheese	245	25	3
French Fat Free	75	0	18
Italian Fat Free	20	0	5
House Ranch	215	21	5
Thousand Island	185	19	4
Desserts:			
Grilled Stickies a la Mode	730	39	81
Ice Cream, 2 scoops	230	12	27
Pies: Per Slice			
Apple	520	27	67
Cherry	520	28	63
Peachberry	390	19	51
Strawberry	295	12	45

Edo Japan® (Sept '09)

Meals: Per Bento Box w/o Teriyaki	C	F	Cb
Beef Yakisoba, 20.28 oz	830	30	102
Chicken Yakisoba, 20.53 oz	800	25	102
Seafood Grill, 23 oz	860	16	129
Sizzling Shrimp, 22.05 oz	800	16	122
Sukiyaki Beef, 20.14 oz	900	28	120
Teriyaki Dishes: *Without Teriyaki Sauce*			
Curry Chicken Bowl, 13.23 oz	500	21	27
Ginger Pork, 14.6 oz	650	23	82
Hawaiian Chicken, 15.52 oz	590	12	85
Seafood Grill, 17.71 oz	570	4	89
Sukiyaki Beef, 14.85 oz	610	16	80
Teriyaki Chicken, 15.1 oz	580	12	80

Einstein Bros®/Noahs® (Sept '09)

Bagels:	C	F	Cb
Asiago Cheese	330	5	59
Blueberry Bagel	290	1.5	64
Chocolate Chip	290	3	60
Garlic Dip'd	290	2.5	60
Onion Dip'd	270	1	59
Cinnamon Sugar Chicago Style	310	2.5	66
Egg Bagel	300	6	52
Everything	270	1.5	56
Honey Whole Wheat; Onion; Plain	270	1.5	60
Poppy Dip'd Bagel	280	3	56
Potato Bagel	260	1	58
Power Bagel, Fruit & Nut	380	6	72
Sesame Dip'd Bagel	280	3	56
Sundried Tomato Bagel	270	1.5	58
Gourmet Bagels: Dutch Apple Bagel	340	7	66
Green Chile Bagel	370	8	62
Spinach Florentine Bagel	360	8	61
Six-Cheese Bagel	350	6	60
Breakfast Sandwiches			
Egg Way: Original	530	20	62
with Bacon	580	24	59
with Black Forest Ham	570	21	62
Spinach Mushr. & Omelette	540	20	65
Bacon & Spinach Panini	860	51	66
Sausage Ranchero Panini	680	29	64
Vegetable Breakfast Panini	730	36	68
Wraps: California Chicken	630	28	63
Chipotle Turkey	730	37	70
Bagel Dogs: With Cheddar Cheese			
Original	550	26	56
Original Asiago	560	27	56
Pizza Bagels: Cheese	420	12	63
Pepperoni	470	16	63
Cream Cheese: Whipped, Per 2 Tablespoons			
Blueberry	70	5	6
Garlic Herb/Garden Veggie/Jalapeno	60	5	3
Honey Almond; Strawberry	70	5	6
Onion and Chive	70	6	3
Plain	60	5	2
Smoked Salmon; Sun Dried Tom. Basil	60	6	2
Salads: With Dressing			
Bros Bistro	820	68	38
Bros Bistro with Chicken	940	71	39
Chipotle	590	38	53
Chicken Chipotle	710	41	54
Caesar Salad with Chicken	820	66	20
Coffee, Specialty: Per Regular, 12 fl.oz			
Café Latte, Regular	140	5	13
Cafe Latte, Non-Fat	100	1	14
Cappuccino, Whole Milk	150	8	13
Mocha Whole Milk	270	9	38
Espresso, Regular 2 fl.oz	1	0	0
Americano Regular 8 fl.oz	1	0	0

Updated Nutrition Data ~ www.CalorieKing.com
Persons with Diabetes ~ See Disclaimer (Page 24)

El Pollo Loco® (Sept '09)

	C	F	Cb
Burritos:			
Classic Chicken	550	17	69
Twice Grilled	840	39	56
Ultimate Grilled	710	23	86
BBQ Chicken: With Sauce			
Breast, 5 oz	245	9	5
Leg, 2 oz	90	4	2
Thigh, 4 oz	230	15	4
Wing, 2 oz	95	5	2
Flame-Grilled Chicken:			
Breast	220	9	0
Leg	90	4	0
Thigh	220	15	0
Wing	90	5	0
Bowls: Chicken Caesar	490	22	44
The Original Pollo	690	10	106
Ultimate Pollo	1050	34	110
Loco Value Menu: Chicken Taquito	230	12	20
Chips & Guacamole, 2.6 oz	250	14	26
Cheese Quesadilla	210	13	35
Loco Salad with Cilantro Dressing	170	14	7
Taco al Carbon	150	5	17
Mexican Favorites:			
Grilled Chicken Nachos	810	40	70
Tacos: Crunchy Chicken	190	8	16
Soft Chicken	260	12	18
Sliders: With Dressing			
Chicken: BBQ, 3 oz	180	5	24
Classic, 4 oz	515	32	40
Spicy, 4 oz	485	28	41
Salads: Chicken Tostada	825	42	72
Garden Salad, small	125	7	10
Sauce & Dressings: Per Packet			
Creamy Cilantro, 3 oz	440	46	3
Light Creamy Cilantro, 2 oz	70	5	6
Light Italian, 2 oz	20	1	2
Ranch, 2 oz	230	24	2
Thousand Island, 2 oz	220	21	6
Condiments			
Guacamole, 1.3 oz	70	6	3
Salsa: Avocado, 1.5 oz	40	3.5	2
House, 1.5 oz	10	0	2
Pico de Gallo, 1.5 oz	15	1	2
Sides			
Corn Cobbette, 5 oz	90	0.5	19
French Fries, 6 oz	330	17	42
Fresh Vegetables w/ Marg., 4.1 oz	60	3	8
Macaroni & Cheese, 5.5 oz	280	17	28
Mashed Potatoes with Gravy, 6 oz	120	1.5	25
Pinto Beans, 6 oz	200	4	29
Refried Beans with Cheese, 6.3 oz	270	7	36
Spanish Rice, 4½ oz	220	2	45
Desserts: Caramel Flan, 5.1 oz	260	12	34
Churros (2)	300	18	32

For Complete Nutritional Data ~ see CalorieKing.com

Fatburger® (Sept '09)

	C	F	Cb
Burgers: Baby Fat	400	21	37
Sausage & Egg Sandwich	780	53	47
Grilled Chicken Sandwich	430	14	42
Fatburger	590	31	46
Kingburger	850	41	69
Turkey Burger	480	21	50
Shakes (16 fl.oz): Chocolate	910	45	115
Strawberry	880	44	111
Vanilla	890	44	113
Fries & Sides: Chili Cup, 7.6 oz	200	11	10
with Cheese & Onions	320	20	12
Fat Fries, 8 oz	380	18	47
Skinny Fries, 5.5 oz	390	15	58
Onion Rings, 5.5 oz	540	29	64

For Complete Nutritional Data ~ see CalorieKing.com

Fazoli's® Italian Food (Sept '09)

	C	F	Cb
Pasta Bowl: Per Serving			
Fettuccine w. Alfredo, 19.9 oz	900	27	126
Fettuccine w . Marinara, 20.5 oz	660	3	129
Ravioli with Marinara Sce, 12.3 oz	490	15	69
Ravioli with Meat Sauce, 13.1 oz	570	21	70
Spaghetti w/ Marinara Sce, 20.5 oz	660	3	129
Sampler Platter: Per Serving			
Classic Sampler Platter, 22.8 oz	880	30	110
Ultimate Sampler Platter, 29.9 oz	1130	34	153
Oven-Baked Pasta: Per Serving			
Chicken Parmagiano, 21.6 oz	1000	39	108
Baked Spaghetti, 15.5 oz	640	22	80
with Italian Sausage, 18.5 oz	950	46	85
with Meatballs, 18.5 oz	890	39	86
Creamy Chicken Florentine, 18.3 oz	890	42	73
Fazoli's Deep Dish Pasta, 19.5 oz	850	40	85
Penne w. Creamy Basil Chkn, 18.7 oz	970	51	73
Rigatoni Romano, 17.3 oz	880	44	76
Tortellini Robusto, 17.6 oz	1020	50	80
Twice-Baked Lasagna, 18.4 oz	700	39	47
Pizzas: Per Slice			
Cheese, 4 oz	270	11	32
Pepperoni, 4.3 oz	310	14	32

Continued next page...

Fazoli's® cont... (Sept '09)

Submarinos	C	F	Cb
Club Italiano, 13 oz	780	36	68
Fire-Roasted Pepper Chkn, 10.9 oz	640	21	59
Ham 'n' Swiss Supremo, 12.1 oz	690	31	68
Italian Beef Gorgonzola, 12.7 oz	750	38	72
Italian Four Chse & Tomato, 11.1 oz	690	35	58
Smoked Turkey Basil, 12.8 oz	750	37	68
Salads: *Without Dressing*			
Antipasto	260	15	11
Caesar Side Salad, 4.2 oz	40	2	4
Chicken Caprese	370	10	9
Cranberry & Walnut Chicken	390	14	27
Crispy Chicken BLT	480	26	31
Grilled Chicken Artichoke	240	4.5	11
Italian Side Salad, 4.2 oz	80	4.5	4
Salad Dressing: *Per 1.5 oz*			
Caesar	230	25	1
Italian	160	14	7
Fat Free	25	0	6
Honey French	220	18	14
Ranch	220	24	2
Lite Ranch	120	12	2

For Complete Nutritional Data ~ see CalorieKing.com

Firehouse Subs® (Sept'09)

Subs: Per Medium	C	F	Cb
Chicken Salad	760	46	63
Engine Company	390	6	52
Engineer	380	5	55
Ham	410	7	58
Hero	430	7	54
Hook & Ladder	410	7	68
Italian	560	25	55
NY Steamer	410	12	48
Roast Beef	410	6	48
Tuna Salad	610	28	62
Turkey	370	4	54
Veggie	300	5	56
Chili and Salads: *Includes Meat, Cheese and Egg, w/o Dressing*			
Chili	370	28	17
Chief's Salad: with Chicken Salad	740	58	16
with Tuna Salad	610	40	16
with Ham	360	18	16
with Turkey	300	15	12
Desserts: Brownie (1)	420	18	63
Choc Chip Cookie	290	14	37

Five Guys (Sept '09)

Burgers	C	F	Cb
Bacon Burger	780	50	39
Bacon Cheeseburger	920	62	40
Cheeseburger	840	55	40
Hamburger	700	43	39
Little: Bacon Burger	560	33	39
Bacon Cheeseburger	630	39	40
Cheeseburger	550	32	40
Hamburger	480	26	39
Dogs			
Bacon Dog	625	42	40
Bacon Cheese Dog	695	48	41
Cheese Dog	615	41	41
Hot Dog	545	35	40
Fries: Regular 8.6 oz	620	30	78
½ Regular Order	310	15	39

Freshens® (Sept '09)

Frozen Yogurt: Per Serving	C	F	Cb
Soft Serve Yogurt, 1 oz	35	0.5	7
Smoothies: *100% Juice (21 fl.oz)*			
Acai Energy Smoothie	320	3	72
All That Razz	360	0	79
Berry Breeze	305	0	77
Caribbean Craze	290	0	73
High Test Energizer	300	0	74
Jamaican Jammer	355	0	78
Mango Beach	90	0	48
Maui Mango	290	0	74
Mystic Mango	355	3	82
Orange Passion	135	3	37
Orange Sunrise	355	3	81
Peach Sunset	270	0	67
Peachy Pineapple	335	0	73
Peanut Butter Energizer	475	10	83
Pineapple Paradise	330	4	77
Strawberry: Oasis	90	0	49
Shooter	245	0	64
Squeeze	315	0	68
Sunrise	155	0	35
Active Nutrition at Energy Zone: *Per 4 oz Muffin*			
Banana Nut Muffin	440	22	53
Blueberry Cranberry Muffin	460	22	58
Fudge Brownie, 3½ oz	380	17	48

Frisch's Big Boy® (Aug '09)

	C	F	Cb
Breakfast, **HealthSmart, Egg Beaters:**			
Plain Omelette	310	8.5	38
Scrambled	310	8.5	38
Vegetarian Omelette	340	8.5	45
Health Smart Meals: Tossed Salad	45	0.5	6
Grilled Chicken Breast	325	10	22
Lemon Baked Cod	490	4.5	72
Spaghetti Marinara	420	6.5	76
Vegetable Stir-Fry	610	3.5	134
Sandwiches: Big Boy	600	26	35
Brawny Lad	420	21	30
Buddie Boy	760	34	80
Fish Sandwich	690	48	41
Small Hamburger	445	30	30
Super Big Boy	830	66	35
Swiss Miss	635	44	28
Sides: Chili	315	18	19
French Fries	360	19	45
Onion Rings	580	41	45
Tartar Sauce	370	40	1
Trio Salad	620	46	18
Soups: HealthSmart Cabbage Soup	50	0.5	9
Beverages: HealthSmart Shake	160	0	33

Gold Star Chili® (Sept '09)

Meals	C	F	Cb
Bowls: Low Carb Coney, 10.5 oz	570	47	7
Veggie Chili, 9 oz	160	2	29
Coney, 5.15 oz	285	14	30
Cheese Coney, 5.64 oz	345	18	31
Chili: 8 oz	215	12	8
Tex Mex, 8 oz	210	9	17
Chili Cheese Nachos, 8.47 oz	410	25	30
Regular: 2-Way	420	11	58
Bean	490	12	71
Onion	435	11	62
Onion Bean	505	12	75
Regular 3-Way	650	30	59
Regular 4-Way	665	30	63
Regular 5-Way	735	30	76
Super 5-Way	1140	51	109
Sandwiches: Chili	210	5	32
Chili Cheese	290	12	30
Sides: Fries, 5 oz	365	19	44
Garlic Bread: Without Cheese, 2 oz	215	13	19
w. Cheese, 2½ oz	270	18	19

Gino's East® (Sept '09)

	C	F	Cb
Deep Dish Pizza: Medium 11" ~ Per Slice (⅙ Pizza)			
Cheese	410	11	58
Crumbled Sausage	420	21	38
Pepperoni	450	15	57
Spinach	410	11	59
Deep Dish Pizza: Small 6" ~ Per Whole Pizza			
Cheese	720	16	116
Crumbled Sausage	800	22	116
Pepperoni	780	20	116

Golden Corral® (Sept '09)

Meals	C	F	Cb
Bourbon Street Chicken, 3.5 oz	210	11	5
Cajun Style Fish Filet, 3.5 oz	210	10	18
Cajun Whitefish, 3 oz	110	7	0
Fresh Fried Chkn, Leg or Thigh (1)	250	19	2
Meatloaf, 3.5 oz	190	10	10
Sirloin Steak, 3 oz	220	13	0
Steakburger, 6 oz	860	55	0
Turkey Breast w. Wing, 2 oz	70	3	1
Vegetables: Glazed Sesame Carrots	260	16	27
Fresh Vegetable Trio, ½ cup	25	0	5
Ranch Style BBQ Beans, ½ cup	130	3	20

Godfather's™ Pizza (Sept '09)

Golden Pizza: Per Slice	C	F	Cb
Cheese: Medium, ⅛ pizza	220	8	25
Large,¹⁄₁₀ pizza	250	9	28
Combo: Medium, 1/8 pizza	290	13	27
Large, slice, ¹⁄₁₀ pizza	330	15	30
Original Pizza			
Cheese: Mini, ¼ pizza	150	4	20
Medium, ⅛ pizza	260	7	34
Jumbo, ¹⁄₁₂ pizza	350	10	44
Combo: Mini, ¼ pizza	200	8	21
Medium, ⅛ pizza	350	14	36
Jumbo, ¹⁄₁₂ pizza	480	20	47
Thin Pizza			
Cheese: Medium, ⅛ pizza	170	8	15
Large, ¹⁄₁₀ pizza	210	10	17
Combo: Medium, ⅛ pizza	240	13	17
Large, ¹⁄₁₀ pizza	280	16	20
Sides			
Breadstick (1)	110	2	20
Cheesestick,1 piece, ⅙	130	3.5	18
Potato Wedges, 4 oz	175	8	24

209

Fast - Foods & *Restaurants*

(The) Great American
Bagel Co® (Sept '09)

Bagels:	C	F	Cb
4-Grain Honey	390	4	80
Apple Cinnamon Oat Bran	370	4	73
Apple Cinnamon Sugar	390	4	78
Apple Crumb	620	11	118
Asiago	520	16	72
Banana Nut	410	9	69
Blueberry	370	3.5	75
Cheddar Bacon	600	23	71
Chocolate Chip	420	8	78
Cinnamon Delight	640	18	108
French Toast	430	8	77
Jalapeno Cheddar	370	7	63
Onion	380	4	74
Plain; Pumpernickel; Salt	360	4	71
Strawberry	380	3.5	76
Stuffed Pepperoni	570	17	78
Stuffed Spinach	640	20	86
Sun-Dried Tomato Basil	390	4	74
Tomazzo	520	13	77
Veggie	310	3.5	61

Green Burrito (Sept '09)

Burritos:			
Bean & Cheese	820	37	100
Grilled Chicken	1070	53	91
Meat Bean & Cheese: Chicken	720	29	80
Ground Beef	860	42	83
Steak	750	31	83
The Green Burrito w. Steak	930	34	122
Specialties:			
Enchiladas, Cheese (2)	480	33	29
Super Nachos: Chicken	950	50	94
Ground Beef	1080	63	97
Taco Salad: Chicken	830	45	74
Ground Beef	970	58	76
Steak	860	48	76
Tacos: Fish	320	15	36
Hard: Chicken; Steak, average	195	9	15
Ground Beef	270	16	16
Soft: Chicken	200	7	17
Ground Beef	290	15	19
Sides: Chips, 2 oz	300	17	35
Chips & Cheese, 5 oz	700	42	62
Guacamole, 1.4 oz	60	5	3
Pinto Beans & Cheese, 8.5 oz	320	16	43
Rice, 7 oz	340	10	58
Sour Cream, 1.4 oz	50	3.5	3

(The) Great Steak & Potato Company® (Sept '09)

Breakfast Sandwiches	C	F	Cb
Bacon, Egg & Cheese	600	36	39
Egg and Cheese	500	29	39
Ham and Cheese	430	22	41
Ham, Egg and Cheese	570	32	42
Sausage, Egg and Cheese	700	47	39
Steak, Egg & Cheese	600	34	40
Breakfast Sides:			
Potatoes: Deluxe Home	390	23	44
Fresh Cut Home	380	23	42
Sandwiches: 7"			
Chicken Philly	620	22	62
Great Steak Cheesesteak	740	37	62
Ham Delight	710	33	71
Ham Explosion	710	34	70
Philly Cheesesteak	650	26	62
Reuben	690	33	61
Super Steak Cheesesteak	750	37	64
Veggie Delight	610	31	66
Sides			
Chicken Nuggets, Kids, 2.8 oz	165	9	10
Great Fry: Kids, 6.17 oz	270	13	36
Regular, 10.3 oz	440	20	60
Large, 12.42 oz	540	25	72
Potato Skins, 6.46 oz	390	26	24
Baked Potato, Plain, 6 oz	160	0	36
Meat: Per 4 oz Serving, without Sides			
Chicken	140	3	0
Corned Beef	135	8	0
Gyro	210	12	5
Ham	120	4	6
Steak	160	7	0
Turkey	90	1	2
Salads: Without Dressing			
Chef Salad	260	11	15
Garden	60	1	13
Grilled Steak	400	23	18
Sauces: Buffalo 1 oz	10	0	2
Teriyaki, 1 oz	25	0	3
Tzatziki, 1 oz	50	4	2
Breads/Pita			
Bread, 12"White, 7 oz	420	4	82
Bread, 7"Wheat, 4 oz	310	4	56
Pita, 2.8 oz	220	5	38

Fast - Foods & *Restaurants*

Haagen-Dazs® (Sept '09)

Ice Cream: Per ½ Cup	C	F	Cb
Baileys Irish Cream	260	17	21
Banana Split	280	16	31
Butter Pecan	310	23	21
Caramel Cone	320	19	32
Cherry Vanilla	240	15	23
Chocolate	270	18	22
Chocolate Chip Cookie Dough	310	20	29
Chocolate Chocolate Chip	300	20	26
Coffee	270	18	21
Cookies & Cream	270	17	23
Creme Brulee	280	19	23
Dulce de Leche	290	17	28
Mango	250	14	28
Pineapple Coconut	230	13	25
Pistachio	290	20	22
Reserve: *Per ½ Cup*			
Fleu de Sel Caramel	280	17	28
Pomegranate Chip	280	16	31
Toasted Coconut Sesame Brittle	300	18	31
Light Ice Cream: Dutch Chocolate	190	5	33
Sorbet: Chocolate, Low-Fat	130	0.5	28
Fat-Free: Orchard Peach	130	0	33
Raspberry/Strawberry	120	0	31
Zesty Lemon	110	0	28
Frozen Yogurt: Per ½ Cup			
Vanilla Honey & Granola	200	4	32
Wildberry	180	2	34
Low-Fat: Coffee/Vanilla	200	4.5	31
Dulce de Leche	190	2.5	35
Vanilla Raspberry Swirl	170	2.5	32

Ice Cream Bars ~ See Page 111

Hardee's® (Sept '09)

Breakfast	C	F	Cb
Biscuits: Bacon, Egg & Cheese	560	38	37
Biscuit 'N' Gravy	530	34	47
Chicken Fillet	600	34	50
Cinnamon 'N Raisin	280	12	40
Country Ham	440	26	36
Country Steak	620	41	44
Loaded Omelet	640	44	37
Made from Scratch	370	23	35
Monster	710	51	37
Sausage	530	38	36
w. Egg	610	44	36
Smoked Ssge w. Egg & Cheese	750	56	38

Hardee's® cont... (Sept '09)

Breakfast Bowls:	C	F	Cb
Loaded Biscuit 'N' Gravy	770	54	49
Low Carb	620	50	6
Breakfast Burritos: Loaded	780	51	38
Breakfast Croissants:			
Sunrise: w/ Bacon	450	29	28
w/ Ham	430	26	28
w/ Sausage	550	38	29
Breakfast Sandwiches, Frisco	420	20	37
Texas Toast: Bacon, 4.73 oz	380	21	31
Ham, 6.35 oz	390	18	31
Sausage, 5.5 oz	480	30	32
Breakfast Sides:			
Country Potatoes, Small, 3.5 oz	200	9	27
Medium, 5 oz	290	12	39
Large, 8.3 oz	480	21	64
Grits, 5 oz	110	5	16
Burgers:			
Big Shef 7.5 oz	660	46	36
Cheeseburger: ⅓ lb	680	39	52
Double, 6.55 oz	510	26	38
Regular, 4.62 oz	350	16	36
Hamburger, 4.15 oz	310	12	36
Thickburger: Original, ⅓ lb	910	64	53
Bacon Cheese, ⅓ lb	910	64	50
Chili Cheese, 12 oz	990	62	56
French Dip, 9.45 oz	650	33	47
Little Thickburger ¼ lb	620	40	38
Low-Carb ⅓ lb	420	32	5
Monster, ⅔ lb	1420	108	46
Mushroom & Swiss ⅓ lb	720	42	48
Six Dollar Burger, ½ lb	950	59	58
Sandwiches:			
Chicken: BBQ Chicken	340	4	40
Big Chicken Fillet	800	37	76
Charbroiled Chicken Club	560	30	32
Fish, Supreme	630	38	51
Ham, Big Hot Ham 'N' Cheese	520	24	40

Continued next page...

Fast - Foods & *Restaurants*

Hardee's® cont... (Sept '09)

	C	F	Cb
Salads: With Sauce, includes Tortilla Bowl			
Southwest Chicken, 14.14 oz	**1090**	80	68
Chicken Strips: Without Sauce			
Strips, 5 Strips, 8.5 oz	**630**	34	45
Sides			
Beer Battered Onion Rings, 4.3 oz	**410**	24	45
Kids Meals: Incl. Kid's Fries & Small Drink			
Cheeseburger	**600**	27	68
Crispy Chicken Strips (2), w/o sce	**500**	25	50
Hamburger	**560**	24	67
Fries:			
Bacon Ranch:	**710**	46	63
Crispy Curls: Small 3 oz	**260**	13	33
Medium 4.66 oz	**410**	20	52
Large 5.4 oz	**480**	23	60
Natural Cut: Small, 4.27 oz	**320**	14	45
Medium, 5.68 oz	**430**	19	60
Large, 6.2 oz	**470**	21	65
Desserts: Apple Turnover	**290**	15	36
Drinks: Hot Chocolate	**150**	3	18
Malts: Per 16 fl.oz			
Chocolate	**780**	35	97
Orange Cream	**680**	33	82
Oreo Cookie	**790**	39	91
Strawberry	**775**	35	98
Vanilla	**710**	35	97
Shakes: Per 16 fl.oz			
Chocolate	**700**	34	85
Orange Cream	**680**	33	82
Oreo Cookie	**720**	37	79
Strawberry	**700**	33	86
Vanilla	**710**	33	87

Harvey's® (Sept '09)

Sandwiches & Burgers	C	F	Cb
Angus Burger	**560**	26	47
Angus Burger w. Cheese	**640**	32	49
Angus Patty, 1 patty	**320**	23	4
Cheeseburger	**460**	23	39
Hamburger	**380**	16	37
Grilled Chicken Sandwich	**290**	5	28
VeggieBurger	**290**	10	33
Hot Dog, (1)	**300**	13	32

Harvey's® cont... (Sept '09)

	C	F	Cb
Breakfast:			
Bacon, 3 Strips	**40**	2	0
Extra Egg (1)	**90**	6	0
Homefries	**300**	19	29
Sandwich: Breakfast Club	**400**	19	36
Breakfast Club Deluxe	**530**	28	39
Toast, White, 2 slices	**180**	2	35
Sides:			
Chicken Strips, 3 pieces	**320**	15	27
French Fries: Regular, 4.23 oz	**320**	13	49
Large, 5.3 oz	**410**	16	61
Value, 3.1 oz	**240**	10	37
Onion Rings: Regular, 2.8 oz	**270**	15	33
Large, 5.1 oz	**550**	29	65
Garnishes:			
Barbecue Sauce, 1 oz	**50**	0	12
Canadian Cheddar Cheese, 1 slice	**80**	6	1
Ketchup, 0.3 oz	**10**	0	2
Light Mayonnaise, ½ oz	**45**	5	1
Relish, 0.71 oz	**20**	0	5
Dipping Sauce: Barbecue. 1.52 oz	**90**	0	21
Honey Mustard, 1.52 oz	**160**	12	13
Plum, 1.52 oz	**80**	0	21
Sweet n' Sour, 1.52 oz	**80**	0.5	17

Heavenly Ham® (Sept '09)

Meats: Per 3 oz Serving	C	F	Cb
Bone-In Hams: Glazed	**190**	11	4
Fat Removed	**160**	3	4
Boneless Hams: Glazed	**120**	4	4
Fat Removed	**90**	1	4
Turkey			
Boneless Brst, Glazed Roasted;Smoked	**60**	0	3
Whole: Roasted	**160**	10	0
Smoked	**145**	8	1
Classic Sandwiches: Roast Beef	**635**	36	50
Swiss Philly	**700**	46	36
Salads: Without Dressing			
Chicken	**260**	17	14
Taste of Italy	**310**	20	21
Bread: Croissant	**230**	12	27
French Batard	**210**	0.5	46
Multigrain Batard	**250**	3.5	46
Sliced Wheat Bread	**300**	5	54
Sauces: BBQ, 1.75 oz	**260**	26	4
Bistro, 0.75 oz	**120**	13	1
Dill, 1.5 oz	**170**	19	1
Mayonnaise, 1 oz	**200**	24	0
Ranch, 1.5 oz	**220**	23	2
Spicy Brown Mustard, 1 oz	**30**	0	0
Sweet Café Spread, 1 oz	**100**	10	4
That Mustard, 1 oz	**150**	0	30

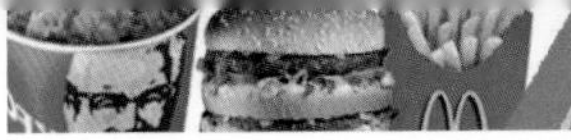

Hot Dog on a Stick® (Sept '09)

Menu Items	C	F	Cb
Beef Hot Dog on a Bun	460	29	37
Turkey Hot Dog on a Stick	240	11	28
Veggie Dog on a Stick	250	5	35
American Cheese on a Stick	270	14	26
Pepperjack Cheese on a Stick	260	13	25
French Fries, 4.48 oz	390	15	60
Lemonade (16 fl.oz): Original	150	0	38
Sugar Free Lemonade	15	0	3
Cherry	210	0	52

Hungry Howie's Pizza® (Sept '09)

Pizzas: Per Slice	C	F	Cb
Cheese: Small, ⅙ pizza	160	3.5	20
Medium, ⅛ pizza	190	5.5	23
Large, ⅒ pizza	210	5	25
X-Large, ⅛ pizza	395	9	42
Oven Baked Subs: Per ½ Sub			
Deluxe Italian	505	18	61
Ham & Cheese	475	15	61
Steak & Cheese	490	15	64
Turkey	555	15	63
Vegetarian	530	21	64
Sides: Chicken Tenders, 2 pieces	140	4.5	11
Howie Wings, 5 wings	180	13	0
Salads: Per Small, without Dressing			
Antipasto (2)	230	15	6
Chef (2)	230	13	8
Garden (2)	40	0.5	6
Greek (2)	250	15	16
Dressings: Creamy Italian, 1 oz	120	12	2
Greek, 1 oz	110	11	2
Ranch, 1 oz	180	19	1
Thousand Island, 1 oz	140	14	4

In-N-Out Burger® (Aug '09)

	C	F	Cb
Burgers: Hamburger w/ Onion	390	19	39
w. Mustard/Ketchup, w/o Spread	310	10	41
Protein Style w. Lettuce Wrap, w/o Bun	240	17	11
Cheeseburger w/ Onion	480	27	39
w. Mustard/Ketchup, w/o Spread	400	18	41
Protein Style w. Lettuce Wrap, w/o Bun	330	25	11
Double Double® w/ Onion	670	41	39
w. Mustard/Ketchup, w/o Spread	590	32	41
Protein Style w. Lettuce Wrap, w/o Bun	520	39	11
French Fries, 4.4 oz	400	18	54
Drinks: Milk, 10 fl.oz	180	6	18
Coca-Cola®,16 fl.oz	200	0	54
Lemonade, 16 fl.oz	180	0	40
Root Beer,16 fl.oz	220	0	60
Shakes: Choc., 15 fl.oz	690	36	83
Strawberry, 15 fl.oz	690	33	91

IHOP® (Aug '09) *(Author Estimates)*

Pancakes: (Syrup/Butter extra)	C	F	Cb
Buttermilk (1), 1.7 oz	110	3	17
Short Stack, 3	330	9	51
Full Stack, 5	550	15	85
Harvest Grain 'N Nut: (1) 2¼ oz	180	9	20
Combo	1035	65	80
Crepe-Style, 2 oz	120	6	14
IHOP For Me: Buttermilk Trio (3), 5 oz	330	9	51
w. Marg. & ¼ c. sugar-free syrup	470	20	63
Syrup: Regular, 1 Tbsp	50	0	12
Sugar-Free, 1 Tbsp	10	0	3
Whipped Butter/Margarine, 1 T.	80	9	0
Waffles (Plain), Belgian, reg. (1), 4 oz	390	19	48
Breakfast: Per Serving			
Classic Combos: Cntry Fried Steak/Eggs	1530	105	73
Signature: Rooty Tooty	855	45	84
T-Bone Steak & Eggs	1310	86	63
Omelette Feast			
Colorado Omelette: No pancakes	790	68	5
with 3 buttermilk pancakes	1205	83	66
The Big Steak Omelette: No pancakes	910	72	14
with 3 buttermilk pancakes	1325	87	75
Burgers & Sandwiches			
Chicken Clubhouse Stacker w. Fries	1710	98	132
Ham & Egg Melt w. Onion Rings	1350	70	121
Patty Melt w. Fries	1480	72	145
Tuscan Chicken Griller: w/o Fries	720	28	67
with French Fries, 4 oz	1070	46	111
Entrees: Old Fashioned Pot Roast	765	48	30
with Mashed Potatoes	965	53	65
Balsamic-Glazed Chicken w. Sides	490	20	36
Grilled Tilapia Hollandaise w. Sides	1380	100	66
Top Sirloin Steak, w. Topping & Sides	1780	121	95
Crispy Chicken Salad: w/o Sides	680	42	36
with 3 oz Dressing & Garlic Bread	1200	78	76

Jack's® (Sept '09)

	C	F	Cb
Sandwiches: Big Bacon Burger	610	41	31
Big Jack Burger	530	33	35
Cheeseburger	380	21	31
Chicken Fillet Sandwich	500	25	43
Double Big Jack Cheese Burger	850	59	35
Double Cheeseburger	540	34	31
Grilled Chicken Sandwich	380	16	32
Hamburger	340	18	31
Chicken: Chicken Fingers, 3 pieces	420	23	28
Fries, regular	310	13	42
Breakfast, Egg & Cheese Biscuit	360	21	31
Additional Listings ~ see CalorieKing.com			

Jack in the Box® (Sept '09)

Sandwiches & Burgers	C	F	Cb
Bacon Ultimate Cheeseburger	980	67	52
Hamburger: with Cheese	320	15	30
w/o Cheese	280	12	29
Deluxe: w. Cheese	430	25	33
w/o Cheese	340	18	31
Jumbo Jack: Original	580	33	51
with Cheese	670	40	53
Junior Bacon Cheeseburger	400	23	30
Sirloin Cheeseburger	950	60	61
Sourdough Jack	680	46	41
Ultimate Cheeseburger	920	63	52
Chicken & Fish			
Bacon Chicken Sandwich	440	24	38
Chicken Breast Strips, crispy (4)	500	25	36
Chicken Fajita Pita, no salsa	320	11	33
Chicken Sandwich	400	21	38
Fish & Chips, small, 8.47 oz	630	35	61
Jack's Spicy Chicken Sandwich	550	24	59
w. Cheese	630	30	61
Sourdough Grilled Chicken Club	530	28	34
Tacos			
Beef Taco (1), Regular	160	8	15
Breakfast			
Biscuit: Bacon, Egg & Cheese	440	26	37
Homestyle Chicken Biscuit	520	26	52
Sausage, Egg & Cheese	590	40	38
Breakfast Jack: Regular	290	12	29
w. Sausage	450	28	29
Croissant: Sausage	580	39	37
Supreme	450	25	36
Sandwiches: Sourdough	420	24	31
Ultimate	570	27	49
Extreme Sausage Sandwich	670	48	31
Hash Brown Sticks (5)	230	16	20
Meaty Burrito, without salsa	610	36	39
Snacks & Sides: Crispy Chicken (1)	390	19	39
Egg Rolls (3)	400	19	44
Fish (1)	380	19	39
Grilled Chicken (1)	310	13	31
Stuffed Jalapenos, (3)	230	13	22
Stuffed Jalapenos, (7)	530	30	51

Jack in the Box® cont... (Sept '09)

Snacks & Sides (cont)	C	F	Cb
Natural Cut Fries: Medium, 6 oz	460	24	55
Kids, 2.72 oz	210	11	25
Seasoned Curly Fries, med., 4.6 oz	420	24	46
Pot. Wedges, Bacon Cheddar, 9.17 oz	760	52	53
Onion Rings (8), 4.2 oz	500	30	51
Teriyaki Bowls			
Chicken, 17 oz	580	5	106
Sirloin Steak, 17 oz	650	10	106
Salads: No Dressing or Condiments			
Asian Chicken w. Gr. Chicken	180	1.5	22
Chicken Club w. Gr. Chicken	320	16	12
Side Salad	50	3	5
Southwest Chicken w. Gr. Chkn Strips	310	12	28
Sauces & Dressings			
Dipping Sauce: Barbecue, 1 oz	45	0	11
Buttermilk House, 1 oz	130	13	3
Frank's Red Hot Buffalo, 1 oz	10	0	2
Sweet & Sour, 1 oz	45	0	11
Tartar, 1½ oz	210	22	2
Sauce: Mayo-Onion, ½ oz	90	10	1
Soy, 0.3 oz	5	0	1
Taco, 0.3 oz	0	0	0
Cheese: American, 1 slice	45	3.5	1
Real Swiss, 1 slice	70	8	0
Condiments			
Ketchup, 1 pkt	20	0	5
Mustard, 0.2 oz	5	0	1
Sour Cream, 1 oz	60	5	2
Desserts			
Cheesecake, 3.6 oz	310	16	34
Chocolate Overload Cake, 3.3 oz	300	7	57
Ice Cream Shakes: Per Regular, 16 fl.oz			
Chocolate Ice Cream	750	36	95
Oreo Cookie Ice Cream	760	40	87
Strawberry Ice Cream	730	35	90
Vanilla Ice Cream	650	35	70

For Complete Nutritional Data ~ see CalorieKing.com

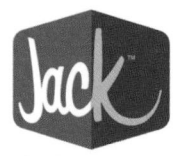

in the box

Updated Nutrition Data ~ www.CalorieKing.com
Persons with Diabetes ~ See Disclaimer (Page 24)

Jamba Juice® (Sept '09)

	C	F	Cb
Breakfast			
Ideal Meals: Berry Topper, 16 fl oz	540	11	88
Chunky Strawberry, 16 fl oz	590	18	95
Mango Peach Topper, 16 fl oz	560	11	106
Hot Oatmeal: With Fruit & Sugar			
Apple Cinnamon	290	4	60
Blueberry/Blackberry	290	3.5	59
Grab N Go Food:			
California Flat Bread: With Dressing			
Four Cheesy, 4.2 oz	330	13	35
Mediterrane Yum, 4.34 oz	250	8	37
Smokehouse Chicken, 4.52 oz	300	8	41
Tomato Artichoko, 4.59 oz	310	11	44
Wraps: With Sauce			
Asian-Style Chicken, 10.55 oz	430	7	72
Chimichurri Chicken, 10.41 oz	560	25	67
Greek Goodess, 11.22 oz	550	26	70
Greens & Grains, 10.86 oz	640	14	108
Salads: With Dressings/Mayonnaise			
Caesar The Day, 7.5 oz	330	22	15
Couscous and Produce, 10.86 oz	480	19	72
Gobble'icious, 9.28 oz	570	28	49
All Fruit: Original, 24 fl oz			
Mega Mango	360	1	91
Peach Perfection	340	0.5	84
Pomegranate Paradise	380	1	95
Strawberry Whirl	340	1	85
Blended With A Purpose: Per 16 fl.oz			
Acai Super-Antioxidant	290	4.5	59
Coldbuster	270	1.5	63
Pomegranate Heart Happy	300	0.5	72
Protein Berry Workout w. Whey	290	1	55
Strawberry Energizer	300	1	71
Classics: Per 16 fl.oz			
Aloha Pineapple	300	1	70
Caribbean Passion	270	1	63
Mango-a-go-go	310	1	72
Strawberry Surf Rider	330	1	80
Creamy Treats: Per 16 fl oz			
Chocolate Moo'd	460	6	93
Orange Dream Machine	350	1.5	75
Peanut Butter Moo'd	490	11	85
Fresh Squeezed Juices: Per 16 fl oz			
Carrot	130	0.5	30
Orange	220	1	52
Light: Per 16 fl oz			
Berry Fulfilling	160	0.5	34
Mango Mantra	170	0.5	36
Strawberry Nirvana	170	0	36
Shots: Single			
Matcha Energy Shot-Soymilk, 4 fl.oz	70	0	14
Wheatgrass, 1 fl oz	5	0	0.5

Jersey Mike's Subs® (Sept '09)

	C	F	Cb
Cold Subs: Regular, on Wheat, w/o Oil or Mayo Unless Indicated			
#1 BLT	530	24	55
#2 Jersey Shore Favorite	520	16	59
#3 American Classic	520	16	57
#5 Super Sub	540	17	59
#6 Roast Beef & Provolone	680	23	56
#7 Turkey Breast & Provolone	500	14	56
#8 Club Sub w. Mayonnaise	850	50	58
#9 Club Supreme w. Mayonnaise	900	50	58
#10 Albacore Tuna	870	57	58
#13 Original Italian	640	25	60
#14 Veggie	680	31	57
Hot Subs/Cheese Steaks: Per Regular on Wheat Roll			
#15 Meatball & Cheese	850	50	64
#17 Chicken Philly	590	23	57
Steak Philly	580	22	56
#43 Chipotle Cheese Steak	860	53	58
#43 Chipotle Chicken	870	54	60
#18 Chicken Parmesan	610	20	69
#19 BBQ Beef	670	14	75
#20 Pastrami Reuben	540	16	52
#56 Big Kahuna Cheese Steak	630	26	57
#56 Big Kahuna Chicken	640	27	58
Cold Wraps: With Flour Tortilla, w/o Vin./Oil or Mayo			
#1 BLT	590	29	60
#2 Jersey Shore Favorite	580	22	64
#3 American Classic	580	22	63
#5 Super Sub	600	22	65
Salads: Without Dressing			
Chef, 16 oz	240	10	12
Grilled Chicken Caesar, 12.5 oz	510	35	11
Tossed, 12 oz	50	0.5	11
Tuna, 18 oz	690	60	15
Dressings: Per 2 Tbsp, 1 oz			
Caesar	150	15	2
Chipotle Mayo	180	20	0
Golden Italian	110	11	3
Ranch	120	12	2
Russian	160	16	4
Condiments: Oil, regular, 1 oz	270	30	0
Chipotle Mayo, 1 oz	180	20	0
Mustard, ½ oz	0	0	0
Cookie, Choc Chip, 1.5 oz	200	11	24
Brownie, Chocolate, 4 oz	440	20	60
Drinks: Mountain Dew, 22 oz	310	0	84
Mug Root Beer, 22 oz	290	0	79
Tropicana Twister Orange, 22 oz	360	0	96

Jimmy John's® (Sept '09)

Subs (8")   **C** **F** **Cb**

Figures Based on French Bread w/ Standard Toppings, Dressing & Mayo

	C	F	Cb
#1 Pepe	685	37	55
#2 Big John	565	27	54
#3 Totally Tuna	500	20	57
#4 Turkey Tom	555	26	54
#5 Vito	580	25	56
#6 Vegetarian	640	36	57
JJBLT	660	35	54

Giant Club Sandwiches: Figures Based on French Bread w/ Standard Toppings· Dressing & Mayo

	C	F	Cb
#7 Gourmet Smoked Ham	850	40	76
#8 Billy	865	40	77
#9 Italian Night	975	52	77
#10 Hunter's	855	38	76
#11 Country	840	38	75
#12 Beach	795	37	78
#13 Gourmet Veggie	855	46	77
#14 Bootlegger	720	28	74
#15 Club Tuna	720	29	77
#16 Club Lulu	790	34	74
#17 Ultimate Porker	845	41	73

Plain Slims: Figures Based on French Bread w/o Toppings, Dressing or Mayo

	C	F	Cb
Slim 1 Ham & Cheese	540	12	72
Slim 2 Roast Beef	420	1.5	71
Slim 3 Tuna Salad	575	19	72
Slim 4 Turkey Breast	405	0.5	70
Slim 5 Salami Capicola & Cheese	625	21	72
Slim 6 Double Provolone	590	20	71
The J.J. Gargantuan	1010	55	60

Low Carb Options: With Standard Toppings, Dressing & Mayo, w/o Bread

	C	F	Cb
Hunter's Club Unwich	520	39	8
The JJ Gargantuan Unwich	770	55	11

Low-Fat Options: W/o Standard Toppings, Dressing or Mayo

	C	F	Cb
#4 Turkey Tom	310	1	51
Slim 4 Turkey Breast	405	1	70

Sides

	C	F	Cb
Jimmy Chips: BBQ, 1 oz	160	9	17
Jalapeno, 1 oz	150	7	18
Regular, 1 oz	160	8	18
Sea Salt & Vinegar, 1 oz	140	8	16
Skinny, 1 oz	130	5	19
Pickle: Spear	5	0	1
Whole	15	0	3
Cookies, average	420	16	64

Johnny Rockets® (Sept '09)

Original Hamburgers   **C** **F** **Cb**

	C	F	Cb
Hamburger #12	900	59	55
Original Burger	820	53	52
Chili Cheese	850	50	53
Patty Melt	690	37	49
Rocket: Single	710	44	45
Double	1020	63	52
Route 66	920	60	55
Smoke House: Single	950	55	68
Double	1360	80	99
St Louis	990	56	53
Streamliner	410	8	57

Sandwiches: Chicken Club

	C	F	Cb
Chicken Club	930	51	58
Grilled Breast of Chicken	560	25	47
Grilled Cheese	540	29	48
Philly Cheese Steak	715	46	48
Tuna Melt	900	62	40
Tuna Salad	800	50	41

Other Favourites

	C	F	Cb
Chicken Tenders without Sauce	610	33	39
Chili Dog	810	55	48
Hot Dog	370	20	34
Extras: Bacon, 2 slices, 0.6 oz	90	7	1
Chili, 3 oz	155	12	5
Grilled Mushrooms, 1 oz	35	3	1
Grilled Peppers & Onions, 1 oz	20	1	3

Starters

	C	F	Cb
Chili Bowl, 13 oz	870	73	24
American Fries, 8 oz	550	22	78
Cheese Fries, 10 oz	780	44	72
Chili Fries, 15 oz	1010	62	85
Onion Rings, 8 oz	790	36	80
Rocket Wings, 9 oz	640	36	26
Desserts: Apple Pie, 10 oz	800	33	119
A la Mode, scoop, 4 oz	250	16	25
Super Sundae, 13 oz	1110	74	120

Beverages: 20 fl.oz

	C	F	Cb
Root Beer	170	0	49
Coke	170	0	28
Sprite	170	0	45
Lemonade	170	0	49

Shakes: Original, 16 fl.oz

	C	F	Cb
Chocolate	890	44	102
Strawberry	750	44	77
Vanilla	840	44	100

Updated Nutrition Data ~ www.CalorieKing.com
Persons with Diabetes ~ See Disclaimer (Page 24)

KFC® (Sept '09)

Original Recipe

	C	F	Cb
Breast: 1 piece, 5.85 oz	370	21	7
w/o skin or breading	140	2	1
Drumstick, 1 piece, 1.85oz	110	7	2
Thigh, 1 piece, 3.5oz	260	19	6
Whole Wing, 1 piece, 1.5	110	7	3
Extra Crispy: Breast, 1 pce, 6.4 oz	490	31	17
Drumstick, 1 piece, 2 oz	150	9	6
Thigh, 1 piece, 3.9 oz	370	27	12
Whole Wing, 1 piece, 1.75 oz	150	10	6

Grilled Chicken:

	C	F	Cb
Breast, 4.2 oz	180	4	0
Drumstick, 1.38 oz	70	4	0
Thigh, 2.29 oz	140	9	0
Wing, 1.16 oz	80	4	0

Chicken Strips:

	C	F	Cb
Crispy, 2 Strips	250	15	8
3 Strips	380	22	12
Original, 3 Strips	310	15	11
Popcorn Chicken: Kids, 3 oz	290	19	16
Individual, 4 oz	400	26	22
Large, 5.6 oz	550	35	30

Sandwiches: With Sauce

	C	F	Cb
Double Crunch			
with Original Recipe Strip	470	23	35
with Crispy Strip	510	27	36
Crispy Twister:			
with Original Recipe Strip	540	26	48
with Crispy Strip	580	30	49
Filet Sandwich, Original Recipe	480	23	38
Tender Roast Sandwich	400	15	29

Toasted Wraps:

	C	F	Cb
with Original Recipe Strip	340	18	27
with Crispy Strip	360	20	27
with Tender Roast Filet	310	14	24

KFC Snackers: With Crispy Strip

	C	F	Cb
Regular	300	14	28
Buffalo	260	9	30
Ultimate Cheese	280	11	29

Wings:

	C	F	Cb
Fiery Buffalo; Honey BBQ (1)	80	5	4
Boneless: Fiery Buffalo (1)	80	3.5	6
Honey BBQ (1)	80	3.5	7
Hot Wings: Regular (1)	70	5	3
Fiery Buffalo (1)	80	5	5
Honey BBQ (1)	90	5	7

KFC® cont... (Sept '09)

Dipping Sauces

	C	F	Cb
Fiery Buffalo, 1 oz	25	0	6
Creamy Ranch, 1 oz	140	15	1
Garlic Parmesan, 1 oz	130	13	2
Honey BBQ, 1 oz	40	0	9
Honey Mustard, 1 oz	120	10	6
Sweet & Sour, 1 oz	45	0	12

Sides: Per Single Portion

	C	F	Cb
BBQ Baked Beans, 4.6 oz	200	1.5	39
Biscuit, 2 oz	180	8	23
Cole Slaw, 4.6 oz	180	10	22
Corn on the Cob (3"), 3 oz	70	0.5	16
Macaroni & Cheese, 4.8 oz	180	9	20
Mashed Potatoes with Gravy, 5.4 oz	130	4.5	20
Mean Greens, 4.5 oz	30	0	4
Potato Wedges, 3.6 oz	260	13	33

KFC Famous Bowls & Pot Pie

	C	F	Cb
Chicken Pot Pie	690	40	57
Mashed Potato with Gravy, 18.5 oz	700	32	77
Rice w. Gravy, 1 reg. bowl, 18 oz	790	28	106

Salads: Without Dressing or Croutons

	C	F	Cb
Crispy Chicken BLT	340	19	14
Crispy Chicken Caesar	320	19	12
House Side Salad	15	0	2
Roasted Chicken BLT	200	7	7
Roasted Chicken Caesar	190	6	5

Dressings:

	C	F	Cb
Original Ranch Fat Free, 1½ oz	35	0	8
Creamy Parmesan Caesar, 2 oz	260	26	4
Light Italian, 1 oz	10	0.5	2
Croutons, Parm. Garlic, Pouch (1)	70	3	8

Desserts:

	C	F	Cb
Lil' Buckets Parfait Cups:			
Chocolate Cream, 4 oz	280	14	37
Lemon Creme, 4.5 oz	390	14	60

Kilwin's® ~ see CalorieKing.com

Koo♦Koo♦Roo® ~ see CalorieKing.com

Kohr Bros® ~ see CalorieKing.com

Kolache® ~ see CalorieKing.com

Fast - Foods & *Restaurants*

Krispy Kreme® (Sept '09)

Doughnuts	C	F	Cb
Apple Fritter	380	20	47
Caramel Kreme Crunch	380	19	49
Chocolate Glazed Cruller	290	15	37
Chocolate Iced Cake	280	14	36
Chocolate Iced Custard Filled	300	17	35
Chocolate Iced Glazed	250	12	33
Chocolate Iced Kreme Filled	350	20	39
Chocolate Iced with Sprinkles	270	12	38
Cinnamon Apple Filled	290	16	32
Cinnamon Bun	260	16	28
Cinnamon Twist	240	15	23
Dulce de Leche	300	18	31
Glazed: Chocolate Cake	300	15	42
Cinnamon	210	12	24
Cruller	240	14	26
Kreme Filled	340	20	39
Lemon Filled	290	16	35
Maple Iced	240	12	32
Original	200	12	22
Raspberry Filled	300	16	36
Sour Cream	300	13	43
Powdered: Cake	290	14	37
Strawberry Filled	290	16	33
Sugar Doughnut	200	12	21
Traditional Cake Doughnut	230	13	25
Doughnut Holes: Orig. Glazed (4)	200	11	25
Glazed Cake, Regular/Choc. (4)	210	10	29

Chiller Beverages: No Cream Topping
Fruity Chillers:

	C	F	Cb
Average all flavors,12 fl.oz	175	0	43
20 fl.oz	295	0	71

Kremey Chillers: Includes Whipped Cream Topping

	C	F	Cb
Orange & Kreme: 12 fl.oz	630	28	92
20 fl.oz	970	40	150
Lemon Sherbert: 12 fl.oz	630	28	95
20 fl.oz	980	40	155
Choc./Mocha: Avg. 12 fl.oz	670	29	104
average 20 fl.oz	1050	41	171
Lotta Latte: 12 fl.oz	670	28	49
20 fl.oz	1050	40	79

For Complete Nutritional Data ~ see CalorieKing.com

Krystal® (Sept '09)

Burgers/Sandwiches	C	F	Cb
B.A. Burger	470	27	39
w. Cheese	530	32	40
B.A. Double Bacon Cheese	800	53	41
Krystal: Burger	160	7	17
Double Burger	260	13	24
Bacon Cheese	190	10	16
Cheese Burger	180	9	17
Double Cheese	310	16	26
Chik Burger	240	11	24
Pups: Chili Cheese Pup	210	12	17
Corn Pup	260	19	19
Plain Pup	170	9	15
Sampler Combo: Krystal, Chik,			
Pup, Fries + 16 fl.oz drink	1330	54	170

French Fries	C	F	Cb
Regular, 4.2 oz	470	20	53
Chili Cheese Fries, 7.3 oz	540	28	59

Sides	C	F	Cb
Krystal Chili	200	7	22
Chik'n Bites, Small, 4 oz	310	19	16
Chik'n Bites Salad	290	20	12
Kryspers	190	13	17

Breakfast Items	C	F	Cb
Krystal Sunriser Sandwich	240	14	14
Biscuit: Bacon, Egg & Cheese	390	23	33
Biscuit & Gravy	280	14	34
Chik Biscuit	360	15	40
Plain Biscuit	270	13	33
Sausage Biscuit	480	33	33
Country Breakfast	660	42	46
Scrambler, 11 oz	440	26	33
4-Carb Scrambler: Bacon	370	29	4
Sausage	600	51	3
Desserts: Apple Turnover, fried	220	10	31
Lemon Icebox Pie	260	9	41

Drinks: Per 16 fl.oz with ¼ ice

	C	F	Cb
Coca-Cola Classic	130	0	36
Diet Coke	0	0	0
Sprite	125	0	39

For Complete Nutritional Data ~ see CalorieKing.com

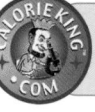

**For Menu Updates,
Check Author's Website
www.CalorieKing.com**

La Rosa's Pizzeria® (Sept '09)

	C	F	Cb
Focaccia Style: Per Slice, ⅒ of Medium Pizza			
Florentine	240	13	24
Roma	300	18	23
Hand Tossed: Per Slice, ⅒ of Medium Pizza			
Deluxe Topper	290	12	29
Buddy Topper	310	14	29
Cheese	230	8	29
Meat Topper	320	15	29
Pepperoni Topper	300	14	29
Veggie Topper	265	10	30
Pan Crust: Per Slice, ⅒ of Medium Pizza			
Buddy Topper	310	14	29
Cheese	300	16	30
Deluxe Topper	370	21	31
Pepperoni Topper	370	22	30
Stuffed Pizza Pie: Per Slice			
Cheese, 4.02 oz	340	14	40
Meat, 8.4 oz	790	53	44
Traditional Crust: Per Slice, ⅒ of Medium Pizza			
Buddy Topper	275	15	20
Cheese	200	10	19
Deluxe Topper	270	16	20
Meat Topper	300	18	20
Pepperoni Topper	280	16	20
Calzones: Per Calzone, No Dipping Sauce			
3 Meat & 3 Cheese	1080	55	102
3 Veggie & 3 Cheese	860	34	105
Cheese & Pepperoni	960	45	101
Cheese	840	34	101
Philly Cheese Steak	870	39	90
Sausage Pelucci	1040	52	92
Pasta Dinner: No Sides			
Cheese Ravioli	660	26	80
Lasagna w. Meat Sauce	735	38	61
Spaghetti: & Meatballs	870	28	119
with Alfredo Sauce	975	50	104
with Meat Sauce,	700	18	104
with Traditional Sauce	640	12	113
Ziti Chicken Alfredo	980	42	102
Ziti Sausage Pelucci	765	20	115
Appetizers			
Chicken Tenders	540	31	30
Four Taste Sampler	1570	99	82
French Fry Basket w. Provolone	860	56	73
Mozzarella Cheese Sticks	635	43	36
Onion Twists, Regular, no Sauce	460	27	48
Boneless Wings: Hot (1)	80	5	6
BBQ (1)	75	3	8

For Complete Nutritional Data ~ see CalorieKing.com

La Salsa Fresh Mexican Grill® (Sept '09)

	C	F	Cb
Appetizers: Salsa & Chips, 14.5 oz	700	32	87
w/ Guacamole, 14.5 oz	970	55	103
Nachos:			
Black Beans: with Carnitas	1570	83	141
with Chicken	1600	83	148
with Steak	1580	84	142
Pinto Beans: with Carnitas	1560	83	139
with Chicken	1590	83	146
with Steak	1565	84	139
Burritos: Black Beans w. Cheese	1100	48	132
with Carnitas	1205	51	132
with Chicken	1240	52	139
Pinto Beans with Cheese	1070	48	115
with Chicken	1200	52	122
with Steak	1175	54	115
Baja Fish Burrito	875	53	58
California Steak & Black Beans	820	35	91
Overstuffed Grilled Burrito:			
with Chicken	1260	59	110
with Carnitas	1200	59	108
with Steak	1290	66	109
Grande, Black Beans:			
with Carnitas	810	34	91
with Chicken	810	33	93
with Steak	820	35	91
Tacos: Baja Fish	395	22	29
Baja Shrimp	320	19	30
Guadalajara Carnitas	320	15	30
Quesadillas: With Chips unless indicated			
Classic: Carnitas	1160	68	82
Chicken	1155	67	83
Steak	1165	69	82
Grande, Pinto Beans:			
with Carnitas	1335	71	114
with Chicken	1330	71	116
with Steak	1330	72	115
Favorites: Without Chips			
Stuffed Fajita Quesadilla:			
with Carnitas	855	51	53
with Chicken	865	52	56
with Steak	885	55	53
with Shrimp	800	49	54
Fire Roasted Bowl			
Black Beans: with Chicken	730	32	74
with Steak	735	34	73
w/o meat	630	29	71
Pinto Beans: with Chicken	730	32	73
with Steak	720	34	70
w/o meat	620	29	69

Fast - Foods & *Restaurants*

Little Caesars® (Sept '09)

14" Pizza: Per Slice, ⅛ Pizza

	C	F	Cb
3 Meat Treat	350	18	30
Ultimate Supreme	310	14	31
Vegetarian	270	10	32
Deep Dish:			
Just Cheese	320	13	38
Pepperoni	360	16	38
Hot-N-Ready: Cheese Only	240	9	30
Pepperoni	280	11	30
Hula Hawaiian: with Ham	270	9	33
with Canadian Bacon	280	9	34
Baby Pan! Pan!, Single	360	18	33
Caesar Wings: Barbecue, 1 wing	70	4	3
Mild/Hot, 1 wing	60	4.5	1
Oven, Roasted, 1 wing	50	3.5	0
Caesar Dips: Per 1.5 oz Container			
Buffalo	140	14	4
Buffalo Ranch	230	24	3
Buttery Garlic	380	42	0
Cheezy	210	21	3
Chipotle	220	24	2
Ranch	250	26	3
Bread: Per Piece			
Crazy Bread, 1 stick	100	3	15
Crazy Sauce, 4 oz	45	0	10
Churros, 1 stick, 1.5 oz	150	4	25
Churros Sauces, avg.	90	2.5	16

Lone Star Steakhouse® (Aug '09)

Starters

	C	F	Cb
Amarillo Chse Fries, ¼ order, 8 oz	660	38	89
Chicken Tenders	1090	66	91
Lone Star Wings	950	62	15
Spinach Artichoke Dip	490	40	13
Texas Rose	1260	38	108
Texas Rose Sauce	155	17	1
Tostado Tortilla Chips	390	22	46
Steaks: Cajun Ribeye	820	52	6
Chopped Steak	710	52	0
Five Star Filet, 6 oz	335	18	2
Garlic Medallion & Shrimp	370	11	0
Lunch Steak, plain	390	27	1
NY Strip Steak	525	28	0
Sirloin Steak & Lobster	335	8	10
Texas Ribeye	700	40	6

Lone Star® cont... (Aug '09)

Seafood

	C	F	Cb
Fried Shrimp (5)	290	15	30
Grilled Shrimp (5)	190	7	17
Lobster Tail, grilled	85	0.5	8
Mesquite Grilled Shrimp: Dinner	230	8	17
Entree	310	18	0
Sweet Bourbon Salmon	240	11	0
Mesquite-Grilled Specialties: Sides not included			
Baby Back Ribs	400	26	5
Bubba (BBQ) Chicken Breast	165	1.5	5
Grilled Chicken	170	4	0
Grilled Pork Chop	320	16	0
Mesquite Grilled Shrimp Dinner	230	8	17
Superstar Combo	645	29	5
Burgers & Sandwiches			
Bubba Chicken Sandwich	170	2	5
Lone Star Cheeseburger	900	45	50
Steak Sandwich	640	22	55
Swiss & Mushroom Burger	845	38	52
Salads: Cobb	685	37	23
Chicken Caesar Salad	480	24	19
El Paso Salad	350	19	25
Steakhouse Salad	710	53	2
Dressings: Bleu Cheese	95	9	2
Catalina Dressing	90	5	9
Creamy Caesar Dressing	100	9	3
Honey Mustard Dressing	145	14	5
Lemon Butter	230	25	0
Ranch Dressing	110	11	2
Steakhouse Dressing	70	6.5	2
Texas Ranch Dressing	105	11	28
Thousand Island Dressing	65	4	5
Whipped Honey Butter	315	30	11
Sides & Partners:			
Baked Potato, plain	230	0.5	50
Chili: Cup, 4 oz	140	7	5
Bowl, 10 oz	345	18	14
Garlic Lovers Medallions & Shrimp	370	11	0
Sauteed Mushrooms	140	9	11
Sauteed Mushrooms & Onions	140	7	15
Sauteed Onions	85	2.5	14
Steak Fries, 8oz	610	26	86
Sweet Potato, plain	330	0.5	76
Soups: Steak Soup, Bowl, 10 oz	65	7	11
Chicken Pot Pie, Bowl, 10 oz	50	5	12

220

Long John Silver's® (Sept '09)

Sandwiches & Burgers: Includes toppings and condiments

	C	F	Cb
Chicken, 4.8 oz	410	22	39
Fish, 6.2 oz	470	23	49
Ultimate Fish, 7 oz	530	28	50

Seafood

Alaskan Flounder, 1 piece, 3.7 oz	250	11	26
Baked Cod, 1 piece, 3.6 oz	120	4.5	0
Battered Fish, 1 piece, 3.2 oz	260	16	17
Battered Shrimp, 8 pieces, 4 oz	360	25	21
Breaded Clam Strips, 3 oz	240	13	22
Buttered Lobster Bites, 1.75 oz	130	4.5	13
1 snack box, 3.5 oz	250	9	27
1 platter portion, 3.5 oz	250	9	27
Lobster Stuffed Crab Cake, 2.2 oz	170	10	16
Popcorn Shrimp, 1 snack box, 2.9 oz	270	16	23
Shrimp Scampi, 8 pieces	110	5	1

Chicken

Chicken Plank, 1 piece, 1.8 oz	140	8	9

Bowls:

Salmon: without Sauce, 13.5 oz	380	8	47
with Sauce, 15 oz	460	8	65
Shrimp: without Sauce, 11.8 oz	300	4.5	46
with Sauce, 13.3 oz	380	4.5	64

Freshside Grille: Served with Rice & Vegetable Medley

Grilled Pacific Salmon, 2 filets	255	6.5	24
Grilled Tilapia, 1 filet	215	4	23

Sauces & Condiments:

Ginger Teriyaki Sauce, 1 pkt	80	0	18
Louisiana Hot Sauce, 1 tspn	0	0	0
Ketchup, 1 pkt	10	0	2
Malt Vinegar, ½ oz	0	0	0

Sides

Breadstick, 2 oz	170	3.5	30
Broccoli Chse Soup, 1 bowl, 7.4 oz	220	18	8
Cole Slaw, 4 oz	190	14	15
Corn Cobbette w. Butter Oil, 3.4 oz	150	10	14
Crumblies, 1 oz	170	13	14
Fries: Regular, 3 oz	230	10	33
Large, 4 oz	310	14	45
Hushpuppies, 1 pup, 0.8 oz	60	3	9
Rice, 5 oz	180	1.5	37
Veggie Bites:			
Broccoli Cheese, 5 pieces, 3.1 oz	220	12	23
Jalapeno Cheddar, 5 pcs, 3.1 oz	250	14	24

Dipping Sauces: Per 1 oz

Cocktail	25	0	6
Tartar	105	9	4

For Complete Nutritional Data ~ see CalorieKing.com

Macaroni Grill (Sept '09)

Appetizers: Inc. Sauce & Garnish

	C	F	Cb
Calamari Fritti	960	81	30
Crab-Stuffed Mushrooms	580	42	26
Romano's Sampler, 3 Choices	1200	71	96
Tomato Bruschetta	630	15	96

Meals

Amore De Le Grill: *Includes Sides*

Grilled Pork Chops	1380	77	96
Grilled Salmon	750	35	55
Honey Balsamic Chicken: Lunch	540	13	54
Dinner	640	15	54

Classico Italian: *Lunch*

Chicken Marsala	1050	61	97
Chicken Scaloppine	1280	103	64
Eggplant Parmigiana	1110	61	101
Parmesan-Crusted Sole	1190	71	101
Spaghetti Bolognese	840	50	63

Classico Italian: *Dinner*

Chicken Marsala	1180	70	101
Chicken Scaloppine	1410	112	68
Parmesan-Crusted Sole	1710	105	131

Mediterranean Grill: *Includes Sides*

Bistecca Filet	450	17	26
Calabrese Strip	720	35	35
Grilled Chicken Spiedini	360	10	17
Jumbo Shrimp Spiedini	230	5	15

Handcrafted Pasta

Capellini Pomodoro	390	14	55
Carmela's Chicken Rigatoni, lunch	1130	68	85
Lobster Ravioli	650	39	46
Pasta Milano, lunch	1210	77	95
Penne Rustica, dinner	1590	92	93
Pollo Caprese	550	20	45
Shrimp Portofino	560	34	37
Seafood Linguine	615	20	60

Pizzas: Per Pizza

Brick Oven: BBQ Chicken	1090	24	150
Pesto Chicken	1550	72	148
Sicilian	1390	60	133

Salads: Includes Dressing

Chicken Florentine	1020	76	47
Insalata Blu with Chicken	750	59	12
Parmesan-Crusted Chicken	960	63	49
Scallops & Spinach	390	19	18

Salad Dressings & Condiments: Per 1 fl.oz

Parmesan Peppercorn Ranch	120	12	2
Roasted Garlic Lemon Vinaigrette	120	11	4
Low-Fat Caesar	30	2	3

Desserts: Per Serving

Italian Sorbetto with Biscotti	220	2	48
Tiramisu	1120	80	88

For Complete Nutritional Data ~ see CalorieKing.com

McDonald's® (Sept '09)

Burgers/Sandwiches	C	F	Cb
Hamburger	250	9	31
Cheeseburger	300	12	33
Double Cheeseburger	440	23	34
Big Mac	540	29	45
Big N'Tasty	460	24	37
Big N'Tasty w. Cheese	510	28	38
Quarter Pounder:	410	19	37
with Cheese	510	26	40
Double with Cheese	740	42	40
Angus: Bacon & Cheese	790	39	63
Deluxe	750	39	63
Mushroom & Swiss	770	40	59
Filet-O-Fish	380	18	38
McChicken	360	16	40
McRib	500	26	44
Southern Style Chicken Sandwich	400	17	39
Premium Chicken Classic Sandwiches:			
Crispy Chicken	530	20	59
Crispy Chicken Club	630	28	60
Crispy Chicken Ranch BLT	580	23	62
Grilled Chicken	420	10	51
Grilled Chicken Club	530	17	52
Grilled Chicken Ranch BLT	470	12	54
Snack Wraps:			
Chipotle BBQ: w. Grilled Chicken	260	9	28
with Crispy Chicken	330	15	35
Honey Mustard: w. Grilled Chicken	260	9	27
with Crispy Chicken	330	16	34
Ranch: with Grilled Chicken	270	10	26
with Crispy Chicken	340	17	33
French Fries:			
Small, 2.5 oz	230	11	29
Medium, 4.1 oz	380	19	48
Large, 5.4 oz	500	25	63
Ketchup, 1 pkg	15	0	3
Chicken McNuggets® & Sauces			
Chicken McNuggets: 4 pieces	190	12	11
6 pieces	280	17	16
10 pieces	460	29	27
Chicken Selects® Breast Strips			
Strips: 3 pieces	400	24	23
5 pieces	660	40	39
Sauces: Barbecue, 1 oz	50	0	12
Creamy Ranch, 1.5 oz	200	22	2
Spicy Buffalo, 1.5 oz	70	7	1
Sweet 'N Sour, 1 oz	50	0	12
Tangy Honey Mustard, 1.5 oz	70	2.5	13

McDonald's® cont... (Sept '09)

Breakfast Menu	C	F	Cb
Biscuit: Regular	260	12	33
Large	320	16	39
Bacon Egg & Cheese: Regular	420	23	37
Large Biscuit	480	27	43
Sausage with Egg: Regular	510	33	36
Large Biscuit	570	37	42
Southern Style Chicken, Regular	410	20	41
Big Breakfast, Regular Biscuit	740	48	51
Deluxe Breakfast, Regular Biscuit	1090	56	111
English Muffin	160	3	27
Grape/Strawberry Jam	35	0	9
Hash Brown (1), 2 oz	150	9	15
Hotcakes: Plain (3)	350	9	60
w. Margarine (2 pats), no Syrup	430	18	60
w. Margarine (2 pats) & Syrup (1)	610	18	105
McGriddles: Bacon, Egg & Cheese	420	18	48
Sausage	420	22	44
Sausage, Egg & Cheese	560	32	48
McMuffin: Egg	300	12	30
Sausage	370	22	29
Sausage with Egg	450	27	30
McSkillet: Burrito with Sausage	610	36	44
Burrito with Steak	570	30	44
Sausage, 1.4 oz patty	170	15	1
Sausage Burrito	300	16	26
Scrambled Eggs (2)	170	11	1
Happy Meals			
with Chicken McNuggets (4):			
+ Small Fries + Apple Juice	520	23	63
+ Small Fries + Low Fat Milk	520	25	52
+ Apple Dipper/ Dip + Choc Milk	464	15	60
with Hamburger:			
+ Small Fries + Apple Juice	580	20	83
+ Small Fries + Sprite (12 oz)	590	20	88
+ Apple Dippers/Dip + Low-Fat Milk	455	12	66
with Cheeseburger:			
+ Small Fries & Apple Juice	630	23	85
+ Small Fries + Low-Fat Milk	630	26	74
+ Apple Dippers/Dip & Choc Milk	575	16	82
Mighty Kids Meals			
with Chicken McNuggets (6 pc):			
+ Small Fries + Apple Juice	610	28	68
+ Apple Dippers/Dip + Choc Milk	555	21	65
with Double Cheeseburger:			
+ Small Fries + Apple Juice	770	34	86
+ Apple Dippers/Dip + Low-Fat Milk	645	26	69

McDonald's® cont... (Sept '09)

Salads: Without Dressing	C	F	Cb
Bacon Ranch Salad: No Chicken	140	7	10
with Crispy Chicken	370	20	20
with Grilled Chicken	260	9	12
Caesar Salad: No Chicken	90	4	9
with Crispy Chicken	330	17	20
with Grilled Chicken	220	6	12
Southwest Salad: w. Crispy Chicken	430	20	38
with Grilled Chicken	320	9	30
Fruit & Walnut, Snack Size, 1 pkg	210	8	31
Side Salad	20	0	4
Butter Garlic Croutons, ½ oz	60	1.5	10
Salad Dressings: Per Package			
Newman's Own: Ranch, 2 fl.oz	170	15	9
Creamy Caesar, 2 fl.oz	190	18	4
Creamy Southwest, 1.5 fl.oz	100	6	11
Low-Fat: Balsamic Vinaigrette	40	3	4
Family Recipe Italian, 1.5 fl.oz	60	2.5	8
Desserts/Cookies			
Apple Dippers: 1 pkg. 2.4 oz	35	0	8
withLow-Fat Caramel Dip	105	0.5	23
Baked Hot Apple Pie, 2.7oz	250	13	32
Cinnamon Melts, 4 oz	460	19	66
Cookies: Chocolate Chip Cookie, (1)	160	8	21
McDonaldland® Cookies, 2 oz	260	8	43
Oatmeal Raisin (1), 1.1 oz	150	6	22
Sugar Cookie (1), 1.1 oz	160	7	21
Fruit 'n Yogurt Parfait: Reg., 5.3 oz	160	2	31
without Granola, 5 oz	130	2	25
Ice Cream: Kiddie Cone, 1 oz	45	1	8
Vanilla Reduced-Fat Cone, 3.2 oz	150	3.5	24
McFlurry™: M&M® Candies, 12 fl.oz	620	20	96
Oreo® Cookies, 12 fl.oz cup	550	17	88
Sundaes: Hot Caramel Sundae, 6.4 oz	340	8	60
Hot Fudge Sundae, 6.3 oz	330	10	54
Strawberry Sundae, 6.3 oz	280	6	49
Peanuts (for Sundaes), 0.3 oz	45	3.5	2
Triple Thick Shakes: Average all Flavors:			
12 fl.oz cup	425	10	74
16 fl.oz cup	565	14	98
21 fl.oz cup	750	18	130
32 fl.oz cup	1125	27	197
Fruit Juice			
Apple Juice, 6.8 fl.oz box	100	0	23
Orange Juice: Small, 12 fl.oz	140	0	33
Medium, 16 fl.oz	180	0	42
Large, 21 fl.oz	250	0	57

McDonald's® cont... (Sept '09)

Sodas	C	F	Cb
Coca-Cola or Sprite: Without Ice			
Child, 12 oz cup	110	0	29
Small, 16 fl.oz cup	150	0	40
Medium, 21 fl.oz cup	210	0	58
Large, 32 fl.oz cup	310	0	86
Diet Coke	0	0	0
Hi-C Orange Lavaburst: Without Ice			
Child, 12 fl.oz cup	120	0	32
Small, 16 fl.oz cup	160	0	44
Medium, 21 fl.oz cup	240	0	64
Large, 32 fl.oz cup	350	0	94
Powerade Mountain Blast: Without Ice			
Child, 12 fl.oz	70	0	20
Small, 16 fl.oz	100	0	27
Medium, 21 fl.oz	150	0	39
Large, 32 fl.oz	220	0	58
Milk: 1% Low-Fat, 8 fl.oz	100	2.5	12
1% Chocolate, 8 fl.oz ctn	170	3	26
Hot Chocolate, w. Non-Fat Milk, 12 fl.oz	250	5	43
Iced Tea, no added sugar	0	0	0
Coffee Drinks, Black, 16 fl.oz	0	0	0
Coffee Cream 1 pkg, 0.4 fl.oz	20	2	0
Sugar Packet (1), 4 g	15	0	4
Iced Coffee:			
Regular or flavors:			
Small, 8 fl.oz	130	5	21
Medium, 11.5 fl.oz	190	8	29
Large, 17 fl.oz	270	11	45
with Sugar-Free Vanilla Syrup:			
Small, 8 fl.oz	60	5	8
Medium, 11.5 fl.oz	90	8	11
Large, 17 fl.oz	120	11	16
McCafe Coffees			
Cappuccino			
Whole Milk: Small 12 fl oz	120	7	9
Medium 16 fl oz	140	8	11
Large 20 fl oz	180	10	13
Nonfat Milk: Small 12 fl oz	60	0	9
Medium 16 fl oz	80	0	12
Latte			
Whole Milk: Small 12 fl oz	150	8	11
Medium 16 fl oz	180	10	13
Nonfat Milk: Small 12 fl oz	90	0	13
Medium 16 fl oz	110	0	15
Mocha			
Whole Milk: Small 12 fl oz	280	11	40
Medium 16 fl oz	330	12	48
Nonfat Milk: Small 12 fl oz	240	5	41
Medium 16 fl oz	280	6	50

Extra Listings ~ www.CalorieKing.com

223

Manhattan Bagel® (Sept '09)

Bagel (East Coast): Per Bagel

	C	F	Cb
Blueberry, 3.8 oz	270	1	60
Chocolate Chip, 3.8 oz	290	2.5	58
Cinnamon Raisin, 4.1 oz	330	1	70
Egg, 4.1 oz	320	2	67
Jalapeno Cheddar, 4.1 oz	320	1.5	67
Pumpernickel, 3.6 oz	250	1.5	55
Salt, 4.3 oz	320	1	68
Spinach, 4.1 oz	320	1	67
Sundried Tomato, 4.1 oz	310	1	66
Cream Cheese: Reduced-Fat, 1.75 oz	150	12	5

For Complete Nutritional Data ~ see CalorieKing.com

Max & Erma's® (Sept '09)

Appetizers	C	F	Cb
Black Bean Roll-Ups	575	10	95
Entrees:			
Caribbean Chicken (lunch)	535	20	60
Salads: No Breadstick			
Hula Bowl with Dressing	585	10	78
Half Hula Bowl with Dressing	320	5	45
Baby Greens Salad, no dressing	120	11	6
Sides			
Fruit Salad, 4.5 oz	55	0	17
Garlic Breadstick (1)	150	6	20
Fruit Smoothie	125	0.5	28
Dressings: Per 2 Tablespoons			
Bleu Cheese	200	21	0.5
Italian	110	12	1
Ranch	120	13	0.5
Fat Free, Honey Mustard	50	0	12

For Complete Nutritional Data ~ see CalorieKing.com

Mazzio's® (Sept '09)

Appetizers: Per Serving	C	F	Cb
Cheese Dippers, no sauce, ⅓ order	405	18	47
Cinnamon Sticks, ¼ order	625	36	70
BBQ Chicken Wings, ⅓ order	190	12	7
Nachos: Beef w. Jalapenos, ½ order	485	34	20
Cheddar with Jalapenos, ½ order	425	30	19
Calzones: Per ⅒ Whole			
Ham Bacon & Cheddar, no Sauce	245	7.5	32
Pepperoni	260	10	32

Mazzio's® cont... (Sept'09)

Pastas: Without Garlic Toast	C	F	Cb
Fettuccine Alfredo	1060	56	106
Spaghetti with Marinara Sauce	640	8	120
Lasagna: with Meat Sauce	950	52	64
with Marinara Sauce	705	30	73
with Alfredo Sauce	1265	94	55
Sandwiches: Without Chips or Pickle			
Wheatberry:			
Chicken, Bacon & Swiss	1020	70	48
Ham & Cheddar	745	47	47
Mazzio's Sub	770	49	45
Turkey & Swiss	720	38	46
Tuscan Smash	645	34	45
Hoagie: Chicken, Bacon & Swiss	1360	72	120
Ham & Cheddar	1090	50	119
Mazzio's Sub	1110	52	117
Turkey & Swiss	1060	40	118
Tuscan Smash	985	36	117
Pizzas: Per ⅛ Medium, 12" Pizza			
Cheese: Original Crust	235	9	30
Thin Crust	180	9	18
Chicken Club: Original Crust	260	9	31
Thin Crust	205	9	19
Mazzio's Works: Original Crust	305	14	31
Thin Crust	255	15	20
Meatbuster: Original Crust	285	13	30
Thin Crust	235	13	19
Mexican: Original Crust	315	14	35
Thin Crust	265	14	23
Pepperoni: Original Crust	255	11	30
Thin Crust	200	11	18
Sausage: Original Crust	275	12	30
Thin Crust	225	12	19
Supremebuster: Original Crust	255	10	31
Thin Crust	205	11	19
Veggie: Original Crust	230	8	31
Thin Crust	180	8	19
Sides: Breadsticks, no sce, ¼ order	150	3	26
Garlic Toast, no sce, 1 pce, 1.4 oz	160	10	15
Kosher Pickle Spear, 1 oz	5	0	1
Potato Chips, 1 oz	150	10	15

For Complete Nutritional Data ~ see CalorieKing.com

Updated Nutrition Data ~ www.CalorieKing.com
Persons with Diabetes ~ See Disclaimer (Page 24)

Mimi's Cafe® (Sept '09)

Breakfast

	C	F	Cb
Just Enough: Eggs Ranchero Bowl	785	44	66
Ciabatta Breakfast Sandwich	945	53	77
Gourmet: Brie Chse Lorraine Crepes	550	41	21
Eggs Benedict	810	56	36
Eggs Florentine Benedict	690	50	36
Ham & Cheddar Croissant	1235	84	64
House Specialties: Chipotle Burrito	965	44	84
Huevos y Papas	1245	46	144
Three Egg Omelettes: Caprese	475	38	8
Mardi Gras	620	45	5
Monterey	750	59	7
Tuscan Vegetable	915	73	14

Dinner

	C	F	Cb
Just Enough Dinner:			
Honey Dijon Salmon	500	32	25
Meatloaf Stroganoff	640	27	68
Salisbury Steak, 24 oz	2270	156	60
Santa Fe Shrimp & Chkn Fettuccine	925	55	70
Sweet & Sour Chicken	380	18	31

For Complete Nutritional Data ~ see CalorieKing.com

Miami Subs® (Aug '09)

Burgers

	C	F	Cb
Deluxe Burger	785	59	31
Deluxe Cheeseburger	860	65	32
Deluxe Bacon Cheeseburger	920	69	32
Platters: Chicken Breast	745	41	57
Gyros	1420	93	81
10 Wings w. Fries & Blue Cheese	1020	67	50
Salads: Caesar w. Dressing	460	34	26
Chicken Caesar w. Dressing	610	39	28
Chicken Club	490	25	23
Garden	310	18	21
Greek	285	15	24
Side Greek w. Dressing	80	5	4
Cheesesteaks (6"): Original	410	11	45
Classic	420	11	47
Chicken Philly Classic	550	27	46
Works	530	22	51
Pitas: Gyros	660	39	46
Chicken	390	13	33
Subs(6"): Ham & Cheese	450	18	79
Italian Deli	515	24	49
Meatball	490	22	49
Tuna	470	18	44
Turkey	485	18	51
Sides: Mozzarella Sticks	755	56	34
Onion Rings	870	68	55
Spicy Fries: Regular	530	39	39
Large	1040	72	85

Mr. Goodcents® (Sept '09)

	C	F	Cb
Cold Sub: Per ½ Sub on Wheat Bread			
Centsable	480	20	58
Italian Sub	640	37	55
Mr. Goodcents Original	510	25	56
Oven Roasted Chicken Breast	350	6	55
Penny Club	350	6	57
Pepperoni & Cheese	740	46	55
Roast Beef	350	6	55
Tuna Salad	490	21	63
Veggie Sub	290	4	58
Hot Sub: Per ½ Sub on Wheat Bread w/ Cheese			
Chicken Bacon Ranch w/ Cheddar	630	29	57
Meatball w/ Mozzarella	670	33	65
Philly Jack 'n Cheese	490	16	60
Pasta: Alfredo Sauce	1290	80	106
Chicken Alfredo	1370	70	112
Chicken Parmesan	660	10	100
Red Sauce	520	4	100

Mr. Hero® (Sept '09)

7" Hot Subs & Burgers

	C	F	Cb
Burgers: Cheeseburger	835	54	61
Romanburger	935	62	62
Meatball Sub	810	49	60
Steak Subs: Tuscan	705	31	58
Hot Buttered Cheesesteak	750	43	59
Zesty Bacon & Swiss	675	31	56
7" Deli Subs: Original Italian	715	40	61
Tuna & Cheese	790	54	58
Turkey	530	20	60
Ultimate Italian	770	43	61
4½" Taste Buddies: Per Sandwich			
Bacon Cheeseburger	430	30	33
Grilled Italiano	440	32	32
Tuna 'n Cheese	485	38	31
Zesty Chicken	495	25	48
Pasta, Spag./Rigatoni w/ Meatballs	1115	36	153
Salads: Without Dressing			
Grilled Chicken	165	2.5	13
Tuna Delight	495	48	10
Sides			
Breadsticks (2), 6 oz	445	17	64
Cheese Sauce, 1.5 oz	55	4	4
Jalapeno Poppers. 4.5 oz	430	28	37
Mozzarella Sticks, 8.7 oz	565	43	12
Onion Petals, 5.7 oz	595	37	58
Fries, Potato Waffer, 5.7 oz	430	30	38
Desserts: Oreo Cookie Cheesecake	340	19	38
Strawberry Swirl Cheesecake	290	16	32

Mrs Fields Cookies® (Sept '09)

Brownies: Per 2.6 oz Brownie	C	F	Cb
Butterscotch Blondie	350	14	52
Double Fudge	360	20	45
Pecan Fudge	360	20	46
Special Walnut Fudge & Blondie	330	16	43
Toffee Fudge	360	19	47
Walnut Fudge	360	20	45
Cake			
Chocolate Chip, 3 oz piece	350	17	45
Cookies			
Bite Size Nibblers: Cinn. Sugar (3)	170	8	22
Debra's Special (3)	170	7	23
Peanut Butter (3)	180	10	20
Semi-Sweet Chocolate (3)	170	8	24
Triple Chocolate (3)	170	9	23
White Chunk Macadamia (3)	180	9	23
Butter Cookie (1)	200	8	29
Cut Out Cookie (1)	400	19	56
Debra's Special (1)	200	9	28
Peanut Butter (1)	210	12	24
Semi-Sweet Chocolate (1)	210	10	29
with Walnuts(1)	220	11	29
Triple Chocolate (1)	210	11	28
White Chunk Macadamia (1)	230	12	27
Muffins: Blueberry (1), ¾ oz	70	3	10
Chocolate Chip (1), ¾ oz	80	4	11
Mandarin Orange (1), ¾ oz	80	3	9
Raspberry (1), ¾ oz	70	3	10

For Complete Nutritional Data ~ see CalorieKing.com

Nathan's Famous® (Sept '09)

Burgers	C	F	Cb
Burger with Cheese,10.2 oz	705	43	45
Double Burger w. Cheese, 15.6 oz	1180	84	45
Bacon Cheeseburger, 10.8 oz	785	50	45
Super Cheeseburger, 13.65 oz	985	72	47
Corn Dog with Stick, 3.2 oz	380	21	39
Nathan's Famous Hot Dogs			
All Beef (1), 3.5 oz	295	18	24
All Beef Cheese (1), 4.5 oz	340	21	27
All Beef Chili 5.5 oz	400	23	33
Chicken			
Chicken Tenders (3), 6.2 oz	525	39	24
Chicken Tender Platter, 17.5 oz	1245	90	80
Chicken Wing w. Bleu Chse, 12.9 oz	1240	100	23
Gr. Chicken Breast Platter, 15 oz	840	56	58

Nathan's Famous® (Sept '09)

Sides	C	F	Cb
Fries: French: Medium, 6.5	440	29	36
Large, 9 oz	610	41	50
Super, 14 oz	940	63	78
Cheese: Medium, 8 oz	490	34	41
Large, 9 oz	680	46	56
Super, 17 oz	1070	73	89
Mozzarella Sticks (3), w. sauce, 5.5 oz	385	28	20
Onion Rings, regular, 5.6 oz	545	45	36
Wraps			
Grilled Chicken Caesar	700	34	60
Grilled Chicken Santa Fe	750	39	62

For Complete Nutritional Data ~ see CalorieKing.com

Ninety Nine (Sept '09)

Appetizers: Per Serving	C	F	Cb
Boneless Wings & Skins Sampler	350	21	17
Calypso Coconut Shrimp	150	8	15
Outrageous Potato Skins	280	21	11
Steak & Cheese Spring Rolls w. sce	230	14	16
Sandwiches: Without Sides			
Chicken Parmigiana	880	36	92
Triple-Decker Turkey Club	980	37	107
Steakburger: Bacon & Cheese	940	57	46
Mushroom & Cheese	950	58	49
Steakburger	810	47	45
with Cheese	890	53	46
Sweet & Smokey	1060	61	67
Meals: Without Sides			
Cape Cod Seafood Trio	640	38	20
Captain's Combo Platter	1950	130	131
Fish & Chips	1720	116	108
Grilled Chicken Fajitas	1350	54	101
Smothered Sirloin Tips	820	40	9
Salads			
Boneless Buffalo Wing	510	24	30
King Size	980	47	51
Pecan Crusted Chicken	880	44	80
Wild Bleu Chicken & Spinach	1220	80	57
Sides			
Double Bleu Iceberg Wedge	450	41	9
Garlic Red-Skin Mashed Potatoes	260	12	34
Honey Butter Biscuit w/ Honey Butter	220	12	27
Perfect: Baked Potato	330	6	65
Rice Pilaf, 2 scoops	280	6	51
French Fries, Kids, 5 oz, raw wt.	320	21	30
Desserts: Per Serving			
Apple Fortune	870	39	123
Little Midnight Fudge Hero	440	24	54
Strawberry Mimosa Cake	680	33	85

Noodles & Company® (Sept '09)

Meals: Per Regular Order	C	F	Cb
American: Buttered Noodles	620	16	84
Mushroom Stroganoff	780	31	100
Wisconsin Mac & Cheese	900	31	119
Asian Noodles: Bangkok Curry	490	13	85
Indonesian Peanut Saute	950	23	165
Japanese Pan	690	9	133
Pad Thai	700	20	117
Mediterranean: Pasta Fresca	780	22	111
Penne Rosa	810	26	119
Pesto Cavatappi	910	30	124
Whole Grain Tuscan Fettuccine	770	26	108
Proteins: Braised Beef	190	10	0
Organic Tofu	180	11	4
Parmesan Crusted Chicken	190	8	17
Sauteed Beef	210	12	0
Seasoned Chicken Breast	130	2.5	0
Salads: Caesar	160	14	5
Side: Cucumber Tomato	80	0	18
Tossed Green	60	6	3
Sides: Potstickers, 3 Pieces	200	4.5	31
Ciabatta Roll (1)	160	1.5	31
Soups: Chicken Noodle	110	1	16
Tomato Basil Bisque	130	7	14

Nothing But Noodles® (Sept '09)

Noodle Bowls	C	F	Cb
American: Beef Stroganoff	510	31	33
Buttery Noodles	650	44	46
Santa Fe Pasta	705	54	40
Southwest Chipotle	715	58	41
Spicy Cajun Pasta	660	50	44
Asian: Pad Thai Noodles	600	10	118
Sesame Lo Mein	410	11	64
Spicy Japanese Noodles	420	8	74
Thai Peanut	570	20	89
Italian: Basil Pesto	575	42	36
Cappelini Primavera	500	28	56
Fettuccini Alfredo	725	56	36
Margherita Pasta	475	31	36
Marinara Pasta	485	11	77
Three-Cheese Macaroni	445	21	45
Rice Dishes: General Tso's Chicken	760	44	69
Kung Pao Chicken	935	51	89
Thai Peanut Stir Fry	595	27	59

Extra Menu Items ~ See CalorieKing.com

O'Charley's® (Sept '09)

Appetizers: Per Serving	C	F	Cb
Buffalo Kickin'Wings (10)	1830	147	43
Chicken O'Tenders w. Buffalo Sce (6)	810	53	31
Chips & Salsa	520	18	82
Over-Loaded Potato Skins	1120	81	47
Shredded Beef Quesadilla	1120	67	63
Spicy jack cheese Wedge (;7)	880	60	55
Brunch: Per Serving			
Cinnamon Sugar Donuts (10)	1140	54	139
Omelets: *Without Sides*			
Spinach Mushroom	550	41	9
Ultimate	640	46	13
Brunch Quesadilla	1220	81	65
Texas Toast	210	19	20
Lunch/Dinner: Per Serving			
Chicken: Parmesan Pasta	1500	77	138
Chicken O'Tenders w. Buffalo Sce	810	53	31
Grilled Chicken Dinner	500	17	31
Seafood: Cedar Planked Salmon	590	35	2
Cedar Planked tilapia	280	11	2
Grilled Shrimp Dinner	300	8	33
Steak & Ribs: *Per Serving*			
Filet Mignon, 9 oz	450	28	0
Flame Grilled Top Sirloin, 7 oz	430	28	0
O'Charley's Signature Baby Back Ribs			
1 full rack	1480	96	76
Prime Rib, 10 oz	1020	79	3
Ribeye Steak, 12 oz	810	55	0
Steak Tips Monterey	1000	64	47
Sandwiches: Without Fries/Sides			
Buffalo Kickin'	1060	66	71
Chicken Parmesan	1030	52	86
Club Sandwich	1020	59	83
Roast Beef Ciabatta	910	50	74
Southern Fried Chicken Tacos	720	29	75
Salads: With Dressing Unless Indicated			
Apple Crunch Salad	870	51	75
Black & Bleu Caesar	1000	75	23
Cajun Chicken	740	49	17
California Chicken w/o dressing	710	37	50
Classic chicken Caesar	710	53	15
Pecan Chicken Tender	750	47	48
Sides: Rice Pilaf	200	5	31
French Fries: Junior	310	19	31
Adult	390	24	40
Potato: Plain	240	5	50
Loaded	480	29	54
Smashed	370	12	47

Extra Menu Items ~ See CalorieKing.com

Old Country Buffet® (Sept '09)

	C	F	Cb
Entrees: BBQ Beef Ribs, 5 oz	300	23	7
BBQ Smoked Sausage, 2.8 oz	140	10	9
Carved: Beef Brisket, 3 oz	210	11	2
Ham, 3 oz	140	9	0
Roast Beef, 3 oz	230	15	0
Roast Turkey, 3 oz	170	8	0
Salmon Filet, 3 oz	190	11	0
Chicken Hand Breaded Fried:			
Breast, 5.85 oz	280	12	3
Drumstick (1), 2.65 oz	130	8	1
Thigh (1), 4.3 oz	250	16	3
Wing (1), 2 oz	70	3	1
Chicken, Trad'l Baked: Breast	270	12	0.5
Drumstick (1), 2.65 oz	130	9	0.5
Thigh (1), 4.3 oz	240	16	0.5
Fish: Patties, 1 piece, 2.6 oz	180	9	17
Fried, 1 piece, 1.3 oz	90	4.5	10
Shrimp: Fried, 6 shrimp, 2oz	200	10	22
Butterfly Shrimp, fried (11)	385	17	44
Sausage: 1 link, 2 oz	90	8	0
Smoked Saus. & Sauerkraut (1)	195	17	3
Salads:			
California Coleslaw, 3.5 oz	100	0	24
Macaroni Vegetable Salad, 3.5 oz	240	16	21
Marinated Vegetables, 3.5 oz	50	3.5	5
Seven Layer Salad, 2.6 oz	190	17	4
Tossed Green Salad, 1 cup, 1.6 oz	5	0	1
Three Bean Salad, 1 Tbsp, 3.5 oz	90	4.5	12
Sides: Baked Potato (1), 6.3 oz	180	0	31
Hash Browns, 2.8 oz	100	6	11
Soups: Chili Bean, 4 fl.oz ladle	80	3.5	14
Corn Chowder, 4 fl.oz ladle	130	8	14
Navy Bean Soup, 4 fl.oz ladle	50	0.5	9
Desserts			
Cheesecake, plain, 1 piece, 2.8 oz	230	12	28
Cherry Pie, red. sugar, 1 pc, 3.35 oz	170	10	18
Chocolate Decadence Cake, 1 piece	220	10	30
Cookie, Sugar Free Ranger (1), 0.7 oz	90	5	10
Hot Fudge Sundae Cake, 3 oz	160	3	33
Lemon Cream Pie, 2.3 oz	170	4	32
Pudding: Chocolate, 1 Tbsp, 3 oz	120	4.5	19
Reduced Sugar/Calorie, 3 oz	70	1	12
Vanilla, 1 Tbsp, 3 oz	130	5	19

Olive Garden® (Sept '09)

	C	F	Cb
Appetizers			
Bruschetta	620	13	100
Muscles di Napoli	180	8	13
Sicilian Scampi	500	22	43
Stuffed Mushrooms	410	28	20
Entrees:			
Lunch: Eggplant Parmigiana	620	26	70
Fettuccine Alfredo	800	48	69
Five Cheese Ziti al Forno	770	32	89
Lasagna Classico	580	32	35
Dinner: Chicken Parmigiana	1090	49	79
Fettucini Alfredo	1220	75	99
Manicotti Formaggio	940	46	81
Specials: Grilled Chicken Crostada	1270	75	51
Grilled Steak Crostada	1230	70	56
Garden Fare Selections (Lower Fat)			
Lunch: Capellini Pomodora, 13 oz	480	11	78
Linguine alla Marinara, 10.6 oz	310	4	55
Shrimp Primavera, 19 oz	510	9	79
Venetian Apricot Chicken	280	3	32
Dinner: Capellini Pomodora, 21 oz	840	17	141
Linguine alla Marinara, 17 oz	430	6	76
Shrimp Primavera, 26 oz	730	12	110
Venetian Apricot Chicken	380	4	32
Desserts: Black Tie Mousse Cake	760	48	73
Chocolate Gelato	620	25	89
Tiramisu	510	32	48

(The) Old Spaghetti Factory® (Sept '09)

	C	F	Cb
Appetizers: Serves 4			
Shrimp, Spinach & Artichoke Dip	150	10	10
Sicilian Garlic Cheese Bread	330	19	28
Toasted: Beef Ravioli, 4 oz	200	4.5	30
Cheese Ravioli, 4 oz	210	6	30
Entrees, Lunch/Dinner:			
Classics:			
Spaghetti: w. Clam Sauce, 15 oz	660	14	104
w. Marina Sauce, 15 oz	560	5	108
w. Meat Sauce, 15 oz	610	9	105
w. Sicilian Meatballs, 21 oz	960	31	114
Factory Favorites:			
Chicken Parmigiana, 19 oz	830	32	80
Spinach & Cheese Ravioli, 11 oz	480	16	63
Spinach Tortellini w. Alfredo, 12 oz	930	56	86
Signature Selection: Chkn Penne	910	32	105
Crab Ravioli, 11 oz	810	46	73
Lasagna Vegetariano 20¾ oz	830	48	68
Meatloaf, Italian Style, 18½ oz	1180	68	83

On the Border® (Sept '09)

C F Cb

Lunch Favorites:
Chimichangas: *With Rice, w/o Beans Unless Indicated*

	C	F	Cb
Ground Beef, w/o sauce	1060	62	93
Spicy Chicken, w/o sauce	920	48	92

Tacos: *With Black Beans & Vegetables*

Fajita Chicken	570	9	78
Pico Shrimp	490	5	78

Dinner: With Rice, Without Beans
Enchiladas: Gr. Pepper Jack Chkn

	1210	52	108
Ranchiladas	1430	79	114
Suiza	1090	56	115

Fresh Grill: Includes Sides

Honey Chipotle Chkn	870	26	117
Jalapeno-BBQ Salmon	590	21	45
Mahi Mahi	950	33	102
Spice Crusted Chicken	850	25	114

Salads: Without Dressing Unless Indicated

House	210	12	20
Mexican Chopped w/ Jalap. Vinaig.	230	15	19
Sizzling Fajita Chicken	740	47	26

Sides: Per Serving

Mexican Rice	290	4	56
Pico de Gallo	15	0.5	1
Sauce: Guacamole	40	3.5	3
Sour Cream Sauce	200	20	4
Ranchero Sauce	60	3	8
Dressing: Ranch Dressing	230	23	2
Smoked Jalapeno Vinaigrette	230	23	8
Sour Cream	60	4.5	2

For Complete Nutritional Data ~ see CalorieKing.com

Orange Julius® (Sept '09)

C F Cb

	C	F	Cb
Orange Julius: Small, 16 fl.oz	130	0.5	33
Medium, 20 fl.oz	160	0.5	41
Large, 32 fl.oz	260	1	65

Other Julius Originals: Per 16 fl.oz

Bananarilla	320	7	65
Pina Colada	260	7	52
Raspberry	300	7	59
Strawberry Banana	300	7	60

Premium Fruit Smoothies: Per 20 fl.oz

Blackberry Storm	680	15	128
Mango Passion	370	0	86
Orange Swirl	540	12	103
Raspberry Creme	650	15	118
Strawberry Xtreme	390	0	89
Tropi-Colada	530	10	99
Nutrition Boosts: Fiber Plus, 6g	5	0	4
Heart Health, 4g	15	0	3
Joint Care, 6g	20	0	5
Protein (Soy), 19g	90	3	8

Outback Steakhouse® (Sept '09)

Figures are for Californian Outlets Only and may vary between States.

Aussie-Tizers: With Sauce/Dressing

C F Cb

	C	F	Cb
Alice Springs Chkn Quesadilla, reg.	1840	n/a	72
Aussie Cheese Fries: Small	1210	n/a	81
Regular	2140	n/a	146
Bloomin' Onion, serves 4-6	1560	n/a	185
Crab Stuffed Shrimp, serves 2	565	n/a	28
Gold Coast Coconut Shrimp, serves 4	945	n/a	114
Kookaburra Wings, serves 4	1460	n/a	78
Seared Ahi Tuna	430	n/a	13
Tassie's Buffalo Strips, serves 4	1195	n/a	99

Steaks: Meat Only ~ Add Extra for Sides

New York Strip, 12 oz	625	n/a	1
Outback Special: 6 oz Sirloin	330	n/a	1
9 oz Sirloin	665	n/a	1
12 oz Sirloin	825	n/a	1
Prime Ribs, 8 oz	540	n/a	3
Ribeye, 14 oz	1190	n/a	1
Teriyaki Ribeye, 14 oz	1165	n/a	16
The Melbourne, P/house, 20 oz	1010	n/a	1
Victoria's Filet: Tenderloin, 7 oz	585	n/a	1
Tenderloin, 9 oz	725	n/a	1

Add Extra for Crumb Crust:

Blue Cheese	225	n/a	5
Horseradish	220	n/a	7

Outback Favorites: Per Whole Dish as Per Menu

Alice Springs Chicken w/ Fries	1675	n/a	80
Baby Back Ribs w/ Fries	2580	n/a	127
Grilled Chicken on the Barbie	865	n/a	34
Mum's Chopped Steak	1070	n/a	54
New Zealand Rack of Lamb	1820	n/a	23
No Rules Parmesan Pasta	1040	n/a	103
with Chicken Breast	1480	n/a	120
Fish & Seafood: Atl. Salmon w veg.	760	n/a	19
Shrimp en Fuego w. Fr. Beans	960	n/a	47
Tilapia w. Lump Crab Meat w. veg.	760	n/a	23
Salads: Ahi Tuna Chopped Salad	590	n/a	45
Queensland Salad: w/o Dressing	860	n/a	27
with Ranch Dressing	1075	n/a	33
Side Salads: Caesar Salad	330	n/a	16
Classic Blue Cheese Wedge Salad	360	n/a	26
Soups: French Onion, bowl	845	n/a	105
Clam Chowder, bowl	750	n/a	65
Sides: Aussie Fries	355	n/a	46
Baked Potato: Plain	190	n/a	38
Dressed	390	n/a	39
Fresh Veggies	155	n/a	12
Garlic Mashed Potatoes	370	n/a	33
Sweet Potato	595	n/a	99

Extra Menu Items ~ See CalorieKing.com

Fast - Foods & *Restaurants*

Panda Express® (Aug '09)

Appetizers	C	F	Cb
Chicken Egg Roll, (1), 3 oz	200	12	16
Chicken Potsticker, 3 pieces	220	11	23
Veggie Spring Roll, (2)	160	7	22
Meals			
BBQ Pork, 4.6 oz	360	10	13
Beef & Broccoli, 5.4 oz	150	6	12
Beijing Beef, 4.9 oz	660	41	52
Black Pepper Chicken, 5.5 oz	200	11	11
Eggplant & Tofu, 6.1 oz	310	24	19
Kung Pao Chicken, 6.1 oz	300	20	13
Mongolian Beef, 6.1 oz	200	9	16
Orange Chicken, 5.4 oz	400	20	42
Sweet & Sour Pork, 5.6 oz	400	23	36
Rice & Noodles: Per Serving			
Chow Mein, 8.3 oz	400	12	61
Fried Rice, 10 oz	570	18	85
Steamed Rice, 8.7 oz	420	0	93

Panera Bread® (Sept '09)

	C	F	Cb
Bagels: Blueberry	330	1.5	67
Dutch Apple & Raisin	360	3	77
Plain	290	1.5	59
Spreads: Plain Cream Cheese, 2 oz	180	18	2
Reduced-Fat, average, 2 oz	140	11	6
Salads: With Dressing			
Asian Sesame Chicken, 11.5 oz	410	19	31
Caesar, 9.75 oz	390	27	25
Classic Cafe, 10 oz	170	11	19
Greek, 13.75 oz	440	39	15
Sandwiches: Per Full Sandwich			
Cafe: Sierra Turkey w/ Asiago Chse	970	54	80
Smoked Ham & Swiss on Rye	700	35	55
Smoked Turkey Brst on Country	730	23	92
Tuna Salad on Honey Wheat	750	47	65
Signature: Asiago Rst Beef w. Chse	710	32	57
Bacon Turkey Bravo, on Tom. Basil	840	32	87
Italian Combo, on Ciabatta	1040	45	94
Soups: Per 8oz			
Broccoli Cheddar	190	10	16
Cream of Chicken & Wild Rice	200	12	19
French Onion, no Cheese/Croutons	90	3	13
Low-Fat: Chicken Noodle	100	2	16
Garden Vegetable	110	2.5	18
Muffins: Choc. Chip Muffie, 2.75 oz	270	12	40
Pumpkin Muffie, 2.75 oz	250	10	39
Wild Blueberry Muffin, 4.5 oz	390	15	58

Papa Gino's® (Sept '09)

Appetizers: *Small, Per ½ Serving*	C	F	Cb
BBQ Chicken Tenders, 4 oz	260	9	28
Buffalo Chkn Tenders 4 oz	225	10	18
Cheese Breadsticks, 6.75 oz	485	20	58
Cinnamon Sticks, 3.6 oz	310	10	50
French Fries, 6 oz	270	12	40
Mozzarella Sticks, 5.5 oz	475	30	35
Pastas: Entree Size			
Papa Platter, Penne, Spagh., 19.4 oz	990	32	135
Ravioli, 13.5 oz	590	24	71
Spaghetti & Meatballs, 19.6 oz	890	29	123
Spagh. Chkn Parmigiana, 23.5 oz	1070	39	129
Pizzas: Per Slice			
Large Thin Crust: BBQ Chicken	270	7	38
Buffalo Chicken	240	7	31
Cheese	220	6	31
Chicken and Roasted Garlic	290	10	34
Chicken Pepper	270	9	32
Meat Combo	330	15	32
Papa Roni	320	15	32
Pepperoni	270	11	31
Super Veggie	240	7	35
The Works	300	12	33
Pizza Slices: Per Slice			
Thin Crust: Cheese, 5.6 oz	310	9	42
Pepperoni, 6 oz	380	16	42
Subs: Per Small Sub			
BLT	720	35	71
Italian	910	48	69
Meatball	740	32	76
Meatball Parmesan	840	41	76
Steak	630	25	65
Steak & Cheese	720	32	68
Super Steak	760	32	76
Tuna	740	39	67
Turkey Club	630	23	70
Salads: Without Dressing or Bread Stick			
Buffalo Chicken Tender	330	15	29
Caesar	190	10	19
with Chicken	320	12	14
Chicken Bacon Cheddar	530	33	22
Chicken Tender	320	14	29
Garden	180	8	25
Side: Caesar	70	4	6
Garden	70	3	10
Dressings: Bleu Cheese, 1.1 oz	150	15	2
Caesar, 3 oz	400	44	2
Ranch, 3 oz	280	30	4
Honey Dijon Fat-Free, 1.5 oz	60	0	13

Papa John's® (Sept '09)

Original Crust (14"): *Per ⅛ Pizza*

	C	F	Cb
BBQ Chicken & Bacon, 5.3 oz	340	11	44
Spicy Italian, 5.2 oz	370	11	38
Spinach Alfredo, 4.1 oz	280	11	36
The Meats, 3.7 oz	350	16	38
The Works, 5.5 oz	330	11	39

Pan Crust (12"): *Per ⅛ Pizza*

BBQ Chicken & Bacon, 5.5 oz	430	22	33
Spicy Italian, 5.6 oz	470	21	38
The Meats, 5.36 oz	440	26	37
The Works, 5.89 oz	420	21	38

Thin Crust (14"): *Per ⅛ Pizza*

BBQ Chicken & Bacon, 4 oz	270	13	27
Spicy Italian, 3.9 oz	310	13	22
Spinach Alfredo, 2.8 oz	220	13	19
The Meats, 3.7 oz	280	17	21
The Works, 4.2 oz	260	13	22

Wings: Without Sauce

BBQ, 2 wings, 2.6 oz	160	10	4
Buffalo, 2 wings, 2.6 oz	160	11	1

Dipping Sauces: *Per 1 oz Container*

Barbeque	45	0	11
Blue Cheese	160	16	1
Buffalo	15	0.5	2
Ranch	100	10	1

Sides: *Without Dipping Sauce*

Breadsticks (2)	290	4.5	53
Cheesesticks (4), 4.8 oz	370	16	42
Papa's ChickenStrips (2), 2.6 oz	160	8	10
Cinnamon Sweetsticks (4), 6.8 oz	570	15	98

Papa Murphy's® (Sept '09)

Pizzas: *Per Slice, Family Size*

Original Crust: BBQ Chkn, 1/12 pizza	340	13	37
Cheese, 1/12 pizza	270	11	30
Cowboy, 1/12 pizza	350	18	32
Gourmet: Chicken Garlic, 1/12	320	14	30
Classic Italian, 1/12 pizza	350	18	31
Vegetarian, 1/12 pizza	300	14	31
Hawaiian, 1/12 pizza	290	11	33
Murphy's Combo, 1/12 pizza	360	18	33
Pepperoni, 1/12 pizza	320	15	31
Rancher, 1/12 pizza	330	16	31
Specialty of the House, 1/12, avg.	320	15	32
Vegetarian Combo, 1/12 pizza	300	13	33
Stuffed Pizza: 5 Meat, 1/16 pizza	370	16	39
Big Murphy, 1/16 pizza	370	16	40
Chicago Style, 1/16 pizza	370	16	40
Chicken and Bacon, 1/16 pizza	375	15	38

Papa Murphy's® cont... (Sept '09)

Pizzas Cont:

	C	F	Cb
Thin Crust deLITEs: Cheese, 1/10	140	7	13
Hawaiian, 1/10 pizza	160	7	15
Pepperoni, 1/10 pizza	170	9	13
Veggie, 1/10 pizza	160	9	13

Salads: *Without Dressing or Croutons*

Club	280	16	12
Garden	200	12	16
Italian	280	20	14

Pei Wei Asian Diner (Sept '09)

First Tastes: *Per ½ Dish, One Serving*

Crab Wontons (2)	190	13	9
Crispy Potstickers (2)	130	7	10
Edamame	155	8	12
Minced Chicken w. Lettuce Wraps, w/o Rice Sticks	250	4	31
Spring Rolls (1)	90	5	11

Noodles & Rice Bowls: *Per Bowl, Serves 2*

Dan Dan Noodle, Chicken	780	14	108
Fried Rice: Beef	1260	42	136
Chicken	1050	22	136
Lo Mein Noodles: Chicken	920	22	122
Beef	1140	42	122
Pad Thai: Beef	1340	60	126
Chicken	1120	40	122
Teriyaki Bowl:			
with Brown Rice: Beef	1160	34	132
Chicken	920	14	128
with White Rice: Beef	1120	32	124
Chicken	880	12	120
Shrimp	980	34	120
Thai Blazing Noodles: Beef	1260	64	110
Chicken	1040	44	110
Shrimp	965	44	110

Signature Dishes: *Per ½ Bowl, One Serving*

Honey Seared: Chicken	420	15	45
Shrimp	370	14	43
Sweet & Sour: Chicken	440	13	61
Shrimp	390	11	59

Salads: *Per Dish, Serves 2, Without Dressing*

Asian Chopped Chicken	400	16	20
Spicy Chicken	420	5	46

Sauces & Dressings: *Per 2 oz Serving*

Lime Vinaigrette	230	20	13
Sesame Ginger	170	16	5
Sauces: Lettuce Wrap	70	4.5	2
Sweet Chile	140	0	34
Thai Peanut	170	11	15
Soup, Hot & Sour, 1 bowl	500	28	37
Cookies: Chocolate Chip (1)	340	14	53
Fortune Cookie (1)	30	0	7

Pepe's Mexican® (Sept '09)

Burritos:	C	F	Cb
Beef & Bean	510	24	52
Beef & Bean Suizo	640	34	55
Chicken & Bean	480	21	51
Chicken & Bean Suizo	610	31	54
Pork & Bean	470	19	51
Pork & Bean Suizo	600	29	54
Flauta: Beef, plain	160	9	10
Beef w. cheese & sauce	190	12	11
Chicken, plain	190	10	16
Chicken w. cheese & sauce	230	13	17
Tacos: Beef Crisp	210	11	16
Beef Soft Corn	250	10	28
Beef Soft Flour	250	11	24
Chicken Crisp	190	9	15
Chicken Soft Corn	230	8	27
Chicken Soft Flour	230	9	23
Pork Crisp	170	6	16
Pork Soft Corn	220	6	27
Pork Soft Flour	220	7	24
Tostada			
Beef & Bean	380	23	26
Beef & Bean Suiza	440	29	26
Chicken & Bean	360	21	21
Chicken & Bean Suiza	410	26	25
Pork & Bean	350	20	26
Pork & Bean Suiza	410	25	26
Taco Salads			
Beef w/ 4 oz salsa	550	26	52
w/o Taco Shell	330	19	20
Chicken w/ 4 oz salsa	520	23	51
w/o Taco Shell	300	16	19
Pork w/ 4 oz salsa	500	20	52
w/o Taco Shell	290	13	19

Perkin's® Family Restaurant (Aug '09)

Entrees	C	F	Cb
Chicken Dinner	620	13	60
Fish Dinner	470	7	60
'Lite & Healthy'	105	2	15
Omelettes: Country Club	930	79	6
Deli Ham & Cheese	960	79	8
'Everything' Omelette	695	54	9
Granny's Country Omelette	940	82	7
w. 9 oz Hash Browns	1245	90	57
Salads: Chef's, Mini	215	11	7

Perkin's® Family Restaurant cont... (Aug '09)

Muffins:	C	F	Cb
Banana	650	33	78
Blueberry; Pumpkin	550	26	78
Bran Muffin	550	16	94
Carrot	455	26	55
Chocolate Chips	620	26	81
Cranberry Nut	585	29	75
Lemon Poppyseed	685	33	88
Oat Bran	455	15	68
Peaches & Cream; Apple, avg.	520	23	72
Raspberry & Cream	585	26	81
Pancakes: Buttermilk (1), no syrup	140	4.5	20
Short Stack (3), no syrup	425	14	60
Regular Stack (5), no syrup	705	24	100
Pies, Per Slice: Apple Pie, ⅙ pie	375	15	56
Wildberry, ⅙ pie	390	16	66
Bundt Cake, w. Icing (sugar free)	385	17	70
Fruit Cup	50	0.5	12

For Complete Nutritional Data ~ See CalorieKing.com

Peter Piper® Pizza (Sept '09)

Pizza: Per Slice	C	F	Cb
Original Crust: *Per ⅛ of 14" Pizza*			
Cheese	300	9	37
Ham & Pineapple	280	7	38
Pepperoni	300	10	36
Hand-Tossed Crust: *Per ⅛ of 14" Pizza*			
Cheese	290	9	38
Ham & Pineapple	280	7	39
Pepperoni	290	10	37
Pan Crust: *Per ⅛ of 14" Pizza*			
Cheese	290	9	38
Ham & Pineapple	310	7	46
Pepperoni	330	10	44
Specialty			
Original Crust: *Per ⅛ of 14" Pizza*			
5 Meat Supreme	350	13	38
Chicago Classic	300	10	38
New York 3 Cheese w. Pepperoni	380	16	38
Smokehouse	370	15	38
The Werx	320	11	38

Updated Nutrition Data ~ www.CalorieKing.com
Persons with Diabetes ~ See Disclaimer (Page 24)

P.F. Chang's® (Sept '09)

Starters/Small Plates:	C	F	Cb
Crab Wontons w/o Plum Sauce (2)	170	11	13
Egg Roll (1)	175	8	22
Lettuce Wraps: Chicken (1)	155	7	15
Vegetarian (1)	135	7	10
Peking Dumplings: Pan-Fried (1)	95	5	7
Steamed (1)	65	3	6
Shrimp Dumplings: Pan-Fried (1)	70	2	8
Steamed (1)	60	1	8
Spare Ribs: Northern, ¼ dish, 4 oz	340	19	11
Changs BBQ, ¼ dish, 4 oz	345	24	7
Spring Rolls (2)	315	16	34
Meals: Per Whole Dish without Rice, 1.5-5 Servings			
Beef: A La Sichuan, 12 oz	775	33	60
Mongolian, 12 oz	705	38	50
Orange Peel, 13.5 oz	815	36	63
Chicken: w. Black Bean Sce, 22oz	1090	60	60
Chang's Spicy, 13.5 oz	900	36	87
Kung Pao Chicken, 24 oz	1180	66	72
Mu Shu w/o Pancakes, 16 oz	465	24	26
Orange Peel Chicken, 15.75 oz	1030	53	74
Philip's Better Lemon, 22 oz	1145	50	115
Sesame Chicken, 24 oz	1120	48	93
Sweet & Sour Chicken, 13.5 oz	830	39	87
VIP Duck, 24 oz	1485	54	174
Seafood: Cantonese Scallops, 16 oz	595	28	50
Cantonese Shrimp, 16 oz	525	20	36
Chang's Lemon Scallops, 18 oz	750	12	80
Kung Pao Scallops, 24 oz	805	36	48
Kung Pao Shrimp, 24 oz	775	36	48
Lemon Pepper Shrimp, 16 oz	455	20	32
Shrimp w/ Candied Walnuts, 24 oz	1235	78	90
Vegetarian Plate:			
Buddha's Feast, steamed, 20 oz	405	7.5	60
Coconut Curry Vegetables, 24 oz	885	63	48
Ma Po Tofu, 20 oz	650	37	45
Lunch Bowls: Served on White Rice			
Moo Goo Gai Pan	835	24	109
Sesame Chicken	1025	25	148
Shrimp w. Lobster Sauce	720	20	103
Sides: Small			
Garlic Snap Peas, 5 oz	100	3	12
Green Tea Soba Noodles, 23 oz	410	18	51
Shanghai Cucumbers, 6 oz	65	3	5
Sichuan Asparagus, 6 oz	105	5	11
Spicy Green Beans, 5 oz	95	5	10
Spinach Stir-Fried w. Garlic, 7 oz	90	5	8
Soups: Hot & Sour, 1 bowl	510	19	54
Egg Drop Soup: 1 cup	70	3	10
1 bowl	400	15	58
Wonton: 1 cup	60	2	10
1 bowl	695	24	49
Desserts: Banana Spring Rolls	990	45	145
Great Wall of Chocolate Cake	1440	61	231
Tiramisu Mini Dessert	235	17	17

Piccadilly Cafeteria® (Sept '09)

Meals: W/o Sides	C	F	Cb
Beef: Chopped Steak Fried, 4.5 oz	415	33	6
Roast Leg, small, 4 oz	350	22	2
Steak: Filet Mignon, 6 oz	340	20	1
New York Strip, 10 oz	875	71	1
Ribeye, 10 oz	1040	91	2
Chicken: Breast, Mesquite Smoked	210	8	1
Baked Cajun, Boneless Breast	430	27	9
Fish: Catfish Cajun Baked	405	28	6
Catfish Filet Stuffed	550	40	9
Tilapia Baked	210	11	10
Trout Almondine Baked, large	490	22	11
Trout Cajun Baked	520	27	7
Trout Filets Baked	465	19	10
Pork Loin, Bone in Roast, 5 oz	375	13	10
Shrimp, Fried	460	19	34
Turkey Breast, Carved, 5.5 oz	265	10	5
Salads			
Caesar Salad, 3 oz	145	11	7
Chef's Salad, Small, 6 oz	145	9	4
Italian Coleslaw, 3.7 oz	165	16	5
Louisianne Bowl	45	3	2
Mexican	60	3	8
Piccadilly Bowl	25	0	6
Shrimp Remoulade	515	28	33
Dressings			
Au Jus, 3 fl.oz	5	0	1
Blue Cheese, 2 Tbsp	160	18	1
Cheese Sauce, 2 fl.oz	35	1	5
French, 2 Tbsp	130	13	5
Italian, 2 Tbsp	160	17	1
Ranch, 2 Tbsp	150	17	1
Ranch Fat-Free, 2 Tbsp	35	0	7
Thousand Island, 2 Tbsp	170	18	2
Soups: Per 9.5 oz (No Rice)			
Gumbo: Chicken	100	2	11
Chicken & Sausage	225	15	10
Extras			
Broccoli w. Cheese Sauce	105	7	9
Cabbage: Buttered, Steamed	70	5	6
Bacon Seasoned	105	8	6
Cauliflower, Buttered	90	6	8
Greens: Collard Mustard & Turnip	135	10	3
Turnip w. Diced Turnips, 3.2 oz	150	12	4
Okra Creole	80	4	9

Pita Pit (Sept '09)

Breakfast Pitas: Includes white pita and standard toppings.
Add extra for cheese & sauce

	C	**F**	**Cb**
Awakin' with Bacon	610	27	57
Chicken Classic	565	19	60
Ham n' Eggs	510	16	59
Meat the Day	570	24	59
Morning Glory	505	18	61
Sausage Sunrise	530	20	59

Meat Pitas: Includes white pita bread.
Add extra for toppings and sauces

Black Forest Ham	320	2.5	45
B.L.T.	455	19	44
Chicken Breast	310	5	44
Chicken Caesar	395	11	45
Chicken Crave	370	6	46
Chicken Souvlaki	355	10	42
Dagwood	390	6	46
Gyro	600	35	51
Philly Steak	310	4	42
Roast Beef	360	7.5	45
Tuna	330	2.5	41
Turkey	300	2.5	43

Veggie Pitas: Includes white pita bread. Add extra for
toppings and sauces

Babaganoush	270	5.5	47
Cheddar	420	19	41
Falafel	455	4	65
Feta	320	8.5	43
Garden	200	0.5	41
Hummus	300	7.5	49
Pita: White (1)	200	0.5	41
Toppings: Avocado	45	4	2
Babaganoush	35	2.5	3
Hummus	50	3.5	4
Pineapple	10	0	2
Salad Veggies, average	20	0	4
Sauces: BBQ	50	0	14
Caesar	140	15	0
Hot Sauce	0	0	0
Mayo	70	7	2
Ranch	80	8	2
Sour Cream	60	6	2
Teriyaki	35	0	8
Tzatziki	45	4	2
Cheeses: American Swiss	50	4.5	1
Cheddar	220	18	0
Feta	120	8	2
Smoothies: Berry Go Round	300	0.5	69
Banana Very Berry	270	0	63
Mango Tango	280	0	65

Pizza Hut® (Aug '09)

Thin 'n Crispy (12"): Per Whole Pizza

	C	**F**	**Cb**
All Natural: Ital. Sausage & Onion	1760	80	184
Pepperoni	1600	72	168
Pepperoni & Mushroom	1520	56	176

Thin 'n Crispy (12"): Per ⅛ Pizza

Cheese Only, 2.6 oz	190	8	22
Ham & Pineapple, 3 oz	180	6	23
Meat Lover's, 3.7 oz	290	17	22
Supreme, 3.6 oz	230	11	23
Veggie Lover's, 3.5 oz	180	6	23
All Natural:			
Italian Ssg & Onion, 3.3 oz	220	10	23
Pepperoni, 2.6 oz	200	9	21

Fit n' Delicious (12"): Per Slice, ⅛ Pizza

Chicken, Mushrooms & Jalapeno	180	4.5	22
Chicken, Onion & Green Peppers	180	4.5	24
Ham, Pineapple & Tomato, 3.4 oz	180	4.5	24

Hand-Tossed Style (12"): Per Whole Pizza

All Natural: Ital. Sausage & Onion	1920	80	216
Pepperoni, 25.6 oz	1840	80	200
Pepperoni & Mushroom, 28 oz	1680	64	208

Hand-Tossed Style (12"): Per Slice, ⅛ Pizza

Cheese Only, 3.2 oz	220	8	26
Ham & Pineapple, 3.5 oz	200	6	27
Meat Lover's, 4.3 oz	310	17	26
Supreme, 4.1 oz	260	12	26
Veggie Lover's, 3.9 oz	200	7	27
All Natural:			
Italian Sausage & On.,3.8 oz	240	10	27
Pepperoni, 3.2 oz	230	10	25
Pepperoni & Mushroom, 3 oz	210	8	26

P'Zone: Per ½ P'Zone

Classic, 9 oz	630	23	77
Meaty, 9.4 oz	740	33	76
Pepperoni, 8.3 oz	630	24	76

Pan (12"): Per Slice, ⅛ Pizza

Cheese Only, 3.4 oz	230	9	27
Ham & Pineapple, 3.6 oz	220	8	28
Meat Lover's 4.4 oz	330	18	27
Supreme, 4.2 oz	280	13	27
Veggie Lover's, 3.9 oz	220	8	28
All Natural:			
Italian Sausage & On., 3.9 oz	260	11	27
Pepperoni, 3.3 oz	250	11	26
Pepperoni & Mushroom, 3.6 oz	230	9	27

The Edge (12"): Per 2 Slices, ⅛ Pizza

Combo	240	12	24
Meaty	330	20	22
Pepperoni	220	11	22

Updated Nutrition Data ~ www.CalorieKing.com
Persons with Diabetes ~ See Disclaimer (Page 24)

Fast - Foods & Restaurants

Pizza Hut® cont... (Aug '09)

Personal Pan (6"): Per Pizza

	C	F	Cb
Cheese Only, 9 oz	590	24	69
Ham & Pineapple, 9.2 oz	550	20	71
Meat Lover's, 12 oz	850	47	69
Supreme, 10.9 oz	720	35	70
Veggie Lover's, 9.9 oz	550	20	70
All Natural: Pepperoni, 8.8 oz	610	27	68
Pepperoni & Mushroom, 9.2 oz	570	23	68

Pizza Mia (12"): Per Slice, ⅛ Pizza

	C	F	Cb
Cheese Only, 2.9 oz	200	7	24
Pepperoni, 2.8 oz	200	8	24

Stuffed Crust (14"): Per Slice, ⅛ pizza

	C	F	Cb
Cheese Only, 5 oz	340	14	39
Ham & Pineapple, 5.5 oz	330	13	41
Meat Lover's, 6.7 oz	480	26	39
Supreme, 6.3 oz	410	20	40
Veggie Lover's, 6 oz	330	13	40
All Natural: Ital. Sausage & Onion	390	18	40
Pepperoni, 5.2 oz	380	18	39
Pepperoni & Mushroom, 5.5 oz	350	15	39

The Natural (12"): Per Slice, ⅛ Pizza

	C	F	Cb
All Natural Pepperoni	230	9	26
Cheese Only	220	8	26
Classicana	260	11	27
Veggie Lover's, w/o Olives	190	6	27

Appetizers

	C	F	Cb
Breadsticks (1), 1.8 oz	140	6	18
Cheese Breadsticks (1), 2.2 oz	180	7	20
Wings: Hot w/o dipping sce, 2 pcs	120	7	1
Mild w/o dipping sce, 2 pieces	110	7	1

Pastas, Tuscani: Per ¼ Order

	C	F	Cb
Bacon Mac N Cheese, 12.4 oz	520	22	54
Chicken Alfredo, 11.9 oz	640	33	56
Lasagna, 11.53 oz	570	30	45
Meaty Marinara, 11.4 oz	510	24	48

Sauces

	C	F	Cb
Dipping: Blue Cheese, 1.5 oz	230	24	2
Marinara, 3 oz	60	0	12
Ranch, 1.5 oz	220	23	3

Desserts

	C	F	Cb
Cinnamon Sticks, 2 pieces, 1.9 oz	170	6	26
Hershey's Chocolate Dunkers, 2 pcs, with choc. sauce, 1.5 oz	320	12	50
Dipping Cup, White Icing, 2 oz	190	0	47

Pizza Ranch® (Sept '09)

Pizzas, 12": Per Slice (⅛ Pizza)

	C	F	Cb
Original: Beef	170	6	21
BBQ Chicken	170	5	23
Bacon Cheeseburger	190	7	21
California Chicken	210	10	22
Canadian Bacon, avg.	170	6	21
Cheese; Chicken Broccoli, av	180	7	21
Garlic Cheese	190	9	21
Italian Sausage; Pepperoni	180	8	21
Prairie; Sweet Swine, av	170	6	22
Roundup	190	8	22
Stampede	210	9	22
Texan	200	8	26
Skillet: Beef	180	6	23
BBQ Chicken	180	5	24
Bacon Cheeseburger	200	7	23
Bronco; California Chicken, av	220	10	24
Cheese; Chicken Broccoli, av	190	7	23
Garlic Cheese	200	9	22
Italian Sausage; Pepperoni, av	190	8	23
Prairie; Sweet Swine	180	6	24
Roundup	200	8	24
Stampede	210	9	24
Texan	210	8	28
Thin: Beef	130	6	12
BBQ Chicken	130	5	14
Bacon Cheeseburger	140	7	12
California Chicken; Bronco, av	165	9	13
Canadian Bacon, av	120	5	12
Cheese; Chicken Broccoli, av	135	7	12
Garlic Cheese	140	9	11
Italian Sausage; Pepperoni, av	140	7	12
Prairie; Sweet Swine, av	130	6	13
Roundup	150	8	13
Stampede	160	8	13
Texan	160	7	17
Broasted Chicken: Breast, 1 pce	440	23	4
Leg, 1 piece	190	12	2
Thigh, 1 piece	370	26	4
Wing, 1 piece	190	13	2
Sides: Potato Wedges (1)	60	0	13

For Complete Nutritional Data ~ see CalorieKing.com

Fast - Foods & *Restaurants*

Planet Smoothie® (Sept '09)

Cool Blended Smoothies
Per 22 fl.oz Unless Otherwise Stated

	C	F	Cb
Captain Kid, 12 fl oz	180	0	46
PB & J	780	32	115
Shag-a-delic	410	0	99
The Last Mango	340	1	85
Twig & Berries	340	0	82
Vinnie del Rocco	370	0	92

Energy Smoothies: Per 22 fl.oz

Berry Bada-Bing	400	0.5	94
Chocolate Elvis	630	16	115
Frozen Goat	370	0	89
Grape Ape	440	0	112
Road Runner	330	0	84
Spazz	280	0	73

Workout Smoothies: Per 22 fl.oz

Big Bang with Boost	380	0	90
Chocolate Chimp, protein blast	400	0	92
Merlin's Mix, Pineapple, 32 fl oz	330	2	29
Strawberry, 32 fl oz	460	2	65

Pollo Tropical® (Sept '09)

Chicken:	C	F	Cb
Dark Meat: with skin	270	17	0
without skin	180	9	0
White Meat: with skin	350	17	0
without skin	230	7	0

Tropichop:
Chicken, White Rice/Black Beans:			
Regular	530	10	90
Large	1090	27	142
Chicken, Yellow Rice/Vegetables:			
Regular	330	5	51
Large	840	22	93
Pork, White Rice/Black Beans: Reg.	680	22	92
Large	1260	49	145
Pork, Yellow Rice/Vegetables: Reg.	490	18	54
Large	1000	44	97
Vegetarian:Regular	580	12	110
Large	950	21	178

Fajita: With Sides, Toppings, Tortillas
Chicken; Steak, av.	1145	38	153
Salad, Caribbean Cobb	950	41	57

Tropical Favorites:
Cheesy Yuca Bites, 6 pieces	290	14	32
Fried Yuca, 5 pieces	500	24	69
Sweet Plantains, 5 pieces	310	8	63
Wraps: Chicken Caesar	790	39	65
Cuban	680	29	61
Pork	740	25	73

Popeye's® (Sept '09)

	C	F	Cb
Chicken: Chkn Breast, Mild/Spicy avg.	355	21	8
Chicken Leg, Mild/Spic, avg.	105	6	3
Chicken Thigh, Mild/Spicy, avg.	290	22	7
Chicken Wing, Mild/Spicy, avg.	145	10	5
Big Deals: Delta Mini (1), 3.6 oz	300	13	30
Chicken Biscuit, 3.6 oz	350	20	30
Loaded Chicken Wrap, 6 oz	400	17	44
Sides: Biscuit, 2.1 oz	240	13	26
Cajun Rice, regular, 4.1 oz	170	6	22
Coleslaw, regular, 5 oz	260	23	14
Corn on the Cob (1), 7.8 oz	190	2	37
French Fries, 3 oz	310	17	35
Mashed Potatoes: no Gravy, reg.	100	3	17
w. Gravy, regular, 5 oz	120	4	18
Red Beans & Rice, regular, 6 oz	320	19	31
Desserts: Cinn. Apple Turnover, 3 oz	250	12	34

Port of Subs® (Sept '09)

Figures Based on West Coast Outlets
Light Submarine: Per 5" Sub (Five Grams of Fat or Less)

	C	F	Cb
#2 Ham Turkey	330	5	46
#5 Smoked Ham & Turkey	320	5	46
#6 Vegetarian, no Cheese	240	2	44
#7 Roast Beef	315	4	43
#8 Turkey	315	4	47
#9 Peppered Pastrami	295	4	44
#10 Roasted Chicken Breast	305	3	44
#14 Smoked Ham	300	4	44
#18 Roast Beef & Turkey	315	4	45

Cold Submarine S'wiches: Per 5" Sub w/o Mayo/Mustard

#1 Ham, Salami, Capicolla			
& Pepperoni w. Provolone	530	26	45
#2 Ham & Turkey w. Provolone	435	15	46
#3 Salami & Turkey w. Provolone	465	20	46
#4 Ham & Salami w. Provolone	470	21	45
#5 Smkd Ham & Turkey w. Cheddar	430	15	47
#6 Vegetarian w. Avocado & Olives	600	33	49
#7 Roast Beef w. Provolone,	420	14	43
#8 Turkey w. Provolone	420	14	47
#9 Peppered Pastrami w. Swiss	440	17	44
#10 Rstd Chicken Brst w. Provolone	410	13	45
#11 Ham w. American	380	20	45
#12 Salami w. Provolone	480	25	45
#13 Peppered Pastrami Turkey Swiss	510	26	44
#14 Smoked Ham w. Swiss	445	17	45
#15 Salami & Pepperoni w. Prov.	510	27	45
#16 BLT Sandwich	520	30	43
#17 Tuna no Cheese	420	18	45
#18 Rst Beef & Turkey w. Provolone	420	14	45

Updated Nutrition Data ~ www.CalorieKing.com
Persons with Diabetes ~ See Disclaimer (Page 24)

Port of Subs® cont... (Sept '09)

Figures Based on West Coast Outlets

Grillers: 5" Serving

	C	F	Cb
BBQ Pork Griller	780	18	104
Grilled Chicken	520	13	58
Hot Pastrami	540	15	58
Italian	555	21	58
NY Steak & Cheese	615	18	57

Tortilla Wrap: Per Wrap, 12" Tortilla

Chicken Caesar	630	34	35
Hot Grilled Chkn & Smokey Cheddar	485	18	35
Turkey & Bacon Ranch	590	38	34
Tortilla (1)	200	7	27

Fresh Salads:

Caesar Salad with Dressing: 6 oz	335	30	7
with Grilled Chicken, 13 oz	540	34	15
Chefs Salad w/ Oil & Vinegar, 11 oz	390	25	13
Garden Salad w/ Oil & Vinegar, 8 oz	95	5	10
Grilled Chicken w/ Oil & Vin. 13 oz	300	10	16
Macaroni Salad, 8 oz	440	30	36
Potato Salad, 8 oz	360	26	54
Tuna Salad w/ Oil & Vinegar, 11 oz	310	23	12

Dessert:

Brownie, 5 oz	300	10	48

Pret A Manger® (Sept '09)

	C	F	Cb

Sandwiches

Avo'cado & Parmesan	570	27	59
Balsamic Chicken & Avocado	500	20	64
Chicken & Bacon	460	13	58
Classic Turkey Club	520	21	59
Smoked Salmon	460	14	48
Slims: Avocado & Parmesan	285	14	30
Balsamic Chicken & Avocado	250	11	32
Chicken & Bacon	230	13	29
Classic Turkey Club	260	11	30

Baguettes:

Chicken Mozzarella	510	14	77
Ham & Swiss	620	16	68
Roasted Beef Arugula & Parm.	670	13	65
Slims: Chicken Mozzarella	255	7	39
French Brie & Basil	265	10	33
Ham & Swiss	310	8	34
Wraps: Jalapeno Chicken, Hot	400	21	46
Spicy Falafel Hot	540	24	61
Swedish Meatball Ragu, Hot	720	37	49

Soup: Per Medium 12 oz Serving

Pasta Fagioli	285	9	35
Spicy Chicken Chowder	390	4	23
Thai Chicken Curry	330	15	36
Tomato Basil	120	5	12

Pret A Manger® cont... (Sept '09)

Salads: Per Pack, w/o Dressing

	C	F	Cb
Cobb & Greens	430	24	30
Grilled Chicken & Avocado	430	28	41
Grilled Chicken Caesar	400	16	24
Red, White & Greens	300	17	1
Summer Salad	440	25	18
Bakery: Banana Cake	420	24	48
Carrot Cake	460	29	47
Chocolate Brownie	390	20	51
Chocolate Cake	470	19	71
Raspberry Bar	390	18	55

For Complete Menu ~ See CalorieKing.com

Pretzelmaker® (Sept '09)

Pretzels:

	C	F	Cb
Bites: Small (1), 5.3 oz	450	11	80
Medium (1), 7½ oz	640	16	112
Large (2) 11½ oz	1020	26	176
Cinnamon Sugar, 6 oz	520	12	95
Pretzel Dog	440	27	34
Pretzels: Caramel Nut	390	7	74
Cinnamon Sugar	370	8	68
Garlic	350	7	64
Original	340	7	61
Parmesan	360	9	61
Plain	290	2	61
Ranch	240	7	63

Sauces: Per 1.5 oz Container

Caramel	140	0	35
Cheddar Cheese	70	5	6
Cream Cheese	200	20	4
Cream Cheese Icing,	180	9	22
Ketchup	20	0	4
Mustard	5	0	1
Nacho Cheese	80	5	7
Pizza	30	0.5	6

Beverages: Per 20 fl.oz

Breezer: Coffee	640	21	107
Mocha	620	20	106
Peach	650	20	117
Raspberry	650	20	117
Strawberry Banana	650	20	115
Lemonade: MCF, 20 fl.oz	160	0	92
MCF, 32 fl.oz	270	0	147
Diet Coke, 20 fl.oz	0	0	0

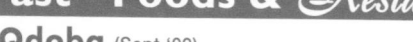
Qdoba (Sept '09)

Signature Burritos: *With 13" Flour Tortilla, Cilantro-Lime Rice, Pinto Beans, Corn Salsa, Cheese & Sour Cream & Standard Sauce*

	C	F	Cb
Ancho Chile BBQ w/ BBQ Sce	1150	32	176
Grilled Vegetable w/o sauce	940	29	133

Burritos: *With 13" Flour Tortilla, Cilantro-Lime Rice, Black Beans, Salsa Verde, Sour Cream*

Chicken	970	28	125
Pork	930	22	134
Shredded Beef	970	26	129

Tacos: *With Cheese & Sour Cream, Lettuce, Pico de Gallo*

Crispy Shell: Chicken	170	10	8
Ground Sirloin	210	13	8
Pork	180	8	11
Shredded Beef	190	10	10

Taco Salads: *With Crispy Taco Salad Shell, Black Bean Corn Salsa, Picante Ranch Dressing, Cheese & Sour Cream*

Chicken	780	44	53
Ground Sirloin	830	50	53

Quesadillas: *With 13" Four Tortilla, 4 oz. Cheese, Pico de Gallo*

Chicken	970	54	57
Shredded Beef	970	52	61

3-Cheese Nachos: *With Chips, 3-Cheese Queso, Pinto Beans, Sour Cream, Salsa Verde*

Regular: with Chicken	1150	57	111
with Ground Sirloin	1210	64	111
with Pork	1130	52	120

Breakfast Items: *With 10" Flour Tortilla*

Breakfast Burrito: *With Eggs, Potato & Chorizo*

with 3-Cheese Queso Sauce	540	26	54
with Fajita Ranchero Sauce	480	20	53

Condiments: 3-Chse Queso, 4 oz

3-Chse Queso, 4 oz	200	16	6
Black Bean Corn Salsa, 2 oz	60	0.5	11
Chips, 4 oz	560	26	75
Guacamole, 3 oz	130	11	7
Mango Salsa, 4 oz	60	0	14
Sour Cream, 2 oz	60	4	3

Quizno's Subs® (Sept '09)

Based on Quizno's Standard Portion Sizes. Figures may not apply for Denver, Boise, Des Moines, Baltimore, Springfield, Raleigh, Cleveland.
Subs *Regular: With Cheese & Dressing Unless Indicated*

Every-Day Value Subs:

Honey-Cured Ham & Swiss	820	46	72
Oven Roasted Turkey & Cheddar	780	41	70
Primo Meatball	770	36	78
Roast Beef & Cheddar	790	41	71
The 5 Meat Stack	900	52	68
Tuna Melt	1230	92	67

Quizno's Subs® cont... (Sept '09)

Based on Quizno's Standard Portion Sizes. Figures may not apply for Denver, Boise, Des Moines, Baltimore, Springfield, Raleigh, Cleveland.
Subs *Regular:*
With Cheese & Dressing Unless Indicated

	C	F	Cb
Signature Classics: Italian	950	47	72
Classic Club	920	54	71
Tuscan Turkey	670	26	75
Turkey, Bacon & Guacamole	840	42	74
Turkey, Ranch & Swiss	660	27	74
Veggie	860	42	71
Premium Subs:			
Baja Chicken w. Bacon	800	35	73
Black Angus Steak	810	27	83
Chicken Carbonara w. Bacon	860	41	68
Honey Mustard Chicken	880	43	73
Mesquite Chicken w. Bacon	820	38	69
Prime Rib & Peppercorn	990	58	75
Prime Rib Cheesesteak	1070	67	74
Torpedos: Beef Bacon Cheddar	700	30	77
Big Kahuna Tuna	880	53	73
Italian	695	32	74
Pesto Turkey	585	21	76
Turkey Club	735	35	75

Flatbread Sammies:
With Cheese & Dressing Unless Indicated

Alpine Chicken	295	15	25
Bistro Steak Melt	280	13	26
Cantina Chicken, w/o Cheese	205	4	29
Italiano	305	18	24
Roadhouse Steak, w/o Cheese	195	4	29
Sonoma Turkey	280	14	26

Kids Sammies: *With Cheese w/o Dressing*

Ham Melt	200	7	25
Just Cheese; Tasty Turkey, avg.	190	6	24

Breakfast Sandwiches:

Black Angus, Steak & Cheddar, small	390	18	36
Egg & Cheddar	350	20	36
Ham, Egg & Cheddar	350	17	37
Garden Vegetable w. Cheddar	310	16	38

Soups: *Per Bowl*

Broccoli Cheese, with 3 Crackers	360	22	28
Chili, with 3 Crackers	360	15	36
Bread Bowls: Chili	760	22	107
Country Fresh Chicken	760	26	103

Flatbread Salads: *With Cheese & Dressing*

Black & Bleu	670	22	86
Chicken Caesar	1020	69	61
Classic Cobb w Ranch Dressing	910	58	61
Rstd Chicken w. Honey Mustard	1070	71	69

Updated Nutrition Data ~ www.CalorieKing.com
Persons with Diabetes ~ See Disclaimer (Page 24)

Fast - Foods & *Restaurants*

Rally's/Checkers® (Aug '09)

Burgers/Sandwiches	C	F	Cb
Bacon Double Cheeseburger	650	42	32
Big Buford	570	36	31
Chili Cheeseburger	320	15	30
Crispy Fish Sandwich	430	19	51
Grilled Chicken Sandwich	370	9	40
Philly Cheesesteak Burger	500	26	38
Rallyburger	390	22	32
with Cheese	420	24	33
Triple Cheeseburger	690	43	33
Fries:			
Chili Cheese Fries, 7.76 oz	550	34	48
French: Medium, 4.23 oz	420	27	40
Large, 6 oz	590	38	57

Ranch 1® (Sept '09)

	C	F	Cb
Sandwiches: Chicken & Cheese	390	12	39
Chicken Philly, 9.2 oz	410	13	40
Crispy Chicken, 11.4 oz	710	39	60
Crispy Spicy Chicken, 11.4 oz	545	17	68
Grilled Spicy Chicken, 10.3 oz	365	7	46
Ranch 1 Classic, 9.4 oz	685	47	37
Bowls: Chicken Teriyaki, 19.3 oz	505	7	78
Fajitas, Chicken, 10 oz	540	24	53
Chicken, Rice, 10.9 oz	275	6	28
Popcorn Chicken: Small, 5.5 oz	325	12	30
Large, 7.5 oz	420	15	38
Kids Meal, 2 oz	110	4	10
Salads: Complete			
Grilled Chicken Caesar, 13.2 oz	430	30	14
Mandarin Chicken, 19.3 oz	815	43	78
Southwest Chicken, 17.5 oz	745	50	44
Fries: Medium, 5.8 oz	380	21	43
Large, 8 oz	530	29	58
Kids Meal, 4 oz	280	15	31
Cheese: Regular, 9 oz	495	27	54
Large, 14 oz	755	42	80

Red Hot & Blue® (Aug '09)

BBQ Platters	C	F	Cb
Five Meat Treat	1160	85	15
Memphis Half Chicken	1510	103	11
Pulled Chicken	365	24	7
Pulled Pork	485	34	7
Smoked Sausage	950	67	36
BBQ Sandwiches: Regular			
Carolina Chopped Pork	460	23	34
Pulled Chicken	390	17	36
Pulled Pork	470	23	37
Ribs, Half Slab: Dry	1350	100	32
Sweet	1315	95	40
Wet	1260	95	26

Red Hot & Blue cont... (Sept '09)

Salads	C	F	Cb
Grilled Chicken Caesar	755	45	45
RH & B Chopped Salad	935	55	54
Smokehouse Salad	770	45	44
Southern Fried Chicken	690	31	58
Soup: Corn Chowder, 1 bowl	320	18	22
Kids: Chicken Tenders Meal	305	14	20

Red Lobster® (Sept '09)

Lunch	C	F	Cb
Starters:			
Chilled Jumbo Shrimp Cocktail	120	1	9
Crispy Calamari & Vegetables	1520	98	116
Pan Seared Crab Cakes	360	22	15
Southwestern Lobster Rolls	870	51	74
Fish, Grilled/Broiled: Per ½ Portion, Served w. Broccoli			
Flounder	195	1.5	9
Rainbow Trout	225	10	6
Salmon	265	8.5	8
Tilapia	205	3	9
Classics: Per ½ Portion			
Cajun Chkn Linguini Alfredo	630	27	45
Crab Linguini Alfredo	560	25	47
Crunchy Popcorn Shrimp	280	15	26
Dinner			
Starters: Clam Strips	370	22	31
Lobster, Artichoke & Seafood Dip	1200	74	101
Parrot Bay Coconut Shrimp	590	33	54
Ultimate Fondue	1490	80	124
Entrees: Live Main Lobster, 1¼ lb	45	0.5	0
Gr. Scallops, Shrimp & Chicken	600	13	42
North Pacific King Crab Legs	390	3	3
Steak, Lobster & Shrimp Oscar	990	60	20
Walt's Favorite Shrimp	700	40	52
Sides: Fries	330	17	40
Home-Style Mashed Potatoes	180	9	22
Garden Salad	90	3	13
Garden Salad with Shrimp	105	3	13
Dressings & Dips: Per 1 oz			
Cocktail Sauce	25	0	6
Sweet & Spicy Glaze	90	0	21
Tartar Sauce	130	13	4
100% Pure Melted Butter	230	25	1

For Complete Nutritional Data ~ see CalorieKing.com

Red Robin® (Aug '09)

Entrees	C	F	Cb
Arctic Cod Fish & Chips	1120	67	83
Chicken Fajitas	970	38	77
Chicken Parmigiano Pasta	1480	56	166
Clucks & Fries: Regular Style	1390	85	105
Buffalo Style	1635	113	105
Ensenada Chicken Platter	780	45	22
Jumbo Shrimp & Slaw Platter	1240	56	146
Red's Rice Bowl	810	8	140
Shrimp & Cod Duo	1415	83	131
Southwest Chicken Pasta	1485	83	118
Sandwiches & Burgers			
Chicken Burger: Blackened	750	41	49
California	945	57	49
Crispy	930	56	71
Jamaican Jerk'd	705	36	53
Teriyaki	905	49	61
Whiskey River BBQ,	965	53	68
Classic Gourmet Burgers:			
A.1. Peppercorn Burger	1435	97	92
Bacon Cheeseburger	1030	70	48
Blackened Bayou	845	56	41
Bleu Ribbon	1050	63	69
Gourmet Cheeseburger	850	49	58
Guacamole Bacon	1160	77	52
Monster	1150	69	57
Natural	570	25	48
Royal	1190	83	48
Santa Fe	1095	68	66
Sauteed 'Shroom	960	57	55
The Banzai	1035	63	65
Whiskey River BBQ	1115	69	68
Insanely Delicious Burgers:			
Bruschetta Chicken	830	48	53
Chili Chili Cheeseburger	965	55	54
Prime Rib Dip	1000	55	72
Other Favorites: Crispy Fish	605	30	58
Grilled Salmon	855	50	53
Grilled Turkey	695	43	49
Lettuce-Wrapped Your Burger	420	27	8
The Garden Burger	540	23	62
Wraps: Caesar's Chicken	850	43	69
Whiskey River BBQ Chicken	1110	62	84
Shareable Starters			
Bueno Con Queso	1435	89	106
Crmy Artichoke & Spinach Dip	1205	73	101
Fresh-Fried Cheese Sticks	1170	67	90
Guacamole, Salsa & Chips	810	47	88
Just-in-Quesadilla	1070	55	69
RR's Buzzard Wings	1075	84	4
Towering Onion Rings	1820	122	160

Rita's® (Sept '09)

	C	F	Cb
Italian Ice: Kids, 7.5 oz	200	0	50
Regular, 12 oz	320	0	80
Large, 19 oz	500	0	126
Sugar Free: Chocolate, 3 oz	50	0	11
Mango-Peach; Pineapple	35	0	8
Other flavors, 3 oz	5	0	2
Cream Ice: Kids, 7.5 oz	240	3	53
Regular, 12 oz	380	5	85
Large, 19 oz	600	8	134
Custard: Kids, 4 oz	230	12	28
Regular, 5.75 oz	330	17	40
Large, 7.5 oz	430	22	52
Gelati: Per 10 oz			
w/ Italian Ice, avg. all flavors	390	12	68
Light: Mango-Peach/Pineapple	230	0	51
Other flavors	170	0	37
Misto: Per 15.5 oz			
w/ Italian Ice: Chocolate	510	7	106
Vanilla	480	8	103
w/ Cream Ice, avg. all flavors	560	13	111
Light Pretzel Blendini: Per 11 oz			
Chocolate	420	1.5	90
Mango-Peach/Pineapple	400	1	86
Light M&Ms, Oreo Blendinis: Per 11 oz			
Chocolate	440	8	86
Mango-Peach/Pineapple	420	6	82

For Complete Nutritional Data ~ see CalorieKing.com

Robeks (Aug '09)

Smoothies: Per 12 fl.oz	C	F	Cb
Acai Energizer	165	1	36
Cardio Cooler	215	1	44
Cranberry Quest	175	0	40
Dr. Robeks	180	1	40
Guava Lava	180	1	42
Mahalo Mango	175	1	42
Malibu Peach	155	0	36
Passionfruit Cove	170	1	38
Pomegranate Passion	195	0	48
Pomegranate Power	210	0	50
Raspberry Romance	170	0	42
Robeks Rejuvenator	195	1	43
Robeks MuscleMax	200	1	38
Strawnana Berry	180	0	44
Venice Burner	230	1	46
Zen Berry	190	1	45
Light Smoothies: Banana-Mango	155	0	40
Pineapple-Mango	160	0	41
Raspberry-Banana	160	0	39
Strawberry-Pineapple	125	0	32

Updated Nutrition Data ~ www.CalorieKing.com
Persons with Diabetes ~ See Disclaimer (Page 24)

Rocky Rococo® (Sept '09)

Pastas: Per Serving

	C	F	Cb
Can't Decide, 14 oz	465	9	77
Fettuccine w. Alfredo Sauce:			
Regular, 14 oz	460	14	66
Light, 7 oz	230	7	33
Spaghetti w. Meatballs: Reg., 15 oz	630	16	89
Light, 7.5 oz	315	8	45
Spaghetti w. Tomato Sauce: Reg.	470	4	87
Light, 7 oz	235	2	44

Pizzas: Per Slice, ⅛ Pizza

	C	F	Cb
Cheese	380	9	54
Garden	390	10	56
Pepperoni	425	13	54
Sausage	495	19	54
Sausage Mushroom	500	19	55

Sides

	C	F	Cb
Breadsticks: w. Marinara Sce (6)	420	7	72
w. Jalapeno Cheese Sauce (6)	530	18	72
Wheat Muffin (1)	200	4	38

Roly Poly® (Sept '09)

	C	F	Cb

Wraps: Per Small Whole Wheat Bread Wrap

Baked Ham & Roast Pork:	C	F	Cb
BarBQ Pork Melt	300	10	26
Italian Classic	330	12	28
Key West Cuban Mix	320	12	27
Peachtree Melt	325	11	28
Porky's Nightmare	310	12	26
Chicken: Basil Cashew Chicken	290	11	27
Catalina Chicken Salad	305	12	27
Chicken Caesar	310	12	28
Chicken Cordon Bleu	305	11	27
Chicken Fajita	310	13	27
Chicken Popper	280	9	29
Cobb Salad	320	14	28
Delhi Chicken	320	12	32
Hickory Chicken	335	11	27
Oriental Chicken	260	6	31
Santa Fe Chicken	305	12	27
Seafood: Popeye's Tuna	310	4.5	30
Classic Tuna Melt	335	18	26
Texas Tuna Melt	310	13	26
Thai Hot Tuna	325	13	27
Tuna Luau	325	15	29

Round Table® Pizza (Aug '09)

Appetizers	C	F	Cb
Buffalo Wings, 6 pieces	420	30	6
Garlic Bread, 6 pieces	420	21	54
with Cheese, 6 pieces	600	36	54
Garlic Parmesan Twists, 3 pieces	510	15	78
Honey BBQ Wings 6 pieces	480	27	12

Pizzas (Large 14"): Per Slice, 1/12 Pizza

Original Crust: Cheese	230	9	25
Chicken & Garlic Gourmet	250	11	25
Chicken Smokehouse	270	12	26
Gourmet Veggie	240	10	27
Guinevere's Garden Delight	220	8	26
Hawaiian	220	8	27
Italian Garlic Supreme	270	14	25
King Arthur Supreme	270	13	26
Maui Zaui, with Polynesian Sce	260	10	29
Montague's All Meat Marvel	290	15	25
Pepperoni	240	11	24
Smokehouse Combo	290	14	26
Pan Crust: Cheese	300	11	38
Chicken & Garlic Gourmet	340	13	39
Chicken Smokehouse	360	14	40
Gourmet Veggie	320	12	41
Guinevere's Garden Delight	300	10	39
Hawaiian	300	10	40
Italian Garlic Supreme	360	16	39
King Arthur Supreme	340	14	39
Maui Zaui with Polynesian Sce	340	12	43
Montague's All Meat Marvel	360	15	38
Pepperoni	320	13	38
Skinny Crust: Cheese	190	9	18
Chicken & Garlic Gourmet	220	11	18
Chicken Smokehouse	240	12	19
Gourmet Veggie	200	10	20
Guinevere's Garden Delight	180	8	19
Hawaiian	190	8	20
Italian Garlic Supreme	240	14	18
King Arthur Supreme	240	13	19
Maui Zaui with Polynesian Sce	220	10	22
Montague's All Meat Marvel	260	15	18
Pepperoni	210	11	18
Sandwiches:			
Chicken Club	800	43	59
Ham Club	740	40	60
RT Pizza	410	18	78
Turkey Club	720	38	59
Turkey Sante Fe	730	40	57

For Complete Nutritional Data ~ see CalorieKing.com

Fast - Foods & Restaurants

Roy Rogers® (Sept '09)

Breakfast Items	C	F	Cb
Biscuit & Sausage Gravy	865	48	85
Creamed Chipped Beef on Biscuit	425	22	43
Sourdough Ham, Egg & Cheese	440	21	37
Sandwiches & Burgers:			
Bacon Cheeseburger	520	33	32
Double-R-Bar Burger	735	43	42
Gold Rush Chicken Filet	560	30	51
Hamburger	345	18	32
Quarter Pound Cheeseburger	480	29	32
Roy's Real Roast Beef	330	10	29
Fried Chicken:			
Breast	370	15	29
Leg	170	7	15
Tenders (5)	1020	38	75

Rubio's Mexican Grill®

(Sept '09)

	C	F	Cb
Burritos:			
Fish Burrito	710	40	71
Grilled Mesquite Shrimp Burrito	710	34	72
Grilled Veggie Burrito	630	29	73
Mahi Mahi Burrito	700	42	49
Big Burrito Especial: Chicken	830	32	99
Steak	870	38	99
Health Mex: Chicken Burrito	500	10	70
Mahi Mahi Burrito	510	15	68
Tacos: Carnitas Rajas	210	11	23
Grilled Chicken	280	15	22
Fish, Especial	330	20	30
Health Mex: Chicken	150	1.5	21
Mahi Mahi	160	4	21
Grilled Mesquite Shrimp	230	12	22
Grilled Steak	220	10	22
Street: Chicken	100	4	9
Steak	120	6	9
World Famous Fish	270	14	29
Quesadillas: Cheese	1070	67	85
Chicken	1190	69	87
Salads: Includes Dressing/Sauce			
Chicken Chipotle Ranch	520	35	24
Chicken Chopped	570	33	34
Chicken Fiesta	590	46	13
Chicken Grilled Grande Bowl	700	33	61
Chicken Tropical	410	23	25

Ruby Tuesday® (Sept '09)

	C	F	Cb
Appetizers: Per ¼ Order without Sides or Sauce			
Asian Dumplings	110	5	12
Cheddar Fries	315	18	26
Fire Wings	160	9	2
Jumbo Lump Crab Cake	70	4	4
Quesadillas: Chicken	140	7	10
Fresh Avocado	215	14	13
Thai Phoon Chicken Strips	260	18	13
Burgers & Sandwiches: Without Sides			
Handcrafted Burgers:			
Bacon Cheeseburger	1225	86	65
Bison Bacon Cheeseburger	1105	71	65
Buffalo Chicken	1125	82	80
Classic Cheeseburger	1160	81	65
Jumbo Lump Crab	820	54	59
Smokehouse	1435	97	89
Turkey	890	48	65
Veggie	950	53	98
Prime Burgers Triple Prime	1000	69	50
Triple Prime Cheddar	1160	83	50
Sandwiches:			
Blackened Fish	860	53	46
Chicken BLT	1145	67	80
The Ultimate Chicken	1160	66	61
Feature Menu Items: Without Sides			
Asian Salmon & Shrimp	465	28	7
Lobster Entree	225	7	0
Shrimp Scampi & Steak	1050	54	79
Steak & Lobster Tail	410	19	2
Fork-Tender Ribs: Without Sides			
Classic BBQ: Full-Rack	985	65	29
Half-Back	495	32	14
Memphis Dry Rub: Full-Rack	1075	80	7
Half-Rack	540	40	3
Ribs & Louisiana Fried Shrimp	915	49	55
Triple Play	1095	56	59
Specialties: Without Sides			
Chicken & Broccoli Pasta	1165	55	101
Chicken Bella	385	17	6
Chicken Fresco	425	22	9
Chicken Tender Dinner	650	25	40
Louisiana Fried Shrimp	425	17	40
Parmesan Chicken Pasta	1450	76	117

Ruby Tuesday® (Sept '09)

	C	F	Cb
Steak Dinners: *Without Sides*			
Bayou Sirloin	385	16	5
Cowboy Rib Eye	930	56	32
Peppercorn Mushroom Sirloin	415	18	10
Salads: *Without Dressing*			
Carolina Chicken	1130	71	36
Club House	840	53	9
Signature House	390	30	22
Sauces & Dressings: *Per 1 oz*			
Dressings: Balsamic Vinaigrette	35	2	4
Blue Cheese	170	18	1
Ranch: Regular	95	10	1
Light	45	5	1
Signature Parmesan Dressing	150	16	1
Sauces: Asian Barbecue	60	3	7
Lemon Butter	90	9	1
Marinara	15	1	2
Orange Peanut	60	3	8
Parmesan Cream	60	5	1
Sweet Chile	170	17	2
Signature Sides			
Baked Potato: Plain, Oil-Coated	330	2	66
Loaded	670	31	68
Brown Rice Pilaf	225	7	35
Creamy Mashed Cauliflower	135	8	14
Fries	360	13	57
Onion Straws	300	21	24
Sauteed Baby Portabella Mushr.	75	4	6
White Cheddar Mashed Potatoes	130	7	17
Soups			
Broccoli & Cheese	405	29	22
White Bean Chicken Chili	320	11	40
Desserts			
Blondie for One	625	27	88
Chocolate Tallcake	1275	60	175
Cookie: Chocolate Chip	320	15	42
White Choc. Macadamia Nut	340	20	39
Double Chocolate Cake	990	50	124
Strawberries & Ice Cream	900	50	102

For Complete Menu ~ see CalorieKing.com

Runza® (Sept '09)

	C	F	Cb
Sandwiches			
BBQ Chicken Sandwich, grilled	390	9	46
Buffalo Chicken Sandwich, grilled	440	13	36
Cheese Sandwich	560	21	66
Deluxe Chicken, crispy	480	19	51
Original Sandwich	500	17	65
Polish Dog	420	26	30
Smothered Chicken, grilled	380	10	41
Swiss Cheese Mushroom	590	25	68
Burgers			
Junior: Cheeseburger	330	17	28
Cheeseburger Runza	310	14	30
Swiss Mushroom	380	21	26
Legendary: ¼ lb Cheeseburger	430	21	32
½ lb Double Cheeseburger	640	32	37
¼ lb Bacon Cheeseburger	510	29	36
¼ lb Legend Supreme	770	37	62
¼ lb Swiss Cheese Mushroom	450	25	36
Sides			
French Fries: Small, 3.1 oz	280	15	31
Medium, 4.55 oz	410	23	46
Large, 6.9 oz	630	35	70
Frings, 6.3 oz	540	28	64
Onion Rings: Medium, 4.1 oz	370	20	41
Large, 6.5 oz	590	32	66
Onion Ring Dip, 2.1 oz	90	6	4
Salads: *No Dressing*			
Sweet Berry Chicken	410	16	20
Tossed Salad w. Crispy Chicken	440	27	29
Tossed Salad w. Grilled Chicken	280	13	13
Dressing: Asian Sesame Ginger, 2.4 oz	300	26	14
Fat-Free Hidden Valley Ranch	60	0	15
Raspberry Vinaigrette, 2 oz	25	0	6
Soups: *Per Bowl*			
Boston Clam Chowder	320	23	33
Broccoli Cheese	360	27	35
Cauliflower Cheese	330	26	32
Chicken Noodle	170	5	21
Homemade Chili	310	10	26
Potato w. Bacon	310	20	40
Vegetable Cheese	330	22	28
Wisconsin Cheese	430	35	36
Kids Meals: *Includes Small Fries*			
Mini Corn Dogs (5)	550	32	56
Chicken Strips (2)	460	25	42
Desserts & Drinks			
Chocolate Chip Cookie (1)	310	16	34
Shakes: Cappuccino, reg., 12 f.loz	470	18	65
Vanilla, regular, 12 fl.oz	470	16	69
Pepsi Slushie, medium, 18 fl.oz	220	0	60

Ryan's® Grill, Buffet & Bakery (Sept '09)

Main Courses: *Sides Not Included*	C	F	Cb
BBQ Ribs, 3.6 oz	180	12	7
BBQ Chicken, 2.75 oz	150	6	9
Carved Turkey Breast, 2 oz	90	3.5	0
Chicken Fried Steak (1), no gravy	210	13	15
Chicken Fried Steak (1), w. gravy	220	13	16
Chicken Pot Pie, 4.4 oz	290	18	24
Fried Breaded Catfish, 6.3 oz	340	16	12
Fried Fish (1), 1.6 oz	90	5	4
Fried Shrimp (11)	150	8	16
Fried Tilapia, 0.9 oz	70	2.5	4
Grilled Chicken Breast, plain, 4 oz	180	4	0
Grilled Pork Chop: Plain (1), 3 oz	170	9	0
BBQ; Teriyaki, avg., 1 chop	190	10	4
Grilled Teriyaki Chicken Thighs, 1 oz	60	2.5	4
Macaroni and Cheese, 3.5 oz	120	2.5	19
Meat Lasagne, 6.15 oz	250	11	22
MealLoaf, 2 oz	100	6	6
Mexican Casserole, 4.4 oz	190	9	21
Pizza: Cheese, 1 slice, 3 oz	200	8	21
Pepperoni, 1 slice, 3 oz	250	13	21
Rotisserie Chicken: Breast, 4.8 oz	280	13	0.5
Leg, 2.65 oz	120	9	0.5
Thigh, 4.3 oz	250	16	1
Sirloin Steak, 3 oz	1809	9	0
Spaghetti, 3 oz	130	2.5	23
Spaghetti Sauce, with Meat, 2 oz	140	8	10
Taco Meat, 1.4 oz	70	4	3
White Turkey w. gravy, 4.23 oz	90	2	4
Sides: Baked Potato, plain, 6.35 oz	180	0	31
Baked Beans, 3.88 oz	90	1	20
Breaded Fried Okra, 3 oz	220	12	28
Brussel Sprouts, 2.8 oz	40	2	6
Corn Cobbet (1) 2.68 oz	90	6	11
Garlic Mashed Potatoes, 3 oz	90	4	11
Glazed Baby Carrots w. Sce, 1.9 oz	60	3	7
Gr. Vegetables w. Broccoli, 1.75 oz	40	3	2
Pinto Beans, 3.25 oz	70	1	14
Rice Pilaf, 1.5 oz	60	1	12
Steamed Cabbage w. Bacon, 1.75 oz	60	5	2
Yellow Squash w. Onions, 1.75 oz	40	3.5	2
Desserts: Cheesecake, plain, 1 sl.	370	19	45
Ice Cream Cone (flat bottom)	15	0	3
Key Lime Pie, 1 slice, 2.65 oz	280	12	39
Lemon Creme Cake, 1 slice	170	15	9
Cookies: Oatmeal Raisin (1)	120	5	16
Sugar Cookie (1)	120	5	17

7-Eleven® (Aug '09)

Breakfast Sandwiches	C	F	Cb
Big Bite Breakfast Sandwich	430	27	29
Croissant: w. Bacon, Egg & Chse	400	33	34
w. Ham, Egg & Chse	390	22	34
Engl. Muffin w. Saus., Egg, Chse	450	24	37
Sausage, Egg & Cheese Biscuit	500	31	34
Sausage, Egg & Twister Roll	430	27	29
Hot Dogs (Big Bite)			
¼ Pound Hot Dog, no bun	360	34	6
⅓ Pound Hot Dog, no bun	480	45	3
Spicy Bite, 1 link, 4 oz	425	38	2
Reynaldo's Jumbo Burritos (10 oz)			
Beef & Bean; Beef & Potato	590	20	82
Red Hot Burrito	640	20	88
Green Burrito	710	26	93
Sandwiches (7-Eleven)			
Black Forest Ham	380	6	59
Chicken Salad, 7.3 oz	500	28	44
Chicken w. Ancho Lime Spread	500	26	47
Classic Chicken Caesar, 8.3 oz	590	27	45
Classic Sub on Roll, 7.6 oz	380	6	49
Ham & Swiss, 4.9 oz	330	11	39
Pastrami & Swiss on Wheat	480	21	48
Turkey & Ham on White Bread	350	6	53
Tuna Salad, 7.5 oz	540	27	45
Bakery Stix™ Treats: *Per Stick (3.5 oz)*			
Grilled Cheese	270	11	30
Ham & Cheese	280	12	32
Pepperoni & Cheese	340	18	30
Salads			
Tuna Macaroni Salad, 8 oz	270	8	29
Reser's Coleslaw, 3½ oz	130	7	17
Reser's Macaroni Salad, 3½ oz	220	15	20
Reser's Potato Salad, 3½ oz	200	10	19
Go-Go Taquitos			
Beef Taco & Cheese, 3 oz (1)	250	11	30
Fiesta Chicken, 3 oz (1)	220	12	23
Jalapeno & Cream Cheese, 3 oz	240	13	27
Monterey Jack Chkn, 3 oz (1)	280	14	30
Donuts: Blueberry Cake (1)	330	22	31
Chocolate Iced (1)	250	11	35
Glazed (1)	250	16	24
Jelly (1)	420	16	66
Sour Cream Donut (1)	450	19	65
Muffins: Banana Nut, 7 oz	660	26	97
Blueberry, 5.6 oz	310	8	54
Brownies: Original, 5 oz	570	28	83
Peanut Butter Cup Brownie, 4.4 oz	560	20	55
Walnut Brownie, 5 oz	600	31	78

Updated Nutrition Data ~ www.CalorieKing.com
Persons with Diabetes ~ See Disclaimer (Page 24)

7-Eleven® cont... (Aug '09)

Fountain Drinks (Fig. Assume ⅓ Ice)	C	F	Cb
Coca-Cola/Pepsi/Dr.Pepper/7Up:			
Gulp, 20 oz	195	0	51
Big Gulp, 32 oz	310	0	82
Super Gulp, 44 oz	430	0	112
Double Gulp, 64 oz	625	0	163
Diet Coke/Diet Pepsi, 16 oz	1	0	0
Slurpees: Average All Flavors,			
12 oz size	95	0	24
22 oz size	175	0	44
28 oz size	220	0	56
40 oz size	315	0	80
Hawaiian Punch; Dr Pepper, avg.,			
12 oz size	180	0	48
22 oz size	330	0	88
28 oz size	420	0	112
40 oz size	600	0	160
Cafe Select Coffee: 12 fl.oz	8	0	2
16 fl.oz size	10	0	2
20 fl.oz size	14	0	3
Hot Drinks: Hot Chocolate, 8 fl.oz	180	3	36
French Vanilla Cappuccino, 8 fl.oz	160	6	26

Saladworks® (Sept '09)

Salads: Per Container	C	F	Cb
Autumn Harvest Salad	240	8	33
B.L.T.	200	7	10
Bently	275	14	10
Chicken Caesar	265	8	19
Cranberry Spinach	260	16	21
Fire Roasted Fiesta	295	14	26
Greek	185	9	15
Mandarin Chicken	230	7	37
Newport	150	4	10
Nicoise	245	7	70
Southwest Crispy Chicken	320	18	23
Spensa	440	14	150
Tivoli	430	20	73
Turkey Club	215	5	71
Panini:			
Fromano	890	55	63
Smokey T	1090	67	73
Wraps: Buffalo Chicken	620	33	59
Chicken Caesar	590	30	52
Tuna Salad	580	28	56
Turkey Club	485	23	53
Soup: Per 3.5 oz Container			
Chicken Orzo	60	2	6.5
Chicken Pot Pie	105	4.5	12
Cream of Broccoli	55	3.5	4.5
Maryland Crab	35	0.5	6

Samurai Sam's® (Sept '09)

Bowls: With White Rice	C	F	Cb
Low-Carb, regular	230	4	16
Spicy Beef 'n Broccoli: Regular	620	13	97
Large	930	16	152
Sweet & Sour White Chicken: Reg.	580	4.5	96
Large	820	6	136
Teriyaki Dark Chicken, regular	540	10	79
Teriyaki Steak: Regular	530	8	86
Large	750	11	123
Teriyaki Veggie: Regular	365	1	81
Large	525	1	117
Yakisoba Bowls: Shrimp	675	10	110
Steak	810	20	112
White Chicken	795	14	114
Veggie	510	8	110
Wraps: With White Rice			
Teriyaki White Chicken	640	11	96
Teriyaki Steak	650	14	101
Teriyaki Veggie	510	8	94

Sandella's Flatbread Cafe (Aug '09)

Wraps	C	F	Cb
Buffalo Chicken	455	17	53
Chicken Fajita	445	13	54
Pacific Chicken	420	11	56
Pesto Turkey	480	18	58
Sweet & Spicy Chicken	355	4	55
Paninis			
Chicken Delicato	535	22	51
Spinach, Ham & Swiss	510	19	53
Turkey & Mozzarella	495	19	54
Tuscan Chicken	580	25	56
Quesadillas			
California	410	16	53
Chicken Fajita	385	8	52
Mediterranean	470	24	55
Grilled Flatbread			
Aloha	570	20	70
Brazilian Chicken	460	15	51
Pesto Chicken	665	33	57
Spinach & Bacon	680	41	52
Vegetarian	685	19	61
Chopped Salads			
Aloha	295	11	36
Greek	305	9	18
Rice Bowls			
Black Bean & rice	705	7	133
Chicken Fajita	630	9	102

For Extra Menu Items ~ see CalorieKing.com

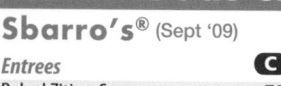

Sbarro's® (Sept '09)

Entrees	C	F	Cb
Baked Ziti w. Sauce	700	41	43
Chicken Parmigiana	520	22	16
Meat Lasagna	650	37	36
Spaghetti w. Sauce	820	28	120
Pizza: *Per Slice (Thin Crust)*			
Cheese	460	13	60
Pepperoni	730	37	61
Sausage	670	31	60
Supreme	630	27	63
Stuffed Pizza: *Per Slice*			
Spinach & Broccoli	790	34	89
Pepperoni	960	42	89

Schlotzsky's® (Sept '09)

	C	F	Cb
Oven-Toasted Sandwiches: *Per Medium Sandwich*			
Angus: Beef & Provolone	760	29	81
Corned Beef Reuben	910	40	80
Corned Beef	580	13	78
Pastrami Reuben	910	39	80
Pastrami & Swiss	905	36	83
BLT	560	21	74
Chicken & Pesto	570	14	73
Chicken Breast	515	6	78
Chipotle Chicken	550	14	68
Dijon Chicken	575	11	79
Homestyle Tuna	565	16	73
Santa Fe Chicken	620	15	76
Smoked Turkey Breast	520	9	77
Smoked Turkey Reuben	895	38	84
Turkey & Guacamole	565	13	82
Turkey Bacon Club	785	32	77
Original Style: The Original	770	34	78
Cheese	790	38	76
Ham & Cheese	735	27	80
Turkey	830	35	80
Panini: Classic Swiss & Tomato	625	26	63
Grilled Chicken Romano	570	16	62
Italiano	735	32	67
Mozzarella & Portobello	485	15	63
Smoked Ham Crostini	645	23	67
Smoked Turkey & Guacamole	600	21	69
Wraps: Asian Chicken	535	11	80
Feta & Portobello	620	39	55
Grilled Chicken & Guacamole	695	36	59
Homestyle Tuna	455	17	55
Mediterranean Tuna	420	12	57
Parmesan Chicken Caesar	650	33	56

Schlotzsky's® cont... (Sept '09)

8" Pizzas: *Per Pizza*	C	F	Cb
BBQ Chicken & Jalapeno	715	16	99
Baby Spinach Salad	455	7	80
Bacon, Tomato & Portobello	615	22	76
Combination Special	640	25	76
Double Cheese	595	21	74
Fresh Tomato & Pesto	555	19	73
Grilled Chicken & Pesto	685	22	85
Mediterranean	560	20	74
Pepperoni & Double Cheese	685	30	74
Smoked Turkey & Jalapeno	655	21	78
Thai Chicken	725	23	85
Vegetarian Special	540	17	74
Salads: *Without Dressing/Croutons Unless Indicated*			
Baby Spinach & Feta	195	15	10
Caesar Salad	105	5	10
Chicken Salad	290	15	12
Garden Salad	50	1	12
Greek Salad	135	8	13
Gr. Chicken Caesar w. Dress./Croutons	220	8	12
Ham & Turkey Chef Salad	255	13	14
Pasta Salad	70	3	12
Potato Salad	240	13	29
Side Salad	25	1	7
Turkey Chef Salad	310	8	14
Kid's Meals: *Without Cookie or Drink*			
Cheese Pizza	480	13	73
Cheese Sandwich	395	15	48
Ham & Cheese Sandwich	425	16	49
Pepperoni Pizza	525	17	73
Turkey Sandwich	300	5	49
Desserts			
Brownie	415	24	54
Carrot Cake	715	42	80
New York Style Cheesecake	350	23	30
Cookies: Chocolate Chip	160	7	24
Fudge Chocolate Chip	160	7	23
Oatmeal Raisin	145	5	24
Sugar	150	6	23
White Choc Macadamia	165	8	23

Second Cup® ~ *see CalorieKing.com*

Shakey's® (Sept '09)

	C	F	Cb
Pizzas (12"): Per ⅒ Pizza			
Cheese: Pan Crust	185	6	26
Thin Crust	150	6	18
Firehouse: Pan Crust	260	12	27
Thin Crust	220	12	19
Garden Veggie: Pan Crust	185	6	27
Thin Crust	150	5	19
Margherita: Pan Crust	175	5	26
Thin Crust	135	4.5	18
Rustic Garlic Chicken: Pan Crust	190	5.5	26
Thin Crust	155	5.5	18
Shakey's Special: Pan Crust	210	6.5	31
Thin Crust	195	10	18
Texas BBQ Chicken: Pan Crust	205	5	29
Thin Crust	170	5	21
Ultimate Meat: Pan Crust	280	14	26
Thin Crust	245	13	18
Additional Toppings: Beef	35	3	0
Cheese	15	1	0.5
Chicken	15	0.5	0
Ham	10	0.5	0
Pepperoni	25	2.5	0
Sausage	45	4	0.5
Sharables: Per Serving			
Chicken Strips (5)	620	31	48
Mojo Potatoes (5)	215	11	25
Mojo Supreme, serves 4-6	1950	120	160
Shakey's Spicy Wings (6 pces)	495	29	28
Shakey's Famous Chicken: Per Piece			
Fried Chicken: Breast	475	26	16
Leg	170	19	6
Thigh	350	24	10
Wing	130	9	3.5

Sheetz® (Sept '09)

	C	F	Cb
M.T.O Breakfast: Plain Bagel, Cheese if Indicated, w/o Condiments or Dressing			
Shmagels: Bacon, Egg & Egg	530	26	54
Egg & American Cheese	445	18	52
Ham, Egg & Provolone	525	20	56
Shmiscuits: Bacon & Egg	540	34	40
Egg & American Cheese	455	26	38
Ham, Egg & Swiss Cheese	540	28	42
Sausage, Egg & American Chse	630	43	38
Shmuffins: Bacon & Egg	410	24	30
Egg & American Cheese	325	16	28
Ham & Egg	310	10	31
Sausage, Egg & Cheddar Cheese	495	33	28
Steak & Egg	395	15	28

Sheetz® (Sept '09)

	C	F	Cb
M.T.O Cold Subz: Per 6" White Sub (No Cheese/Toppings or Condiments Unless Indicated)			
American Cheese	375	10	52
BLT	460	18	54
Chicken Salad with Tomatoes	515	22	61
Club Turkey w. Lettuce, Tom., On.	325	3	56
Deli	400	12	53
Ham, w. Swiss, Lettuce, Tomato	440	11	57
Italian	380	9	53
Rst Beef w. Lettuce, Tom., Olives., On.	325	4	56
Tuna Salad w. Lettuce, Tom., Pickles	480	17	63
Turkey & Provolone	410	11	54
M.T.O® Hot Subz: Per 6" White Sub			
Chicken & American Cheese	490	14	52
Meatball w. Marinara Sauce	395	12	55
Pepperoni	455	19	51
Steak & Swiss Cheese	540	17	53
M.T.O Deli Bagel: No Cheese Unless Indicated			
Chicken Salad	500	24	58
Deli Combo with Provolone Cheese	540	26	53
Ham & Swiss Cheese	445	14	54
Italian w. Lettuce, Tomato & Onion	430	14	55
Roast Beef w. Lettuce & Tomato	315	5	52
Tuna Salad w. Lettuce, Tom., Pickles	475	19	60
Turkey w. Provolone, Lettuce & Tom.	410	13	54
M.T.O Hot Dogz: Without Cheese			
Deli Dogz w. Ketchup & Mustard	655	35	58
Hot Dogz w. Chili & Onions	310	19	27
M.T.O Nachos: With Jalapinos			
Nachos Bueno w. Nacho Cheese	510	23	66
M.T.O Salads: No Cheese/Dressing Unless Indicated			
Chef Salad	150	4	12
Crispy Chicken	270	8	30
Garden Salad with Jack Cheese	140	9	8
Grilled Chicken	145	4	7
Steak Salad	210	8	8
Taco Salad	255	10	38
Sides			
Fryz: Bag, 3.2 oz	160	6	23
Cup, 5.1 oz	260	10	36
Cheese, 14.3 oz	650	30	81
Smokehouse, 15.3 oz	975	52	103
Coffeez™: Per 16 fl.oz			
Hot Chocolate, medium	250	4	52
Cupo'ccino®: Per Medium (16 fl.oz)			
Capo'ccino: Creme Brulee	280	8	40
Fat-Free French Vanilla	140	0	34

Fast - Foods & *Restaurants*

Shoney's® (Sept '09)

Breakfast	C	F	Cb
All Star, no Sides	190	15	1.5
Big Eater Steak, no Sides	630	41	1.5
Country Fried Steak	995	66	49
Biscuits, biscuit	310	14	41
Biscuits & Gravy, serving	685	32	88
Biscuits, Sausage, biscuit	540	34	42
Black/Blueberries, ¼ cup, 1.3 oz	20	0	5
Half Stack Pancake Platter	930	14	187
Sunrise Breakfast	975	60	88
Burgers: All American	690	32	44
A A Bacon Cheeseburger	890	49	45
Famous Patty Melt	945	60	40
Half-O-Pound Burger	1350	53	130
Mushroom Swiss	970	58	49
Sandwiches: Blackened Chicken	885	21	122
Charbroiled Chicken, sandwich	895	22	122
Chicken Parmesan, sandwich	750	30	80
Corned Beef Reuben, sandwich	795	53	37
Fish, sandwich	825	17	127
Fried Chicken, sandwich	560	15	77
Hot Roast Beef w. Potatoes & Gravy	770	24	95
Hot Turkey w. Potatoes & Gravy	840	30	94
Original Slim Jim	1005	34	123
Raymond's French Dip	500	15	54
Turkey Club	950	53	47
Ultimate Grilled Cheese	895	47	77
Beef: BBQ Ribs	1520	78	125
Choice Sirloin	1225	51	128
Half-O-Pound: w. Mushrooms	1315	53	128
with Grilled Onions	1335	52	133
Southwest	1305	69	83
Ribeye	1480	75	128
T-Bone	1810	100	128
Rib Combos:			
¼ Rack & BBQ Chicken w. Fries	1230	54	104
¼ Rack & Fried Shrimp w. Frie	1145	51	114
¼ Rack & Gr. Shrimp w. Fries	1125	53	103
¼ Rack & Tenderloins w. Fries	1370	70	121
Surf & Turf: Ribeye & 5 Fried Shrimp	1640	82	139
Ribeye & 6 Grilled Shrimp	1590	81	128
Sirloin & 5 Fried Shrimp	1380	58	139
Sirloin & 6 Grilled Shrimp	1330	57	128
T-Bone & 5 Fried Shrimp	1965	107	139
T-Bone & 6 Grilled Shrimp	1920	106	128

Shoney's® cont... (Sept '09)

Blue Plate Specials	C	F	Cb
Baked Whitefish	505	8.5	58
Cajun Whitefish	480	11	56
Grandma's Meatloaf w. Glaze	1090	47	93
Grandma's Meatloaf w. Gravy	1090	49	88
Grilled Liver & Onions	710	22	80
Ham Steak Dinner	665	26	60
Original Country Fried Steak	1150	62	103
Roast Beef Platter	880	30	96
Chicken: Chicken Stir-Fry	1200	35	172
Charbroiled Blackened Chicken	830	26	100
Charbroiled Chicken Breast	795	23	99
Fried Chicken Tenderloins	1155	61	121
Monterey Chicken	910	40	84
Smothered Chicken	890	35	90
Seafood: Fried Fish Platter	1050	39	123
Grilled Salmon	750	19	95
Grilled Shrimp	720	20	96
Lite: Grilled Cod, serving	200	4	1
Grilled Salmon	180	4	0
Grilled Shrimp	320	9	30
Shrimp Stir-Fry	875	19	131
Shrimper's Feast	1030	40	128
Pastas: Chicken Alfredo	1705	78	171
Italian Feast	1435	46	204
Pasta Ya Ya	1845	81	176
Shrimp Alfredo	1780	85	172
Kids Menu: Junior Chicken	190	10	12
Junior Fish & Chips	310	12	30
Sides: Baked Potato, Plain,	345	6.5	68
French Fries, 4 oz	215	11	26
Macaroni & Cheese, ½ cup	240	15	18
Mashed Potatoes & Gravy	225	10	30
Onion Rings (7)	500	15	83
Sweet Potato Casserole, 4 oz	245	6	44
Turnip Greens, 4 oz	45	3.5	4
Desserts			
Cheesecake, 1 slice, 4 oz	365	26	23
Pies: Apple a la Mode	1205	53	174
Cherry Nutrasweet	465	18	66
Original Strawberry	330	17	45
Peach Nutrasweet	480	21	68
Sundaes: Caramel	620	27	83
Hot Fudge	600	30	75
Strawberry,	610	28	86
Ultimate Hot Fudge Cake	875	37	127
Walnut Brownie a la Mode	575	34	61
Milk Shakes: Chocolate	1080	52	142
Strawberry	1115	50	151
Vanilla	1075	50	139.5

Updated Nutrition Data ~ www.CalorieKing.com
Persons with Diabetes ~ See Disclaimer (Page 24)

Sizzler® (Sept '09)

Burgers & Sandwiches:	C	F	Cb
Burgers: Mega Bacon Chseburger	1010	61	48
Sizzler Burger: ⅓ lb	620	30	47
½ lb	760	40	47
Sandwiches: Crispy Chicken	590	27	61
Grilled Chicken Club	665	31	48
Malibu Chicken	645	32	57

Hot Entrees: *W/o Sides, Dipping Sauces & Condiments Unless Indicated*

	C	F	Cb
Chicken: Hibachi Chkn Breast (1)	200	7	7
with Hibachi Sauce, 1 oz	245	7	17
Lemon-Herb Chicken Breast	215	11	1
with Lemon Herb Sauce, 1 oz	260	15	2
Malibu Chicken Patty, each	300	20	10
with Malibu Sauce, 1.5 oz	570	15	10
Seafood: Gr. Salmon w. Rice Pilaf	530	20	40
Fish 'n Chips	1035	49	111
Fisherman's Platter	820	34	82
Gr. Shrimp Fettuccine Alfredo	985	55	64
Shrimp: Grilled Skewers (2)	545	26	42
Fried: 6 only	215	6	24
12 only	435	12	48
Shrimp, Shrimp, Shrimp	970	41	92
Steaks: Bacon Wrapped Sirloin Filets	555	35	5
Classic: 6 oz	255	12	2
8 oz	320	14	2
Porterhouse, 18 oz	1365	107	1
Rib Eye, 12 oz	950	62	1

Prepared Salads: *Per 6 oz Serving w/out Dressing*

Ambrosia	125	8	4
Caesar	50	4	2
Carrot Raisin	110	6	12
Creamy Cole Slaw	70	4	6
Greek	45	4	1
Macaroni	225	12	27
Potato	325	27	18
Seafood	160	11	11

Salad Dressings: *Per 2 Tbsp, 1 oz*

Honey Mustard	110	8	9
Italian, Low Fat	40	3	6
Ranch	115	12	1
Signature Blue Cheese	105	11	1
Thousand Island	95	9	5

Sizzler® cont... (Sept '09)

Salad Bar Items:	C	F	Cb
Bacon Bits, 2 oz	110	6	6
Cottage Cheese, 2 oz	50	2	2
Eggs, Chopped, 2 oz	100	8	0
Garbanzo Beans, 2 oz	50	0	8
Kidney Beans, 2 oz	50	0	8
Peas, 2 oz	30	0	6
Turkey Ham, 2 oz	70	6	2

Sides: *W/o Condiments/Toppings*

Baked Potato, 1.5 oz	90	0	23
Brocoli, 5 oz	50	0	7
Cheese Toast, 1 slice	235	19	13
French Fries, 5 oz	285	13	42
Rice Pilaf, 5 oz	225	4	39
Smashed Red Potatoes, 6 oz	160	6	24

Soups: *Per 6 oz Bowl*

Broccoli Cheese	305	19	28
Chicken Noodle	100	2	14
Clam Chowder	325	18	35
French Onion	55	2	6
Menudo	70	1	14
Minestrone	70	1	14

Dessert Bar: Chocolate Syrup, 1 oz

Chocolate Syrup, 1 oz	90	0	21
Choc/Vanilla Soft Serve, 4 oz	135	4	24
Strawberry Topping, 1 oz	70	0	18
Whipped Topping, 1 Tbsp	10	1	1

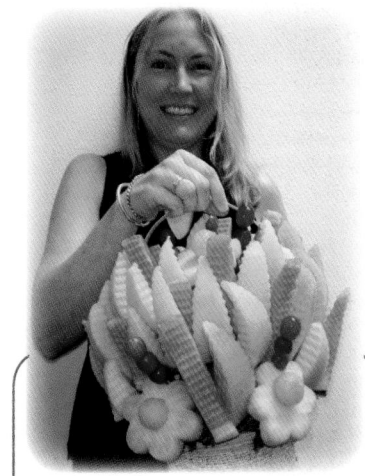

Balance eating out with fruit and veggies
(EdibleArrangements.com)

Skyline Chili® (Sept '09)

Burritos	C	F	Cb
All Chili Burrito	560	30	37
All Chili Deluxe Burrito	650	35	45
Salads: *Without Dressing*			
Buffalo Chicken Salad	150	7	7
Classic Chicken Salad	150	7	8
Garden Salad	80	5	6
Greek Chicken Salad	170	8	9
Greek Salad	60	3.5	5
Southwestern Chkn w. Tortilla Chips	760	44	66
Meals: *Per Regular Serving*			
Coney w. Cheese	340	22	17
Coney, no Cheese	220	12	17
Black Bean & Rice, 3-Way	800	40	74
Black Bean & Rice, 4-Way	810	40	77
Black Bean & Rice, 5-Way	880	40	89
Black Bean & Rice, Spaghetti	490	12	79
Bowls:			
Chili	270	16	6
Chili Bean	270	12	17
Chili Cheese	440	30	6
Coney	870	69	9
Loaded Chili	580	40	18
Vegetarian Black Beans & Rice	320	9	46
Chili Spaghetti:			
Regular	450	18	43
w. Bean & Onion	530	17	64
w. Bean	520	17	61
Steamed Potatoes:			
Plain	310	0	72
Cheddar	740	41	72
Chili	440	8	74
Sour Cream	570	27	72
Wraps: *Without Dressing*			
Buffalo Chicken	520	21	55
Classic Chicken	510	21	55
Greek Chicken	510	21	54
Southwest Chicken	670	30	85
Sides:			
Cheese	230	19	1
Chili	130	8	3
Crackers	100	3	20
French Fries	630	33	79

For Complete Nutritional Data ~ see CalorieKing.com

Smoothie King® (Sept '09)

Fruit Smoothies: Per 20 fl.oz Cup

Figures Include Turbinado. Without Turbinado, deduct 100 calories and 23 carbs.

	C	F	Cb
Build Up, High Protein Smoothies:			
Almond Mocha	365	9	42
Banana	320	9	32
Chocolate	365	9	42
Lemon	370	9	44
Pineapple	320	9	29
Get Energy: Acai Adventure	435	5	92
Go Goji	435	0	104
Green Tea Tango	305	4	54
Indulge: Banana Boat	550	14	95
Pina Colada Island	600	10	110
Snack Right: Banana Berry Treat	370	0	88
Berry Punch	365	0	93
Fruit Fusion	360	0	84
Grape Expectations	550	0	133
Stay Healthy: Cranberry Cooler	495	0	120
Cranberry Supreme	555	1	130
Mangosteen Madness	385	0	94
Orange Ka-BAM	465	0	117
Trim Down: Angel Food	355	0	84
Blackberry Dream	365	1	88
Island Impact	310	0	73
MangoFest	285	0	72
Muscle Punch	365	1	84
Passion Passport	395	0	96
Peach Slice	315	0	72
Pineapple Pleasure	280	0	66
Raspberry Collider	345	0	88
Raspberry Sunrise	390	0	95
Slim-N-Trim: Chocolate	295	2	57
Orange Vanilla	215	1	46
Strawberry	375	1	84
Strawberry Kiwi Breeze	375	0	90
Youth Fountain	255	0	61
The Shredder: Chocolate	310	3	36
Youth Fountain	255	0	61

32 fl.oz Cup: Multiply 20 fl.oz figures by 1.5
40 fl.oz Cup: Multiply 20 fl.oz figures by 2

Updated Nutrition Data ~ www.CalorieKing.com
Persons with Diabetes ~ See Disclaimer (Page 24)

Smoothie King® cont... (Sept '09)

Kids Kup Smoothies	C	F	Cb
Berry Interesting	275	0	69
Choc-A-Laka	250	3	45
Gimme-Grape	265	0	64
Smarti Tarti	200	0	49

Snappy Tomato (Sept '09)

Pizza: Per Slice , ⅛ of Pizza	C	F	Cb
Buffalo Grilled Chicken	250	8	32
Cheese Pizza	220	7	30
Hawaiian Pizza	370	18	33
Meat Topper	430	23	31
Pepperoni Pizza	340	17	31
Ranch Pizza	370	21	31
Snapperoni Pizza	390	22	31
Supreme Pizza	340	17	32
Veggie Pizza	240	8	33

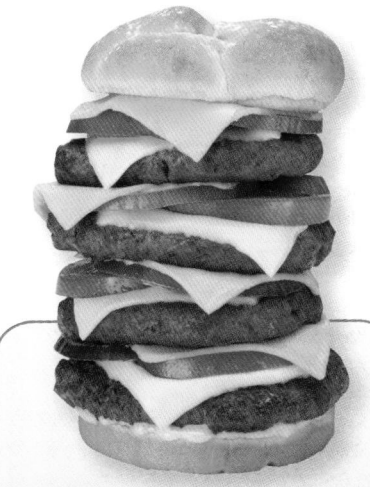

*This **Quadruple Bypass Burger**® is offered by Heart Attack Grill in Chandler, Arizona.*

With some 5000 calories, it contains 2 lbs beef, 4 fried eggs, 8 slices cheese, mayo and garnish – all in a large bun dipped in pure lard.

Definitely not for anyone with a heart!
(Photo: Ken Epstein)

Sonic Drive-In® (Sept '09)

Burgers	C	F	Cb
Sonic Burger w. Mayonnaise	650	37	55
Sonic Burger w. Mustard	560	26	54
Sonic Cheeseburger w. Mayo	720	42	56
Sonic Cheeseburger w. Mustard	620	31	55
Sonic Bacon Cheeseburger	780	48	57
Super Sonic Chseburger: w. Mayo	980	64	58
w. Mustard	890	53	57
Jr. Burger	310	15	30
Jr. Double Cheeseburger	570	35	33
Sandwiches/Coneys/Wraps			
Coney: Extra-Long Chili Cheese (1)	600	39	55
Corn Dog (1)	210	11	23
Toaster Sandwiches: Chkn Club	740	46	55
Bacon Cheeseburger	670	39	52
Wraps: Crispy Chicken	480	21	54
Grilled Chicken	400	14	39
Chicken			
Chicken Strip Dinner	930	43	100
Jumbo Popcorn Chicken:			
Small, no Sauce, 4 oz	380	22	27
Large, no Sauce, 6 oz	560	32	41
Salads: No Dressing			
Grilled Chicken	250	10	12
Jumbo Popcorn Chicken	420	25	32
Santa Fe Grilled Chicken	310	12	22
Salad Dressings: Per 1½ oz Serving			
Honey Mustard	180	16	10
Italian Fat-Free	40	0	10
Original Ranch	190	20	2
Original Ranch Light	110	5	14
Popcorn Chicken Sauces: BBQ	45	0	11
Honey Mustard	90	7	7
Ranch	150	16	1
Sides			
French Fries: Plain, medium, 4 oz	330	13	48
w. Cheese, medium, 4.95 oz	420	21	51
w. Chili & Cheese, med., 7.1 oz	490	27	54
Fritos Chili Cheese Pie, med. 4.9 oz	470	32	36
Mozzarella Sticks, no sauce, 4.95 oz	440	22	40
Onion Rings, medium, 5½ oz	440	21	55
Tater Tots: Plain, medium, 3.95 oz	320	21	32
w. Cheese, medium, 4.9 oz	420	28	35
w. Chili & Cheese, med., 7.5 oz	490	34	48

Sonic Drive-In®cont... (Sept '09)

Breakfast	C	F	Cb
Burritos: Bacon, Egg & Cheese	450	27	38
Sausage, Egg & Cheese	480	31	38
SuperSonic	570	36	48
French Toast Sticks: w. Syrup (4)	580	31	70
no Syrup (4)	500	31	49
Breakfast Sandwiches			
CroiSonic: Bacon, Egg & Cheese	510	26	39
Sausage, Egg & Cheese	600	46	29
Toaster: Bacon, Egg & Cheese	530	32	40
Sausage, Egg & Cheese	620	42	40
Desserts: Per Regular			
Banana Split	420	9	80
Vanilla Cone	180	6	30
Vanilla Dish	240	9	36
Cream Pie Shakes: Reg., Banana	590	19	98
Chocolate	660	19	114
Coconut	580	20	93
Strawberry	620	19	106
CreamSlush:			
Lemon-Berry; Strawb., avg.	455	12	85
Other varieties, average	440	13	79
Floats: Diet Coke; Diet Dr Pepper	220	8	33
Coca-Cola	290	8	54
Shakes: Chocolate	540	16	89
Banana; Vanilla, avg.	470	17	74
Pineapple; Strawberry, avg	505	16	82
Sonic Blast: Butterfinger	580	22	88
M&M's	600	24	88
Reese's Peanut Butter Cups	560	19	89
Single Topping Sundaes: Choc.	410	13	67
Hot Fudge	440	18	63
Pineapple; Strawberry	375	13	60
Drinks: Barq's Root Beer, 20 fl.oz	190	0	52
Cranberry Juice: Regular	170	0	46
Large, 20 fl.oz	210	0	56
Fruit Smoothies: Strawberry, reg.	540	0	35
Strawberry-Banana, regular	440	0	110

For Complete Nutritional Data ~ see CalorieKing.com

Souper Salad® (Sept '09)

Soups: Per 5 oz Serving	C	F	Cb
Adobe Rice & Chicken	100	5	10
Black Bean	80	2	20
Cherokee Joe's Cornbread	70	1.5	13
Chicken Noodle	80	3	9
Chicken Tortilla	60	2	7
Holiday Harvest	90	6	5
Mama Mia Minestrone	80	3	8
Minestrone	70	1	13
Mr. B's Hot & Sour Chicken	60	1.5	8
Pasta Tortellini	100	3.5	14
Red French Onion, no Crouton	40	1	6
Seafood Bisque	120	8	8
Spicy Meatballs with Rice	100	4.5	10
Vegetable Lentil	70	0	16
Vegetarian Vegetable	50	0.5	11
Signature Salads: Per ⅓ Cup			
Edamame	70	4.5	4
Fisherman's Kettle	120	8	9
Paco's Taco	100	5	12
Roasted Mushroom, Artichoke, Feta	40	3	3
Tropical Tuxedo	60	3	7
Tuna Skroodle Pasta	130	9	10
Bread			
Blueberry Bread, piece	110	2	22
Cheese Drop Biscuit, piece	70	3	8
Cornbread, piece	130	3.5	23
Garlic Breadstick, piece	130	4.5	18
Gingerbread, piece	130	4.5	22

For Complete Nutritional Data ~ see CalorieKing.com

Souplantation® (Sept '09)

Soups: Per Cup	C	F	Cb
Low Fat: Chicken Tortilla	100	3	11
Classical Minestrone	120	2	20
Vegetable Medley	90	1	14
Regular Soup: *Per Cup*			
Chesapeake Corn Chowder	290	17	30
Cream of Mushroom	290	24	15
Irish Potato Leek	260	16	23
Marvellous Minestrone w. Bacon	220	8	31
Minestrone w. Italian Sausage	220	12	17
New Mexican Corn	200	10	19
Vegetarian Harvest	200	10	23
Breads: Sourdough	150	0.5	27
Buttermilk Cornbread, 1 pce	140	2	27
Focaccia: Garlic Asiago	160	8	19
Old World Greek	190	9	24
Tossed Salads: Per Cup			
Aztec Taco w. Turkey	130	9	7
Caesar Salad Asiago	270	22	10
Won Ton Chicken Happiness	170	9	15

Updated Nutrition Data ~ www.CalorieKing.com
Persons with Diabetes ~ See Disclaimer (Page 24)

Souplantation® cont... (Sept '09)

Prepared Salads: Per ½ Cup	C	F	Cb
Aunt Doris' Red Pepper Slaw	70	0	18
Baja Bean & Cilantro	180	3	29
BBQ Potato	170	9	21
Carrot Raisin	90	3	17
Dijon Potato w. Garlic Dill Vinegar	150	12	9
Greek Couscous w. Feta Cheese	210	10	25
Oriental Ginger Slaw w. Krab	70	3	8
Southern Dill Potato	120	3	20
Thai Noodle w. Peanut Sauce	190	10	19
Zesty Tortellini	230	15	20
Dressing & Croutons: Per 2 Tbsp			
Balsamic Vinaigrette	180	19	1
Blue Cheese Dressing	130	13	3
Honey Mustard Dressing	150	13	8
Fat Free	25	0	7
Italian Dressing, Fat-Free	25	0	7
Ranch Dressing	150	15	4
Fat Free	50	0	2
Thousand Island Dressing	90	9	3
Croutons, Garlic Parmesan, 5 pces	80	5	6
Hot Tossed Pastas: Per Cup			
Bruschetta	260	4	41
Creamy Bruschetta	360	16	43
Garden Vegetable w. Meatballs	310	10	44
Italian Vegetable Beef	290	9	43
Vegetarian Marinara w. Basil	260	4	44
Muffins: Chocolate Brownie	180	8	26
Fruit Medley Bran	130	0.5	29
Georgia Peach Poppyseed	150	6	20
Tangy Lemon	140	4	24
Wildly Blue Blueberry, small	140	5	22
Desserts: Per ½ Cup			
Apple Cobbler	360	10	67
Apple Medley	70	0	18
Banana Royale	80	0	20
Rice Pudding	110	2	20
Vanilla Pudding	150	4	27
Cookies & Cake: Choc. Chip Cookie	90	4	13
Chocolate Lava Cake, ½ cup	330	8	62
Syrup/Topping: Choc. Syrup, 2 T	110	3	20
Granola Topping, 2 Tbsp	110	4	16

For Complete Nutritional Data ~ see CalorieKing.com

Southern Tsunami® (Sept '09)

Sushi: Per Pack	C	F	Cb
Blue Crab Roll, 8.85 oz	455	14	63
Classic Miso Roll, 10.8 oz	465	9	64
California Roll w/ Brown Rice, 9.5 oz	305	7	53
Cream Cheese Roll, 9.8 oz	530	20	64
Crunchy Shrimp Roll, 10.3 oz	520	20	69
Dragon Roll: (Seawater Eel), 10.15 oz	470	14	72
Eel Roll (Freshwater Eel), 9.9 oz	505	16	69
Eel Roll (Sea Eel), 9.9 oz	450	11	71
M&M Roll: Shrimp & Avocado, 7.55 oz	335	5	62
Tuna & Cucumber, 7.87 oz	320	1	60
Marina Plate, 7.7 oz	380	7	57
Meteor Special, 9.26 oz	395	3	73
Nigiri: Fish Roe, 1 piece,1.35 oz	60	0	10
Fresh Salmon, 1 piece, 1.3 oz	70	1	9
Fresh Water Eel, 1 piece, 1.5 oz	100	4	11
Octopus, 1 piece, 1 oz	60	1	9
Sea Eel, 1 piece, 1.5 oz	85	3	11
Shrimp, 1 piece, 1 oz	45	0	9
Smoked Salmon, 1 piece, 1.87 oz	95	1	16
Tilapia, 1 piece, 1.13 oz	50	1	9
Tuna, 1 piece, 1 oz	50	0	7
Yellowtail, 1 piece, 1.2 oz	55	1	9
Ocean Crab Roll, 10 oz	415	8	66
Orange Roll, 10.55 oz	405	6	71
Rainbow Roll, 12.45 oz	500	8	70
Spicy Roll: Salmon, 9.82 oz	485	14	64
Baby Shrimp, 10 oz	420	8	68
Tuna, 10 oz	460	9	64
Tempura Roll, 11.1 oz	540	11	87
Tsunami Roll, 9.15 oz	470	12	74
Vegetable Combo: 12 pieces, 9.4 oz	355	6	68
Roll n' Wrap: Avocado Salad, 5 oz	200	9	30
Smoked Salmon Salad, 4 oz	180	8	20
Combinations: Fullmoon, 9.9 oz	435	12	69
Seaside: Tuna & Salmon, 8.4 oz	410	4	63
Tuna, Salmon, Shrimp, Eel, 6.9 oz	395	7	59
Shoreline, 11.23 oz	480	7	82
Stardust, 12.4 oz	555	9	103

Spaghetti Warehouse® (Aug '09)

Lunch	C	F	Cb
Minestrone Soup	80	1.5	12
Grilled Chicken Marinara	530	8	65
Seafood Marinara	385	5	65
Spaghetti: w. Tomato Sauce	425	5	82
w. Marinara Sauce #12	440	5	84
Spicy Marinara Sce Spaghetti	280	4	52
Vegetable Primavera	340	4	65
Dinner			
Minestrone, 1 bowl	110	2	18
Grilled Chicken Marinara	640	10	85
Grilled Halibut Dinner	880	14	106
Grilled Marinated Chicken Breast	910	17	116
Marinara Sauce #12	520	6	99
Seafood Marinara	520	8	86
Spaghetti w. Tomato Sauce	525	6	101
Spicy Marinara Sce Spaghetti	330	6	60
Vegetable Primavera	610	8	116

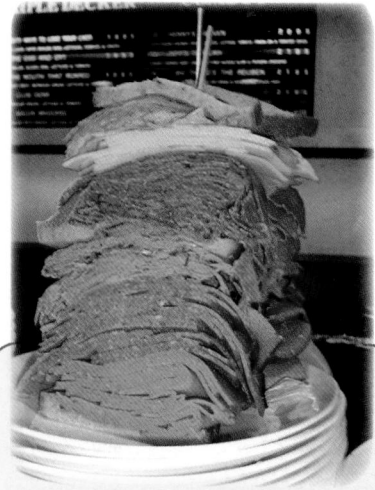

This Triple Decker (Carnegie Deli, New York) contains up to 3 lb meat and 8 oz cheese ~ approx. 4000 calories and 300 grams fat.

Note: Only half the sandwich is shown – the other half is hidden behind!

Carnegie's Challenge: Eat one Triple Decker ... get the second one free!

Starbucks® (Sept '09)

Figures Based on 16 fl.oz Grande w/o Whip

Classic Favorites	C	F	Cb
Apple Juice	250	0	64
Apple Juice, Steamed	230	0	56
Hot Chocolate	300	9	47
White Hot Chocolate	410	12	61
Brewed Coffee			
Caffe Misto/Au Lait: w. Whole Milk	130	7	9
w. Nonfat Milk	70	0	10
w. Soy Milk	100	3	12
Espresso Hot			
Caffe Americano	15	0	3
Caffe Latte: w. Whole Milk	220	11	18
w. Nonfat Milk	130	0	19
w. Soy Milk	170	4.5	23
Caffe Mocha: w. Whole Milk	290	12	40
w. Nonfat Milk	220	2.5	42
w. Soy Milk	250	6	45
Cappuccino: w. Whole Milk	140	7	11
w. Nonfat Milk	80	0	12
w. Soy Milk	110	3	15
Caramel Macchiato: w. Whole Milk	270	10	34
w. Nonfat Milk	190	1	35
w. Soy Milk	230	5	38
Cinn. Dolce Latte: w. Whole Milk	290	10	39
w. Nonfat Milk	210	0	41
w. Soy Milk	250	4	44
Cinn. Dolce Latte, w. Sug.-Free Syrup:			
w. Whole Milk	210	11	17
w. Non-Fat Milk	130	0	19
w. Soy Milk	170	4.5	24
Espresso: 1 doppio, 2 fl.oz	10	0	2
1 solo, 1 fl.oz	5	0	1
Espresso Iced			
Caffe Americano	15	0	3
Caffe Latte: w. Whole Milk	150	7	12
w. Nonfat Milk	90	0	13
w. Soy Milk	120	3	17
Caffe Mocha: w. Whole Milk	220	8	35
w. Nonfat Milk	170	2.5	36
w. Soy Milk	200	4.5	38
White Choc. Mocha: w. Whole Milk	360	11	55
w. Nonfat Milk	310	6	55
w. Soy Milk	330	8	58
Espresso Truffle	250	11	34

Updated Nutrition Data ~ www.CalorieKing.com
Persons with Diabetes ~ See Disclaimer (Page 24)

Starbucks® cont... (Sept '09)

Figures Based on Grande (16 fl.oz)
Without Whip Unless Indicated

Frappuccino Blended Coffee	C	F	Cb
Caffe Vanilla	310	3	67
Caramel	270	3.5	53
Cinnamon Dolce	260	3	52
Coffee	240	3	48
Espresso	190	2.5	38
Java Chip	340	8	64
Mocha	260	3.5	54
White Chocolate Mocha	300	4.5	59
Frappuccino Blended Creme			
Double Chocolaty Chip	400	8	75
Mint Chocolaty Chip	400	6	80
Pumpkin Spice	360	2.5	71
Strawberries & Creme	440	2.5	92
Tazo: Chai	330	2	67
Green Tea	380	2.5	78
Vanilla Bean	350	2.5	72
Frappuccino Light Blended Coffee			
Caffe Vanilla	190	1	42
Caramel	160	1.5	30
Cinnamon Dolce	140	0.5	29
Coffee	130	0.5	25
Espresso	110	0.5	20
Java Chip	200	4.5	36
Mocha	140	1	29
White Chocolate Mocha	180	2	34
Frappuccino Juice Blend			
Lemonade	250	0	63
Vivanno Blends: Per 16 fl.oz			
Banana Chocolate w. 2% Milk	270	4.5	48
with Espresso shot	250	4	44
Orange Mango Banana w. 2% Milk	260	2	51
Strawberry Banana w. 2% Milk	280	1.5	56
Drink Extras			
Flavored Syrup: 1 pump, 0.35 oz	20	0	5
Sugar-Free, 1 pump, 0.35 oz	0	0	0
Mocha Syrup, 1 pump, 0.6 oz	25	0.5	6
Topping: Caramel, 0.53 oz	15	0.5	2
Chocolate, 1 serving, 0.14 oz	5	0	1
Sprinkles, 1 serving	0	0	0.5
Whipped Cream Topping:			
Cold Beverage, 1 venti, 1.2 oz	110	11	3

Starbucks® cont... (Sept '09)

Breakfast Specialities	C	F	Cb
Bacon, Gouda, Cheese Frittata	380	20	31
Egg White, Spinach, Feta Wrap	280	9	35
Egg White/Turkey Bacon S'wich	340	10	47
Ham, Egg, Cheese Frittata	370	16	32
Portobello Mushroom Piadini	370	18	39
Sausage Piadini	500	32	36
Sandwiches: Cobb Salad	460	18	42
Egg Salad	450	26	36
Tarragon Chicken Salad	490	12	62
Turkey Cranberry Pesto	400	19	35
Bars & Brownies: Blueberry Oat Bar	250	10	35
Double Chocolate Brownie	410	24	46
Marshmallow Dream Bar	210	4	43
Rich Toffee Pecan Bar	380	22	42
Strawberry Rhubarb Crumble	290	14	38
Cookies: Chocolate Chunk	360	17	50
Outrageous Oatmeal	370	14	56
Starbucks Indulgent	320	19	40
Croissants: Butter Croissant	310	18	32
Chocolate Croissant	300	17	34
Mini Chocolate Croissant	140	8	16
Loaves & Coffee Cakes:			
Banana Nut Bread	480	19	73
Marble/Pumpkin Loaf, av.	325	12	50
Red. Fat Coffee Cakes:			
Banana Chocolate Chip	380	7	77
Cinnamon Swirl	290	7	55
Very Berry	320	9	54
Starbucks Classic Coffee Cake	420	19	59
Muffins: Apple Bran	350	9	64
Blueberry Streusel	360	11	59
Low Fat Raspberry Sunshine	340	6	65
Zucchini Walnut	490	28	52
Scones: Blueberry	460	22	61
Cinnamon Chip/Maple Oat, av.	470	20	64
Petite Vanilla Bean	140	15	21
Raspberry	490	22	65
Sweet Rolls & Danishes:			
Apple Fritter	420	20	59
Cheese Danish	420	25	39
Double Iced Cinnamon Roll	490	20	70
Morning Bun	350	16	45
Parfaits: Strawberry/Blueberry	350	4.5	66
Yogurt & Honey	290	12	43

Ice Cream & Ice Cream Bars ~ See Page 35, 38
For Bottled Drinks ~ See Page 164

Steak Escape® (Sept '09)

Sandwiches & Burgers	C	F	Cb
7" Sandwiches: Cajun Chicken	410	5	58
Classic Italian Sub	470	11	60
Vegetarian	310	1	65
Turkey Club	380	2	62
Wild West BBQ	455	6	60
12" Sandwiches: Cajun Chicken	630	10	80
Classic Italian Sub	760	22	85
Vegetarian	440	2	93
Turkey Club	580	3	88
Wild West BBQ	730	12	84
Kids Sandwiches: Chicken	205	7	29
Ham	185	1	31
Steak	210	3	29
Turkey	185	1	31
Salads			
Grilled Side: Salad	40	0.5	8
w. Chicken	175	5	11
w. Ham/Turkey	130	2	8
w. Steak	185	6	11
Sides			
Fresh Cut Fries:			
Kids Meal Fries, 3 oz	250	13	34
12 oz cup	500	26	67
16 oz cup	650	34	87
25 oz cup	920	48	123
32 oz cup	995	52	134
Loaded French Fries:			
Bacon & Cheddar, 10.85 oz	905	44	88
Ranch & Bacon, 10.85 oz	1045	71	84
Kids Chicken Tenders (2)	240	11	21
Portions: Chicken, 8 oz	240	0	8
Ham, 6 oz	150	1	6
Steak, 8 oz	260	0	10
Turkey, 6 oz	150	1	6
Smashed Potatoes: Plain, 13.8 oz	245	0	53
w. Chicken, 20 oz	385	4	56
w. Ham, 20 oz	340	2	59
w. Steak, 20 oz	395	5	56
w. Turkey, 20 oz	340	2	59

For Complete Nutritional Data ~ see CalorieKing.com

Steak 'n Shake® (Sept '09)

Sandwiches & Burgers	C	F	Cb
Cheddar 'n Bacon Steakburger	570	28	39
Frisco Melt Sandwich	980	72	42
Grilled Cheese & Bacon Sandwich	750	54	41
Grilled Chicken Breast Sandwich	240	7	29
Original Dbl Steakburger w. Cheese	410	21	26
Original Single w. Cheese	310	15	26
Philadelphia Steakburger	595	32	44
Triple Steakburger	450	22	26
Turkey Melt Sandwich	915	64	47
Sides:			
Chicken Fingers, without fries	260	18	14
Chili 3-Way	825	45	65
Chili 5-Way	1120	69	74
Chili Deluxe, 6 oz cup	540	38	21
Fries:			
French: Regular, 5 oz	450	23	57
Large, 7.25 oz	645	34	82
Cheddar Cheese, regular, 9 oz	615	36	64
Salads: *Without Dressing:*			
Apple Walnut Gr. Chicken	335	10	38
Beef Taco	1000	69	66
Classic Grilled Chicken	465	25	23
Fried Chicken	700	53	20
Soups: *Per 6 fl.oz Cup, without Crackers or Toppings*			
Chicken Gumbo	80	2	14
Chicken Noodle	80	1.5	10
Broccoli & Cheese	90	4.5	10
Vegetable Beef	60	1.5	12
Breakfast: Bacon Bagel	460	17	51
Biscuit & Sausage Gravy	655	38	59
Classic Stack O' Cakes (4)	320	4	62
Cheddar Scrambler	1150	80	72
Sourdough Sausage Melt	1040	85	35
Sourdough Steakburger Melt	810	57	33
Desserts: Outrageous Parfait	830	43	103
Berry Berry Cobbler a la mode	650	29	92
Brownie Fudge Sundae	862	44	112
Strawberry Shortcake	575	27	76
Shakes: *Per Regular*			
Banana, Mocha, Vanilla, avg.	720	22	116
Chocolate	745	22	122
Chocolate Mint, large	930	29	148
Frozen Yogurt Vanilla	695	16	126
Fruit & Frozen Yogurt, Strawberry	545	13	97
Orange Freeze	685	20	113

Updated Nutrition Data ~ www.CalorieKing.com
Persons with Diabetes ~ See Disclaimer (Page 24)

Sub Station II® (Sept '09)

Sandwiches: *Per ½ Sub, 6" Hoagie, Includes Oil, Lettuce, Tomato, Onion*

	C	F	Cb
All Cheese	700	49	40
Bologna & Cheese	660	47	44
Cheese, Turkey & Ham	605	37	49
Cheese, Pepperoni & Ham	720	49	48
Ham & Cheese	580	36	48
Ham, Turkey & Cheese	605	37	49
Roast Beef & Cheese	630	40	44
Roast Beef, Turkey & Cheese	605	38	41

Lite: *Per ½ Sub, 6" Hoagie, Incudes Lettuce, Tomato, Onion, without Cheese or Oil*

	C	F	Cb
Bologna	355	15	43
Genoa Salami & Pepperoni	485	26	42
Ham	275	4	48
Ham & Genoa Salami	375	14	45
Ham & Turkey	300	5	48
Roast Beef	325	8	43
Turkey	295	5	47

Submariner® (Sept '09)

Sub Classics, 6": *Includes Wheat Bread, Provolone, w/o Sides or Condiments*

	C	F	Cb
Combo Cheese	730	49	45
Ham & Turkey	415	15	45
Oven Roasted Chicken	400	14	44
Pepperoni	650	40	47
Roast Beef	440	17	46
Salami	620	37	47

Sub Favorites, 6": *Includes Wheat Bread, Cheese, w/o Sides or Condiments*

	C	F	Cb
Albacore Tuna	780	54	48
Avocado, Rst Beef w/ Smoked Cheddar	490	24	49
California Sub	550	27	48
Chicken/Turkey Club	480	21	45
Italian Sub	600	34	47
Triple Play	440	17	45

Sub Melts, 6":

	C	F	Cb
Chicken Breast Filet	400	13	44
Hot Pastrami	370	16	44
Meatball	860	14	56

Subway® (Sept '09)

6" Sandwiches (6g Fat or Less) C F Cb
Figures based on 9-grain wheat bread and toppings: lettuce, onion, tomato, onion, green peppers, olives and pickles. **Cheese, oil or mayo not included.**

	C	F	Cb
Black Forest Ham	290	4.5	47
Oven Roasted Chicken Breast	320	4.5	49
Roast Beef	310	4.5	46
Subway Club	320	5	47
Sweet Onion Chicken Teriyaki	380	4.5	60
Turkey Breast	290	3.5	47
Turkey Breast & Black Forest Ham	300	4	47
Veggie Delite	230	2.5	45

6" Sandwiches: *Figures based on 9-grain wheat bread, lettuce, tomato, onion, green peppers, pickles and olives.* **Cheese, oil or mayo not included.**

	C	F	Cb
Big Philly Cheesesteak	520	18	53
BLT	360	13	45
Chicken & Bacon Ranch	570	28	49
Cold Cut Combo	410	16	48
Italian B.M.T.	450	20	48
Meatball Marinara	580	23	70
Spicy Italian	520	28	47
Steak & Cheese	390	10	50
Subway Melt	380	11	49
The Feast	540	22	50
Tuna	530	30	46

Flatbread Sandwiches (8g Fat or Less): *Figures based on flatbread, lettuce, tomatoes, onions, green peppers, pickles, olives.* **Cheese, oil or mayo not included.**

	C	F	Cb
Black Forest Ham	320	7	47
Oven Roasted Chicken Breast	350	7	48
Roast Beef	340	8	45
Subway Club	350	8	47
Sweet Onion Teriyaki	410	7	59
Turkey Breast	310	6	47
Turkey Breast & Black Forest Ham	330	7	47
Veggie Delight	260	5	44

Low-Fat Footlong Sandwiches: *Figures based on 9-grain wheat bread, lettuce, tomato, onion, green peppers, pickles and olives.* **Cheese, oil or mayo not included.**

	C	F	Cb
Black Forest Ham	570	9	94
Oven Roasted Chicken Breast	640	9	97
Roast Beef	630	9	91
Subway Club	640	10	95
Sweet Onion Chicken Teriyaki	760	9	120
Turkey Breast & Black Forest Ham	590	8	95
Veggie Delight	460	4.5	90

4" Mini Sandwiches: *Kids Pak Figures based on 9-grain wheat bread, lettuce, tomatoes, onions, green peppers.*

	C	F	Cb
Black Forest Ham	180	2.5	31
Roast Beef	200	3	30
Turkey Breast	190	2.5	31

Subway® cont... (Sept '09)

6" Breakfast Sandwiches: Figures based on 9-grain wheat bread and toppings: lettuce, tomato, onion, green peppers, olives and pickles.

	C	F	Cb
Cheese	420	18	46
Double Bacon & Cheese	520	25	47
Mega	720	45	47
Steak & Cheese	490	20	48
Western with Cheese	450	19	48

6" Regional Subs: Figures based on 9-grain wheat bread, lettuce, tomatoes, onions, green peppers and cucumbers. Additional condiments specified.

Barbecue Chicken	310	5	53
Big Pastrami, w/ Cheese	590	29	49
Buffalo Chicken, w/ Ranch Dressing	420	15	47
Turkey Bacon Avocado, w/ cheese	420	15	51
Tuscan Chicken	370	9	48
Veggie Patty	390	7	57

Salads (6g Fat or Less)
Includes lettuce, tomato, onions, green peppers, olives, carrot, cucumber. **No Dressing or Croutons.**

Ham	110	3	12
Oven Roasted Chicken Breast	130	2.5	10
Roast Beef	140	3.5	10
Subway Club	140	3.5	12
Sweet Onion Chicken Teriyaki	200	3	25
Turkey Breast & Ham	120	3	12
Turkey Breast	110	2	12

Sandwich Components: For 6" Sub or Salad

Cheese: American, 0.4 oz	40	3.5	1
Monterey Cheddar, 0.5 oz	50	4.5	1
Natural Cheddar, 0.5 oz	60	5	0
Pepperjack; Provolone, 0.5 oz	50	4	0
Swiss, 0.5 oz	50	4.5	0
Meats: Bacon, 2 strips, 0.3 oz	45	3.5	0
Chicken Strips, 2.5 oz	80	1.5	0
Ham, 2 oz	60	2	3
Roast Beef, 2.5 oz	80	2.5	1
Seafood Sensation, 2.5 oz	190	16	7
Subway Club, 3 oz	90	2.5	2
Tuna, 2.5 oz	260	24	0

Sauces & Dressings:

Chipotle Southwest, 1½ Tbsp	100	10	1
Honey Mustard, Fat-Free, 1½ Tbsp	30	0	7
Mayonnaise: 1 Tbsp, ½ oz	110	12	0
Light, 1 Tbsp, ½ oz	50	5	0.5
Mustard, Yellow or Deli Brown. 2 tsp	5	0	0.5
Olive Oil Blend, 1 tsp	45	5	0
Ranch Dressing, 1¼ Tbsp	110	11	1
Sweet Onion, Fat-Free, 1¼ Tbsp	40	0	9

Subway® cont... (Sept '09)

Soups: Per Bowl

	C	F	Cb
Chicken & Dumpling	170	5	23
Chicken Tortilla	110	1.5	11
Chili Con Carne	340	11	35
Chipotle Chicken Corn Chowder	140	3	22
Cream of Potato with Bacon	240	13	26
Fire-Roasted Tomato Orzo	130	1	24
Golden Broccoli & Cheese	180	11	16
Minestrone	90	1	17
New England Style Clam Chowder	150	5	20
Roasted Chicken Noodle	80	2	12
Rosemary Chicken & Dumpling	90	1.5	14
Spanish Style Chicken with Rice	110	2.5	16
Tomato Garden Vegetable w. Rotini	90	0.5	20
Vegetable Beef	100	2	17
Wild Rice with Chicken	230	11	26

Cookies & Desserts

Apple Slices, 1 pkg, 2.5 oz	35	0	9
Chocolate Chip Cookie, 1.6 oz	210	10	30
Dannon Light & Fit Yogurt, 6 oz	80	0	16
Oatmeal Raisin Cookie	200	8	30

Sweet Tomatoes®
~ Same Menu & Data as Souplantation (See Page 253) ~

Swiss Chalet® (Aug '09)

Burgers/Sandwiches/Wraps: Without Sides

Bacon Cheese Burger	890	54	46
Classic Chicken S/wich, white meat	380	6	29
Hamburger	710	39	43
Veggie Burger	330	12	52
Chicken on a Kaiser, white meat	440	6	42
Chicken Quesadilla, w/o sour cream	620	23	72

Starters:

Garlic Cheese Loaf, 9 oz	860	53	77
Chalet Chicken Wings (8), w/ sauce	550	34	23
Cheese Perogies (7)	420	10	69
Caesar Salad with Dressing	420	37	16

Rotisserie Chicken: *Meat Only*

Double Leg w. Skin	630	38	4
Half Chicken, w. Skin	610	31	5
Quarter Chicken: Leg, no Skin	220	10	0
Leg meat with Skin	310	19	2
Breast meat w/o Skin	180	3.5	0
Breast meat with Skin	300	11	3
Chicken Pot Pie, 1 pie	550	34	63
Chicken Stir-Fry: with Rice	750	30	89
without Rice	430	26	26

From the Grill: Without Sides

BBQ Ribs: Half Rack	650	42	6
Full Rack	1300	85	11

Updated Nutrition Data ~ www.CalorieKing.com
Persons with Diabetes ~ See Disclaimer (Page 24)

Swiss Chalet® cont... (Aug '09)

Entree Salads:	C	F	Cb
Bacon Ranch, with 2 oz chicken	530	37	22
Chalet Chopped, with 2 oz chicken	440	27	29
Spinach Chicken Salad, w/o tortilla	170	2	14
Dressing/Sauce:			
Caesar Dressing, ½ oz	90	9	1
Chalet Dressing, 1 Tbsp, ½ oz	80	7	3
Chalet Dipping Sauce, 3.5 oz	25	0.5	5
Greek Dressing, ½ oz	70	7	1
Sides: Baked Potato, 10 oz	220	0	48
Creamy Coleslaw, 6.4 oz	200	14	15
French Fries, 6 oz	530	27	64
Gravy, 4 oz	45	1.5	7
Mashed Potatoes, 5 oz	150	4	27
Sauteed Mushrooms, 6 oz	220	16	11
Seasoned Rice, 6 oz	240	3.5	48
Desserts/Pies: Apple Pie	440	19	65
Caramel Fudge Cheesecake	660	41	68
Chocolate Lava Cake	430	23	53
Coconut Cream Pie	540	33	57
Cranberry Raspberry Yogurt	110	2	22
Lemon Meringue Pie	400	11	73
Old Fashioned Fudge Cake	720	44	81
Pecan Pie	590	29	79

Taco Bell® (Sept '09)

Burritos	C	F	Cb
½ lb Beef & Potato	510	22	66
½ lb Beef Combo	450	17	51
½ lb Cheesy Bean & Rice	470	21	60
7-Layer	490	17	67
Grilled Chicken	440	20	48
Supreme: Beef	410	15	52
Chicken	390	12	51
Steak	380	12	50
Fiesta: Beef	380	14	50
Chicken	360	10	49
Steak	350	11	48
Fresco Style: Bean	330	7	55
Fiesta, Chicken	340	8	50
Supreme, Chicken; Steak	335	8	50
Grilled Stuft: Beef	690	30	79
Chicken	650	23	76
Steak	630	24	75

Taco Bell® cont... (Sept '09)

Chalupas	C	F	Cb
Baja: Beef	410	26	31
Chicken; Steak, avg.	385	23	29
Nacho Cheese: Beef	370	21	32
Chicken; Steak, avg.	345	18	31
Supreme: Beef	370	21	31
Chicken; Steak, avg.	345	18	30
Gorditas:			
Baja: Beef	360	21	30
Chicken; Steak, avg.	335	18	29
Nacho Cheese: Beef	320	16	31
Chicken; Steak, avg.	295	13	30
Supreme: Beef	320	16	30
Chicken	300	13	29
Steak	290	13	29
Nachos: Regular	330	21	31
BellGrande	760	42	77
Supreme	430	24	41
Tacos:			
Crunchy Supreme	200	12	15
Double Decker	320	13	38
Double Decker Supreme	350	15	40
Soft Taco: Grilled Steak	250	14	20
Ranchero Chicken	270	14	21
Fresco Style: Crunchy	150	7	13
Soft: Beef	180	7	22
Ranchero Chicken	170	4	22
Specialities:			
Crunchwrap Supreme	540	21	71
Enrichito: Beef	360	17	35
Chicken; Steak, avg.	335	14	33
Grilled Taquitos, Chicken; Steak	315	11	37
MexiMelt	280	14	23
Quesadillas: Chicken	520	27	41
Steak	510	28	41
Taquitos, Chicken/Steak, average	315	11	37
Taco Salads: Fiesta: with Shell	820	43	81
without Shell	460	22	41
Fully Loaded Taco Salads:			
Chicken Ranch	960	57	78
Chipotle Steak	950	59	76
Volcano: Burrito	800	42	81
Taco	240	17	14

Continued Next Page

Taco Bell® cont... (Sept '09)

Sides	C	F	Cb
Cheesy Fiesta Potatoes, 4.75 oz	270	16	28
Guacamole, 1½ oz	70	6	4
Mexican Rice, 3 oz	130	3.5	21
Pintos 'n Cheese	170	6	18
Salsa, 1½ oz	10	0	2
Sour Cream, 1½ oz	60	4	4
Why Pay More!™			
Bean Burrito	350	9	54
Caramel Apple Empanada	310	15	39
Cheese Roll-Up	200	10	19
Cheesy Double Beef Burrito	470	20	54
Cinnamon Twists	170	7	26
Crunchy Taco	170	10	12
Soft Taco, Beef	210	9	21
Triple Layer Nachos	340	18	38

Note: Nutritional data for New York residents may vary slightly. Please check Taco Bell website

Taco Cabana® (Sept '09)

Burritos			
Bean & Cheese	690	35	71
Black Bean	370	7	68
Stewed Chicken	620	25	68
Flameante Chicken: Per Serving			
¼ Chicken Dark Dinner	920	41	82
¼ Chicken White Dinner	770	22	81
½ Chicken Dinner	1220	54	83
Sizzling Fajitas: Chicken Dark	700	21	92
Chicken White	710	20	93
Steak	730	24	93
Tacos:			
Crispy: Beef	180	10	11
Chicken	160	7	13
Soft: Bean & Cheese	300	14	31
Beef	230	9	21
Black Bean	180	4	30
Carne Guisada	90	4.5	2
Chicken	210	7	23
Sides: Per Serving			
Black Beans	40	1	6
Borracho Beans	110	3	16
Guacamole, small	110	9	7
Queso, small	200	15	5
Refried Beans	250	13	24
Rice	120	0.5	25
Salsa, all types	10	0	2
Sour Cream, small	160	14	3
Tortillas: 6" Flour	130	3.5	22
6" Table Corn	70	1	11

Taco John's® (Sept '09) C F Cb

Burritos: Super Burrito	450	18	54
Meat & Potato Burrito	500	23	58
Chicken & Potato Burrito	470	19	56
Crunchy Chicken & Potato Burrito	600	28	65
Bean Burrito	380	9	58
Beefy Burrito	440	20	45
Beef Grilled Burrito	600	32	52
Combination Burrito	400	14	50
Chicken Grilled Burrito	590	29	50
Tacos:			
Soft Shell Taco	220	11	21
Taco Bravo	340	13	40
Taco Burger	270	12	28
10 Grams of Fat or Less:			
Crispy	180	10	13
Chili	160	6	17
Soft Shell	190	8	20
Specialties: Taco Salad w/o dress.	520	33	37
Chicken Taco Salad w/o dressing	480	27	35
Crunchy Ckn Taco Salad w/o dress.	660	40	47
Super Nachos: Small	450	27	38
Regular	810	48	74
Super Potato Oles: Small	620	39	53
Regular	1030	65	87
Cheese Quesadilla	450	23	43
Chicken Quesadilla	500	24	44
Crunchy Chicken w/o sauce	450	27	24
Snacks: Chips & Queso	430	25	43
Buffalo Chicken Snackarito	290	15	27
Cini-Sopapilla Bites	210	5	37
Ranch Chicken Snackarito	240	12	23
Sides: Potato Oles: Small	430	26	45
Medium	600	36	62
Large	770	46	80
Kid's Meal portion	290	18	31
Refried Beans: with cheese	320	6	47
without cheese	260	1.5	47
Mexican Rice	250	6	45
Condiments: Nacho Cheese, 3 oz	120	9	5
Salsa, 2 oz	20	0	4
Sour Cream, 2 oz	120	12	2
House Dressing, 1.5 oz	70	7	2
Ranch Dressing, 1.5 oz	140	16	3
Desserts: Apple Grande	270	12	39
Choco Taco	390	20	48
Churro	190	7	15

Updated Nutrition Data ~ www.CalorieKing.com
Persons with Diabetes ~ See Disclaimer (Page 24)

Taco Mayo® (Sept '09)

Burritos	C	F	Cb
Bean	495	16	71
Beef	490	23	41
Beef & Bean	495	20	56
Super Burrito, Beef	540	23	57
Super Chicken	405	16	39
Melts			
Tamale	615	34	50
Tostadat	525	32	35
Quesadillas			
Chicken	675	37	46
Fajita Chicken	700	39	47
Fajita Steak	725	40	47
Tacos			
Crispy Taco, Beef	160	10	10
Soft Taco: Beef	230	11	17
Chicken	185	6	16
Salads			
Acapulco: Chicken Salad	680	50	35
Steak	705	51	35
SalsaLita Steak	305	8	33
Taco Steak	445	25	30
Sides			
Mexicali Rice	160	1	36
Refried Beans	295	9	43
Potato Locos, Small	380	24	36

Taco Time® (Sept '09)

Burritos	C	F	Cb
Beef, Bean & Cheese	495	17	55
Chicken, B.L.T.	695	39	43
Big Juan: Chicken	575	16	70
Ground Beef	635	23	73
Casita: Chicken	485	17	42
Ground Beef	545	24	46
Crisp Burrito: Chicken	380	17	33
Ground Beef	430	21	36
Pinto Bean	365	14	47
Soft Burrito: Meat	425	16	43
Pinto Bean	370	10	54
Soft Veggie	520	17	73
Tacos			
Soft Tacos: *Per 7 oz*			
Chicken	360	9	40
Ground Beef	420	16	43
Jr Soft Taco, 5.3 oz	315	13	28
Super Soft Taco: Beef, 10.5 oz	590	23	63
Chicken, 10.5 oz	530	16	60
Other Favorites: Cheddar Melt	250	12	25
Nachos Grande	925	43	96
Tostada: Bean	230	13	21
Chicken	315	13	22
Ground Beef	375	20	25

Taco Time® cont... (Sept '09)

Sides	C	F	Cb
Cheddar Fries, med. 7 oz	500	35	39
Mexi Fries®, medium, 6 oz	385	26	38
Mexi-Rice, 3.5 oz	75	1	17
Stuffed Fries, medium, 7 oz	465	28	42
Refritos with Chips, 6 oz	225	7	29
Salads:			
Regular: Chicken Taco, 9.5 oz	315	13	22
Ground Beef Taco, 9 oz	370	20	24
Tostada Delight: Chicken, 9 oz	445	19	35
Ground Beef, 9 oz	485	26	36
Salsas, Sauces & Dressings			
Chipotle Ranch Dressing, 1 oz	165	18	1
Guacamole, 1 oz	50	5	2
Salsa Fresca, 1 oz	10	0	2
Desserts:			
Churro: Plain	205	16	17
with Cinnamon & Sugar	245	16	27
Crustos	295	6	58
Empanada: Apple	235	7	40
Cherry	240	7	41
Pumpkin	255	8	42

Tacone® (Aug '09)

Gourmet Wrapped Sandwiches	C	F	Cb
Campfire, ½ wrap	340	12	41
Malibu Melt, ½ wrap	360	17	25
Pilgrim, ½ wrap	260	14	21
Thai Cone, ½ wrap	300	9	35

For Complete Nutritional Data ~ see CalorieKing.com

Target Food Court (Aug '09)

	C	F	Cb
Breakfast: Pancakes (3) + Syrup	490	4	104
Breakfast Sandwich w. Bacon	380	20	29
Cinnamon Swirl French Toast, 2 slices	230	5	36
Pretzels (Cinnabon): Cinnamon, 5¾ oz	550	9	105
Mega Cinnamon, 6½ oz	650	15	115
Salted Pretzel, 5½ oz	435	3.5	89
Meals: Bowl of Chili, 9 oz cup	300	10	32
Chicken Tenders, 5 strips, 3 oz	280	19	14
Hot Dog Meal: w. Chips & Soda	570	22	84
w. Applesauce & Soda	520	12	93
Hot Dog: Plain, 3½oz	260	12	28
All Beef Meat, 5 oz	350	20	30
Cheddar, 4 oz	310	16	38
Macaroni & Cheese: 8 oz	340	13	41
w. Apple Sauce & Soda Meal	600	13	106
w. Chips & Soda, Meal	650	23	97
Mini Pizza (6"), 5½ oz	360	14	42
Nachos w. Cheese, 40 chips, 4 oz	1100	59	132
Spaghetti O's Meal: w. Chips & Soda	490	11	93
w. Apple Sauce & Soda	440	1	102

For Complete Nutritional Data ~ see CalorieKing.com

TCBY® (Sept '09)

Soft Serve Frozen Yogurt: Per ½ Cup	C	F	Cb
Average all flavors	110	2	23
Golden Vanilla	120	2	23
White Chocolate Mousse	120	2	23
No Sugar Added, Fat Free:			
Average all	90	0	24
Chocolate	80	0	23
No Sugar Added:			
White Chocolate Macadamia	90	0	24
Sorbet: Per ½ Cup			
Classic Tart	90	0	21
Mango	110	0	26
Orange; Strawberry Kiwi	100	0	24
Raspberry	100	0	25
Hand-Scooped Frozen Yogurt			
Butter Pecan: Child, 2 oz	120	6	14
Small, 4 oz	240	12	28
Medium, 6 oz	360	17	42
Large, 8 oz	470	23	56
Chocolate Chocolate: Child, 2 oz	90	2.5	15
Small, 4 oz	190	5	30
Medium, 6 oz	280	8	45
Large, 8 oz	380	10	60
Cookies & Cream: Child, 2 oz	110	3.5	17
Small, 4 oz	210	7	33
Medium, 6 oz	320	10	50
Large, 8 oz	420	13	67
Mocha Almond: Child, 2 oz	110	4	17
Small, 4 oz	230	8	33
Medium, 6 oz	340	12	50
Large, 8 oz	450	16	67
Strawberries & Cream: Child, 2 oz	90	2	15
Small, 4 oz	170	4	30
Medium, 6 oz	260	6	45
Large, 8 0z	350	8	60
Vanilla Bean: Child, 2 oz	90	2.5	14
Small, 4 oz	180	5	29
Medium, 6 oz	270	8	43
Large, 8 oz	370	10	58
No Sugar Added Hand-Scooped			
Choc. Chocolate Swirl: Child, 2 oz	70	0	16
Small, 4 oz	130	0.5	32
Medium, 6 oz	200	1	49
Large, 8 oz	270	1.5	65
Vanilla Fudge Brownie: Child, 2 oz	80	1.5	17
Small, 4 oz	160	3	34
Medium, 6 oz	240	4.5	51
Large, 8 oz	310	6	69

Teriyaki Stix® (Aug '09)

Bowls:	C	F	Cb
Beef Bowl	620	7	102
Chicken Bowl; Hot & Spicy	730	15	101
Chicken Curry	680	17	92
Teriyaki Chicken Salad	360	13	26
Teriyaki Special	740	13	111
Veggie Bowl	440	1	99
Yakisoba	360	4.5	56

The Taco Maker® (Sept '09)

Burritos	C	F	Cb
Regular: Bean	405	16	52
Beef	365	12	44
Chicken	505	20	44
Crispy: Bean	400	26	31
Beef	250	5	41
Soft Shell: Beef	365	13	45
Chicken/Turkey, avg	435	18	45
½ lb Max Burrito, Beef	420	18	51
Nachos: Per Regular			
Cheese	300	23	7
Grande Deluxe: Beef	440	32	13
Chicken	510	37	13
Guacamole	500	40	16
Tacos: Beef	740	42	49
Chicken	550	23	45
Platters:			
Burrito Grande: Beef	430	17	53
Chicken	500	21	53
Fajita Dinner			
Beef/Chicken, avg.	800	38	72
Fiesta Dinner:			
Beef	550	23	54
Chicken	765	36	54
Quesadilla Dinner, Cheese	1100	62	95
Taco Salads: Without Dressing			
Beef	740	42	49
Chicken	550	23	45
Fries: Regular	150	6	21
Baked Potatoes			
Papa Taco: Bean	270	4	54
Beef	445	19	54
Chicken	520	24	54
Potato, Bacon & Cheese	523	27	52
Turkey	505	23	56

Updated Nutrition Data ~ www.CalorieKing.com
Persons with Diabetes ~ See Disclaimer (Page 24)

ThunderCloud Subs® (Sept '09)

Subs: Small, Without Cheese/Mayo/Mustard	C	F	Cb
Classic: Ham & Cheese	375	12	42
Roast Beef	290	6	40
Smoked Chicken	295	4	40
Turkey	280	4	41
Hot Subs: Meatball	650	32	56
Hot Pastrami	430	13	41
Signature Subs: Club	480	19	43
California Club	510	23	45
N.Y. Italian	570	30	42
Office Favorite	850	46	81
Texas Tuna	700	45	44
Veggie Delite, w/ Hummus,	360	10	53

Tim Hortons® (Aug '09)

Sandwiches	C	F	Cb
Tim's Own: Chicken Salad	380	9	54
Egg Salad	390	13	52
Ham & Swiss w. Tim's Own Dress.	440	12	56
Turkey Bacon Club w. Mustard	440	8	63
Soup: Per 10 oz Bowl			
Chicken Noodle	120	2	18
Chili	300	19	17
Cream of Broccoli	160	9	16
Creamy Field Mushroom	150	3	28
Hearty Potato Bacon	250	13	23
Hearty Vegetable	70	0.5	14
Minestrone	120	3	24
Split Pea with Ham	150	2.5	27
Turkey Rice	120	1.5	21
Vegetable Beef Barley	110	1.5	21
Bagels: Plain	260	1.5	52
Blueberry; Cinnamon Raisin	270	1	55
Everything	280	2	53
Onion	260	1.5	53
Poppy Seed	270	2	53
Muffins: Per Muffin			
Blueberry Bran	300	10	53
Cranberry Fruit	350	12	59
Chocolate Chip	430	16	69
Fruit Explosion	360	11	61
Raisin Bran	360	10	65
Strawberry Sensation	350	11	61
Wheat Carrot	400	19	55
Low-Fat varieties	290	2.5	62

Tim Hortons® Cont... (Aug '09)

Timbits: Low-Fat	C	F	Cb
Cake: Chocolate Glazed	70	2.5	10
Old Fashion Plain	70	5	5
Filled, all varieties	60	2	10
Yeast: Apple Fritter	50	1.5	9
Honey Dip	60	2	9
Baked Goods: Per Serving			
Croissant: Plain	200	11	21
Cheese	230	14	19
Tea Biscuit: Plain, 3 oz	250	9	35
Raisin, 3 oz	290	10	45
Cinnamon Roll: Frosted	470	25	57
Glazed	420	23	50
Danish: Cherry Cheese	230	10	27
Chocolate	340	16	42
Maple Pecan	290	12	37
Cookies			
Caramel Chocolate Pecan	230	11	32
Oatmeal Raisin Spice	220	8	35
Peanut Butter	280	16	27
Chocolate Chunk	230	9	35
Triple Chocolate	250	13	31
Donuts: Per Donut			
Cake: Chocolate Glazed	260	10	39
Old Fashion Plain	260	19	20
Sour Cream Plain	270	17	27
Filled: Blueberry	230	8	36
Boston Cream	250	9	38
Canadian Maple	260	9	41
Strawberry	230	8	36
Honey Cruller	320	19	37
Yeast: Apple Fritter	300	11	49
Dutchie Donut	250	10	38
Desserts			
Low-Fat Yogurt: Strawb. w. Berries	140	2.5	27
Creamy Vanilla w. Berries	160	2	33
Beverages: Per Serving			
Cafe Mocha, 10 fl.oz	180	8	27
Cappuccino: Eng. Toffee, 10 fl.oz	240	7	41
French Vanilla, 10 fl.oz	250	8	41
Iced Original:			
with Small Milk, 10 fl.oz	150	1.5	32
with Small Cream, 10 fl.oz	250	11	33
Coffee w. med. sugar/cream, 10 fl.oz	75	3.5	9
Hot Chocolate, 10 fl.oz	240	6	45
Lemon Iced Tea, 12 fl.oz	145	0	38

T.J. Cinnamons® (Aug '09)

Bakery	**C**	**F**	**Cb**
Cinnamon Roll, 5.25 oz	505	10	73
Cinnamon Twist (1), 2½ oz	260	14	33
Pecan Sticky Bun: (1), 6.5 oz	690	22	91
4-Pack	2750	90	363
Sticky Bun Smear w/ Pecans, 1¼ oz	180	12	18
T.J. Cream Cheese Icing, 1 oz	115	5	18
Beverages: Per 12 fl.oz Serving			
Mocha Chill: w/o Whipped Cream	265	4	46
with Whipped Cream	305	7	47

Togo's Eatery® (Sept '09)

Sandwiches: Regular 6" Roll	**C**	**F**	**Cb**
Chef's Creations: BBQ Ranch Chkn	750	27	88
Chipotle Rst Beef w/ Provolone	990	49	66
Pacific Cobb	710	36	68
Pastrami Reuben w/ Swiss	990	55	67
Cold: Albacore Tuna	660	28	73
Black Forest Ham & Cheese	670	31	67
Chicken Salad w. Almonds	650	29	74
Roast Beef & Avocado	720	29	70
The Italian	860	43	71
Turkey & Avocado	640	26	74
Turkey & Bacon Club	680	32	68
Hot: BBQ Beef	670	19	85
Chicken	630	20	72
Hot Pastrami	750	33	69
Meatball	690	27	78
Sicilian Chicken	710	28	73
Vegetarian: Avocado & Cheese	740	40	73
Avocado & Cucumber	560	25	75
Egg Salad & Cheese	750	39	70
Salad Wraps: Asian Chicken	670	32	74
BBQ Chicken Ranch	630	26	77
Cobb w/ Blue Cheese	680	36	63
Farmer's Market w/ Fetta	440	14	72
Santa Fe Chicken w/ Cheddar	800	44	75
Salads: Per Full Salad, without Dressing			
Asian Chicken	200	9	17
BBQ Chicken Ranch	230	3.5	31
Chicken Caesar	210	6	17
Cobb	330	20	12
Taco, includes shell	600	39	36

Tropical Smoothie Cafe (Aug '09)

Sandwiches: Without Cheese & Sauce	**C**	**F**	**Cb**
Cranberry Walnut Chicken Salad	735	40	70
Hummus Among Us	620	21	85
Kinda Cubano	335	5.5	36
Lean Turkey Guacamole	590	8	36
Mambo Italiano	360	5.5	38
Ultimate Club	380	10	36
Wasabi Roast Beef	290	3	32
Wraps:			
Breakfast: Early Bird	465	13	55
Western	505	14	58
Buffalo Chicken	405	9	56
Cool Tuna Wrap	550	19	67
Jamaican Jerk	470	10	69
King Caesar	390	9	54
Sesame Chicken	665	19	92
Totally Turkey	440	9	54
Salads: Without Dressing			
Chef Salad	190	3	10
Garden Classic Salad	60	0.5	10
Sesame Chicken Salad	415	10	53
Thai Chicken Salad	355	4	54
Low Fat Smoothies: With Turbinado			
Blimey Limey; Cool Breeze, avg.	410	0	100
Blue Lagoon	330	1	80
Hawaiian Breeze	360	0	88
Island Fever; Orange Passion, avg.	455	0	111
Rockin Raspberry	515	0.5	125
Strawberry Beach	450	0	109
Sunrise Sunset	390	0.5	96
Power Smoothies: With Turbinado			
Fat Buster	375	0.5	91
Health Nut	620	10	104
Lean Machine	475	0.5	115
Muscle Blaster	595	3	119
Peanut Paradise	810	22	119
Dessert Smoothies: With Turbinado			
Beach Bum Chocolate	565	5	125
Chocolate Chiller	555	7	118
Coconut Royale	730	11	155
Mocha Madness	645	12	127
Peanut Butter Cup	840	24	142
With Splenda, deduct 200 calories & 50g carbs			

Updated Nutrition Data ~ www.CalorieKing.com
Persons with Diabetes ~ See Disclaimer (Page 24)

Fast - Foods & Restaurants

Tubby's® (Aug '09)

Subs: Per Regular Sandwich

	C	F	Cb
Burger Subs: Big Tub	670	56	55
Burger Special	900	59	59
Cheeseburger	910	60	59
Pizza Burger	930	60	62
Taco Burger	825	47	67
Deli Subs: Club Sub	700	41	53
Ham & Cheese	570	30	54
Tubby's Famous	665	39	55
Turkey & Cheese	625	32	51
Turkey Club Sub	850	39	83
Specialty Subs: BLT	635	42	50
Cold Veggie	460	14	66
Italian Sausage	730	45	56
Tuna	415	18	47
Veggie Stir Fry	650	27	89
Chicken Subs:			
Chicken & Broccoli	550	23	56
Chicken & Cheddar	545	23	54
Chicken Club Sub	705	41	53
Chicken Fajita Sub	445	12	57
Grilled Chicken	345	5	52
Steak Subs:			
Mushroom Steak	835	26	52
Pepper Steak	710	46	52
Pizza Steak	985	57	85
Steak & Cheese	825	56	51
Steak Special	745	46	58

Uno Chicago Grill® (Aug '09)

Appetizers:

	C	F	Cb
Pizza Skins, ⅓ pizza, 5 oz	480	31	39
Roasted Vegetable Quesadilla (1)	300	13	36
Shrimp & Crab Fondue, 3.3 oz	220	13	12
Burgers: Sliders (2)	1200	80	52
Uno Burger (2)	1080	72	48
BBQ w/ Bacon & Cheddar (2)	1400	92	64
Entrees: Without Side or Breadstick			
Baked Stuffed Chicken (2)	360	18	6
Chicken Spinoccoli (2)	1340	66	120
Chop House Classic (2)	520	18	0
Fisherman's Platter (2)	1540	110	148
Deep Dish Pizza: Per ⅙ Regular			
Chicago Classic	770	55	40
Numero Uno	640	44	41
Spinoccoli	620	45	40
Flatbread Pizza: Per ⅓ pizza			
Mediterranean	280	15	29
Pepperoni, Gluten-Free Crust	340	17	30
Spicy Chicken	350	16	34

For Complete Nutritional Data ~ see CalorieKing.com

Villa Pizza® (Aug '09)

Pizza (18"): Per Slice (⅙ Pizza)

	C	F	Cb
Neapolitan: Cheese	525	19	60
Sausage and Cheese	675	32	61
Pepperoni and Cheese	635	29	60
Stuffed: Meat	880	42	83
Spinach and Mushroom	790	35	87
Sicilian: Deluxe	945	39	105
Stromboli:			
Sausage and Cheese	880	44	83
Pepperoni and Cheese	745	33	83
Pasta & Italian Specialties:			
Baked Ziti	680	35	63
Meat Lasagna	1235	81	86
Spinach and Cheese Lasagna	1065	60	88
Spaghetti	2710	122	349
Chicken Francais	225	11	4
Chicken Cacciatore	780	68	11
Italian Sausage and Peppers	645	64	3
Sauteed Fresh Vegetables	465	43	19
Salads:			
Caesar	110	8	7
Fresh Mozzarella	310	22	10
Greek	155	11	9

Vocelli Pizza® (Aug '09)

Pizze: Per Slice (⅛ Pizza)

	C	F	Cb
Grand Cheese	260	6	38
Grand Pepperoni	410	20	38
Gourmet: Per Slice (⅛ Pizza)			
Deluxe	390	16	40
Meat Magnifico	490	25	38
Philly Steak	360	13	38
Panini: Per Sandwich			
Chicken	900	38	81
Italian	910	42	77
Vegetarian	750	31	83
Insalata: Per Plate			
Antipasta	630	50	16
Chicken Caesar	220	4.5	4
Mediterranean	270	18	20
Tuscany Chicken	350	16	15
Antipasti: Croutons, 1 package	30	1	5
Bruschetta, 1 slice	150	8	14
Buffalo Wings (10)	560	39	26
BBQ Wings (10)	610	33	31
Pepperoni Sticks, 2½ slices	470	26	36
Dressings: Per 2 oz Packet			
Blue Cheese	230	25	2
Italian	200	21	4
Ranch	260	28	2

Wahoo's Fish Taco® (Sept '09)

	C	F	Cb
Bowls: W/ White Rice & Blk Beans			
Blackened Chicken	860	15	127
Charbroiled Chicken	860	15	126
Charbroiled Fish	930	22	126
Teriyaki Fish	930	22	127
Classic Burrito, A la Carte:			
Carne Asada	480	19	53
Carnitas	605	25	54
Charbroiled/Blackened: Fish, av.	545	23	53
Chicken, average	495	18	52
Mushroom	405	16	55
Shrimp	400	16	54
Veggie w/ White Rice & Black Beans	635	19	98
Tacos, A la Carte:			
Blackened Chicken	185	5	22
Carne Asada	180	5	22
Carnitas	235	8	23
Veggie w/ White Rice & Black Beans	215	4	36
Sides: Brown Rice	350	7	64
White Beans	285	3	54
Salads: Chips Not Included			
Blackened Chicken	415	22	14
Carne Asada	400	23	16
Charbroiled Fish	485	29	14

For Complete Nutritional Data ~ see CalorieKing.com

WAWA® (Aug '09)

	C	F	Cb
Breakfast & Baked Goods			
Bagel: Plain	285	1	60
w. Butter	505	23	64
w. Cream Cheese	430	13	67
Bagel Melts: Ham & Cheese	485	13	66
Pepperoni & Cheese	660	33	59
Pork Roll & Cheese	655	26	77
Breakfast Ciabattas:			
Bacon Strips, Egg & Cheddar 7 oz	425	20	41
Beefsteak, Egg & Cheese, 8.35 oz	425	15	41
Ham, Swiss & Egg, 7.9 oz	385	13	42
Breakfast Bowls: Per Bowl			
Creamed Chipped Beef on a Bisc.	475	23	56
Sausage Gravy on a Biscuit	505	27	56
Hash Brown (1), 2.5 oz	130	8	15
Muffins: Banana Walnut, 6 oz	670	34	83
Blueberry, 6.2 oz	610	30	78
Chocolate Chip, 4 oz	680	34	86
Corn, 6 oz	640	29	87
Sizzli Bagels: Bacon Egg & Chse	410	19	48
Sausage Egg & Cheese	515	28	49
Sizzli Biscuits: Bacon Egg & Chse	535	33	52
Sausage Egg & Cheese	635	42	53
Sizzli Muffins:			
Sausage, Egg & Cheese	460	29	35

WAWA® cont... (Aug '09)

	C	F	Cb
Hot Sandwiches: No Cheese Unless Indicated			
Cheese Steak	450	17	35
Grilled Chicken Caesar w. Cheese	455	12	49
Classics: Cheese Steak	700	25	62
Meatball w. Cheese	695	31	74
Pizza Cheese Steak	700	25	62
Roast Beef Homestyle w. Cheese	740	24	71
Cold Sandwiches: No Cheese Unless Indicated			
Chicken and Salad	540	30	41
Corned Beef	400	9	35
Egg Salad	540	33	41
Ham	335	7	38
Classics: BLT	780	42	62
Roast Beef Classic	595	10	62
Turkey Carolina Honey Smoked	470	6	70
Turkey	470	6	70
Tuna Salad	900	53	74
Veggie	330	3	62
Cold Shortis: American	455	20	46
BLT	495	28	37
Chicken Salad	540	29	49
Egg Salad w. Cheese	640	40	49
Turkey	305	4	49
Hot Shortis: Chicken Steak	560	7	94
Meatball w. Cheese	685	21	103
Roast Beef w. Cheese	715	17	100
Hot Dogs: ¼ lb Beef Frank	385	28	23
All Beef Hot Dog	250	15	22
Big Bacon Cheese Dog	720	49	45
Hot Sausage	310	20	21
Bowls: Beef Stew, 14.8 oz	610	38	59
Chili, 18.7 oz	710	11	129
Homestyle Roast Beef, 16.7 oz	725	42	51
Meatballs, 20 oz	790	18	133
Sides: Per Medium Serve			
Beef Stew, 11.5 oz	275	13	23
Chili, 11.6 oz	230	8	30
Homestyle Chkn & Noodles, 11.5 oz	340	16	26
Macaroni & Beef, 13 oz	365	14	44
Macaroni & Cheese, 11.3 oz	470	22	51
Mashed Potatoes, 11 oz	535	34	53
Meatballs in a Cup, 4 oz	160	11	9
Soups: Per 11 oz Medium Bowl			
Boston Clam Chowder	325	17	30
Chicken Corn Chowder	410	27	34
Cream of Broccoli	280	17	24
Vegetable Beef & Barley	150	5	21
Drinks: Per 12 fl.oz			
Cappuccino	250	8	42
French Vanilla Cappuccino	220	7	38
Low-Fat	180	1	39
Mocha Wakeup, 12 fl.oz	195	7	34

Updated Nutrition Data ~ www.CalorieKing.com
Persons with Diabetes ~ See Disclaimer (Page 24)

Wendy's® (Sept '09)

Sandwiches	C	F	Cb
Burgers: Baconator	830	51	35
Double Stack	360	18	26
Double w/ Cheese	700	40	38
Jr. Bacon Cheeseburger	310	16	25
Jr. Cheeseburger Deluxe	300	14	88
¼ lb. Single	430	20	38
Triple w/ Cheese	970	60	39
Chicken: Chicken Club	550	26	48
Crispy Chicken	360	18	36
Homestyle Chicken Fillet	440	16	47
Spicy Chicken	440	16	49
Ultimate Chicken Grill	320	7	36
French Fries: Kid's, 2.5 oz	210	10	27
Small, 4 oz	330	16	44
Medium, 5 oz	420	20	55
Large, 6.5 oz	540	26	71
Chicken Nuggets, 5 pce	230	16	11
Boneless Chicken Wings: Buffalo	520	18	58
Honey BBQ	580	18	75
Sweet & Spicy Asian	550	18	58
Dipping Sauce: Barbecue	45	0	11
Heartland Ranch	160	17	1
Garden Sensations Salads			
Chicken BLT, no dress./topping	470	27	23
w/ Croutons, Honey Dijon Dress.	790	54	41
Chicken Caesar, no dress./topping	180	4	8
w/ Croutons, Caesar Dressing	370	20	18
Southwest Taco, no dress./topping	400	22	26
w/ Tortilla Strips, Chipotle Ranch Dress.	600	35	42
Caesar Side Salad, no dress./topping	70	4	4
Side Salad no Dressing	35	0	8
Baked Potatoes: Plain 10 oz	270	0	61
Plain w. Buttery Spread	320	5	61
Bacon & Cheese	460	13	67
Broccoli & Cheese	340	3	70
Sour Cream & Chives	320	4	63
Sides: Chili Large, 12 oz	280	9	29
Cheddar Cheese, shredded, 2 Tbsp	70	6	1
Homestyle Garlic Croutons	70	3	9
Mandarin Orange Cup, 5 oz	80	0	19
Frosty: Choc/Van., small, av.	315	8	52
Frosti-cino, small	390	10	62
Shakes: Chocolate, large	540	13	94
Strawb/Vanilla, large, av.	505	13	89
Twisted: M&M's, Choc/Van, av.	555	19	86
Oreo, Choc/Van, av.	445	14	72

For Complete Nutritional Data ~ see CalorieKing.com

Wienerschnitzel® (Sept '09)

Hot Dogs: With Standard Bun	C	F	Cb
Original: BBQ Bacon	380	21	33
Chili	290	13	31
Chili Cheese	340	17	31
Deluxe	270	12	30
Pastrami	510	32	31
Plain	270	13	28
Stadium	370	20	32
Corn Dogs: Regular	250	17	15
Mini (6)	320	22	22
Burgers: Chili	310	9	29
Chili Cheese	350	13	29
Deluxe: Hamburger	400	19	33
Bacon Cheeseburger	530	29	33
Cheeseburger	450	23	33
Double Chili Cheese	560	24	35
Pastrami	510	26	30
Sandwiches: Chicken Deluxe	430	21	37
Italian Sausage	350	17	31
Pastrami	580	34	36
Polish Sausage	490	29	39
Sides: Chili Cheese Fries	540	38	39
Fries: Regular	300	22	25
Large	430	31	35
Jalapeno Poppers (3)	210	11	21
Breakfast:			
Biscuit: Egg, Bacon, Cheese	440	25	36
Egg, Sausage, Cheese	540	34	40
Burrito: Egg, Bacon, Cheese	490	25	39
Egg, Sausage, Cheese	590	34	43
French Toast Sticks	490	29	49
Syrup, 1.1 oz	120	0	31
Desserts:			
Cones: Plain, 6 oz.	300	11	49
Chocolate Dipped, 6 oz.	490	29	57
Floats: Mountain Dew, Root Beer avg.	440	12	84
Tropicana Strawberry Lemonade	450	12	82
Freezees: Butterfinger	620	24	100
Oreo; M&M	630	25	99
Reese's Peanut Butter Cup	630	26	97
Sundaes: Caramel, Hot Fudge avg.	400	15	65
Chocolate	390	14	64
Pineapple; Strawberry	370	14	59
Shakes, avg. all	650	23	110
Drinks: 16 fl.oz, without ice			
Lipton Raspberry Iced Tea	180	0	45
Mountain Dew	230	0	61
Mug Root Beer	210	0	57
Pepsi	200	0	55

Whataburger® (Sept '09)

Burgers/Sandwiches	C	F	Cb
Justaburger	290	15	26
Whataburger: Burger	620	30	58
w. Bacon & Cheese	780	43	59
Double Meat	870	49	58
Triple Meat	1120	68	58
Jr.	300	15	28
Sandwich: Grilled Chicken	470	19	49
Whatacatch	460	29	38
Whatachick'n	550	20	65
French Fries: Small, 3 oz	260	13	31
Medium, 4½ oz	400	20	47
Large, 6 oz	530	27	63
Onion Rings: Medium, 4.3 oz	420	28	36
Large, 6.4 oz	630	42	55
Chicken Strips (2)	380	24	22
Salads: Chicken Strips Salad	430	25	33
w. American Cheese 1 lge slice	520	32	34
Garden Salad	50	1	11
w. American Cheese 1 lge slice	140	8	12
Grilled Chicken Salad	220	8	18
w. American Cheese 1 lge slice	310	15	19
Dressing: Per 3.15 oz			
Ranch Sauce	480	51	4
Malts:			
Chocolate; Strawb.: Small, 15.75 oz	670	15	123
Medium, av. 25.25 oz	1045	25	188
Vanilla: Small, 15.75 oz	600	17	98
Medium, 25.25 oz	940	27	55
Shakes			
Chocolate; Strawb.: Small, 15.75 oz	630	16	111
Medium, 25.25 oz	995	26	171
Vanilla: Small, 15.75 oz	560	17	87
Medium, 25.25 oz	890	28	139
Breakfast: Cinnamon Roll	390	9	71
Hash Brown Sticks (4)	200	12	20
Texas Toast, 1 slice	150	7	20
Biscuit: Plain	300	17	32
w. Bacon	350	20	32
w. Gravy	530	36	52
w. Sausage	540	37	32
Honey Butter Chicken	610	38	51
Biscuit Sandwich: w. Egg & Chse	450	28	33
w. Bacon, Egg & Cheese	500	32	33
w. Sausage, Egg & Cheese	690	49	33

Whataburger® cont... (Sept '09)

Breakfast (Cont)	C	F	Cb
Breakfast On A Bun: w. Bacon	360	21	25
w. Sausage	550	38	25
Breakfast Platter (Biscuit/Eggs/Hash Brown):			
w. Bacon	740	45	53
w. Sausage	930	62	53
Pancakes: Plain (3)	580	8	112
w. Bacon	630	12	112
w. Sausage	820	29	112
Taquito: w. Bacon & Egg	380	21	27
w. Bacon, Egg & Cheese	420	24	27
w. Potato & Egg	430	23	37
w. Potato, Egg & Cheese	470	27	37
w. Sausage & Egg	410	24	27
w. Sausage, Egg & Cheese	450	28	27
Dessert: Hot Apple Pie	230	11	29

White Castle® (Sept '09)

Sandwiches & Burgers	C	F	Cb
Cheeseburger	170	9	15
Double	300	17	23
Whitecastle Hamburger	140	7	14
Double	250	13	22
Sandwiches:			
Chicken Ring w. Cheese	200	10	19
Chicken Breast w. Cheese	195	7	21
Chicken Supreme	230	10	21
Fish with Cheese	185	8	19
Surf & Turf with Cheese	390	22	28
Sides			
Chicken Rings: 6 rings, 3.9 oz	310	20	17
9 rings, 5.8 oz	460	30	25
Clam Strips, 4 oz	250	22	5
Fish Nibblers, 4.1 oz	280	16	24
French Fries, 4.3 oz	355	26	24
Mozzarella Cheese Sticks, 3 sticks	250	14	22
Onion Chips, 4 oz	480	23	62
Onion Rings Homestyle, 3.4 oz	400	21	49
Sauces & Condiments: Per Packet			
Ketchup, 0.3 oz	10	0	3
Lemon Juice, 0.1 oz	0	0	0
Mayonnaise, 0.3 oz	70	7	0
Ranch Dressing, 1 oz	150	17	1
Sauce: BBQ, 0.3 oz	15	0	3
Cheese, 1.5 oz	130	10	6
Seafood, 1 oz	30	0	7
White Castle Zesty Zing, 1 oz	120	11	4

Updated Nutrition Data ~ www.CalorieKing.com
Persons with Diabetes ~ See Disclaimer (Page 24)

Winchell's® (Aug '09)

Baked Products	C	F	Cb
Donuts: *Per Donut*			
Cake Donuts, Chocolate Iced	240	10	36
Old Fashioned, Glazed	410	17	60
Jelly Filled:			
Apple with Cinnamon Crumb	450	18	65
Raspberry with Glaze	480	15	78
Strawberry with Sugar	460	15	74
Raised Round: Choc. Iced; Glazed	220	9	31
Sugared	230	9	34

WingStreet (Sept '09)

Chicken	C	F	Cb
Crispy Bone In Wings: *Per 2 Pieces*			
All American, 1.7 oz	170	13	7
Buffalo, Mild/Med./Hot, 2.3 oz	210	13	14
Cajun, 2.3 oz	210	13	15
Garlic Parmesan, 2.3 oz	280	23	8
Bone Out Wings: *Per 2 Pieces*			
All American, 2.15 oz	190	10	11
Buffalo, Mild/Medium, 2.8 oz	220	11	18
Cajun, 2.8 oz	220	10	19
Garlic Parmesan, 2.75 oz	280	20	12
Traditional Wings: *Per 2 Pieces*			
All American, 1.4 oz	80	5	0
Buffalo, Medium/Hot, 2 oz	120	6	7
Cajun, 2 oz	110	6	8
Garlic Parmesan, 2 oz	180	16	1
Sides: Apple Pies, 2 pies, 3.7 oz	360	18	47
Fried Cheese Sticks (4), 3.4 oz	310	19	25
Taters, ½ order, 8 oz	790	52	74

Woody's Bar-B-Q (Aug '09)

Entrees	C	F	Cb
½ Chicken	840	56	0
Baby Back Ribs, ½ Rack, 14 ribs	520	40	2
Beef Prime Rib	230	19	1
Chicken Breast: 1 piece	250	14	4
Spicy Breaded, 1 piece	200	8	14
Chicken Tenders, 2 pieces	190	7	18
Chicken Wings, 2 pieces	210	13	4
Homestyle Meat Loaf, 4 oz	340	26	10
Hot Dog	330	28	8
Pulled Pork, ½ cup	250	19	4
Sausage, 5 pieces	260	16	20
Shrimp, 6 shrimp	180	1	33
Spare Ribs, ½ slab, 4 oz	270	21	0

For Complete Nutritional Data ~ see CalorieKing.com

Yoshinoya® (Sept '09)

Bowls: Without sauce unless indicated	C	F	Cb
Beef Bowl®: Regular	685	27	81
Large	970	38	116
Beef Bowl® w/ Vegetables, regular	605	20	84
Beef & Chicken Combo, large	985	30	131
Chicken Bowl: Regular	610	12	94
Large	910	17	140
Chicken Bowl w/ Teriyaki Sce, reg.	740	12	125
Shrimp Bowl: Grilled, Regular	505	3	96
with Seafood Sauce	635	3	126
Vegetable Bowl, regular	390	2.5	86
Kids: Beef w/ Vegetables	350	11	49
Chicken w/ Vegetables	360	7	53
Soups: Chicken Vegetable	70	1.5	7
Clam Chowder	210	7	34
Miso Soup	60	1.5	8
Salad, Chicken	360	14	14
Garden	50	0	9
Macaroni	350	21	37
Sesame Wings, 6 pieces	420	27	2

Z Pizza® (Sept '09)

Pizzas: Small 10", Per ⅙ Slice	C	F	Cb
Berkeley Soy Cheese Veggie	180	8	19
California	150	6	19
Casablanca	190	9	18
Greek	150	6	17
Italian	180	8	17
Mexican	180	7	19
Napoli	180	8	18
Provence	160	7	20
Santa Fe	180	7	20
Thai	170	6	19
Tuscan	160	7	18
ZBQ	170	5	21
Sandwiches: Hot Meatball Sub	670	34	45
Pollo Latino Sandwich	350	11	38
Supersub	460	23	34
Turkey Breast Sandwich	400	14	35
Z-Tuna Sandwich	670	32	68
Calzones: Meat Calzone	770	37	77
Veggie Calzone	750	27	102
Salads: Small w/o Dressing			
Arugula	260	20	14
Caesar Side	200	17	8
California	100	6	10
Pear and Gorgonzola Salad	530	44	25
ZBQ Salad	220	11	17

Zaxby's (Sept '09)

Zappetizers	C	F	Cb
Onion Rings, w/o Sce	625	41	55
Spicy Fried Mushroom w/o Sce	430	28	37
Tater Chips, 5.6 oz	795	53	75
Chicken: With Sides, w/o Sauce			
Buffalo Fingerz, 5-pieces	420	20	8
Buffalo Wings, 5-pieces	365	23	0
Chicken Fingerz, 5 fingers, 6 oz	420	20	8
Meal Dealz: Without Sauce or Drink			
Big Zax Snax	765	34	78
Buffalo Wings	735	39	53
Chicken Finger Plate: Regular	1055	50	91
Large	1590	73	147
Chicken Finger S'wich w. Sauce	1265	69	116
Grilled Chickenr S'wich w. Mustard	1070	49	102
Kickin Chkn S'wich w. Dress. & Sce	1205	67	107
Nibbler with Zac Sauce	1295	66	126
Wings & Things: Regular	1140	57	79
Large	1675	80	134
Sandwich Baskets: Includes Fries			
Cajun Club	1185	57	108
Zaxby's Club	1220	69	102
Zax Kidz: Kiddie Cheese	435	20	55
Kiddie Finger	390	17	34
Zalads: With Texas Toast, w/o Dressing			
Blue Zalad: w. Blackened Fillet	590	27	37
w. Buffalo Fingerz w/ Sauce	755	39	46
Caesar Zalad: with Chicken Fingerz	665	34	31
with Grilled Fillet	515	23	24
House Zalad: with Grilled Fillet	605	30	36
with Chicken Fingerz	755	41	43
Zensation, w. Chkn Fingers & Sce	835	39	77
Salad Dressings: Per 1.2 oz Packet			
Blue Cheese	180	19	2
Honey French	150	12	9
Honey Mustard	150	13	6
Lite Vinaigrette	50	2	7
Mediterranean	140	14	4
Ranch	160	16	2
Thousand Island	230	24	3
Sides: Celery Basket, 2.6 oz	5	0	2
Cole Slaw, 2.75 oz	115	8	10
Crinkle Fries, 8 oz	590	25	84
Texas Toast, Dry, 1.2 oz	100	1	19

Zero's Subs® (Sept '09)

Oven Baked 6" Subs:	C	F	Cb
Includes cheese, lettuce, tomato, onions, oil & vinegar			
BLT	410	19	48
BLT, no Mayo	330	12	43
Cosmo Vegetarian	470	23	46
Cosmo Vegetarian Deluxe	490	25	48
Grilled Veggie	395	14	52
Grinder	555	31	48
Grinder, Multigrain	560	32	50
Ham & Cheese	440	19	44
Meatball & Cheese	565	30	50
without Cheese	465	22	50
Pepperoni & Cheese	545	31	42
without Cheese	345	15	41
Roast Beef & Cheese	460	19	45
The Club	515	23	44
Tuna & Cheese	520	26	47
Turkey & Cheese	455	17	44
6" Subs From The Grill			
Hot Italian Sausage & Cheese	665	37	45
Philly Chicken & Cheese	400	10	48
w. Mushrooms/Green Peppers	410	10	49
without Cheese	330	4	47
12" Size Subs: Double the figures for 6" size			

Zoup!® (Sept '09)

Soups: Per 8 fl.oz Cup	C	F	Cb
Chicken Potpie	210	9	24
Cream of Broccoli	230	13	15
Fire Roasted Tomato Bisque	320	24	20
Ginger Butternut Squash	220	11	30
Jamaican Bay Gumbo	130	1.5	19
New England Clam Chowder	160	7	17
Seafood Bisque	190	10	11
Vegetable Bounty	110	1.5	21
Vegetarian Split Pea	230	1.5	40
White Chicken Chili	140	1.5	23
SandwichZ: on Ciabatta, half			
Chicken Greek w. Feta	430	12	50
Southwest Turkey	475	18	52
BLT w. Avocado	340	11	52
Bread: Per Piece			
French, 2 oz	150	2.5	21
Multigrain, 2.4 oz	185	2.5	35

Updated Nutrition Data ~ www.CalorieKing.com
Persons with Diabetes ~ See Disclaimer (Page 24)

Notes on Cholesterol

- **Cholesterol** is a white waxy substance produced mainly by our liver. It is also found in animal food products. Plant foods have no cholesterol.

- **Cholesterol is essential to life.** It is a structural part of every body cell wall and is the building block for vitamin D, sex hormones, and bile acids which help in the digestion of dietary fats.

- **The body makes sufficient cholesterol** for its needs and does not rely on cholesterol in the diet. Dietary fats have a major influence on blood cholesterol levels - more so than dietary cholesterol.

- **A high blood cholesterol level increases** the risk of atherosclerosis - the thickening of arteries that can reduce or block blood flow to the heart, brain, eyes, kidneys, sex organs and other body parts.

  This in turn increases the risk of heart attack, stroke, blindness, kidney failure, impotence and other blood circulatory problems.

  Other risk factors which increase the risk of atherosclerosis include high blood pressure, smoking, obesity and uncontrolled diabetes.

BLOOD CHOLESTEROL

CHECK YOUR RISK!

Total Cholesterol Level (mg/dl)		Risk of Heart Attack
240 and above	~	High Risk
200 - 239	~	Borderline/High
Below 200	~	Desirable

- ♥ Know your cholesterol level, particularly if there is a family history of heart disease or stroke. If level is high, see your doctor.

- ♥ All adults should have their cholesterol, HDL and triglycerides tested at least every 5 years.

HEART ATTACK WARNING SIGNALS

Many victims die before reaching the hospital by ignoring warning signals and delaying medical help.

Symptoms vary and commonly include:

- **Chest pain,** vice-like squeezing or burning sensation in center of the chest or between the shoulder blades, or in the mid-back. Pain may even feel like severe indigestion.
- **Pain** may be felt in the arms, shoulders, neck or jaw.
- **Shortness of breath** often occurs with or before chest discomfort.
- **Other signs,** with or without pain, include a cold sweat, nausea or light-headedness.

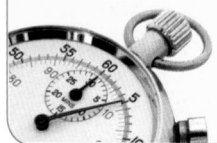

If you experience any of the above symptoms call IMMEDIATELY for medical help. Every minute counts.

Call 9-1-1 or your emergency number

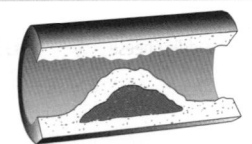

▲ Atherosclerosis can clog arteries and impede blood flow to the heart or other body organs.

▼ A thrombus (blood clot) can form on unstable, festering athero-sclerotic plaque and rapidly block blood flow. A heart attack or stroke can result.

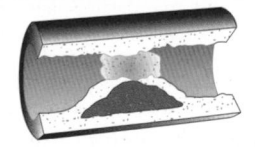

Fats & Cholesterol Guide

The amount and type of dietary fat has the greatest influence on blood cholesterol levels.

Fats in food are a mixture of 3 basic types: saturated, monounsaturated, and polyunsaturated. Animal fats are mainly saturated while plant oils and fish oils are mainly mono- and polyunsaturated.

Saturated fats have subgroups known as long-chain, medium-chain, and short-chain fats. Most of the long chain fats raise blood cholesterol, and increase the risk of blood clots and thrombosis leading to artery blockage.

Long-chain saturated fats are found mainly in full-cream milk, cheese, butter, cream, fatty meats and sausages, and processed foods.

Monounsaturated fats tend to more selectively lower 'bad' LDL cholesterol and maintain the protective 'good' HDL cholesterol in the bloodstream – but only if they replace saturated fats in the diet.

Foods rich in monounsaturates include canola and olive oils, canola margarine, peanuts, and avocados.

Polyunsaturated fats consist of two main classes. **Omega-6** polyunsaturates tend to lower blood cholesterol. Rich sources include safflower, sunflower and corn oils.

Omega-3 polyunsaturated fats can lower blood cholesterol; significantly lower blood triglycerides; and reduce the rise of thrombosis, heart arrythmmia, and artery spasm.

Best practical omega-3 sources include canola oil and margarine, soybean oil and fish.

A balanced intake of the two omega classes is important for optimal health. For most Americans, slightly increasing omega-3 intake would help attain a more ideal balance.

Trans fats from hydrogenated vegetable oils and shortenings should also be avoided. They are common in commercial baked and fried food products such as cakes, muffins, pastries, doughnuts, fried snacks and french fries.

> *Note: All fats are high in calories and need to be limited for weight control.*

DIETARY FATS COMPARISON

■ Saturated Fat ■ Monounsaturated Fat
Polyunsaturated Fats:
□ Linoleic (Omega-6) ■ Alpha-Linolenic (Omega-3)

OILS — PERCENTAGE CONTENT

Oil	Saturated	Monounsaturated	Linoleic	Alpha-Linolenic
CANOLA OIL	7	63	20	10
LINSEED/FLAX OIL	9	19	17	55
SAFFLOWER OIL	9	14	77	
GRAPESEED OIL	10	22	68	
SUNFLOWER OIL	11	23	66	
CORN OIL	14	32	52	2
OLIVE OIL	14	76	10	
SOYBEAN OIL	15	23	54	8
PEANUT OIL	19	45	34	2
COTTONSEED OIL	26	16	58	
PALM OIL	51	39	10	

SPREADS & FATS

Saturated Fat includes 'Trans Fats'   ☐ WATER CONTENT

Spread	Saturated	Monounsaturated	Linoleic	Alpha-Linolenic	Water
LIGHT MARGARINE	14	14	21		51
CANOLA MARGARINE	18	45	12	6	19
POLYUNSATURATED MARG	24	20	36		20
BUTTER	57	18	2		24
LARD	41	47			12
BEEF FAT	44	37	4		15

GOOD SOURCES OF OMEGA-3 FATS

Plant Sources	Omega-3 Fats (Grams)
Canola Oil, 1 Tbsp, ½ fl.oz	1.5g
Flaxseed Oil, 1 Tbsp	8g
Soybean Oil, 1 Tbsp	1.2g
Canola Margarine, 1 Tbsp, ½ oz	1g
Soybeans, cooked, ½ cup, 4 oz	0.5g
Walnuts, ½ oz	0.5g

FISH - *Per 4 oz Serving*

High Content: Salmon (Chinook), Tuna, Trout (Lake), Sardines, Herring, Mackerel — 3g / 3g

Medium Content:
Salmon, (Pink/Red/Coho), 4 oz — 2g

Fair Content: *Per 4 oz Serving*
Bass, Catfish, Cod, Grouper, Hake, Halibut, Kingfish, Perch, Pollock, Shark, Trout (Rainbow), Tuna, Crab, Oysters, Blue Mussels, Shrimp, Squid — 0.5-1g

How Much Is Needed?

As little as 1-2 grams daily of omega-3 fats may benefit general health. High doses of fish-oil supplements should only be taken as directed by your doctor.

Cholesterol in Food

Dietary Cholesterol

Cholesterol in food varies in its effect on blood cholesterol level (BCL) from person to person. Much depends on the amount and type of fat and fiber eaten at the same meal.

Any elevating effect of dietary cholesterol on BCL is more likely to occur when the diet is high in saturated fat. Little elevation, if any, generally occurs when dietary fats are balanced in favor of monounsaturated and polyunsaturated fats (including omega-3 fats).

For example, while fish does contain cholesterol, the omega-3 fats can prevent any increase in BCL. Conversely, a meal containing no cholesterol but rich in saturated fat may result in a significant increase in BCL.

Consequently, the need to be overly-concerned about dietary cholesterol is being de-emphasized in favor of the approach of limiting total fat, saturated fat, and trans fat in particular – and substituting unsaturated fats.

The liver usually cuts back its own cholesterol production in response to cholesterol in the diet. Many people can consume normal amounts of high-cholesterol foods without concern.

However, it is difficult to identify just who is at risk - the so-called 'hyper-responders'. Because over 50% of Americans have a BCL above ideal levels, the **American Heart Association** advises all Americans to be prudent and limit their cholesterol intake to less than 300mg daily, as well as to adopt a heart-healthy diet.

This limitation still allows the inclusion of most foods that are regularly eaten – even the overly-maligned egg.

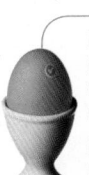

Eggs contain a modest 5 grams of fat per large egg, barely 2 grams of which are saturated, the rest being mono-unsaturated and polyunsaturated.

By comparison, a cup of whole milk has 8g fat of which almost 5g is saturated.

CHOLESTEROL COUNTER

Cholesterol is found only in foods of animal origin. Plant foods contain no cholesterol.
AHA recommends limiting dietary cholesterol to less than 300mg/day.

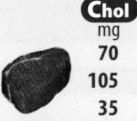

Food	Chol mg
Meat - Average all types:	
Lean Meat, cooked, 4 oz	70
Fatty Meat, cooked, 4 oz	105
Fat, thick strip, 2 oz	35

Note: While lean meat and fat have similar amounts of cholesterol, choose lean meat to limit fat intake.

Food	Chol mg
Chicken/Turkey, average, 4 oz	90
Organ Meats: Liver, fried, 4 oz	500
Brains, beef, pan fried, 3 oz	1700
Sausages: Frankfurter, 1.5 oz	25
Salami, 2 slices, 2 oz	40
Bacon: 3 slices, cooked, 1 oz	20
Fish: Fish fillets, average, ckd, 4 oz	70
Tuna/Salmon, canned, 3 oz	30
Scallops, 9 medium, 3 oz	30
Shrimp, 12 large, raw, 3 oz	130
Oysters, raw, 6 medium, 3 oz	45
Lobster, Crab, raw, 3 oz	80
Eggs (Chicken), 1 large	210
1 medium	180
Egg White, *Egg Beaters*	0
Milk/Yogurt: Whole, 1 cup, 8 fl.oz	35
1% Milk, 1 cup	10
Skim/Non-fat, 1 cup	5
Soy Milk, Tofu, Tempeh	0
Cheese: Natural/Hard/Cream, 1 oz	30
Cottage, lowfat, 4 oz	5
Ricotta, part skim, 4 oz	25
Fats: Butter, 2 Tbsp, 1 oz	60
Margarine, Oils (vegetable)	0
Mayonnaise, 1 Tbsp	10
Cream: Heavy, whipping, 2 T, 1 oz	40
Half & Half/Sour, 2 Tbsp, 1 oz	10
Ice Cream: Regular, ½ cup, 4 fl.oz	30
Fruit, Vegetables, Avocados	0
Nuts, Seeds, Grains	0
Coffee, Tea, Soda, Beer, Wine	0

For Comprehensive Food Listings ~ see CalorieKing.com

Blood Cholesterol ~ Diet Hints

DIETARY HINTS TO LOWER BLOOD CHOLESTEROL

1. **Maintain a healthy weight.**
   If overweight, lose weight with a low-fat meal plan and daily exercise.

2. **Reduce saturated fat intake by:**
   (a) eating less dairy fat. Choose low-fat or fat-reduced varieties of milk, yogurt, soy drinks, cheese, and ice cream.

   (b) replacing saturated fats with fats and oils rich in monounsaturated and polyunsaturated fats. Choose vegetable oils such as canola, olive, sunflower and soybean. Avoid solid frying fats.

   Take Control and *Benecol* (spreads) contain plant stanol esters which can lower total and LDL cholesterol.

   (c) eating less fat from meat and poultry. Choose lean cuts of meat and skinless chicken. Go easy on lunch meats, salami and fatty sausages. Enjoy fish.

   (d) eating less saturated and trans fats from baked and fried fast-foods. Avoid deep-fried foods. Avoid donuts, cakes, pastries and cookies unless made with healthier fats and oils.

3. **Increase your soluble fiber intake.**
   Foods rich in soluble fiber include beans, lentils, chick peas, hummus, nuts, seeds, psyllium-seed husks and psyllium-fiber supplements. Oat bran, rice bran and barley are also good sources, as are fruit, veggies and avocados. (*See Fiber Guide - Page 276-281*).

4. **Eat more soy bean products** such as:
   soy drinks, tofu, tempeh (cultured soy beans), soy flour and soy vegetarian foods. Soy protein in place of animal protein can significantly decrease high blood cholesterol levels as well as 'bad' LDL cholesterol and blood triglycerides while 'good' HDL cholesterol is maintained. For best results, eat at least 25g of soy protein per day (from 3-4 servings).

5. **Eat more fruit, vegetables, and whole grains** in place of high-fat foods. Aim for 2 fruits and 5 servings of vegetables per day. They also contain valuable antioxidants. The fat of avocados (and most nuts) is mainly unsaturated and can lower blood cholesterol levels.

6. **Limit cholesterol to 300mg per day.**
   (Extra Notes ~ See Previous Page)

7. **Avoid brewed unfiltered coffee** (espresso; plunger-style). Several cups per day may raise blood cholesterol. Filtered coffee is fine.

8. **Spread your food intake over the day.** Have 5-6 small meals per day rather than just 2-3 large meals. Nibbling, versus gorging, favors lower blood cholesterol.

ALCOHOL - WINE

Alcohol is a mixed bag. Moderate amounts of 1-2 drinks daily appear to reduce the risk of heart attack and ischemic stroke in older persons.

However, larger amounts increase the risk of high blood pressure, obesity, heart failure and hemorrhagic stroke, and can aggravate hypertriglyceridemia: as well as many other health hazards. (*See Alcohol Guide – Page 25*) The speculative benefits of moderate alcohol intake have been overstated in the media. The overriding harmful effects of excess alcohol do not allow its recommendation for any aspects of health promotion.

Fruit, Vegetables & Tea Also Protect:
Red wine and red grapes (more so than white) contain antioxidants which may help protect cholesterol in the blood from becoming oxidized.

Many fruits, vegetables, grains, nuts and tea also contain protective antioxidants.

Fats in the diet affect more than blood cholesterol levels. They can also strongly influence blood clot formation and thrombosis, as well as blood flow and ultimate oxygen delivery to body parts and organs.

While advanced atherosclerosis can impede blood flow to the heart and other organs, it is thrombosis (complete blockage by blood clots) or arterial spasm which commonly results in a heart attack or stroke.

Plant and fish oils rich in omega-3 fats lessen the risk of blood clots, thrombus formation, and artery spasm by reducing platelet stickiness and adhesion to artery walls. This reduces the risk of atherosclerotic plaque becoming unstable and reactive.

Omega-3 fats also improve blood flow by reducing blood viscosity and increasing the flexibility of red blood cells (RBC) that need to flex and twist on themselves in order to squeeze through tiny narrow capillaries often half their diameter.

A diet high in saturated fats has the opposite effect by stiffening RBC membranes and increasing blood viscosity, thereby hindering blood flow. The stiffening of the RBC membrane also reduces its ability to release vital oxygen to body cells and take up carbon dioxide.

Stiff red blood cells may also form aggregates that resemble coin stacks. In narrow blood vessels, this further impedes blood flow and impairs oxygen release through the much-lessened surface area of red blood cell membranes exposed to blood. (Smoking, lack of exercise, and stress can have similar adverse effects on thrombosis, red blood cell flexibility, and blood flow.)

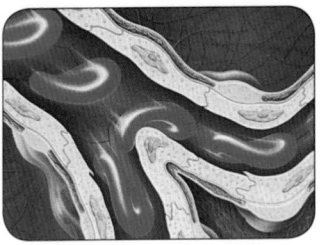

▲ **Picture of Healthy Blood Flow**

Flexible red blood cells twist and slide through tiny capillaries - often half the diameter of red blood cells.

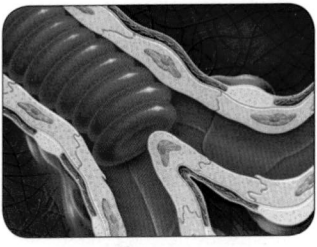

▲ **A Not-So-Healthy Picture!**

Red blood cells have lost their flexibility and ability to twist and slip through capillaries. They are stacked up, thereby impeding blood flow.

A diet high in saturated fats can contribute to this picture - as can smoking, lack of exercise, and stress.

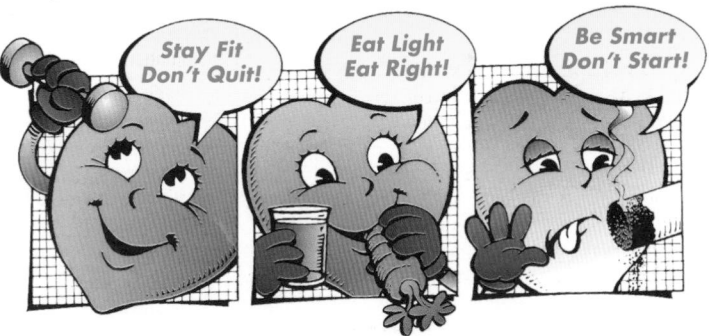

Fiber Guide

Introduction

Fiber is the general term for those parts of **plant** food that we cannot digest (although bacteria in the large bowel partly digests fiber through fermentation). It is not found in foods of animal origin (meats, dairy products).

Fiber promotes intestinal health, bowel regularity, can benefit diabetes and blood cholesterol levels, and may help prevent colon cancer. High-fiber foods also assist weight control.

Most Americans don't eat enough fiber - less than 20 grams/day - instead of a healthier **25 to 35 grams/day.**

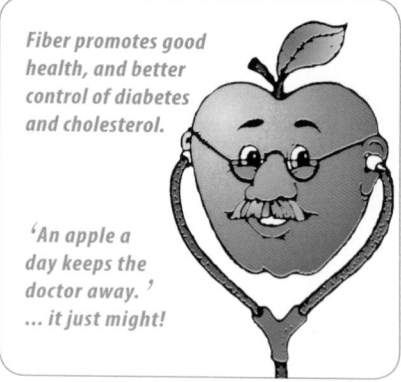

Fiber promotes good health, and better control of diabetes and cholesterol.

'An apple a day keeps the doctor away.' ... it just might!

Types of Fiber

Plant foods contain a mixture of different fibers in varying proportions. Insoluble and soluble fiber categories are based on their solubility in water. All types of fiber are beneficial to the body.

◆ **Insoluble fibers** (cellulose, hemi-celluloses, lignin) make up the structural parts of plant cell walls.

Best food sources are wheat bran, corn bran, rice bran, whole-grain cereals and breads, beans and peas, nuts, seeds, and the skins of fruits and vegetables.

These fibers absorb many times their own weight in water. They create a soft bulk and hasten the passage of waste products through the intestines.

They promote bowel regularity, and aid in the prevention and treatment of uncomplicated forms of **constipation, diverticulosis and hemorrhoids.**

The risk of colon cancer may also be reduced by fiber's diluting effect on potentially harmful substances.

◆ **Soluble fibers** (pectin, gums, mucilages) are found mainly within plant cells, soy milk (whole bean) and products.

Types of Fiber (Cont)

Best Sources of Soluble Fiber: Fruits and vegetables, oat bran, barley, beans and peas, prunes, psyllium and flax seed.

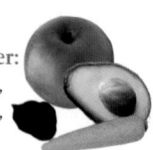

These fibers form a gel which slows both stomach emptying and the absorption of sugars from the intestines. **This helps to control blood sugar levels.**

Weight control is also aided by the slower emptying of the stomach and the feeling of **fullness provided by soluble fiber.**

Some soluble fibers can lower **blood cholesterol** by binding bile acids and excreting them. More body cholesterol must then be broken down to supply bile acids for emulsification of dietary fats. **Rice bran, while not high in soluble fiber, can also lower blood cholesterol.**

◆ **Resistant starch** is that part of starchy foods (approx. 10%) which is tightly bound by fiber and resists normal digestion. Friendly bacteria in the large bowel ferment and change the resistant starch into short-chain fatty acids, which are important to bowel health and may protect against colon cancer.

Starchy foods include bread, cereals, rice, pasta, potatoes and legumes.

Fiber & Weight Control

Fiber can assist weight control in several ways. Fiber-rich foods such as fresh fruit and vegetables, potatoes and whole-grain bread contain few calories for their large volume (due to their low-fat, high-water content).

Their bulk fills the stomach and satisfies the appetite much sooner than fiber-depleted foods. The extra chewing time also contributes to satiety, and gives the stomach time to register a feeling of fullness. Excessive calories are less likely to be consumed.

Fiber-depleted foods and drinks are more concentrated in calories; e.g. fats, sugar, candy, soft drinks, fruit juices, alcohol. They require little or no chewing. Large amounts with excessive calories can be consumed before the appetite is satisfied.

Example: Whereas one fresh apple might satisfy the appetite, an apple juice drink with the equivalent sugars and calories of 2-3 apples only minimally satisfies the appetite. (See illustration below.)

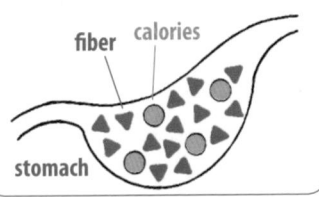

High-fiber foods fill the stomach. Fewer calories are consumed.

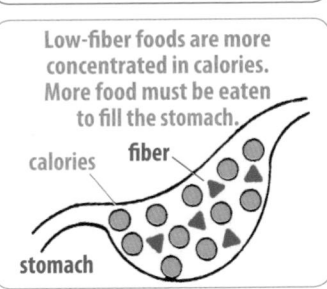

Low-fiber foods are more concentrated in calories. More food must be eaten to fill the stomach.

EFFECTS OF REMOVING FIBER FROM FOOD

2-3 pieces of fresh fruit produces 1 glass of fruit juice. The removal of fiber concentrates the sugar and calories.

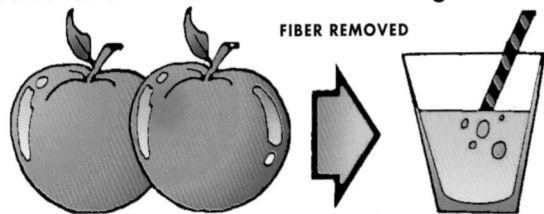

FIBER REMOVED

Fresh Fruit		Fruit Juice
High Fiber	←	Negligible Fiber
Low Calorie Density	←	High Calorie Density
Long Eating Time	←	No Eating Time (Drink)
Satisfies Hunger	←	Does Not Satisfy Hunger
Sugar Slowly Absorbed	←	Sugar More Quickly Absorbed
Less Insulin Required	←	More Insulin Required

Fiber Guide - Constipation

Constipation

Constipation can reasonably be defined as a failure to have a bowel movement at least every second day – and just as importantly, without straining or pain.

Typically, constipated stools are too hard, too narrow and too small.

The **main cause** is simply a lack of dietary fiber. Other contributing factors include insufficient fluids, too little exercise, emotional stress, gastrointestinal disease, lack of proper dentition to chew high-fiber foods, and some medications (e.g. some antacids, antidepressants, pain medications).

Note: Check with your doctor to rule out any underlying medical problem – especially if you have a change in bowel habits in middle-age or later years.

DESIRABLE FIBER INTAKE

Adults: 25-35gm per day
Children (under 18): Age + 5gm
Example: 6-year old (6 + 5)= 11gm

SAMPLE FOOD QUANTITIES
For 35 Grams of Fiber/Day

	Fiber
Breakfast Cereal (higher-fiber)	5g
plus 4 slices whole-grain Bread	6g
plus 3 servings fresh Fruit	9g
plus 1 medium Potato (w. skin)	
or 1 cup Brown Rice	4g
or ½ cup whole-grain Pasta	
plus 3-4 servings Veggies/Salad	6g
plus 1 cup Bean Soup	
or ¼ cup Baked/Soy Beans	
or ½ cup Corn/Peas/Lentils	5g
or 1¼ oz Almonds (natural)	
or 3 medium Figs	

HINTS TO INCREASE FIBER AND AVOID CONSTIPATION

❶ **Breakfast is an important** contributor to daily fiber intake. Eat high-fiber breakfast cereals (bran-based cereals, oatmeal etc.). Add 1-2 tablespoons of unprocessed bran.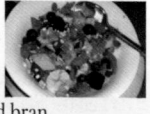
Dried fruits, chopped nuts, soy grits, and seeds are also excellent additions to cereals.
Note: A gradual increase in fiber will prevent bloating, gas or pain. People intolerant to bran may benefit from psyllium-based fiber supplements and cereals.

❷ **Drink adequate water daily.** Fiber works by absorbing many times its own weight in water.

❸ **Eat whole-grain breads,** or fiber-enriched breads. They have over double the fiber of regular white bread.

❹ **Enjoy fruit as fresh fruit** with skin rather than as fruit juice. Enjoy whole-grain pasta, barley, brown rice, nuts and seeds.

❺ **Eat more vegetables,** salads and legumes – especially cooked beans, lentils, potatoes with skins, avocado, broccoli, brussels sprouts, cabbage, carrots, celery, and peas.

❻ **Add bran** (barley/rice/wheat) or soy grits to soups, casseroles, yogurt, desserts, cookies, cakes. Also use whole-meal flour or soy flour in place of white flour. Use nuts, seeds, and ground linseed.

❼ **Snack** on fresh or dried fruits, carrot or celery sticks, popcorn, nuts or seeds, whole-grain crackers, high-fiber bars (low-fat). Limit amounts if overweight.

❽ **Exercise regularly** to strengthen abdominal muscles and stimulate the gut. Keep up water intake, especially in warm weather.

❾ **Avoid** indiscriminate and regular use of harsh laxatives. They can overstimulate the intestinal muscles and may make normal bowel activity impossible. It may take several weeks to restore normal bowel function.

Fiber Guide

FOODS WITH ZERO FIBER

- **Dairy Products (Milk, Cheese, etc)**
- **Meats, Poultry, Fish, Eggs**
- **Fats/Oils, Sugar/Syrups**

  (Only foods of plant origin contain fiber.)

Breakfast Cereals `Fiber`

General Mills:

Basic 4, 1 cup, 2 oz	3
Cheerios (Honey Nut; Multigrain), 1 c., 1 oz	3
Multi-Bran Chex, 1 cup, 2 oz	7
Oatmeal Crisp Almond, 1 cup, 2 oz	4
Raisin Nut Bran, 1¼ cup, 2 oz	5
Total, average all types, ¾ cup, 1 oz	3
Wheat Chex, 1 cup, 2 oz	5
Wheaties ¾ cup, 1 oz	3

Health Valley:

Amaranth Flakes, ¾ cup, 1 oz	4
Crunches & Flakes, ¾ cup, 1.9 oz	4
Fiber 7 Flakes, ¾ cup, 1 oz	4
Golden Flax, ¾ cup, 1.9 oz	6
Granola (Low-Fat), ⅔ cup, 2 oz	6
Healthy Fiber Flakes, ¾ cup, 1.1 oz	4
Oat Bran Flakes, all types, ¾ cup, 1 oz	3
Oat Bran O's, ¾ cup, 1 oz	3
Real Oat Bran, ½ cup, 1.7 oz	5

Kellogg's:

All-Bran, ½ cup, 1.1 oz	10
All-Bran w. Extra Fiber, ½ cup, 1 oz	13
All-Bran Bran Buds, ⅓ cup, 1.1 oz	13
Corn Flakes, Fruit Loops, Smacks 1 cup, 1 oz	1
Cocoa/Rice Krispies Treats, 1¼ cup, 1 oz	0
Complete: Wheat Bran Flakes, ¾ c., 1 oz	5
Oat Bran Flakes, ¾ cup, 1.1 oz	4
Corn Pops, 1 cup, 1.1 oz	0.5
Cracklin' Oat Bran, ¾ cup, 1.7oz	6
Frosted Mini Wheats, 24 bisc., 2 oz	5
Granola w. Raisins, ⅔ cup, 2.1 oz	3
Nutri-Grain Cereal Bars, 1 bar, 1.3 oz	1
Raisin Bran, 1 cup, 2.1 oz	7
Smart Start, Strong Heart, Cinnamon Raisin, 1 cup, 1.8 oz	4
Special K, 1 cup, 1.1 oz	0.5

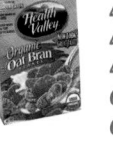
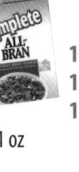
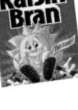

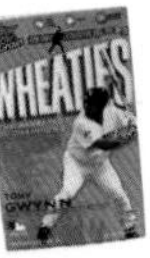

`Fiber` ~ Fiber (grams)

Breakfast Cereals (Cont) `Fiber`

Kashi: GoLEAN Cereal, 1 cup, 1.8 oz	10
GoLEAN Crunch!, 1 cup, 1.9 oz	8
GoLEAN Bars, avg. (1)	4
Good Friends: Original, 1 cup, 1.9 oz	12
Cinna-Raisin Crunch, 1 cup, 1.8 oz	8
Heart to Heart, ¾ cup, 1.2 oz	5
7 Whole Grain Pilaf, ½ cup, cooked, 5 oz	6
7 Whole Grain Puffs, 1 cup, 0.7 oz	1
Quaker: Cap'n Crunch, ¾ cup, 1 oz	1
100% Natural Granola, avg., ½ cup, 1.8 oz	3
Crunchy Corn Bran, 1 cup, 1 oz	5
Life Cereal, ¾ cup, 1.1 oz	2
Oat Bran, ½ cup, 1.4 oz	6
Oatmeal, average, 1 packet	3
Post: 100% Bran, ⅓ cup, 1 oz	9
Alpha Bits, 1 cup, 1 oz	3
Blueberry Morning, 1 cup, 1.9 oz	2
Cocoa/Fruity Pebbles, 1 cup, 1 oz	3
Cranberry Almond Crunch, 1 cup, 1.8 oz	3
Fruit & Bran, 1 cup, 1.9 oz	6
Grape-Nuts, ½ cup, 2 oz	6
Great Grains, ⅔ cup, 1.9 oz	4
Honey Bunches of Oats, ¾ cup, 1.1 oz	2
Shredded Wheat & Bran, ½ cup, 2 oz	6

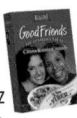
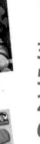
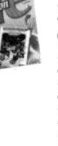
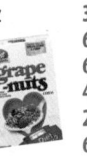

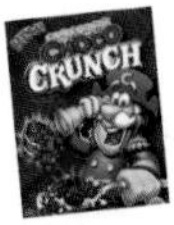

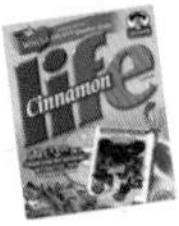

Brans & Supplements, Metamucil

Oat Bran: 1 Tbsp (level)	1
⅓ cup, (5½ Tbsp), 1 oz	5
Rice Bran, raw, ¼ cup, 1 oz	6
Wheat Bran (unprocessed):	
Raw, 1 Tbsp	1.5
2 Tbsp (level), ¼ oz	3
¼ cup, (4 Tbsp), ½ oz	6
Wheat Germ: Raw, ¼ cup, 1 oz	4
Psyllium Seed Husks, 2 Tbsp	8
Fibersure, 1 heaping tsp	5
Metamucil: Orange, 1 rnd Tbsp, 11g	3
Fiber Wafers (2)	6

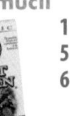
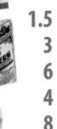
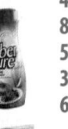

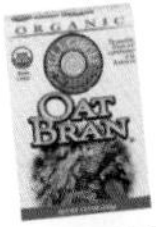

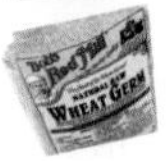

Hot Cereals, Oatmeal

Bulgur (cracked Wheat), ckd, 1 cup	8
Corn/Hominy Grits, dry, 3 Tbsp, 1 oz	0.5
Cream of Wheat, cooked, ¾ cup	1
Oatmeal (uncooked ⅓ cup), ckd, ⅔ cup	3

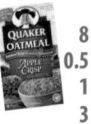

Fiber Guide

Breads & Crackers   `Fiber`

Bread: White, 1 slice, 1 oz — 0.6
Whole-wheat, 1 slice, 1 oz — 1.5
Whole-grain, 1 slice, 1 oz — 2
Rye, Pumpernickel, 1 oz — 1.5
Bagel/Roll/Bun, 1 medium, 2 oz — 1.5
Pita, whole wheat, 6½" pocket — 4.5
Crackers: Graham, average, 2 — 0.4
Saltine, 4 crackers — 0.4
Crispbreads (Rye), average, 2 — 4
Matzo 1 board, 1 oz — 1
Rice Cakes, average, 1 cake — 0.3
Tortilla: Regular, 6" — 0.5
Whole-wheat, 6" — 1.3

Barley, Pasta, Rice & Flours

Barley, pearled, raw, ¼ cup, 1.7 oz — 8
Rice: White, cooked, 1 cup — 0.6
Brown, cooked, 1 cup — 3.5
Rice-A-Roni, average, 1 cup, prepared — 1.5
Spaghetti/Noodles: Cooked, 1 cup — 2
Whole-Wheat, cooked, 1 cup — 4
Flour: Wheat, All-purpose, 1 cup, 4½ oz — 3.5
Whole-Wheat, 1 cup, 4½ oz — 15
Cornmeal, stone ground, 1 cup, 4½ oz — 13
Carob Flour, 1 cup, 3½ oz — 41
Rye Flour, 1 cup, 3½ oz — 15
Soy Flour: Defatted, 1 cup, 3½ oz — 17
Full-fat, raw, 1 cup, 3 oz — 8
Soy Meal, defatted, 1 cup, 4½ oz — 14

Frozen Entrees & Dinners

Average All Brands: Per Serving
Beans/Chili base, average — 6-10
Potato/Pasta base, average — 4-6
Vegetable base, average — 3
Meat/Chicken base, average — 2-3
Pizzas, ¼ large, average — 3
Vegetarian Soy Burgers, 1 pattie — 4

Soups

Chicken Noodle, 1 cup — 0.5
Tomato Soup, average, 1 cup — 0.5
Vegetable Soup, average, 1 cup — 3
Health Valley: Per 1 Cup Serving
Black Bean; Minestrone — 8
Tomato — 1
5-Bean Vegetable; Lentil & Carrots — 10
Mushroom Barley; Vegetable — 4
Split Pea — 8

Fast Foods & Restaurants   `Fiber`

Hamburgers: Small, average — 1.5
Large/Whopper, average — 2.5
Hot Dog, Regular — 1.5
French Fries: Small serving, 2½ oz — 2.5
Regular/Medium, 3½ oz — 3.5
Chicken Nuggets, 6 pack — 0.5
Chicken Sandwich, average — 2
Taco, average — 4
Sundaes, Shakes, Soft Drinks — 0
Arby's: Baked Potato w. Broc. & Cheese — 8
Roast Beef Sandwich, regular — 2
Denny's: Grilled Chicken Salad, no bread — 4
Classic Burger, no fries — 4
Club Sandwich, no fries — 2
Grilled Chicken Sandwich, no fries — 4
Domino's (12"): Classic/Thin, 1 slice — 1
Deep Dish, 1 slice — 3
Feast Pizza, Classic/Thin, 1 slice — 2
McDonald's: Big Mac — 3
Hamburger; Quarter Pounder — 1
Egg McMuffin — 2
Grilled Chicken Caesar Salad — 3
Pizza Hut: Per 1 Slice, Medium
Pan Pizza: Cheese, Pepperoni — 1
Supreme — 2
Thin 'n Crispy, Supreme — 2
Hand-Tossed, average all varieties — 2
Subway: Sandwich, white roll, avg. — 4
w. Honey Wheat Roll, average — 3.2
Footlong w. Wheat Roll, average — 8
Salads, average — 4

Cakes, Cookies, Snack Bars

Apple/Fruit Pie, 1 serving, 4 oz — 2
Cake: w. plain flour, 1 serving, 3.4 oz — 1.5
w. whole-wheat flour, 1 serving — 3
Carrot Cake, 1 serving, 1.2 oz — 2
Cookies, oatmeal, (3 small/1 large) — 1
Donuts, Medium, 1.7 oz — 0.7
Fruit Cake, 1 serving, 1½ oz — 2
Fig Bars, 1 cookie, ½ oz — 0.7
Muffins, Oat Bran (2 small, 1 large), 4 oz — 5
Granola Bars, average, 1 bar — 2
Atkins Advantage Bars, average — 7
Clif Bars, 2.5 oz — 5
Curves, Chocolate Peanut Bar, 25g — 5
Fi-Bar Chewy & Nutty 1 bar — 1
Health Valley: Fruit/Granola Bars — 3
Cereal Bars — 1
Luna Bars, avg., 1.7 oz — 3
Special K, Protein Meal Bar, 1.6 oz — 5

Fiber Guide

Chocolate, Chips, Popcorn — Fiber
Cheese Balls/Curls/Twists	1
Chocolate, Hard Candy, 1 oz	0
Chocolate with nuts/fruit, 2 oz bar	1.5
Mars Bar, 1.8 oz	1
Potato Chips, corn chips, 1 oz	1
Popcorn, 3 cups	3
Pretzels, Twists (6)	1

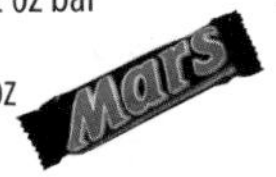

Nuts, Seeds
Almonds: Natural, 25 nuts, 1 oz	3.5
Blanched (skins removed), 1 oz	3
Cashews, Filberts, Pecans, 1 oz	1.7
Peanuts, Mixed Nuts, Coconut, 1 oz	2.5
Peanut Butter, 2 Tbsp, 1 oz	2
Pistachio Nuts, dried, shelled, 1 oz	3
Walnuts, Black/English, dried, 1 oz	2
Seeds: Amaranth, 2½ Tbsp, 1 oz	3.5
Flax Seeds, 3 Tbsp, 1 oz	7
Psyllium Seed Husks, 5 Tbsp, 1 oz	20
Quinoa Seeds, 3 Tbsp, 1 oz	1.7
Sesame Seeds, whole, 1 oz	3.4
Sesame Butter/Tahini, 2 Tbsp, 1.1 oz	1.4
Sunflower kernels, ¼ cup, 1 oz	3.8
Teff Seeds, 1 oz	3.8

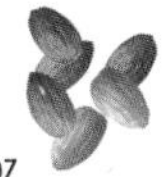

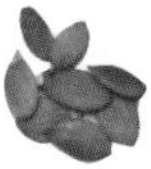

Fruit – Fresh
Apples: 1 medium, 5½ oz (whole)	
with skin + core	3.7
with skin, no core	3.2
without skin, no core	1.7
Apricots, 2 medium, 4 oz	1.5
Avocado, average, ½ medium	6.7
Banana, 1 medium, 6 oz (w. skin)	3
Blueberries, raw, ½ cup, 2½ oz	1.7
Cherries, sweet, raw, 8 fruits, 1.6 oz	1
Grapefruit, average, ½ fruit, 10 oz	1.4
Grapes, 1 medium bunch, seedless, 7 oz	2
Kiwifruit, 1 medium, 2.7 oz	2.3
Mango, 1 medium, 11 oz (whole)	1.6
Melons, Cantaloupe, 4 oz (edible)	1
Nectarine, 1 medium, 4 oz	1.9
Olives, average all types, 7 jumbo, 2 oz	1.5
Oranges, 1 medium (7-8 oz w. skin)	
5½ oz (peeled)	3.8
Passionfruit, 2 medium, 2½ oz	5
Peaches, 1 large, 6 oz	2
Pears, raw, 1 medium, 6 oz	4.5
Pineapple, 1 slice, 3 oz	1.2
Plums, 2 medium, 6 oz	1.8
Strawberries, 6 medium/3 large, 2 oz	1
Watermelon, 4 oz (edible)	0.5

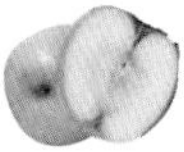

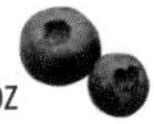

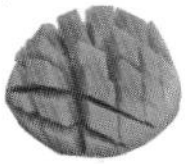

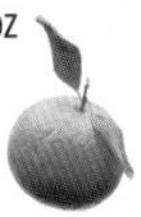

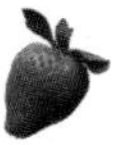

Fruit – Dried, Juice — Fiber
Dried Fruit: Apricots, 8 halves, 1 oz	2.2
Dates (3 med); Raisins (2 Tbsp), 1 oz	1.5
Figs, 3 medium, 1½ oz	5
Prunes, 4 medium, 1 oz	2
Fruit Juice: Orange/Apple etc, 1 glass	<0.5
Prune Juice, 5 oz	1.4
Carrot Juice, 8 oz	1.8

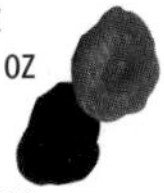

Vegetables
Asparagus, 4 medium spears	1.3
Bean Sprouts, ½ cup, 2 oz	1
Beans: Snap/Green, ½ cup, 2 oz	2
Baked Beans in Tom Sce, ½ c, 4½ oz	5
Dried Beans, ckd, average, ½ cup	7
Beets, ckd, slices, ½ cup, 3 oz	1.7
Broccoli, cooked, ½ cup, 3 oz	2.4
Brussels Sprouts, ckd, ½ cup, 3 oz	3.5
Cabbage: White, ckd, ½ cup, 2½ oz	1
Red, ckd, ½ cup, 2½ oz	2
Carrots, 1 medium (7½"), ½ cup, 3 oz	2.5
Cauliflower, cooked, 3 flowerets, 2 oz	1.5
Celery, raw, diced, 1 cup, 3½ oz	1.6
Chick Peas (Garbanzos), ckd, ½ c., 3 oz	6.5
Corn, kernels, ckd, ½ cup, 2½ oz	2.5
Cream-style, ½ cup, 4½ oz	1.5
Cucumber/Lettuce/Mushrooms, 2 oz	0.5
Eggplant, raw, sliced, ½ cup , 1½ oz	2
Lentils, cooked, ½ cup, 3½ oz	8
Mixed Vegetables, frozen, cooked, ½ cup	3
Onions, Raw, 1 medium, 4 oz	1.5
Spring Onions, chop., ¼ cup, 1 oz	0.7
Peas: Green, Raw, 2½ oz	3.7
Cowpeas (Black-eyed), ckd, ½ cup	10
Split Peas, ckd, ½ cup, 3½ oz	8
Peppers, sweet, raw, 1 large, 6 oz	3
Potatoes: 1 medium, with skin, 5 oz	4
without skin	2.5
½ cup mashed, 3½ oz	1.5
French Fries, small, 2.6 oz	3
Spinach, cooked, ½ cup, 3 oz	2.2
Squash: Summer, cooked, ½ cup, 3 oz	2.5
Winter, cooked, ½ cup, 3½ oz	2.4
Tomatoes: 1 medium, 4½ oz	1.5
Tomato Sauce, 1 cup	0.3
Soybean Products: Miso, ½ c., 5 oz	7.4
Tempeh, cooked, 1 piece, 3 oz	2
Tofu, ½ cup, 4.4 oz	0.4
Salads: Side Salad, average	1
Bean Salad, ½ cup	5
Coleslaw, ½ cup	1
Potato Salad, ½ cup	2

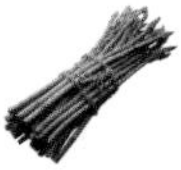

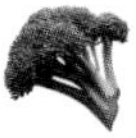

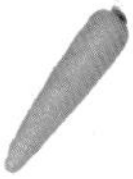

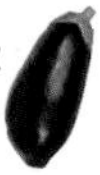

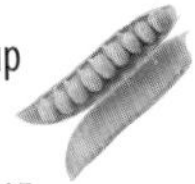

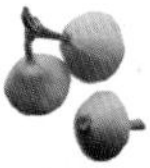

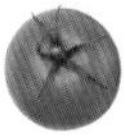

Protein Guide

General Notes

- **Protein has many important body functions.** It builds and repairs muscle, and is the basis of our body's organs, hormones, enzymes, and antibodies to fight infection.

- **Protein is also an emergency fuel** in the absence of sufficient carbohydrate and fats. For this reason, weight loss should be gradual so as to preserve protein levels in muscle, the heart and other body organs.

- **It is easy to obtain sufficient protein,** even if vegetarian. **Plant proteins are not inferior to animal proteins.** In fact, eating more soy and other plant proteins, and less animal protein, may help to build stronger bones and prevent osteoporosis, and may help to control blood cholesterol levels.

- **When changing to a vegetarian diet,** include soybeans, and other beans, soy milk drinks (calcium-enriched), lentils, tofu, tempeh, nuts and whole-grain breads and cereals. Milk, yogurt, cheese and eggs can enhance nutrient intake.

Protein & Muscle

- Although muscles are built of protein, protein is not a special fuel for working muscle cells – carbohydrates and fats are.

- In fact, a diet high in protein (and fat) and low in carbohydrate can significantly reduce the performance of endurance sports athletes. **Carbohydrates** are the best fuel for muscles exercised for long periods.

- Any **extra protein** required by athletes and body-builders can easily be obtained from the extra food eaten to satisfy hunger and energy needs.

- Remember, **excessive protein** intake will not build bigger muscles. Any excess is converted and stored as fat. Excess protein can also strain the kidneys, which excrete the waste products of protein metabolism.

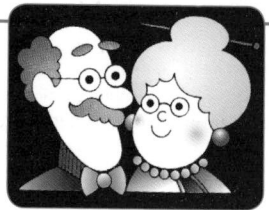

Elderly people (and dieters) must eat sufficient food to ensure adequate protein intake.

Inadequate protein leads to a drop in immune response with greater susceptibility to illness and infections. Muscle strength and muscle mass also drop.

Protein needs are easily met with sensible eating. Athletes who eat enough food for their energy needs can obtain sufficient protein.

RECOMMENDED DAILY PROTEIN INTAKE ~ HEALTHY RANGE ~
(Lower figure is RDA)

		PROTEIN
Children:	1-3 yrs	13g-26g
	4-8 yrs	19g-38g
	9-13 yrs	34g-64g
Males:	14-18 yrs	52g-120g
	19+	56g-120g
Females:	14+	46g-110g
Pregnancy:		71g-120g
Breastfeeding:		71g-120g

Note: On lower-calorie diets, aim for higher amounts of protein within the Healthy Range.

Iron & Anemia Guide

- **Iron deficiency** is one of the most common nutritional deficiencies in women. The risk is increased in dieters who do not eat well-balanced meals. Chronic shortage of iron leads to anemia.

- **Women** between 11 and 50 years of age are at greater risk because of the monthly loss of menstrual blood. Pregnancy, growth, and endurance sports also demand extra iron.

- **In red blood cells**, iron combines with protein to form **hemoglobin** – the red pigment which carries oxygen in the blood. A lack of iron limits the production of hemoglobin and consequently the amount of vital oxygen delivered to body cells.

Note: A blood test will tell you if your Hb and Iron stores (ferritin) are adequate. (Iron stores can be low even when Hb is normal.)

- **Vitamin C** (in fruits/veggies/salads) enhances absorption of 'non-heme' iron in bread, cereals, milk, vegetables, nuts, eggs and iron supplements. Small amounts of meat, fish or poultry also help. (They contain 'heme' iron).

- **Iron absorption is lessened** by up to 60% when high calcium foods are consumed with iron-rich main meals. Tea, coffee, phytates (in bran) and oxalates lessen absorption of non-heme iron.

- **For infants to 1 year,** use iron-fortified milk/soy formula if not breast-feeding. Introduce iron-fortified baby cereals at 4-6 months.

Note: Iron deficiency in children (even without anemia), can result in lethargy, irritability, repeated infections, and developmental problems.

Iron Supplements

- **Most people** can obtain adequate iron from their diet. A **wide variety** of animal and plant foods contain iron. (See Iron Counter)

- **Iron supplements** are only recommended for women with heavy menstrual blood losses or during pregnancy (if tests show a low-iron status), endurance athletes with low blood ferritin (iron stores) and for persons with diagnosed anemia. Check with your doctor.

- While the 5 mg of iron in multi-vitamin/mineral supplements is safe for most people, large amounts can be toxic, (especially for persons with hemochromatosis iron-overload condition).

ANEMIA SYMPTOMS

Anemia reduces the amount of oxygen carried in the blood. The body tissues become starved of oxygen. Symptoms include:

- **Pale skin; brittle fingernails (may turn up into spoon shape)**
- **Excessive tiredness or fatigue**
- **Breathlessness**
- **Feeling of malaise and irritability**
- **Always feel cold**
- **Decrease in attention span**

Note: Other medical conditions may also cause similar symptoms. Check with your doctor.

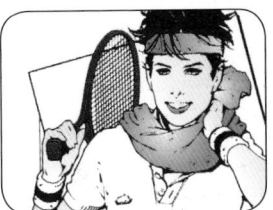

A nutritious diet with adequate iron is important - particularly for women and athletes.

RECOMMENDED DAILY IRON INTAKE (mg)

			Iron
Infants (0-6 mths):			
	Breast-fed	~	0.5mg
	Bottle-fed	~	3mg
	6-12 mths	~	11mg
Children:	1-11 yrs	~	7-10mg
Males:	12-18 yrs	~	11mg
	19+ yrs	~	8mg
Females:	12-18 yrs	~	15mg
	19-50 yrs	~	18mg
	51+ yrs	~	8mg
	Pregnancy	~	27mg
	Breast-feeding	~	12-16mg

Protein & Iron Counter

Pro ~ Protein (grams)   **Iron** ~ Iron (mg)

Meat

	Pro	Iron
Steak: Average all cuts, lean (no fat)		
Small (4 oz raw/3 oz ckd)	23	2.3
Medium (6 oz raw/4¼ oz ckd)	34	3.4
Large (10 oz raw/7¼ oz ckd)	57	5.7
Roast Beef, lean, 2 slices, 3 oz	24	2.5
Ground Beef patty, lean, ckd, 3 oz	21	2
Lamb chop, broiled, 3 oz	22	1.5
Liver, cooked, 3 oz	23	5.5
Veal cutlet, 1 medium	23	1
Pork, cooked, lean, 3 oz	24	1
Bacon, 3 medium slices	6	0.3
Ham, roasted, 2 pieces, 3 oz	18	1
Ham, luncheon, 2 slices, 1½ oz	7	0.3
Pastrami (Oscar Mayer), 3 sl., 1¾ oz	10	1.3
Sausages: Bologna, 2 sl., 2 oz	7	1
Braunschweiger, 2 sl., 2 oz	8	5.3
Pork link, thick, 2 oz	6	0.5
Frankfurter, 1⅓ oz	5	0.5
Salami, hard, 3 slices, 1 oz	7	0.5
Vegetarian (Boca Burger), 1 pattie	13	2

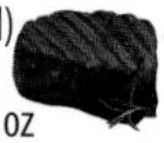

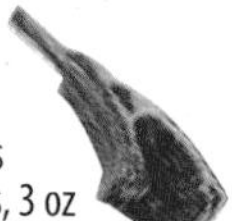

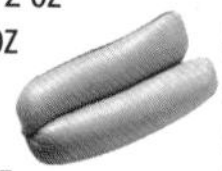

Chicken/Turkey (Without Skin)

	Pro	Iron
Chicken, ckd; Breast, Roasted, 4 oz	36	1.5
Leg/Thigh,Roasted, 2 oz	14	0.5
½ Whole Chicken	60	2.5
Drumstick, Rstd, 1 med., 3 oz	13	0.5
Turkey, cooked: Light meat, 3 oz	28	2
Dark meat, lean, 3 oz	24	2

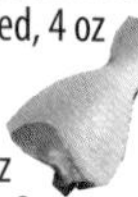

Fish

	Pro	Iron
Fresh Fish: Per 4 oz, cooked		
Cod, Flounder/Sole, Pollock	28	0.5
Catfish, Haddock, Halibut, M/Mahi	28	1.3
Ocean Perch, Swordf., Orange Roughy	28	1.3
Canned Fish: Tuna, Light, 3 oz	25	1.5
White, 3 oz	23	0.5
Salmon, pink, 3 oz	17	0.7
Salmon, red, 3 oz	17	1
Sardines, 3 whole (3"), 1¼ oz	9	1
Anchovies, 1 can, 1½ oz	13	2
Shellfish: Crabmeat, 3 oz	17.5	0.7
Clams, raw, 4 large/9 sml, 3 oz	11	12
Crayfish, cooked, 3 oz	20	2.7
Lobster, cooked, 3 oz	17	0.5
Oysters, raw, 6 medium, 3 oz	7	5
Scallops, 2 lge/5 small, 1 oz	5	0
Shrimp, raw, 6 large, 1½ oz	8.5	1
Fish Products: Fish Sticks, 4 sticks	10	0.5
Fish Portions, in batter, 4 oz	13	0.6
Gefilte Fish, 1 medium ball, 2 oz	8	1

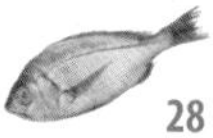

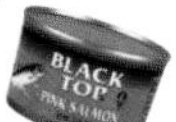

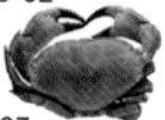

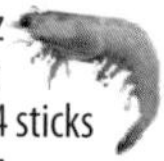

Eggs

	Pro	Iron
1 Large Egg, whole	6	0.7
Egg Yolk	3	0.7
Egg White	3	0
Omelet: Plain, 2 eggs	13	1.7
Ham & cheese	17	3
Egg Substitutes (liquid):		
Egg Beaters, ¼ cup, 2 oz	4.5	1
Better 'n Eggs/Scramblers, ¼ cup, 2 oz	6	0.7

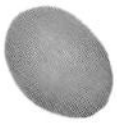

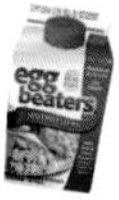

Milk, Yogurt, Ice Cream

	Pro	Iron
Milk: Whole: 2%, 1 cup	8	0
Low-Fat (1%); Fat-Free, 1 cup	8.5	0
Chocolate Milk, 1 cup	8	0.6
Thick Shake, Chocolate, 10 oz	9	1
Vanilla, 10 oz	11	0.3
Soymilk (fortified), average, 1 cup	7	1
Soy Dream Enriched, shelf-stable, 1 cup	7	8
Yogurt: Plain, 6 oz	10	0
Fruit flavors: 6 oz	8	0.3
8 oz	11	0.5
Ice Cream: Rich, ½ cup	2	0
Regular, Vanilla, ½ cup	2.5	0
Sherbet, ½ cup	1	0
Custard, baked, ½ cup	7	0.5

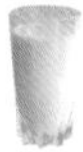

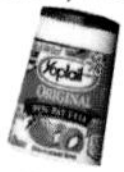

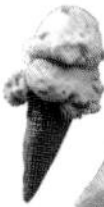

Cheese

	Pro	Iron
Hard Cheeses, average, 1 oz	7	0.2
Cottage Cheese, ½ cup	13	0.3
Cream Cheese, avg., 1 oz	2	0.3
Ricotta, part skim, ½ cup	14	1

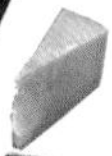

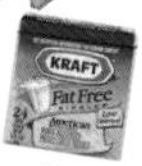

Bread, Bagels, Biscuits

	Pro	Iron
Bread (w. enriched flour): 1 slice, 1 oz	2	1
4 thin slices, 4 oz	8	4
4 thick slices, 6 oz	1.2	6
Bagel, plain 2 oz	6	1.5
Biscuits, 1 oz	2	0.7
Pita Bread, 1 pita, 1½ oz	4	1
Pumpernickel, 1 slice, 1 oz	3	1

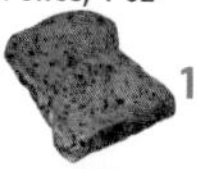

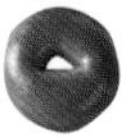

Infant/Baby Foods

	Pro	Iron
Infant Formula Milk:		
Enfamil/Gerber/Similac		
Regular/Low Iron , 5 fl.oz	2.2	0.2
With Iron, 5 fl.oz	2.2	1.8
Isomil/Nursoy/ProSobee	3	1.8
Baby Cereals:		
Average all brands		
Dry, 4 Tbsp, ½ oz	1	7
Jars (w. fruit), 4½ oz	1	7

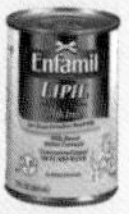

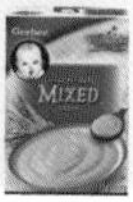

Breakfast Cereals

	Pro	Iron
Hot Cereals, cooked:		
Bulgur, cooked, 1 cup, 5 oz	9	2
Oatmeal: Reg., non-fortified, 1 cup	6	1.5
Instant, fortified, avg., 1 pkt	4	8
Quaker, all flavors, ½ cup	5	18
Corn/Hominy Grits: 1 cup	3	1.5
Quaker: Reg., 3 Tbsp, 1 oz	2	0.8
Instant White, 1 packet	2	8
Cream of Wheat, 1 cup	4	10
Brands ~ Ready-To-Eat		
Arrowhead: Average all varieties, 1 oz	3	1
General Mills: Basic 4, 1 cup, 2 oz	4	4.5
Cheerios, Original, 1 cup, 1 oz	3	8
Cocoa Puffs, 1 cup, 1 oz	1	4.5
Kix, 1⅓ cups, 1 oz	2	8
Multi-Bran Chex, 1 cup, 2 oz	4	16
Country Corn Flakes, 1 cup, 1.2 oz	2	8
Total Raisin Bran, 1 cup, 2 oz	3	18
Wheaties ¾ cup, 1 oz	3	8
Health Valley: Oat Bran O's, ¾ cup, 1 oz	3	0.7
Amaranth Flakes, ¾ cup, 1 oz	3	0.7
Bran Flakes w. Raisins, ¾ cup, 1.1 oz	5	1.5
Low-Fat Granola, ⅔ cup, 2 oz	5	1.4
Real Oat Bran Alm. Crunch, ½ cup, 1.7 oz	6	0.7
Golden Flax, ¾ cup, 1.9 oz	6	1
Kashi: Friends, 1 cup, 1.9 oz	5	1.8
GoLean Crunch!, 1 cup, 1.9 oz	9	1.8
7 Whole Grain Flakes, 1 c., 1.8 oz	6	1.4
Kellogg's: All-Bran, ½ cup, 1 oz	4	4.5
Complete Oat Flakes, ¾ cup, 1.1 oz	3	18
Cocoa Krispies, ¾ cup, 1 oz	1	4.5
Corn Flakes, 1 cup, 1 oz	2	8
Low-fat Granola w. Raisins ⅔ c., 2.1 oz	4	2
Product 19, 1 cup, 1 oz	2	18
Raisin Bran, 1 cup, 2 oz	7	4.5
Rice Krispies, 1¼ cup, 1.2 oz	2	9
Smart-Start Healthy Heart, 1 c., 1.8 oz	6	4.5
Special K: Regular, 1 c., 1.1 oz	6	8
Protein Plus, ¾ cup, 1 oz	10	8
Post: Raisin Bran, ⅔ cup, 2 oz	4	11
Grape Nuts, ½ cup, 2 oz	6	16
Quaker: Crunchy Corn Bran, 1 cup, 1 oz	2	8
100% Natural Granola, ½ cup, 1.7 oz	5	1.4
Life, ¾ cup, 1.1 oz	3	8
Cap'n Crunch, ¾ cup, 1 oz	1	4.5
Oat Bran, ½ cup, 1.4 oz	7	2.7

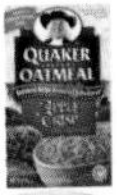

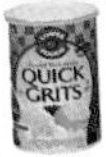

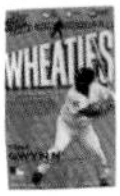

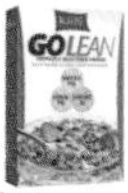

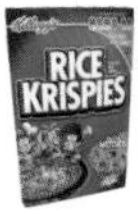

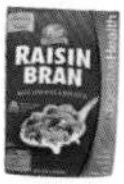

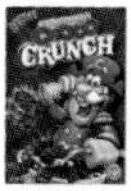

Brans & Wheatgerm

	Pro	Iron
Oat Bran, raw, 1 Tbsp	2	0.5
Rice Bran, raw, 2 Tbsp	1	1
Wheat Bran, unprocessed, 2 T.	1	1
Wheat Germ, 2 Tbsp, ½ oz	4	1.3

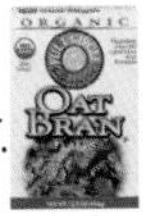

Grains & Flours, Yeast

	Pro	Iron
Amaranth, ½ cup, 3.4 oz	14	7
Barley, ½ cup, 3.2 oz	12	2
Buckwheat Flour: Whole-groat, 1 cup	15	2.7
Carob Flour, 1 cup, 3.6 oz	5	3
Corn Flour, 1 cup, 4 oz	11	2
Corn Meal, 1 cup, 4½ oz	8	3.5
Flour: White, 1 cup, 5.6 oz	9	6
Whole-grain, 1 cup, 4¼ oz	16	5
Millet, whole-grain, 1 cup, 3½ oz	12	7
Rye Flour: Dark, 1 cup, 4½ oz	18	6
Light, 1 cup, 3½ oz	9	1
Soy Flour, full fat, 1 cup, 3 oz	29	5.5
Yeast: Brewers, 2 Tbsp, ½ oz	8	1.5
Nutritional Yeast Flakes *(Red Star)*, 1 heaping Tbsp, ½ oz	8	0.8

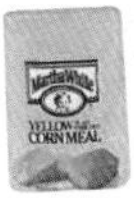

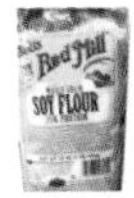

Rice, Spaghetti, Macaroni

	Pro	Iron
Rice: Brown/White, average 1 cup cooked, 6½ oz	5	1
Spaghetti/Macaroni/Noodles (enriched):		
Cooked, 1 cup, 4½ oz	7	2
Canned: in Tomato Sce, ½ c	2	0.5
w. Meatballs, 1 cup, 8 oz	10	2
Macaroni & Cheese, 1 c., 9 oz	8	1

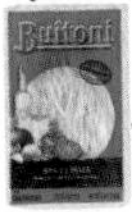

Soups

	Pro	Iron
With Noodles/Vegetables, 1 c.	3	0.5
With Meat/Beans/Peas, 1 c.	8	1.5

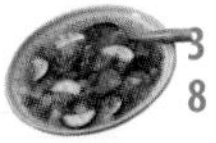

Fruit

	Pro	Iron
Fresh/Canned:		
Average, all types 1 medium/2 small fruit	1	0.5
Avocado, ½ medium	2	1
Dried Fruit: Apricots, 8 halves, 1 oz	1	1.3
Dates, 6 dates, 2 oz	1.5	0.7
Figs, 4 medium figs, 2 oz	2	1.7
Prunes, 5 medium, 1½ oz	1	1
Raisins, 1 oz	1	0.7
Fruit Juice: Average, 1 cup	0.5	0.5
Prune Juice, 6 fl.oz	1	2.5
Tomato Juice, 1 cup, 8 fl.oz	1.5	1

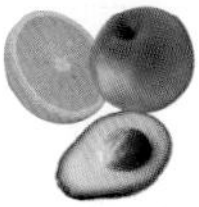

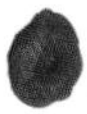

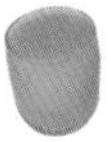

Protein & Iron Counter

Vegetables	Pro	Iron
Beans: Snap/green, ½ cup, 2 oz	1	0.8
Dried: Average all types, cooked, ½ cup	7	2.5
Baked Beans, ½ cup 4½ oz	5	2
Bean Sprouts, mung, 1 c., 4 oz	3	1
Broccoli, 3 raw, ½ cup, 1½ oz	1.5	0.7
Cabbage; Cauliflower, raw, 1 c. 3 oz	1.5	0.6
Corn, raw, ½ cup kernels, 3 oz	2.5	0.3
1 ear trimmed to 3½"	2	0.4
Lentils, cooked, ½ cup, 3½ oz	9	3.3
Mushrooms, raw, ½ c., sliced	1	0.3
Peas: Green, raw, ½ c., 2½ oz	4	1.2
Split Peas, cooked, 1 cup, 7 oz	16	2.5
Potatoes, cooked:		
1 medium, with skin, 5 oz	3.3	2
without skin, 4 oz	2.3	1
French Fries, small, 2.6 oz	2	1
Potato Salad, ½ cup, 4 oz	3.5	2.5
Pumpkin, ½ cup mashed, 4.3 oz	1	1
Seaweed, kelp, 1 oz	<1	2.5
Spinach, cooked, ½ cup, 3 oz	2.7	3.5
Squash, ckd, all types, ½ cup	1	0.3
Tomatoes, 1 medium, 4½ oz	1	0.6
Vegetables, mixed, ckd, 1 cup	2.5	0.7
Soybeans, cooked, ½ cup, 3 oz	14	4.4

Tofu, Tempeh, Miso	Pro	Iron
Tofu, raw, firm, ½ cup, 4½ oz	10	1.5
Tempeh, ½ cup, 3 oz	16	2
Miso, ½ cup, 5 oz	16	4
Miso Soup, 1 cup	3	0.4
Soybean Protein (TVP), 1 oz	18	3

Cakes, Pastries, Pies	Pro	Iron
(Made with enriched flour)		
Carrot w. cream cheese frosting, 4 oz	4	1.3
Cheesecake, 1 piece, 4 oz	6	0.5
Chocolate, 1 piece, 2 oz	4	2
Fruitcake, 1 piece, 3 oz	4	2
Plain, 1 piece, 3 oz	4	1.2
Croissant, plain, 2 oz	5	2
Danish Pastry, 1 pastry, 2¼ oz	4	1.3
Donuts, average, 2 oz	4	1.2
Muffins, average, 1 med., 1½ oz	3	1
Pancakes, 4" diam., two, 2 oz	4	1
Pies: Fruit, 1 piece, 5½ oz	4	1.5
Pecan, 1 piece, 5 oz	7	4.5
Puddings, average, ½ cup, 4½ oz	4	0.3
Waffles, 1 large, 2½ oz	7	1.5

Peanut Butter	Pro	Iron
Regular: 2 Tbsp, 1.1 oz	8	0.5
Peter Pan Plus, 2 Tbsp, 1.1 oz	8	4.5

Sugar, Honey, Jam	Pro	Iron
Sugar: White	0	0
Brown, 1 Tbsp	0	0.3
Molasses: Light/Med., 1 Tbsp	0	1
Blackstrap, 1 Tbsp, ¾ oz	0	3
Corn Syrup, 1 Tbsp, ¾ oz	0	1
Honey, Jams, Jelly	0	0.2

Candy, Chocolate, Carob	Pro	Iron
Candy, sugar-based	0	0
Chocolate: Plain, 2 oz bar	4	0.8
with nuts, 2 oz bar	6	0.8
Carob, plain, 2 oz	6	0.7

Cookies, Crackers, Chips	Pro	Iron
Cookies, average, 4 cookies	2	1
Crackers, Graham, 2½" sq., (2)	1	0
Rice Cakes, average, one	1	0
Corn/Potato Chips, 1 oz	2	0.3

Nuts: Almonds, shelled, 20-25 nuts	Pro	Iron
Almonds, shelled, 20-25 nuts	6	1
Brazil Nuts, 7-8 medium nuts, 1 oz	4	1
Cashews, 12-16 nuts, 1 oz	5	1.5
Macadamias, 1 oz	2	0.5
Peanuts, dry rsted, 40 nuts, 1 oz	6	0.6
Pecans, 24 halves, 1 oz	2	0.5
Walnuts, 15 halves, 1 oz	4	0.7

Seeds: Sesame Seeds, dry, 1 Tbsp	Pro	Iron
Sesame Seeds, dry, 1 Tbsp	2	0.6
Pumpkin Kernels, dry, hulled, 1 oz	7	4.2
Sunflower Seeds, dried, hulled, 1 oz	6	2
Tahini, 1 Tbsp, ½ oz	2.5	1.4

Granola & Food/Protein Bars	Pro	Iron
Granola Bars, avg., 1 bar, 2 oz	2	0.5
Balance Bars, Orig. 1.76 oz	14	4.5
Bariatrix Proti-Bars (1), 1.4 oz	15	0.7
dotFIT: Breakfast Bars, 1.94 oz	15	1
Protein Sticks, 1.76 oz	12	1
Dr Soy Protein Bars, 1.76 oz	11	18
GeniSoy Protein Bar, 1.6 oz	15	6.3
Jenny Craig Bars, 1.8 oz	4	3.6
Met-Rx "Big 100", 3.5 oz	27	7.2
Myoplex Carb Sense Bar, 2.5 oz	26	2
Optifast Peanut Butter, 1.59 oz	8	0.5
Planters Carb Well Bar, 1.2 oz	6	1
PowerBar: Harvest	10	4.5
Performance Bar, 2.3 oz	10	6.3
ProteinPlus, 1 bar, avg., 2.75 oz	24	8
Slim-Fast: High Protein Meal, 1.7 oz	15	2.7
Optima Meal, 2 oz bar	8	2.7
Special K: Protein Meal, 1.6 oz	10	1.8
Protein Snack, 0.9 oz	4	0.7

High Protein Drinks

	Pro	Iron
Atkins Shakes, 11 fl.oz can	18	2.7
Boost High Protein, 8 oz	10	3.5
Carnation Instant Breakfast, 10 oz	13	4.5
Curves Protein Drink, 2 scoops, dry	15	18
dotFIT: FirstString, 4 scoops, 5.2 oz	42	2.5
Meal Replacement,		
Chocolate, 2 scoops, 2.2 oz	20	3.2
WheySmooth, Choc., 2 scoops, 2.2 oz	40	1.8
Ensure Plus, 8 oz can	13	2.3
Gatorade: Nutrition Shake, 11 oz	20	1.8
Protein Recovery Shake, 11 oz	20	0
GeniSoy Shake, 1 scoop, 1.2 oz	14	3.6
Kashi GoLean Shake, 2 sc., 2.1 oz	21	2.7
Lightfull, Chocolate, 8.25 oz	5	2.7
Other flavors, avg. 8.25 oz	5	0.4
Met-Rx RTD 40	40	4.5
Myoplex, Original Nutrition Shake, 1 pkt	42	5.4
Optifast 800, made up, 8 fl oz	14	3.6
Resource (Novartis) Standard, 8 fl.oz	15	4.5
Revival Soy, Plain, 58g pkt	20	3
Slim-Fast Shakes: Meal, 11 oz can	10	2.7
High Protein, 11 oz can	15	2.7
Optima, 11 oz can	10	2.7
Special K20 Protein Water, 16 fl.oz	5	0
Walgreens Slim For Less, 11 oz can	10	2.7
Weider Mass 1000, 4 scoops, 7 oz	34	6

Coffee, Tea, Soda

	Pro	Iron
Coffee, Coffee Substitutes, 1 cup, 8 fl.oz	0	0
Coffee w. 2 oz milk, 1 cup, 8 fl.oz	2	0
Caffe latte, large, 16 fl.oz	12	0
Cappuccino, large, 16 fl.oz	8	0
Frappuccino, avg., 16 fl.oz	6	0
Hot Chocolate,		
with milk, 1 cup, 8 fl.oz	8	1.2
Soft Drinks/Soda	0	0
Tea (all types)	0	0

Beer, Wine, Spirits

	Pro	Iron
Beer, 12 fl.oz	1	0
Wines, red/white, 1 glass	0	0.4
Spirits/Liquor	0	0

Fast-Foods/Burgers

	Pro	Iron
Pancakes: Average all outlets, 3	8	2
Shakes, Chocolate, 16 fl.oz	12	0.4
Sundaes: Average all outlets	7	0.3
Arby's: Roast Beef Sandwich, regular	20	4.6
Chicken Club Salad	32	3.8
Roast Beef Sandwich, Super	21	3.8
Burger King: Whopper S/wich	29	5.4
Bacon Double Cheeseburger	32	4.5
BK Big Fish Sandwich	24	4.5

Fast Foods/Burgers (Cont)

	Pro	Iron
Carl's Jr:		
Famous Star Hamburger	24	2
Charbroiled Chicken Club Sandwich	40	3
Super Star Hamburger	41	3
Domino's Pizza: Deep Dish (12")		
Beef, 2 slices	4	0.7
Cheese, 2 slices	16	3.6
Pepperoni, Sausage, 1 sl.	10	1.8
KFC: Original, Breast	37	1
Crispy Strips, 3 strips	29	1.8
Snacker, Regular	15	2.7
McDonald's: Big Mac	25	4.5
Cheeseburger	15	2.7
Chicken McNuggets (6)	14	0.7
Crispy Chicken Classic Burger	28	3.6
Filet-O-Fish	15	1.8
Hamburger	12	2.7
Quarter Pounder w. Cheese	29	4.5
French Fries: Small, 2.5 oz	3	0.7
Large, 5.4 oz	6	1.5
Salads w. Chicken, average	29	2
Thick Shake, average, 16 fl.oz	13	0.7
Breakfast: Egg McMuffin	18	3.6
Bacon, Egg & Cheese McGriddles	16	2.7
Sausage Burrito	12	2.7
Sausage McMuffin w. Egg	21	3.6
Pizza Hut: Per Medium, 1 slice, 1/8 Pizza		
Thin 'n Crispy, Supreme	11	1
Pan Pizzas, average	10	2
Hand Tossed, Pepperoni	11	1.5
Fit n' Delicious, Ham/Pineapple	8	1
Subway (6" Subs): Roast Beef	19	6.3
Meatball Marinara	24	7.2
Roast Chicken Breast	24	4.5
Subway Club	24	5.4
Sweet Onion Chicken Teriyaki	26	4.6
Taco Bell: Bean Burrito	13	2.7
Chicken Quesadilla	28	1.8
Chicken/Steak Enchirito	21	1.8
Gordita Baja Beef	13	2.7
Steak Burrito Supreme	18	2.7
Taco Supreme	9	1
Tostado	11	1.5
Wendy's: Old Fashioned Single Burger	25	4.5
Chicken Club	34	2.7
Hamburger (Kid's Meal)	15	2.7

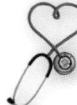

High Blood Pressure

High Blood Pressure

Many American adults have hypertension (high blood pressure), and are unaware of it. It is generally symptomless, so **have your blood pressure checked annually** – particularly if it runs in the family.

Untreated hypertension overworks the heart, damages arteries and promotes atherosclerosis. This in turn greatly increases the risk of heart disease, stroke, blindness, kidney disease and impotence. The earlier hypertension is detected, the sooner it can be brought under control.

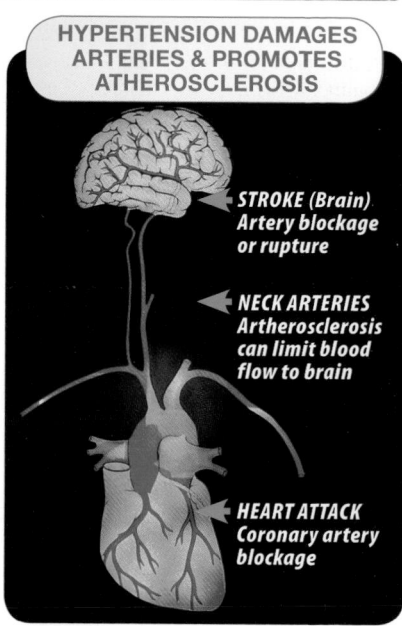

HYPERTENSION DAMAGES ARTERIES & PROMOTES ATHEROSCLEROSIS

STROKE (Brain)
Artery blockage or rupture

NECK ARTERIES
Artherosclerosis can limit blood flow to brain

HEART ATTACK
Coronary artery blockage

BLOOD PRESSURE CLASSIFICATION

For Adults Age 18 & Older ~ Not Acutely Ill or on Medication (American Heart Association)

	DIASTOLIC		SYSTOLIC
Normal ▶	Below 80	and	Below 120
Prehypertension ▶	80-89	or	120-139
Hypertension:			
Stage 1 ▶	90-99	or	140-159
Stage 2 ▶	100 or more	or	160 or more

Treating Hypertension

Prehypertension (in the chart above) means you don't have high blood pressure now but are likely to develop it in the future.

You can take steps to lessen the risk by adopting healthy lifestyle habits such as:
- reducing sodium intake
- eating adequate fruit and vegetables
- losing weight if overweight
- limiting alcohol to 2 drinks or less daily
- quitting smoking
- exercising regularly, managing stress.

Stage 1 hypertension can often be treated with the above lifestyle changes.

Stage 2 hypertension usually requires drug therapy. However, salt restriction, abstaining from alcohol, and the above lifestyle changes will improve the success of drug therapy, and enable smaller drug doses to be prescribed.

STROKE
KNOW THE WARNING SIGNS

Stroke is a medical emergency! If you notice one or more of these signs, call 9-1-1 or your doctor immediately.

These signs may be signalling a possible stroke or transient ischemic attack:

- **Sudden weakness** or numbness in your face, arm, or leg on one side of your body
- **Sudden confusion,** trouble speaking or understanding
- **Sudden trouble seeing,** in one or both eyes
- **Sudden trouble walking,** dizziness, loss of balance or coordination
- **Sudden severe headache** - 'a bolt out of the blue' – with no apparent cause

Salt & Sodium

- **Sodium is a mineral element** most commonly found in salt (sodium chloride). It also occurs naturally in much smaller amounts in animal and plant foods, and water – normally sufficient for our needs without having to add salt to our diet.

- **Sodium is required** for nerve and muscle function, as well as to balance the amount of fluid in our tissues and blood.

  Sodium acts like a sponge to attract and hold fluids in body tissues.

- **Excess sodium** can cause water retention, and increase the risk of developing hypertension. Very high salt intake may also increase the risk of stomach cancer.

- **Too little sodium** may cause low blood pressure (hypotension), and decrease blood flow to the heart, brain and kidneys - especially during exercise. (A certain blood volume is required to sustain the blood pressure needed for adequate blood flow in the capillaries).

Salt-Sensitive Persons

- **Normally, our kidneys** excrete excess dietary sodium. The thirst we feel after a salty meal is the body calling for water to dilute the sodium, and enable the kidneys to flush out excess sodium.

- **However, 'salt - sensitive'** persons (up to 50% of adults) tend to retain excess sodium (above approximately 3000mg daily) instead of excreting it. Such persons are more likely to develop hypertension and would benefit most from sodium restriction. Assume you are susceptible if there is a family history of hypertension.

- **Although not everyone will benefit, all Americans are being asked to moderate their salt and sodium intake** as a public health measure – particularly because so many do not know whether or not they have hypertension, and also because we do not know just who is salt-sensitive.

SAFE SODIUM LEVELS

The American Heart Association recommends a **maximum sodium intake of 2300mg per day** for adults with normal blood pressure. However, people who consume **less than 1500mg sodium** have the lowest blood pressure levels.

Persons with hypertension and kidney ailments are usually restricted to as little as **1000mg sodium per day**. Your doctor will discuss the correct sodium level for you.

Persons with Menière's Disease (chronic attacks of vertigo, dizziness, hearing loss, imbalance), often benefit from lower sodium intake of less than 2000mg/day, as well as even distribution of food and fluids over the day (to prevent fluctuations in body fluids and pressure in the inner ear). Also avoid caffeine and MSG. Limit sugar and alcohol.

further info: www.CalorieKing.com

FINDING HIDDEN SODIUM

On average, **less than one third of our sodium intake comes from the salt shaker.**
The rest is hidden in processed foods that have salt added during manufacture.

Sodium compounds added to food or medicinals can also contribute significant sodium.

Sodium bicarbonate in particular is widely used in antacid tablets (such as Alka Seltzer) and powders. Sodium bicarbonate contains 27% sodium by weight. Each gram contributes 270mg sodium. Large amounts of sodium can be unwittingly consumed – up to 600mg per tablet. (See Antacids ~ Page 293)

Example: 2 Alka-Seltzer Tablets = 1000mg sodium

Other sodium compounds include monosodium glutamate (MSG), sodium ascorbate, sodium nitrite, and sodium citrate.

ALCOHOL DANGER

Excessive alcohol intake contributes to hypertension. Susceptible persons should limit alcohol intake to 1-2 drinks per day.

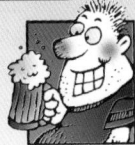

Salt Sodium Guide

Sodium accounts for only 40% of the weight of salt (sodium chloride). Examples:
1 gram (1000mg) Salt has 400mg Sodium
1 teaspoon (5g) Salt has 2000mg Sodium

HINTS TO REDUCE SODIUM

- **Cut down use of the salt shaker.** Start with an easy 50% cut in sodium by using Lite Salt (*Morton*) or *Cardia* Salt. Then gradually cut back until you can leave the salt shaker off the table. Sea salt is still high in sodium.

- **Use fresh herbs**, and salt-free seasonings to add flavor to food.

- **Choose low-sodium**, sodium-free, and reduced-sodium products in place of regular, salted products.

- **Check food labels for sodium levels.** FDA Guidelines for sodium descriptors are:
  - **Reduced Sodium:** At least 25% less sodium than the original product
  - **Low Sodium:** 140 mg or less/serving
  - **Very Low Sodium:** 35mg or less/serving
  - **Sodium Free:** Less than 5mg/serving
  - **No Salt Added:** Made without the salt normally added, but still contains the sodium that is a natural part of the food

- **Use reduced-sodium breads**, butter and margarine. Regular varieties contain up to 2% salt. This is considered high in view of their significant contribution to our diet.

- **Go easy on salty condiments and sauces** such as ketchup, mustard, soy sauce, spaghetti sauces, and salad dressings. Use low-sodium varieties.

- **Limit pizzas and salty fast-foods.** Check *CalorieKing.com* food database.

- **Avoid salty snack foods** such as potato chips, corn chips, salted nuts, pretzels and cheesy-flavored snacks. **Choose unsalted** popcorn, nuts or seeds. Eat more fruit.

- **Don't salt children's food** to your taste.

- **Avoid antacids with** sodium bicarbonate (such as *Alka-Seltzer*). They are high in sodium. Look for low-sodium alternatives.

FOODS HIGH IN SODIUM

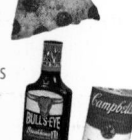

- Cheese, Butter, Margarine
- Pickles, Sauerkraut, Olives
- Condiments, Sauces
- Salad Dressings
- Canned vegetables/salads/beans
- Deli Salads (with dressing)
- Frozen/Packaged Meals/Entrees
- Soups: Canned/dry; bouillon cubes
- Meats: Ham, bacon, sausage, luncheon meats, smoked meats
- Canned Fish (in brine/salt)
- Sea Salt, Garlic/Celery Salt
- Snack Foods (potato chips, pretzels)
- Tomato Juice (Canned), V8 Vegetable Juice
- Fast Foods: Pizza, Burgers, Chicken
- *Alka-Seltzer* Antacid

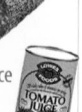

MODERATE SODIUM

- Bread (Reduced Salt)
- Meat, Fish, Poultry - Unprocessed
- Milk, Yogurt, Soy Drinks, Eggs
- Peanut Butter
- Breakfast Cereals (less than 200mg/serving)
- Chocolate Candy, Fruit/Nut Bars
- *Reduced Sodium & Low Sodium Products*

FOODS LOW IN SODIUM

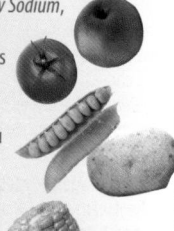

- Products labelled *Very Low Sodium*, or *Sodium Free*
- Fresh fruits and vegetables
- Canned and Dried Fruits
- Potatoes, Rice, Pasta
- Dried Beans & Lentils, Tofu
- Nuts & Seeds (unsalted)
- Corn & Popcorn (unsalted)
- Pepper, Spices, Herbs
- Jam, Honey, Syrup
- Candy, Gum
- Hard & Jelly Candy
- Coffee, Tea, Alcohol
- Fresh Fruit Juices, Water

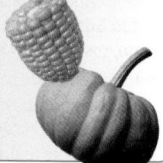

The American Heart Association recommends a sodium intake of **less than 2300mg/day**

Milk & Dairy Products

	Sodium
Milk: Whole/lowfat/skim, average 1 cup, 8 fl.oz	120
Whole, low sodium, 1 cup	5
Choc Milk *(Hershey's)*, 1 cup	130
Soy Milk, 8 fl.oz	30
Buttermilk, cultured, 8 fl.oz	250
Dry/Powder, skim, ¼ cup, 1 oz	110
Yogurt, with fruit average, 8 oz	130
Cheese: Bleu, 1 oz	330
Parmesan, 1 oz	450
Kraft Cheddar, 2% milk, 1 oz	230
Philadelphia Cream Cheese, 1 oz	90
Process Cheese., average,1 oz	430
Swiss, 1 oz	40
Cottage Cheese, ½ cup, 4 oz	450
Ricotta Cheese, ½ cup, 4 oz	150

Ice Cream, Frozen Yogurt

Icecream, average,½ cup	50
Frozen Yogurt, ½ cup	50

Fats/Oils

Butter/Margarine:	
Regular, 2 Tbsp, 1 oz	230
Unsalted, reg., 2 Tbsp, 1 oz	5
Mayonnaise, aver., 2 Tbsp, 1 oz	160
Oils/Lard/Drippings	0
Cream, average, 1 Tbsp	5
Coffee-Mate: Powdered, 1 tsp	2
Liquid, 1 Tbsp	5

Eggs

Whole, 1 large	70
Omelet, 2 egg, plain	220
w. cheese	400
Egg Beaters: Original, ¼ cup	115
Flavors, average, ¼ cup	230

Meats

Meat, average all types, cooked (Beef/Lamb/Veal/Pork), 4 oz	80
Corned Beef, cooked, 3 oz	800
Bacon, cooked, 2 sl., ½ oz	270
Ham, 3 oz	1100

Chicken & Turkey

Chicken/Turkey, cooked, unsalted, 4 oz	80
Stuffing Mixes, average., ½ cup	500

Sodium ~ Sodium (mg)

Sausages & Meats

	Sodium
Bologna, 1 oz	280
Frankfurter, 2 oz	640
Ham, chopped, ¾ oz slice	290
Liverwurst (Braunschweiger), 1 oz	320
Pepperoni, 5 slices, 1 oz	570
Salami, cooked, 1 oz	350
dry/hard, 1 oz	600
Sausage, 1 oz link	220
Pork, 2 oz patty	260
Spam: Classic, 2 oz	790
25% Less Sodium, 2 oz	580
Turkey Roll, 1 oz	160

Fish:

Fresh Fish, average, plain	Sodium
Cooked, 4 oz (no bone)	60
Broiled w. butter, 4 oz	150
Breaded & fried, 4 oz	320
Fish fillets, batter-dipped 3 oz	350
Fish sticks, 1 oz stick	160
Gefilte Fish (w. broth), 1 pce, 1½ oz	220
Herring, pickled, 2 pces, 1 oz	260
Lobster, meat only, 4 oz	180
Oysters, fresh, 6 med., 3 oz	95
Salmon: Canned, 3 oz	460
No Salt Added, 3 oz	65
Smoked fish, average, 3 oz	650
Tuna: Canned, regular, 3 oz	330
No Added Salt, 3 oz	40
Spicy Flavored, 5 oz can	550

Entrees & Meals

Frozen Meals, average	600-900
Lean Cuisine, average	700
Stouffer's, average	580
Dinners, average	900-1200
Side Dishes, average	400-600
Pizza, frozen, ¼ large, 6 oz	800-1200
Microwave Cup Meals	900-1200
Cup O'Noodles, average	1500

Fast-Foods & Restaurants

Cheeseburger	750
Chicken Dinner (3 piece)	2200
Chicken Nuggets w. Sauce	800
Fish/Chicken Sandwich	1000
French Fries, small, 2½ oz	150
Hamburger: Regular	500
Large with cheese	1100
Hot Dog (Frankfurter)	800
Pizza, 2 medium slices	1200
Shake, chocolate	250
Taco	400

Extra Listings ~ see CalorieKing.com

Sodium Counter

Sodium ~ Sodium (mg)

Sodium	
Soups: Condensed, 1 c., 8 oz	800-1000
Low Sodium	70
Chicken Noodle, 1 cup	900
Bouillon Cube, average	950
Cup-A-Soup: Average	850
Lite, average	450
Soup Mixes, average, 1 cup	900

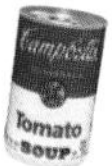

Condiments, Sauces, Dressings

A-1 Sauce, 1 Tbsp	280
Barbecue Sauce, 1 Tbsp	130
Bragg Liquid Aminos, 1 tsp	220
Chili Sauce, 1 Tbsp	230
Ketchup: Tomato, 1 Tbsp	180
Low Sodium, 1 Tbsp	20
Mayonnaise, 1 Tbsp	80
Mustard, 1 tsp	70
Pizza Sauce, ½ cup	700
Salad Dressings, 2 Tbsp, 1 oz	160-400
Spaghetti Sauce, ½ cup	500
Soy Sauce: 1 Tbsp	900
Lite *(Kikkoman),* 1 Tbsp	600
Sweet & Sour, ½ cup	250
Tabasco, 1 tsp	25
Vinegar, Lemon Juice	0
Worcestershire, 1 Tbsp	200
Tomato: Sauce, 1 cup	1200
Paste/Puree (salted), ½ cup	1000
No Salt Added, ½ cup	25

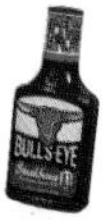

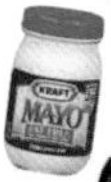

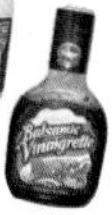

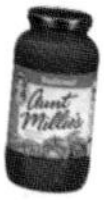

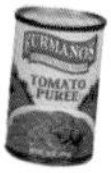

Salt & Salt Substitutes

Table Salt: 1 teaspoon, 6g	2400
Single Serve package, 1 g	400
Cardia Salt, 1 teaspoon	1080
Lite Salt *(Morton),* 1 teaspoon, 6g	1200
Morton Salt Substitute	5
No Salt Salt Substitute, 1 teaspoon	5
Garlic/Seasoned Salt 1 teaspoon, 4g	1300
Sea Salt, 1 teaspoon, 5g	2250

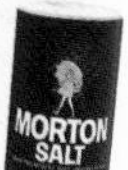

Seasonings, Herbs & Spices

Baking Powder, 1 tsp, 3g	340
Baking Soda (Sodium bicarb), 1 tsp, 3g	810
Accent (Flavor Enhancer), 1 tsp	600
Chili Powder, 1 tsp, 3g	25
Curry Powder	0
Lemon Pepper *(Lawry's),* 1 tsp	340
Meat Tenderizer, 1 tsp, 5g	1750
MSG (Monosodium glutamate), 5g	500
Mrs Dash Blends/Marinades	0
Pepper, Mustard (dry), 1 tsp	1
Yeast, Nutritional, 1 Tbsp	10

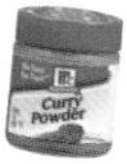

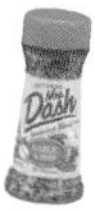

Breakfast Cereals

Sodium	
Kellogg's:	
All-Bran, ½ cup, 1 oz	80
Special K, 1 cup, 1.1 oz	220
Corn Flakes, 1 cup, 1 oz	200
Just Right, ¾ cup, 2 oz	240
Mini Wheats Frosted, 24 bisc., 1.8 oz	5
Health Valley Cereals, 1 serving	5
Quaker: Cap'n Crunch, ¾ cup, 1 oz	200
Crunchy Corn Bran, ¾ cup, 1 oz	230
100% Natural Granola, ½ cup, 1 oz	15
Puffed Rice/Wheat, 2 cups, 1 oz	1
General Mills: Total, ¾ cup, 1 oz	190
Oatmeal: Regular, ¾ cup	1
Instant *(Quaker),* ⅔ cup (1 pkt)	270

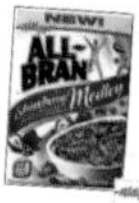

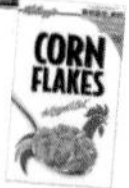

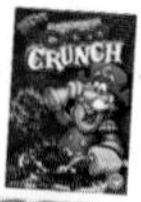

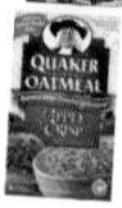

Breads, Bagels, Crackers

Bread: Average all types, 1 oz	140
Low Sodium, 1 oz	10
Bagels: Plain, 2 oz	200
Sara Lee, 3 oz	500
Biscuits, average, 1 oz	180
Bun/Roll, 1 medium, 1½ oz	200
Crackers: Saltine, 2 crackers	70
Low Salt *(Premium),* 2	25
Graham, 2 regular	50
Croissant, average, 2 oz	280
Rice Cakes, average	25
Ritz **Crackers,** Low-Sodium, 1 oz	60
Ry-Krisp Crispbread, Sesame, 2	100

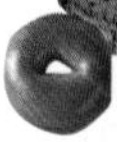

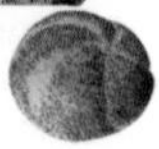

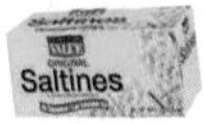

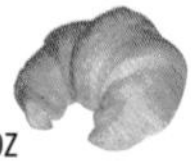

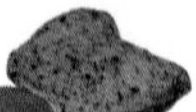

Cookies, Cakes, Desserts

Cookies: Average, 2-3 cookies, 1 oz	100
Mrs Fields', average, 2½ oz	180
Baked Custard, ½ cup	100
Brownie, ¼ oz piece	75
Cake, average, 3 oz piece	250
Cinnamon Sweet Roll, 2 oz	250
Danish, Apple	250
Donut, average	150
Muffins: 1 medium, 2 oz	150
Pancakes, 3 x 4"	360
Pie, average ⅙ of 9" pie	300
Pudding: Average, ½ cup	160
Jell-O (Mix), Instant, ½ cup	400
Waffles:	
Home-made, 7", 2½ oz	350
Frozen: Average, 1¼ oz	260
Aunt Jemima, avg, 2½ oz	565

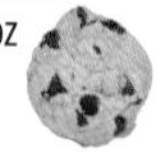

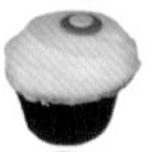

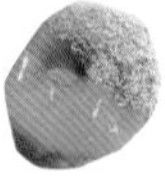

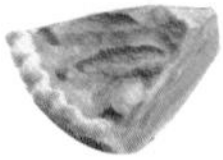

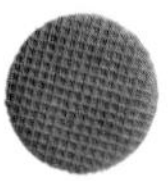

Fruit & Juices | Sodium
Fresh Fruit, average all types, 1 serving	1
Dried/Canned Fruit, ½ cup	1
Fruit Juice: Fresh, sqz'd, 6 fl.oz	1
Commercial, aver., 6 fl.oz	20
Carrot Juice *(Ferraro's)*, 8 fl.oz	230
Tomato Juice *(Campbell's)*, 6 fl.oz	570
Low Sodium (No Salt Added)	20
V8 Vegetable *(Campbell's)*, 6 fl.oz	600
(No Salt Added), 6 fl.oz	45

Vegetables
Fresh/Frozen (No Salt Added): *Per ½ Cup*	
Asparagus, Bean Sprouts, Corn	3
Beets, Carrots, Celery, ½ cup	40
Broccoli, Cabbage, Cauliflower	10
Cucumber, Green Beans, Mushroom, Okra	3
Onions, Peas, Potato, Pumpkin, Squash	3
Peppers, Hot Chili, raw, each	3
Spinach, Turnips, ½ cup, ckd	40
Tomato, 1 medium, 5 oz	10
Canned: Asparagus, 4 spears	300
Beans, baked in tomato sauce	450
Beets, ½ cup, 3 oz	240
Corn Kernels, ½ cup, 3 oz	190
Creamed, ½ cup, 4½ oz	330
Mushrooms w. butter sce, 2oz	550
Peas, ½ cup, 3 oz	250
Sauerkraut, ½ cup, 4 oz	750

Pickles, Olives
Olives, pickled: Green, 1 large	90
Ripe/black, 1 large	40
Pickles: Bread & Butter, 4 sl., 1 oz	200
Dill, 1 pickle, 2½ oz	900
Sweet, 1 gherkin, ½ oz	130

Soybean Products
Miso (Soy Paste), ¼ c., 2½ oz	2500
Soybean Protein Isolate, 1 oz	280
Tempeh, ½ cup, 3 oz	5
Tofu, average, ½ cup, 4 oz	5

Jam, Honey, Syrups
Jam/Jelly, 1 Tbsp	2
Honey/Maple Syrup, 1 Tbsp	1
Log Cabin Syrup, 1 fl.oz	35
Lite, 1 fl.oz	90

Peanut Butter
Peanut Butter: Regular, 2 Tbsp, ½ oz	190
Low Sodium *(Jif)*, 2 Tbsp	65
Unsalted *(Trader Joe's)*, 2 Tbsp	5

Snacks, Nuts | Sodium
Cheese Balls/Curls, 1 oz	280
Corn/Tortilla Chips, average, 1 oz	220
Granola bars, average, 1 bar	80
Nuts: Plain, unsalted, 1 oz	1
Lightly salted, 1 oz	80
Salted or Honey Roasted, 1 oz	160
Popcorn: Plain (unsalted), 1 cup	1
Flavored, average, 1 cup	60
Salt added, 1 cup	180
Potato Chips: Plain, 1 oz	160
Flavored, average, 1 oz	250
Pretzels, regular, 3, 1 oz	450

Candy, Chocolate
Chocolate, milk, 1 oz	30
Fudge, chocolate, 1 oz	55
Candy Bars, average, 1½ oz	60
Hard Candy, Jelly Beans, 1 oz	10
Licorice, 1 oz	30

Beverages, Alcohol
Coffee (& Substitutes), Tea, 1 cup	1
Cocoa, dry, plain, 1 Tbsp	0
Mix, average, 1 envelope	120
Quik *(Nestle)*, 2 tsp	35
Soft Drinks, average, 8 fl.oz	20
Mineral Water, Perrier, 8 fl.oz	5
Gatorade Thirst Quencher, 8 fl.oz	110
Water: Average, 1 cup, 8 fl.oz	5
Drier regions, 1 cup	20+
Alcohol: Beer, average, 12 fl.oz	15
Wines, average, 4 fl.oz	10
Spirits (distilled), 1½ fl.oz	1

Antacids – Alka-Seltzer | Sodium
Alka-Seltzer (Per Tablet):	
Alka-Seltzer P.M., 1 tablet	500
Original (Light Blue Box)	570
Extra Strength (Dark Blue Box)	590
Flavored Lemon/Lime & Cherry	500
Antacid (yellow Box)	310
Gelatine Capsule, 1	0
Alka-Mints, chewable	0
Bromo Seltzer, ¾ capful	760
Rolaids, All types	0
Tums, Regular/Extra Strength	0
Sodium Bicarbonate (27% sodium), 1g	270

Index A - B

A-1 Steak Sauce	148
A&W Cream Soda	53
A&W Float	53
Ahi Tuna	176
Albertson's Sodas	53
Alcoholic Drinks	26
Alcohol Guice	25
Al-Bran: Breakfast Cereal	62
Drink Mix	55
Alligator	175
Almond Breeze	48
Almond Butter	133
Almond Dream	48
Almond Joy	70
Almond Paste	32
Almonds	132
Aloe Vera Juice	163
Alouette Cheese	80
Alta Dena Yogurt	169
Amaranth Flour	100
Amazake	48
AMP Energy Drink	50
Anchovies	97
Ant Eggs/Larvae	181
Antacids	163
Apple Danish	64
Dunkin Donuts	204
Apple Fritter,	
Dunkin Donuts	204
Apple Pie	136
Apple Sauce	82, 104
Applebee's	183
Apples	101
Apricots	101
Arbor Mist Blenders	29
Arbor Mist Wine	28
Arby's	184
Arizona Teas	55
Arroz Con Pollo	181
Asian Foods	175
Panda Express	230
Pei Wei	231
Asparagus	165
Atkins Bars	33
Au Bon Pain	185
Aunt Jemima: Pancakes	134
Waffles	134
Austin S'wich Crackers	155
Avocado	101

Baba Ghannouj	179
Baba Ghannoush	81
Baby Ruth	70
Babybel	78
Bacardi & Coke	30
Bacardi Silver	29
Bacon	128
Bacon Bits	144
Bagel Chips	58
Bagel Dogs	130
Bagel S'wiches:	
Dunkin Donuts	205
Bagel Spreads	58
Bagels	58
Big Apple Bagels	188
Bruegger's Bagels	192
Manhattan Bagel	224
Baileys Irish Cream	31
Baking Ingredients	32
Baking Mix	32
Baking Powder	32
Baklava	64
Balance Bars	33
Ball Park Franks	129
Balsamic Vinaigrette	145
Banana	101
Banana Chips	103
Banana Flakes	103
Banana Split: Denny's	202
Banquet Meals	119
Barbecue Sauce	82
Bariatrix: Drinks	50
Proti-Bar	33
Barley	100
Bars: Breakfast Bars	33
Granola	33-36
Meal/Nutrition	33-36
Protein Counts	286
Bartles & Jaymes	29
Baskin-Robbins	188
Beans	165
Bear Claw	64
Bee Maggots	181

Beef:	126
Beef Ribs	126
Franks	129
Ground Beef	126
Jerky	130
Roast Beef	126
Tallow	96
Beer: Alcoholic	26, 27
Non-Alcoholic	28
Beerwurst	130
Beiglach	178
Ben & Jerry's: Ice Cream	106
Ice Cream Bars	110
Benecol Spread	95
Bernstein's Dressings	145
Best Foods Dressings	145
Betty Crocker: Cake Mixes	67
Muffin Mixes	69
Big Mac	222
Birds Eye, Frozen Veg.	167
Biscotti	83
Biscuits: Burger King	193
Hardee's	211
Jack in the Box	214
McDonald's	222
Bison Steak	128
Blintzes	178
Bloody Mary	30
Bloomin' Onion	229
BLT Sandwich	172
Blue Bunny: FrozFruit	110
Ice Cream	106, 110
Yogurt	169
Blue Cheese Dressing	145
Blue Sky Sodas	53
Bob Evans	190
Boca Burgers	119
Bok Choy	165
Bologna	130
Bolthouse Juice	40
Boost Drinks	50
Borscht Soup	178
Boston Market	191
Boston Pizza	192
Brach's Candy	70
Brain	128
Bran	59
Brandy	29

Bratwurst	130
Braunschweiger	130
Brazil Nuts	132
Bread	56
Bread Crumbs	57
Bread: Buns/Rolls	57
Breadsticks	57
Breakfast Bars	33
Breakfast Cereals	59
Breakfast Meals:	
Denny's	201
Breakfast Sausages	129
Brewer's Yeast	163
Breyers: Ice Cream	106, 110
Yogurt	169
Brioche Cake	175
Broccoli	165
Brownie	64
Brownie mixes	67
Bruegger's Bagels	192
Bruschetta	177
Brussels Sprouts	165
Bubble Tea	175
Bubble Yum	77
Buckwheat:	100
Groats	59
Budweiser Beer	26
Buffalo Wings: Domino's	203
Buitoni Pasta	135
Bulgur: Grain	59, 100
Salad	144
Bumble Bee, Tuna	99
Burger King	193
Burritos: Qdoba	238
Taco Bell	259
Taco John's	260
Taco Mayo	261
Taco Time	261
Butter & Margarine	95
Butter Substitutes	95
Butter Buds	95
Lighter Bake	95
Molly McButter	95
Butterfinger	70
Buttermilk	46
Butterscotch	71

Cabbage 165
Cabbage Rolls 178, 180
Cactus Leaf 165
Caesar Dressing 145
Cadbury Candy 71
Cafeteria Foods 172
Cajun Foods 175
Cake Frosting 67
Cake Mixes 67
Cakes 64
Calamari 97, 176
  Fried, Macaroni Grill 221
Calcium Chews 163
California Pizza Kitchen 138
Calzones, Mazzio's 224
Camembert 78
Canada Dry Sodas 53
Canadian Bacon 128
Candied Fruit 103
Candy 70
Cannelloni 177
Cannoli 64
Cantaloupe 101
Capri Sun 40
Captain Crunch 63
Caramello 71
Caramels 71
Carb Countdown 46
Cardini's Dressings 146
Caribou 128
Carob 77
Carrots 165
Cashews 132
Caterpillars 181
Catfish 97
Catsup 82
Caviar 97
Cereal Drinks 48
Challah Bread 56
Chalupas: Taco Bell 259

Champagne 28
Chapati 56
Cheerios: Cereal 61
  Snack Mix 154
Cheese 78
Cheese Balls 154
Cheese Fries:
  Nathan's Famous 226
Cheese Puffs 154
Cheese Substitutes 80
Cheese Whiz 80
Cheeseburger:
  Burger King 193
  Hardee's 211
  Jack in the Box 214
  McDonald's 222
Cheesecake 64
Cheesecake Factory 195
Cheetos 154
Cheez-It Crackers 154
Chef Boyardee 113
Chef's Salad 144
Cherries 101
Chestnuts 132
Chex Bkfst Cereal 61
Chex Mix 154
Chi Chi 30
Chick Peas 165
Chicken Alfredo 177
Chicken 140
  Chik-fil-A 196
  Church's Chicken 197
  KFC 217
  S'wich, McDonald's 222
Chicken Buffalo Wings:
  KFC 217
Chicken Helper 113
Chicken Katsu 176
Chicken Korma 177

Chicken Kung Pao:
  P.F. Chang's 233
  Panda Express 230
Chicken McNuggets 222
Chicken of the Sea 99
Chicken Strips:
  KFC 217
  McDonald's 222
Chili Cheese Fries: Topz 264
Chili Sauce 82
Chili: Con Carne 179
  Gold Star Chili 209
  Plain 179
  Stagg Meals 117
  Trader Joe's Meals 117
Chili's 196
Chimichangas 179
Chinese Foods 175
Chinese Foods:
  P.F. Chang's 233
Chipotle 197
Chips Ahoy! 87
  Snacks 154
Chocolate Candy 70
Chocolate Baking Chips 32
Chocolate Chip Cookies 83
Chocolate Milk 47
Chocolate Cake 64
Chocolate Éclair 64
Cholent 178
Chopped Liver 178
Chorizo 129
Churros 64
Ciabatta 56
Cider, alcoholic 28
Cinnabon 69, 198
Cinnamon Rolls 64
  T.J.Cinnamons 263
Clam Chowder: 156
  Long John Silver's 221

Clamato Juice 41
Clams 97
Clif Bars 34
Coca-Cola 53
Coca-Cola Zero 53
Cocktail Mixers 30
Cocktails 30
  Premixed 29
Cocoa 37
Cocoa Powder 32
Coconut 101
Coconut Cream 91
Coconut Milk 91
Coconut: Dessicated 132
  Fresh 132
Coffee: 37-39
  Bottled 39
  Biggby coffee 189
  Caribou Coffee 194
  Expresso 38
  Flavored Mixes 37
  Instant 37
  Iced 38, 254
  Irish 38
  Starbucks 39, 254
Coffee-Mate 91
Cola Drinks 53
Coldstone Creamery 198
Coleslaw Dressing 145
Combos 154
Concha 64
Condensed Milk 46
Condiments/Sauces 82
Cookie Dough, Toll House 90
Cookies 83
Cooking Sprays: Pam 96
Cool Whip 91
Coors Beer 26
Coq au Vin 175
Corn 165

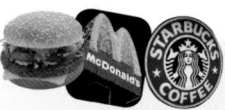

FAST-FOOD RESTAURANTS INDEX
~ SEE PAGE 182 ~

Index C - F

Corn Chips	153	D'Angelo's	199	Ears, Pork	128	Fig Bars	64
Corn Dogs	130	Daiquiri	30	EAS Bars	34	Figs	101
Corn Flakes	60	Dairy Ease	46	Edamame	165, 178	Filet Mignon Steak	125
Corn Grits	100	Dairy Queen	200	Eel	97	Fish	97
Corned Beef	130	Danish Pastry	64	Egg Nog	93	Fish & Chips	97
Cornmeal	100	Dates	103	Eggplant	166	Fish Oil	96
Cornstarch	100	Deer	128	Egg Roll Wrappers	135	Fish Sticks	97
Cosmopolitan	30	Del Taco	201	Egg Rolls	94	Flauta, Pepe's Mexican	232
Cottage Cheese	78	Deli Meats	130	Eggs:	93	Flaxseed	100
Cough/Cold Syrups	163	Denny's	201	Better 'n Eggs	93	Flaxseeds	133
Cough Drops	77	Desserts	92	Egg Beaters	93	Fleischmann's Spread	95
Country Choice Cookies	84	Dibs	110	Egg Whites	93	Flours	100
Cous Cous	179, 100	Diet Coke	53	Eggo: French Toast	134	Focaccia S'wiches,	
Crab	97	Diet Drinks/Shakes	50	Pancakes	134	Mazzio's	224
Crab Cakes	97	Diet Sodas	53	Eggs Benedict	93	Fortune Cookie	175
Cracker Jack	152	DiGiorno Pizzas	138	Empanadas	180	Franks	129
Crackers	83	Dill Pickle	82	Enchilada	179	Frappuccino: Starbucks	255
Cranberries: Dried	103	Dippin' Dots	107, 202	Endive	166	French Foods	175
Fresh	101	Dips/Spreads	81	Energy Drinks	50	French Fries:	166
Crawfish	175	Dolma	176	English Muffins	58	Burger King	193
Cream	91	Domino's Pizza	203	Ensure Drinks	50	McDonald's	222
Cream Cheese	81	Donuts	68	Entenmann's: Cakes	65	French/Italian Dressing	145
Cream of Wheat	59	Tim Horton's	263	Cinnamon Bun	69	French Stick	56
Creamers	91	Winchell's	269	Equal	164	French's Fried Onions	114
Creamsicle	110	dot.FIT: B'kfast Bars	33, 286	Espresso Coffee:	38	Fresca	53
CremaLita	107	FirstString	50, 287	Starbucks	254	Freschetta Pizzas	138
Creole Foods	175	Meal Replacements	50, 287	Evaporated Milk	46	Freshens	208
Crepe Suzette	176	Protein Stick	34, 286	Extra Gum	77	Fried Oreos	174
Crispbreads	90	WheySmooth	50, 287	Fair/Carnival Foods	173	Fried Rice, Panda Express	230
Croissants: Plain	136					Fried Twinkie	174
Sandwiches	172					Fruit Snacks	155
Dunkin Donuts	205	**FAST-FOODS INDEX**				Fruit Spreads	164
Sweet	136	**~ PAGE 182 ~**				Frog Legs	175
Croutons	57					Froot Loops	62
Crunch: Candy (Nestle)	71	Dove: Candy	71	Fajitas	179	Frosting, cake	67
Ice Cream Bar	110	Cookies	84	Chili's	196	Frozen Custard	105
Crunch 'N Munch	152	Ice Cream	107	Famous Amos	84	Frozen Meals	119
Crystal Light	54	Ice Cream Bars	110	Fanta	53	TGI Friday's	123
Cuban Foods	175	Dr Pepper Sodas	53	Fantastic: Cup Meals	114	Trader Joe's	123
Cup-a-Soup	159	Dried Fruit	103	Fat Boy	111	Weight Watchers	124
Cupcakes	64	Dried (Powdered) Milk	46	Feet, Pork	128	Frozen Yogurt	105
Curries, Thai	181	Drippings	96	Falafel	179	FrozFruit	110
Curves: Bars	34	Duck	141	Feta Cheese	78	FRS Energy Drink	50
Protein Drinks	50	Dumplings	175	Fettucine alfredo	177	Frui-A-Freeze	111
Custard, Frozen	105	P.F. Chang's	233	Fibersure	163	Fruit Juices	40
Custards	92	Duncan Hines Cake Mixes	67	Fiddle Faddle	152	Fruit Leather	103
		Dunkin' Donuts	204	5th Avenue	72	Fruit Pies	136
						Fruit Rolls	72

Fruit Sauces	104
Fruit Smoothies	40
Orange Julius	229
Fruit Snack Cups	104
Fruit: Fresh	101
Candied	103
Canned	104
Dried	103
Fruit Leather	103
Sauces	104
Frutzzo	41
Fudge	72
Fudgesicle	111
Full Throttle Energy	50
Funnel Cake	173
Fuze: Energy Drinks	50
Iced Teas	55
Refresh	41
GardenBurger	120
Garlic	166
Garlic Bread	56
Gazpacho Soup	181
Gatorade	50
Gefilte Fish Balls	178
Gelati-da	107
Gelatin	92
Gelatin Parfait	92
Gelato	105
GeniSoy	34
Genisoy Powder Shakes	49
German Foods	176
Ghee	95
Ghirardelli	72
Gin	29
Ginger	166
Glaceau Drinks	50
Glowelle	163
Gluhwein	28
GNC ProCrunch	34
GNC: Pro Performance	51
Gnu Foods	34
Goat Meat	128
Goat's Milk	46
Goat's Milk Cheese	79
Godiva Candy	72
Goji Berries	103

Goldfish	154
Goober P'nut Butter	133
Good Humor	111
Goose	141
Gorditas: Taco Bell	259
Graham Crackers	83
Grains	100
Grandma's Cookies	84
Granola	60
Granola Bars	33
Grapefruit	101
Grapes	101
Gravy	148
Greek Foods	17
Greek Foods:	
Daphne's Greek Café	200
Ground Pork	128
Guacamole	179
Gum	77
Gum Drops	72
Gummi Bears	72
Gyros	176, 200
Haagen-Dazs:	
Bars	111
Ice Cream	107, 211
Haggis	181
Half & Half	91
Halls Drops	77
Ham: Chopped	130
Ham Steak	128
Lunch/Deli	130
Roasted	128
Hamburger Helper	113
Hamburger:	
Carnival/Fair	173
Jack in the Box	214
McDonald's	222
Hansen's: Energy Drinks	50
Iced Teas	55
Juices	41
Sodas	53
Hardee's	211
Hash Browns	94
Burger King	193
Dunkin Donuts	205
McDonald's	222

Hawaiian Foods	176
Head Cheese	128
Heath Candy	72
Health Valley Cookies	84
Healthy Choice: Meals	120
Pizzas	138
Heart	128
Hebrew National Links	129
Heineken Beer	26
Herbalife Bars	34
Shapeworks	51
Herring	98
Hershey's: Candy	72
Cookies	85
Choc Milk	47
Chocolate Mix	37
Hidden Valley Dressings	146
Hoagies: Davanni's	200
Mazzio's	224
Honey	164
Honeycomb	73
Honeydew	101
Horchata	179
Don Jose	48
Horseradish	82, 166
Hostess: Cakes	65
Donuts	68
Muffins	69
Sweet Buns/Rolls	69
Hot & Sour Soup	181
Hot Chocolate	37
Hot Dogs/Franks:	130
A&W	183
Carnival	173
WAWA	266
Wienerschnitzel	267
Hot Dog On A Stick	212
Hot Dog Toppings	130
Hot Pockets	121
Hotcakes, McDonald's	222
Hubba Bubba	77
Hummus	81, 176
Hunt's Snack Pack	92

Ice Cream	105
Ice Cream Bars:	110
Butterfinger	110
Drumstick	111
Klondike	111
Oreo	111
Slim-a-Bear	111
Ice Cream: Carvel	195
Dippin' Dots	202
Starbucks	108
Ice Cream Toppings	164
Iced Tea	55
Mixes	55
Icee Drinks	54
IHOP	213
Indian Foods	177
Italian Dressing	145
Italian Foods	177
Fazoli's	207
Macaroni Grill	221
Mazzio's	224
Italian Sausage	130
Jack In The Box	214
Jam	164
Jamba Juice	215
Jambalaya	175
Japanese Foods	178
Edo Japan	206
Yoshinoya	269
Java Monster Energy	51
Jellies	73
Jell-O: Fruit Passions	92
Gel Snacks	92
Gelatin Mixes	92
No bake Cheesecake	67
Puddings	92
Jelly Beans	73
Jenny Craig	34
Jif Peanut Butter	133
Jolly Rancher	73
Jolt: Cola/Sodas	54
Enrgy Drinks	51
Junior Mints	73

Kahlua 31
Kahlua Mudslide 30
Kaiser Roll 57
Kalua Chicken 176
Kashi GOLEAN 34
   Shakes 51
Kashi TLC: Bkfst Cereals 61
   Cookies 85
   Crackers 85
   Pizzas 138
Keebler: Cookies 85
   Crackers 85
Kefir Cheese 79
Kefir Milk 46
Kellogg's: Breakfast Bars 33
   Breakfast Cereals 62
   Pop Tarts 33
KFC 217
Kid Cuisine 121
Kidneys 128
Kielbasa 130, 180
Kimchee 179
Kind Bars 34
Kisses 73
Kit Kat 73
Kiwifruit 101
Knish 178
Knudsen Yogurt 170
Kombucha Drink 51
Kool-Aid 54
Korean Foods 179
Kosher Deli Foods 178
Krackel 73
Kraft: Cheese 80
   Dressings 146
   LiveActive Cheese 80
   Mayonnaise 96
   Meals 115
Krispy Kreme Donuts 68
Kudos 35
Lactaid 100 46
Lactose-Free 46
Lamb 127
Lamb Pilaf 177
Land O'Lakes Spread 95

Lard 96
Lasagna: Villa Pizza 265
   Meat, Fazoli's 207
Latkes, Potato Patty 178
Lau Lau 176
Lean Cuisine 122
   French Bread Pizza 138
Lean Pockets 122
Lebanese Foods 179
Lecithin Granules 59
Lemon 101
Lemon Cake 64
Lemon Crème 136
Lettuce 166
Lettuce Wraps: P.F.Chang's 233
   Pei Wei 231
Licorice 73
Life Breakfast Cereal 63
Lifesavers 73
Lighter Bake 32

Limes 102
Lindora Bars 35
Lindt 74
Linguine & Seafood 177
Lipton Brisk 55
Lipton Iced Tea 55
Liqueur, Coffee 31
Liqueurs 31
Liquor 29
Little Caesar 220
Little Debbie: Cakes 65
   Cookies 86
   Donuts 68
   Honey Buns 69
Liver 128
Liver Pate 131
Liver, Chopped 178
Liverwurst 131
Lobster 98
Lochshen 178
Locusts 181

Lollipops 74
Lox 98
Luna Bar 35
Lunch Bucket 115
Lunchables 115
Lunchmakers 115
M & M's 74
Macadamia Nuts 132
Macaroni & Cheese 135
Macaroni Salad 144
Mamey Apple 102
Manapua 176
Mandarin 102
Mandelbrot 178
Mango 102
Manhattan Clam Chowder:
   Nathan's Famous 226
Manischewitz 86
Marathon Bars 35
Marble Cake 64

Margarita 30
Marie Callender's Dinners 122
Marie's Dressings 147
Marsala 28
Marshmallows 74
Maruchan Noodles 116
Masa 179
Matzos 90
   Balls 178
   Ball Soup 178
Mayonnaise 96
Mazola Spray 96
McDonald's 222
McMuffin 222
Meals: 113
   Canned/Packaged 113
   Frozen 119
   Knorr Lipton 115
   South Beach Diet 123
   Thai Kitchen Meals 117
   Tyson 124
Meat Snacks 130
Meat Spreads 131

Meats 126
Melon 102
Mentos 74
Meringues 92
Met-Rx: Bars 35
   Shakes 51
Metamucil 163
Mexican: Cakes 180
   Carnival 173
   Cheese 79
Mexican Foods 179
   Pepe's Mexican 232
Michelob Beer 27
Middle Eastern Foods 179
Mike's Hard Lemonade 29
Milk: Canned 46
   Dried 46
   Flavored 46
   Plain 46
Milky Way 74
Miller Beer 27
Millet 100
Minestrone Soup 177
Mint Julep 30
Mints 74
Minute Maid: Juices 42
   Lemonade 54
Minute Rice 116
Miracle Whip 96
Miso Soup 178
Mocha Mix 91
Mojo Bar 34
Molasses 164
Mori Nu Tofu Cheese 80
Morningstar Farms 122
Mounds 74
Mountain Dew 54
Moussaka 176
Mozzarella Cheese 79
Mr Goodbar 74
MRM Protein Drinks 51
Mrs Dash Marinade 150
Mrs Fields Cookies 226
Mud Cake 64
Muffin Mixes 69

FAST-FOODS INDEX
~ PAGE 182 ~

Muffins 69
  Dunkin Donuts 204
Mulled Wine 28
Munchies 154
Muscle Milk 51
Mushrooms 166
Mussels 98
Naan Bread 177
Nachos 179
  Chili's 196
  Qdoba 238
  Taco Bell 259
Naked Juice 42
Nathan's Famous 226
Nature's Path Bars 35
Nayonaise 96
Nectarines 102
Nesquik 37, 47
Nestea, Iced Tea 55
New England Clam Chowder:
  Nathan's Famous 226
Newman's Own: Cookies 88
  Dressings 147
  Juice 43
Newtons Cookies 87
Nigiri, Sthn. Tsunami 253
Nilla Cakesters 65
Nissin Noodles 116
No Fear Energy 51
Noni Juice 51
Noodle Cups 116
Noodles 135
  Pei Wei 231
Noodles & Company 227
Nopal Cactus Salad 179
Nopales 166
Nothing But Noodles 227
Nouriche Yogurt 171
Nut Butter Cookies 87
Nut Spreads 133
Nutella 133
Nutri-Grain Bkfst Bars 33

Nutrilite: Bars 35
  Protein Drinks 51
NutriSystem: Bars 35
  Breakfast Cereals 63
Nuts 132
Oat Bran 59
Oatmeal 59
Oatmeal Raisin Cookies 83
Oats 100
Ocean Spray, Juice 43
Odwalla: Bars 35
  Energy Bars 35
Oils: Fish 96
  Vegetable 96
Okra 166
Old El Paso: Dinner Kits 116
  Dip 81
  Refried Beans 116
  Salsa 81
Olive Garden 228
Olive Loaf 131
Olives 102
Omelets 93
  Farmers Market 94
  Ham & Cheddar 94
  Perkin's 232
  Western Omelette 94
Onion Flower 173
Onions 166
Onion Rings: Burger King 193
  Dairy Queen 200
  Jack in the Box 214
  Zaxby's 270
Optifast: Bars 35, 286
  Shakes 51, 287
Orange Juice 40
Orange Julius 229
Oranges 102
Orangina 54
Oreo: Cakesters 66
  Cookies 87
  Snacks 154
Ostrich 128
Outback Steakhouse 229
Ovaltine 37
Oyster & Soup Crackers 83
Oysters 98

Pad Thai 181
  Pei Wei 231
Paella 181
Pakistani Foods 177
Palmier Cookie 64
Pancakes 134
  IHOP 213
Pancreas 128
Panda Express 230
Panera Bread 230
Paninis 177
  Sandella's 245
  Vocelli Pizza 265
Papaya 102
Papaya Spears 103
Pappadum 177
Parfait 92
Parkay Spread 95
Parmesan Cheese 79
Parsnip 166
Passionfruit 102
Pasta 135
  Macaroni Grill 221
  Pizza Hut 235
Pasta Roni 116
Pasta Sauces 148-151
Pastrami 131
Pastries 64
Pastry Crust 136
Pate 131
PayDay Bar 74
Peach Melba 64
Peaches 102
Peanut Butter Cookie 83
Peanut Butter Cups:
  Newman's Own 74
  Reese's 75
Peanut Butter: 133
  & Jelly S/wich 133
Peanuts 132
Pears 102
Peas 166
Pecan Pie 136
Pecans 132
Pepperidge Farm: Cakes 66
  Cookies 88

Peppermints 75
Peppers 166
Pepsi 52
Pepsi Max 54
Pepsi One 54
Perrier Water 54
Persimmons 102
Pez 75
Philadelphia 81
Philadelphia Cheese Steak
  Sandwich 172
Pickles & Relish 82
Pie Crust 136
Pie Fillings 32, 136
Pierogi 180
Pies 136
Pilaf 179
Piloncillo Sugar Cone 179
Pina Colada 30
Pine Nuts 132
Pineapple 102
Pirate's Booty 154
Pistachios 132
Pita 56
Pizza Hut 234
Pizzas: Frozen 138
  Ready-To-Eat 137
Planters, Peanuts 132
Plums 102
Poi 176
Poke Salad 180
Polenta 100
Polish Foods 180
Pom: Juices 43
  Pomegranate Teas 55
Pomegranate 102
Popcorn: Plain 152
  Caramel 152
  Orville Redenbacher's 152
Popcorn Chicken: KFC 216
  Sonic Drive-In 251
Pops 110

Pork: Meat 127
  Bindaloo Curry 177
  Cracklings 180
  Rind 154
  Sausages 129
  Spareribs 127
Port Wine 28
Porterhouse Steak 125
Post Cereals 63
Potato Salad 144
Potatoes: 166
  Carnival 173
  Baked: Wendy's 267
  French Fries 166
PowerAde 52
Power Bar 35
  Shakes 52
Pralines 75
Pretzelmaker 237
Pretzels: 153
  Rold Gold 153
Prickly Pear 102
Probiotics 171
Progresso Soup 160
Promise Spread 95
Proscuitto 131
Protein Drinks/Shakes 50
Prunes 103
Psyllium Husks 59, 100
Puddings 92
Pumpkin Pie 136
Pumpkin Seeds 133
Pumpkin 167

Qdoba 238
Quadruple Bypass Burger 251
Quail 141
Quaker: Bars 33, 36
  Breakfast Cereals 59, 63
Quakes, Rice Snacks 155
Quarter Pounder 222
Quesadilla 179
  Qdoba 238
Quiche 93
Quinoa 100

Rabbit 128
Radish 167
Raisin Bran 60
Raisin Bread 56
Raisinets 75
Raisins 103
Ramen Noodles 116
Rambutan 102
Ranch Dressing 145
Raspberries 102
Ravioli 135, 177
  Fazoli's 207
Red Bull & Vodka 30
Red Bull Energy 52
Reddi-Wip 91
Red Mango Frozen Yogurt 108
Reese's 75
Refried Beans 116
Relishes 82
Reuben Sandwich 172
Revival Soy Shakes 49
Rice 143
Rice Bran 100
Rice Cakes 58
Rice Crackers 83
Rice Dream 48
Rice Drinks 48
Rice Krispies 62
Rice Noodles 135
Rice Snacks 155
Rice, Sticky Thai 181
Rice-A-Roni 116
Ricola 77
Ricotta Cheese 79
Rite Aid, Nutrit'l Drinks 52
Ritz: Bits 155
  Crackers 88
Rockstar Energy 52
Rogan Josh 177
Rolo 75
Root Beer 53
Rugulah 64
Rum 29
Russell Stover Candy 75
Rye Bread 56
Rye Flour 100

Sake 28
Salad Dressings 145
Salad Toppings: 144
  Bacon Bits 144
Salads: Deli 144
  Packaged 144
Salami 131
Salmon 98
Salsa 82
Saltines 83
Sandwiches: Cosi 198
  D'Angelo's 199
  Denny's 201
  Einstein Bros 206
  Mr. Hero 225
  Schlotzsky's 246
  Subway 257
Sara Lee: Bagels 58
  Croissants 136
  Frozen Cakes 66
  Pies 136
Sardines 99
Sashimi 178
Satay Chicken 18
Sausages 129
Sauces: 148
  Prego Pasta Sauces 150
  Ragu 151
  Worcestershire Sauce 150
Sbarro's 246
Scallops 99
Scone, Fruit 64
Scotch 29
Screwdriver 30
Seagram's Coolers 29
Seaweed 163
See's Candies 75
Seeds 132
Semolina 100
Sesame Butter 132
Sesame Seeds 133
7-Eleven 244
7-UP 54
Shakes 47
Shasta Sodas 54

Shaved Ice 105, 176
Shawourma 179
Shellfish 97
Sherry 28
Shoney's 248
Shooters 30
Shrimp 99
Silk: Creamer 91
  Soy Drinks 49
Simply Asia, Meals 117
Sirloin Steak 125
Sizzler 249
Skippy Peanut Butter 133
Skittles 75
Skyline Chili 250
Slammers 47
Slim-Fast: Bars 36, 286
  Shakes 52, 287
Slurpees, 7-Eleven 245
Smart Balance Spread 95
Smart Beat Spread 95
Smart Start Bars 36
Smarties 75
Smirnoff Ice 29
Smoked Sausage 129
Smoothies 47
  Freshens 208
  Jamba Juice 215
  Smoothie King 250
  Tropical Smoothie Café 264
Smucker's Goober 133
Snacks 152-155
  Cheese Balls 154
  Cheese Puffs 154
  Cheetos 154
Snackwell's, Cookies 89
Snails 181
Snake 181
Snapple 44, 52, 55
Snickers 76
SoBe: Energy Drinks 52
  Iced Tea 55
Soft Drink Mixes 54
Soft Drinks/Soda 53
Sonic Drive-In 251
Sopapillas Pastry Puffs 180
Sopes 179
Sorghum 100

Soul Foods	180
Soups	156
Sour Cream	91
Sourdough Bread	56
Soup:	156-161
Campbell's	157
Cup-a-Soup	159
Progresso	160
South Beach: Bars	36
Meals	123
Southern Comfort	31
Souvliaki	176
Soy Dream: Ice Cream	108
Soy Drinks	49
Soy Flour	100
Soy Milk/Drinks	48
Soy Nuts	132, 155
Soy Powder Mix	49
Soybeans	167
Soyco Cheese	80
Spaghetti Warehouse	254
Spaghetti: & Meat Sauce	177
& Meatballs	177
Cooked	135
Dry/Fresh	135
Meatballs, Rocky Rococo	241
Old Spaghetti Factory	228
Spam: Canned	131
Musubi	176
Spanish Foods	181
Spareribs	127
P.F. Chang's	233
Sparks Energy	29
Special K: Bars	36
Cereals	62
Special K₂O Protein	55
Spreads	95
Spices & Herbs	163
Spinach	167
Spirulina	163
Splenda	164

Spring Roll: Chinese	175
Panda Express	230
Pei Wei	231
Sprite	54
Squash	167
Squaw Bread	56
Squid	99
Stadium Foods	174
Stagg Chili Meals	117
Starbucks: Coffee	254
Ice Cream	108
Starburst	76
Starkist	99
Steak Subs, Mr. Hero	225
Steaks	125
Chili's	196
Lone Star	220
Outback Steakhouse	229
Ruby Tuesday	242
Shoney's	248
Western Sizzlin	267
Steaz Energy	52
Steaz Iced Teas	55
Stella D'Oro, Cookies	89
Stevia	164
Stouffer's	123
Strawberries	102
String Cheese	79
Stromboli: Donato's Pizza	202
Villa Pizza	265
Stonyfield Farm Yogurt	170
Strudel	64
Stuffing Mix	57
Subway	257
Succotash	180
Sugar	164
Sugar Substitutes	164
Sukiyaki	178
Summer Sausage	131
Sundaes	105
McDonald's	223

Sunflower Seeds	133
Sunkist, Sodas	54
SunnyD	44
Sunsweet: Lighter Bake	95
Prune Juice	44
Surimi	99
Sushi	178
Southern Tsunami	253
Swanson Dinners	123
Sweet 'N Low:	164
Candy	76
Sweet Buns/Rolls	69
Sweetbreads	128
Sweet Potatoes	167
Swiss Miss: Drinks	37
Pudding Snacks	92
Swordfish	99
Syrups	164
TAB Soda	54
Tabouli	179
Tacos	179
Qdoba	238
Taco Bell	259
Taco Salads: Qdoba	238
Taco Shell	58, 179
Tahini	132
Tahini Sauce	179
Take 5	76
Tamales	179
Tamarillo	102
Tamarind	102
Tandoori Chicken	177
Tang	44, 54
Tangelo	103
Tangerine	103
Tapioca	100
Taramasolata	176
Tartar Sauce	82
Tasti D-Lite	109
TCBY	109, 262

Tea	55
Tempura	178
Teppan Yaki	178
Tequila	29
Tequila Sunrise	30
Teriyaki: Beef	178
Chicken	178
Salmon	178
Thai Foods	181
Thai Kitchen Meals	117
Thick Shakes, McDonald's	223
Thousand Is. Dressing	145
3 Musketeers	76
Tia Maria	31
Tilt Energy	29
Tim Hortons	263
Tiramisu	64
Toblerone	76
Tofu:	162
Mori-Nu-Tofu	162
Tofu, fried: Panda Express	230
Tofurky Meals	117
Tofutti	109
Tofutti Cheese	80
Tom Yam Soup	181
Tomatillos	103, 167
Tomato: Fresh	103
Ketchup	145
Paste/Puree	148
Sauce	148
Sundried	148
Tombstone Pizzas	139
Tongue	128
Tony's Pizzas	139
Torte	176
Tortellini	135
Tortilla	58
Tortilla Chips:	153
Doritos	153
Tostada	179

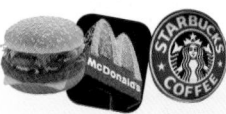

FAST-FOOD RESTAURANTS INDEX
~ SEE PAGE 183 ~

Tostado Bowl	58
Tostitos	153, 155
Tostitos Dip	81
Trader Joe's: Bars	36
Breakfast Cereals	63
Cakes	66
Cookies	89
Frozen Desserts	66
Frozen Meals	123
Ice Cream	109
Juice, Refrigerated	44
Yogurt	170
Trail Mix	132, 155
Tripe	128
Tuna	99
Turkey	141
Turkey Breast, Deli	131
Turkey Loaf	131
Turkey Pastrami	131
Turnip	167
Turnovers, Fruit	64
Twinkies	65
Twisted Tea	229
Twix	76
Twizzlers	76
Tzatziki	176
Udon Noodles	135
Uncle Ben's Meals	118
V8 Juice	45

Vault Energy	52
Veal	127
Veal Parmigiana	177
Vegetable Juices	40
Vegetable Oils	96
Vegetable Shortening	96
Vegetables	165-168
Frozen:	167
Canned/Bottled	168
Vermouth	28
Viactiv Chews	163
Vienna Sausage	180
Vietnamese Foods	181
Vitasoy Soy Drinks	49
Vodka	29
Vodka Tonic	30
Waffles	134
Walgreens: Nutrit'l Drinks	52
Sodas	54
Walnuts	132
Wasabi Peas	155
Water Crackers	83
Water Chestnuts	167
Watermelon	103
Seeds	133
WAWA	266
Weetabix	63
Weider Powders	52

Weight Watchers:	
Candy	76
Frozen Meals	124
Pizzas	139
Smart Ones: B'kfasts	134
Cakes	66
Yogurts	171
Weiners	129
Wendy's	267
Werther's	77
WestSoy: Rice Drinks	48
Soy Milk	49
Wheat Germ	59, 100
Wheat Thins	87
Wheatables	155
Whipped Toppings	91
Whipping Cream	91
Whiskey	29
White Wave	118
Whitman's	77
Wienerschnitzel	267
Wine	28
Wishbone Dressings	147
Wolfgang Puck, Pizzas	139
Wonton Wrappers	135

Wonder Bread	56
Wonka	77
Worthington	118
Wraps, Sandella's	245
Wrigley's	77
Wyder's Cider	28
Yakisoba:	
Samurai Sam's	245
Yams	167
Yeast	32
Yogurt	169
Yogurt Drinks	171
Yogurt Parfait	169
Yogurt Raisins	155
Yonique Yogurt	171
Yoo-Hoo	47
York Peppermint Pattie	77
Yucca Root	167
Yves Veggie Cuisine	118
Zatarain's	118
Zima	29
Zingers	65
Ziti: Fazoli's	207
Zola Acai Drink	52
Zone Perfect Bars	36
Yoplait	171
Zucchini	167

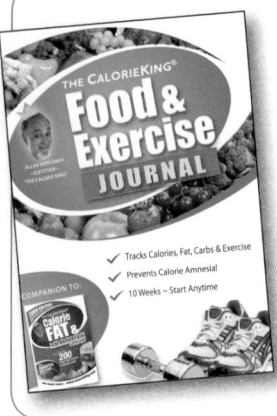
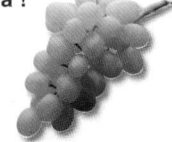

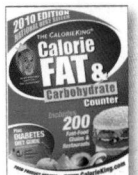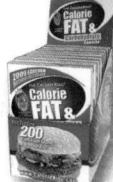
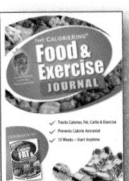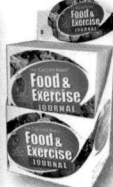
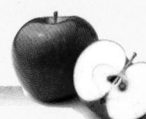
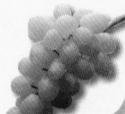
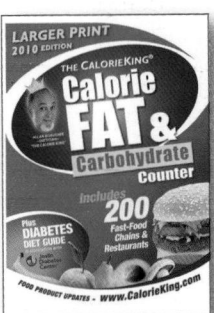

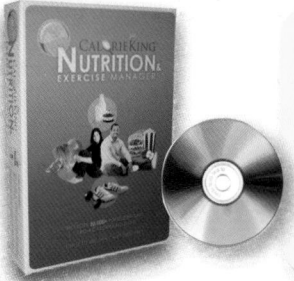

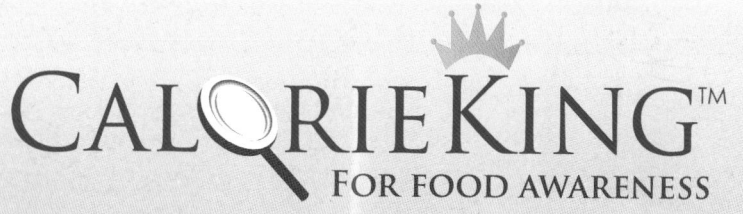

CALORIE KING™
FOR FOOD AWARENESS

Visit us at www.CalorieKing.com
and change your life!

We'll show you how with the Online
CalorieKing Program for weight control.

Get started today with
these useful resources!

Search our food database
Gives you calorie counts on foods
you eat every day

Visit our store
To find weight control aids to help
you fight weight gain

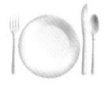

**Record activity in our Food &
Exercise Diary (members only)**
It does all of the math for you

**24/7 support from our diverse
online community(members only)**
Discuss problems, make new friends
and get motivated.

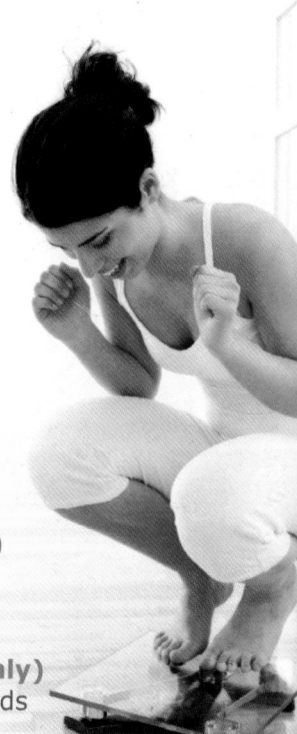